TRANSCULTURAL NURSING

Concepts, Theories, Research, and Practice

THIRD EDITION

Notice

Medicine is an ever-changing science. As new research and clinical experience broaden our knowledge, changes in treatment and drug therapy are required. The author and the publisher of this work have checked with sources believed to be reliable in their efforts to provide information that is complete and generally in accord with the standards accepted at the time of publication. However, in view of the possibility of human error or changes in medical sciences, neither the author nor the publisher nor any other party who has been involved in the preparation or publication of this work warrants that the information contained herein is in every respect accurate or complete, and they disclaim all responsibility for any errors or omissions or for the results obtained from use of such information contained in this work. Readers are encouraged to confirm the information contained herein with other sources. For example and in particular, readers are advised to check the product information sheet included in the package of each drug they plan to administer to be certain that the information contained in this work is accurate and that changes have not been made in the recommended dose or in the contraindications for administration. This recommendation is of particular importance in connection with new or infrequently used drugs.

TRANSCULTURAL NURSING

Concepts, Theories, Research, and Practice

THIRD EDITION

Madeleine Leininger, PhD, LHD, DS, CTN, RN, FAAN, FRCNA

Professor Emeritus
College of Nursing
Wayne State University
Detroit, Michigan

Adjunct Faculty Member
College of Nursing
University of Nebraska Medical Center
Omaha, Nebraska

Founder and Leader of Transcultural Nursing
and Leader of Human Care Research
Omaha, Nebraska

Marilyn R. McFarland, PhD, MSN, CTN, RN

Adjunct Faculty Member
Crystal M. Lange College of Nursing and Health Sciences
Saginaw Valley State University
University Center, Michigan

McGraw-Hill
Medical Publishing Division

New York • Chicago • San Francisco
Lisbon • London • Madrid • Mexico City
Milan • New Delhi • San Juan • Seoul
Singapore • Sydney • Toronto

McGraw-Hill

A Division of The **McGraw·Hill** *Companies*

Transcultural Nursing: Concepts, Theories, Research, and Practice, Third Edition

34567890 DOCDOC 09876543

ISBN 0-07-135397-6

This book was set in Times Roman by TechBooks.
The editors were Andrea Seils and John M. Morriss.
The production supervisor was Catherine H. Saggese.
Project management was provided by Andover Publishing Services.
The cover designer was Aimee Nordin.
The index was done by Andover Publishing Services.
R.R. Donnelley & Sons, Crawfordsville, was printer and binder.

This book is printed on acid-free paper.

Library of Congress Cataloging-in-Publication Data

Leininger, Madeleine M.
    Transcultural nursing : concepts, theories, research & practice /
authors, Madeleine Leininger, Marilyn R. McFarland. — 3rd ed.
        p. ; cm.
    Rev. ed. of: Transcultural nursing. 2nd ed. c1995.
    Includes bibliographical references and index.
    ISBN 0-07-135397-6
    1. Transcultural nursing.   I. McFarland, Marilyn R.   II. Transcultural nursing.   III. Title.
    [DNLM: 1. Transcultural Nursing. 2. Cross-Cultural Comparison. 3. Cultural
Diversity. 4. Philosophy, Nursing. WY 107 L531t 2002]
RT86.54 .L44   2002
610.73—dc21
                                                            2001042559

ABOUT THE AUTHORS

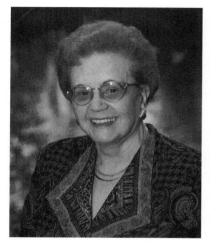

Madeleine Leininger, PhD, LHD, DS, CTN, RN, FAAN, FRCNA, is the founder and leader of the academic field of transcultural nursing with focus on comparative human care, theory, and research. She is Professor Emeritus, College of Nursing, Wayne State University, Detroit, Michigan and Adjunct Professor, College of Nursing, University of Nebraska Medical Center, Omaha, Nebraska. Dr. Leininger is an internationally known transcultural nursing lecturer, educator, author, theorist, administrator, researcher, and consultant in nursing and anthropology. She is a fellow and distinguished Living Legend of the American Academy of Nursing and an Emeritus Member of the American Association of Colleges of Nursing. She was one of the first graduate professional nurses prepared with a PhD in cultural anthropology. She initiated the Nurse Scientist and several transcultural nursing programs in the early 1970s and 1980s. She has done in-depth field studies of fifteen Western and non-Western cultures. Dr. Leininger initiated and was Editor of the *Journal of Transcultural Nursing* and started the Transcultural Nursing Society. She has been a Distinguished Professor and Lecturer in over 90 universities and has given over 1200 public addresses in the USA and overseas. She is author and editor of 28 books and has published over 220 articles. She published the first qualitative nursing research book (1985), an early psychiatric nursing book (1960), and the first Culture Care Diversity and Universality Theory book. Presently, Dr. Leininger resides in Omaha, Nebraska and is active as a worldwide transcultural nursing consultant, educator, lecturer, and writer.

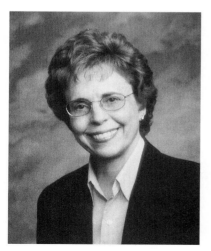

Marilyn R. McFarland, PhD, MSN, CTN, RN, is an adjunct faculty member at the Crystal M. Lange College of Nursing and Health Sciences, Saginaw Valley State University, at University Center, Michigan, where she is currently serving as the coordinator of a special project (OPEN, "Opportunities for Professional Education in Nursing") to recruit, engage, and retain culturally diverse students in nursing. She received her PhD in nursing with a focus on transcultural nursing under Dr. Madeleine Leininger at Wayne State University in Detroit in 1995. Dr. McFarland, a Certified Transcultural Nurse, has focused her professional work on the care and study of elders from diverse cultures in the United States and has presented her research findings about the culture care of elders worldwide. She is a former editor of the *Journal of Transcultural Nursing* and is an active member of the Transcultural Nursing Society, to which she has made many significant contributions. Dr. McFarland has also been a mentor to many students in the United States and abroad, making transcultural nursing meaningful and important in people care. She has received many prestigious awards, including the Leininger Award presented by the Transcultural Nursing Society. She is an outstanding transcultural nursing researcher and educator who has helped to make transcultural nursing an exciting and relevant discipline.

CONTENTS

CONTRIBUTORS

Joanna Basuray, PhD, MS, RN
Associate Professor in Nursing
Director of the Multicultural Institute
Towson University
Towson, Maryland
USA

Anita Berry, PhD, CTN, RN
Professor Emeritus
College of Nursing
San Bernadino Valley College
San Bernadino, California
USA

Elizabeth Cameron-Traub, PhD, BA, RN
Professor and Dean of Health Sciences
Australian Catholic University
New South Wales
Australia

Lenny Chiang-Hanisko, PhD(C), RN
Research Fellow
School of Nursing
Boston College
Boston, Massachusetts
USA

Joanne T. Ehrmin, PhD, MSN, RN
Associate Professor
School of Nursing
Medical College of Ohio
Toledo, Ohio
USA

Rauda Gelazis, PhD, CS, CTN, RN
Associate Professor of Nursing
Ursuline College
Pepper Pike, Ohio
USA

Jody Glittenberg, PhD, FAAN, HNC, RN
Professor of Nursing, Anthropology & Research
Professor of Psychiatry
College of Nursing
University of Arizona
Tucson, Arizona
USA

Beverly Horn, PhD, CTN, RN
Associate Professor Emeritus
School of Nursing
University of Washington
Seattle, Washington
USA

Faye Hummel, PhD, CTN, RN
Associate Professor
School of Nursing
University of Northern Colorado
Greeley, Colorado
USA

Judith Kilmer Lamp, PhD, CNM, RN
Associate Professor
Medical College of Ohio
Toledo, Ohio
USA

Bernard J. Leininger, MD, FACS
Assistant Clinical Professor of Surgery
Loyola University School of Medicine
Chicago, Illinois
USA

Madeleine Leininger, PhD, LHD, DS, CTN, RN, FAAN, FRCNA
Professor Emeritus
College of Nursing
Wayne State University
Detroit, Michigan
and
Adjunct Faculty Member
College of Nursing
University of Nebraska Medical Center
Omaha, Nebraska
USA

Cheryl J. Leuning, PhD, CTN, RN
Associate Professor
Augustana College
Sioux Falls, South Dakota
USA

Linda J. Luna, PhD, MA, MSN, CTN, RN
Interim Chief of Nursing Affairs
King Faisal Specialist Hospital
Jeddah
Saudi Arabia

Joan MacNeil, PhD, MHSc, BScN, RN
Senior Technical Officer
Family Health International
Asia Regional Office
Bangsue, Bangkok
Thailand

Jan Hoot Martin, PhD, GNP, RN
Professor
School of Nursing
University of Northern Colorado
Greeley, Colorado
USA

Grace Mashaba DLH/ET/Phil, RN†
Professor of Nursing
Department of Nursing Science
University of Zululand
Republic of South Africa

Marilyn R. McFarland, PhD, MSN, CTN, RN
Adjunct Faculty Member
Crystal M. Lange College of Nursing and
    Health Sciences
Saginaw Valley State University
University Center, Michigan
USA

Marjorie G. Morgan, PhD, CNM, CTN, RN
Department of Health and Environmental Control
Myrtle Beach, South Carolina
USA

Akram Omeri, PhD, CTN, MCN, RN, FRCNA
Senior Lecturer
Faculty of Nursing
The University of Sydney
Sydney, New South Wales
Australia

Diane Peters, PhD, CTN, RN
Professor and Assistant Director
School of Nursing
University of Northern Colorado
Greeley, Colorado
USA

Louis F. Small, DNSc, RN
Senior Lecturer
Faculty of Medical and Health Sciences
University of Namibia
Windhoek
Republic of Namibia

Rani H. Srivastava, MScN, RN
Director of Clinical Resources
Faculty of Nursing
University of Toronto
Toronto, Ontario
Canada

Lillian Tom-Orme, PhD, MS, MPH, RN, FAAN
Research Assistant Professor
Health Research Center
Department of Family and Preventive Medicine
University of Utah
Salt Lake City, Utah
USA

Agnes van Dyk, D.Cur., RN
Professor and Dean
Faculty of Medical and Health Sciences
University of Namibia
Windhoek
Republic of Namibia

Nancy White, PhD, RN
Professor
School of Nursing
University of Northern Colorado
Greeley, Colorado
USA

FOREWORD

The Augustinian monk Gregor Mendel (1823–1884) is credited with being the first scientist to explain genetic similarities and differences. After years of research, he used the knowledge he had gained to formulate a genetic theory that ultimately enabled future generations to unlock the mystery of the human genome. Although Mendel's work is now recognized as the very foundation of modern genetics, it was so brilliant and unprecedented at the time it took decades for the rest of the scientific community to realize the revolutionary importance of his work. Thanks to Mendel, we now know that all people of the world are genetically 99.9% alike, with human similarities and differences being explained by a coded quartet of chemical letters: adenine (A), thymine (T), cytosine (C), and guanine (G). Three billion pairs of these chemicals are harmoniously combined, sounding the common notes that make us all alike, but also responsible for striking the fewer than one percent of chords that produce a symphony of diversity. When something goes awry, the cacophonous sounds of disease resonate.

But if everyone is genetically humming the same notes, why do people from different cultures and nations sing different melodies? Why do people from various cultures view health and illness differently? Why do they seek different healers and treatments to promote health and treat disease? Why do people's expectations of care and caring vary so widely? What role does culture play in people's expectations of professional nurses and nursing? While searching for the answers to these questions, Professor Madeleine Leininger formulated a transcultural nursing theory to advance nursing and health care knowledge that is as significant and far-reaching as Mendel's work was in genetics.

Nearly fifty years have passed since Professor Leininger first noted the importance of cultural similarities and differences in nursing and health care. She envisioned and established the field of transcultural nursing. She recognized that the goal of nursing science is not merely to accumulate data, so she theorized about the interconnections of the concepts, theories, research, and practice of nursing, culture, and health care. After decades of research in many different cultures, she used the knowledge she had gained to establish the discipline of transcultural nursing. Dr. Leininger's creative *Theory of Culture Care Diversity and Universality* with the *Sunrise Model* and the ethnonursing research method were major breakthroughs in nursing. She also established the Transcultural Nursing Society and the International Association of Human Care, and was the founder of the *Journal of Transcultural Nursing*, serving as Editor from 1989 to 1995. Like Mendel, Dr. Leininger worked patiently for decades while members of the scientific and health care community gradually began to grasp the profound implications of her teaching, research, theory, and findings, and watched as other disciplines began embracing or imitating it. Along the way, Dr. Leininger gave of her time to mentor many students and faculty, enabling them to use her theory in their own areas of clinical practice, education, research, and consultation. During the past five decades, transcultural nursing has reached all continents of the world and Dr. Leininger is recognized as the founder and foremost authority and leader in the discipline.

Among the many students whom Dr. Leininger has mentored is co-author Dr. Marilyn R. McFarland, who earned her doctorate in transcultural nursing at the College of Nursing, Wayne State University. Currently a faculty member at Saginaw Valley State University, Dr. McFarland is a highly respected transcultural nurse leader whose research has focused on the care of the elderly in diverse cultures. From 1995–1998 Dr. McFarland served as editor of the *Journal of Transcultural Nursing*, and she has lectured and consulted on transcultural nursing within and outside the United States of America.

In this third edition of *Transcultural Nursing*, Dr. Leininger and Dr. McFarland have provided the most comprehensive, contemporary, and current opus on transcultural nursing and health ever published. This definitive text is the culmination of nearly fifty years of theory development, teaching, and practice in transcultural nursing, and showcases the work of some of the top national and international scholars in the field. Although Dr. Leininger and Dr. McFarland crafted many substantive chapters themselves, they also invited twenty-four transcultural nurse experts to contribute their knowledge and expertise to this comprehensive text.

The third edition of *Transcultural Nursing* is a *must-have* text for the professional library of nurses and health care providers in other disciplines who strive to provide care to clients of diverse and similar cultures in meaningful, safe and beneficial ways—commonly referred to as *culturally congruent* or *culturally competent* care. Nursing and others in health-related fields will find a wellspring of information that will guide them in their quest for knowledge, understanding, and care of people from various cultures around the world. It is an authoritative, substantive, comprehensive text with both theoretical and practical information on transcultural nursing that will be useful for nurses and other health care providers in clinical practice, education, research, administration, and consultation.

Margaret M. Andrews, Ph.D., R.N., C.T.N.
Chairperson and Professor
Department of Nursing
Nazareth College
Rochester, NY
Former President of the Transcultural Nursing Society and Leader in the Discipline

PREFACE

As the world continues to change in many geographic locations, so professional nurses need to become aware and increasingly knowledgeable about these changing events, issues, and human concerns from a transcultural nursing perspective. Nurses also need to keep abreast of transcultural developments and information in the busy world of care. This third edition of *Transcultural Nursing* has been prepared to update nurses and other interested health personnel on some of the most significant developments, trends, and knowledge in transcultural nursing. Indeed, this edition reflects many new areas of transcultural nursing knowledge that have developed since the first interdisciplinary book, *Nursing and Anthropology: Two Worlds to Blend*, was published in 1970, and since the appearance of the first book on transcultural nursing in 1978. This third edition also shows an advancement of knowledge from the second edition of *Transcultural Nursing* published in 1995. Over these past five decades the discipline of transcultural nursing has been growing steadily and gaining significant relevancy worldwide.

Most assuredly, transcultural nursing is no longer a new idea, as it has been in existence since I launched the field in the mid 1950s. However, there are still nurses and health professionals discovering the field and legitimately concerned that their educational programs failed to prepare them for this important discipline and practice area. Nurses also realize that prior to the establishment of transcultural nursing, there were no formal educational programs to prepare nurses to function as specialists or generalists to care for the culturally different. Moreover, there was no identified body of knowledge or faculty mentors to guide nurses to practice in culturally knowledgeable and competent ways. But today the concept I coined four decades ago of "culturally competent congruent care" as the goal of my theory is being used worldwide.

During the past several decades, this cultural evolution has transformed nursing and health care so that clients of diverse cultures can benefit from transcultural nursing in many places in the world. This whole movement has been a significant development created by a small cadre of committed leaders, with limited financial support from the government and from nursing professional organizations. Nevertheless, considerable progress has been made over the past five decades in developing a body of transcultural nursing knowledge with concepts, principles, and research findings to guide nurses in working with the culturally different. Transcultural nursing theories supported by research findings are gradually being used in the care of people from many different cultures in sensitive and knowledgeable ways.

As the founder and leader of this major cultural movement, it has been most encouraging to see these developments. Granted, there have been many hurdles and challenges to make transcultural nursing a reality, such as shifting nurses' interests, values, and knowledge from largely a unicultural dominant focus to a multicultural one. It was also a challenge to get nurses to study humanistic caring with diverse cultures and to hold culture care as the essence of nursing. Persuading nurses to value and use qualitative research to tap culture care was another major hurdle. Gradually a wealth of new or unknown knowledge was discovered and a new appreciation for human caring within a cultural context was developed. These discoveries and new ways to provide care to clients of diverse and similar cultures in meaningful, safe, and beneficial ways has been a major breakthrough in the profession. Nonetheless, a moral obligation and major challenges are necessary to provide safe, meaningful, and compassionate care to diverse cultures.

The *purpose* of this third edition is to present a wealth of substantive knowledge based on transcultural research, along with important concepts, principles, theories, and other knowledge areas to guide nurses in providing culturally congruent and competent care to people of many diverse and similar cultures. The reader will discover an increasing number of theoretically-based research studies of Western and non-Western cultures with many new and valuable findings to provide creative and practical care to different cultures. This book demonstrates the tremendous importance of transcultural nursing worldwide. The book has been prepared for undergraduate and graduate nursing students and for nursing staff, practitioners, administrators (academic and clinical), faculty, and consultants. Health personnel and scholars from other disciplines will also find this book most valuable as they begin their journey to the study and practice of transculturalism. They will need, however, to use content in appropriate ways to fit *their unique discipline and professional perspectives*. Other health care professionals, such as physicians, dentists, pharmacists, social workers, physical therapists and others, have already found transcultural nursing publications most useful while developing transcultural health services relevant to their discipline. At the same time, they learn anew about the nature, practice, and importance of transcultural nursing in health care services.

In general, this third edition has been prepared as one of the *most substantive, definitive, comprehensive, and holistic books on transcultural nursing knowledge and practices* building upon five decades of knowledge. It is a book that will guide staff nurses and educators to use transcultural knowledge to help people of diverse cultures in meaningful ways. Many nursing service personnel are realizing the critical need to provide direct care to clients of many different cultures in clinics, hospitals, homes, and new health services, and that one cannot rely on "common sense" but one needs to use specific culture care knowledge to guide actions and decisions. Nursing administrators, researchers, and consultants especially need this content to support and advance their work with cultures and to prevent gross ethnocentrism, racism, and a host of other negative outcomes. The research findings in this book from nearly sixty Western and non-Western cultures is important holding and reflective knowledge to guide nurses' thinking and actions. This book crosses geographic borders to help readers learn about many

diverse cultures. The authors are interested in preventing stereotyping and other negative or destructive practices that are cultural taboos in transcultural nursing.

Most important, this book is unique in that research findings are derived from well-conceived theoretical perspectives and domains of inquiry with in-depth emic and etic cultural data derived from key and general informants. These data are essential to provide culture-specific direct care and avoid cultural imposition practices. It is also unique in that there is a historical build-up of transcultural nursing knowledge from the early 1960s to the present time. A major challenge remains to continue to expand, refine, and document positive outcomes as a consequence of using transcultural nursing knowledge and research in creative and purposeful ways in all areas of nursing education and practice.

This third edition has thirty-six chapters, including seventeen new theoretical and research-based studies. In addition, several original and classic chapters have been updated since transcultural nursing began in the 1950s as a formal area of study and practice. These chapters, along with the new ones are essential content for the discipline and practice of transcultural nursing. Twenty-five transcultural nurse scholars and experts have contributed their research and creative work to the book. The unique feature is that practically all contributors have been prepared through graduate courses or programs in transcultural nursing and have conducted theoretically-based research studies in Western or non-Western cultures. Most have used the Culture Care Theory to demonstrate the importance of understanding the totality of humans as an essential and sound basis to arrive at culture-specific and general ways to assist clients of diverse or similar cultures. These contributors have found the theory of Culture Care Diversity and Universality and the ethnonursing research method extremely valuable to discover culturally congruent care and a wealth of largely unknown nursing and health knowledge about cultures and their care and health needs. The contributors show how to use the theory with the Sunrise Model and to arrive at holistic care based on culture-specific care practices with the theoretical modes of action and decision. Such knowledge provides a major shift today from the medical model of focusing on diseases, management of symptoms, and often biased professional diagnoses. Focusing on the cultural human conditions and needs is another major and important feature of the book. Such comparative findings take into account social structure factors of individuals, groups, and families, each with their economic, religious, kinship, cultural beliefs and values, education, language, ethnohistory, and environmental context—all holistic influencers that cannot be overlooked in modern health care practices today. This breakthrough approach in transcultural nursing knowledge is encouraging and imperative to help nurses expand their health care assessments and practices and to grasp the larger lifeworld of clients as well as preventing ethnocentric and superficial knowledge about cultures.

Thus this book builds upon an evolving body of grounded and comparative theoretically-derived transcultural knowledge within transcultural nursing as a scientific and humanistic discipline. The reader will discover the tremendous importance of using theory to guide nurses' thinking and research with one of the *oldest* and most holistic theories of nursing, namely the Culture Care Theory. They also show the value of using one of the first nursing research methods, namely, ethnonursing with enablers that are designed to fit the theory along with other theoretical views and research methods.

The diverse studies of Western and non-Western cultures with special contemporary topics and issues related to history, ethical and moral cultural care, home therapies, transcultural mental health, nutrition, and complementary generic and professional care are presented to help the reader grasp the trends, scope, nature, and importance of transcultural nursing worldwide. Suggestions of ways to teach, practice, and offer sound consultation services are discussed along with critical issues related to student-faculty exchanges in unfamiliar cultures and administrative practices. The references and other source materials will be valuable to nurses and to other professionals. The reader will gain new insights and knowledge, and builds confidence in one's ability to practice transcultural nursing. Such knowledge will help to prevent unfavorable or non-therapeutic practices.

The book has been purposefully organized into five major sections. The first one focuses on the essential concepts, definitions, historical developments, importance of transcultural nursing, theory and research methods with findings, culturalogical assessment, and other major transcultural nursing knowledge domains. These chapters are followed with a section on the scope and major characteristics of transcultural nursing. The third section contains in-depth knowledge of many specific cultures with theory and research findings. The last two sections of the book are focused on teaching, administration, research, consultation, reference sources, and a look at the future of transcultural nursing.

In sum, this third edition builds upon an accumulation of essential transcultural nursing knowledge from several early publications to the present time. The book reflects the work of some of the top scholars in the discipline of transcultural nursing. The extensive experiences and active sustained leadership of the editors along with other expert contributors' work in this book make it a substantive, authoritative, and credible book in transcultural nursing. Transcultural nursing continues to be heralded by many astute and creative scholars within and outside of nursing as one of the most significant in this third millennium and beyond, and is viewed as essential for human health care and well-being and for survival in a growing and complex transcultural world. So although some nurses have been slow to study and use transcultural nursing in the mid twentieth century, they are now realizing how valuable, relevant, and essential it is for quality culturally-based competent care today. Indeed, my vision to establish transcultural nursing has often been said to have been "ahead of its time," but today it is clearly "of the time" and viewed as a moral and practice necessity. Transcultural nursing must remain a *global imperative* to study and practice. It signifies to me a lifelong career and contribution to humanistic people care. Unquestionably it has been most rewarding to see the discipline and practice of transcultural nursing unfold into a highly relevant and major worldwide development that must be integrated into all aspects of health care services. Since this will be my last major revision of the book, I have confidence that Dr. McFarland, a scholar, colleague, and friend, and other transcultural nursing scholars will carry forth future publications so that the culture care needs of people in the world will be met by nurses who are knowledgeable and competent to provide meaningful, congruent, and compassionate care to many cultures.

Madeleine Leininger

DEDICATION AND ACKNOWLEDGEMENTS

This third edition is dedicated to the many nursing students, clinicians, faculty, researchers, and leaders who have been active and committed to make transcultural nursing knowledge and practices a reality in human caring. These students and colleagues have shown futuristic thinking and risk-taking efforts to carve a new pathway in using research-based transcultural nursing knowledge along with major concepts, principles, and practices in order to establish some relevant ways to provide cultural care. A core of dedicated transcultural nursing leaders, advocates, and creative followers have been willing to change and develop nursing practices to fit the culturally different in Western and non-Western cultures. Their thoughtful review, genuine interest, and suggestions for this book have been much appreciated.

The book is also dedicated to our families, who have been so understanding and caring to us as we spent many days and nights on this major publication. We thank them for their patience, support, and tolerance of this work.

Very special thanks go to our outstanding contributors. Twenty-five transcultural nurse experts have shared their knowledge and practices to make this book truly a definitive, major and substantive publication. The contributors' scholarship and expertise are clearly evident in their work, which draws upon their extensive in-depth experiences and use of theoretically-based research knowledge to demonstrate the use and practice of transcultural nursing.

Our special thanks go to Angela LeFevre and to Jan Ohlinger for their most valuable assistance in preparing many of these chapters. Their help with this manuscript was very important and appreciated. We are also grateful for the encouragement and help of John Dolan, Sally Barhydt, and their colleagues at McGraw-Hill Our thanks to all of you.

We are also most grateful to Dr. Margaret Andrews for her willingness to write the foreword to this book amid her very busy schedule. Her colleagueship, leadership, and friendship for more than twenty years in transcultural nursing have been deeply and warmly treasured.

Finally, we thank the many cultural informants in Western and non-Western cultures who have been our inspiration and true teachers of their cultures and have supported the field of transcultural nursing education and practices. This book presents over one hundred cultures that have stimulated the authors and editors to establish the new discipline of transcultural nursing and to inspire quality care to diverse cultures worldwide.

Madeleine Leininger
Marilyn McFarland

TRANSCULTURAL NURSING

Concepts, Theories, Research, and Practice

THIRD EDITION

Transcultural Nursing: Essential Knowledge Dimensions

1

Transcultural Nursing and Globalization of Health Care: Importance, Focus, and Historical Aspects

Madeleine Leininger

If human beings are to survive and live in a healthy, peaceful and meaningful world, then nurses and other health care providers need to understand the cultural care beliefs, values and lifeways of people in order to provide culturally congruent and beneficial health care. LEININGER, 1978

Globalization and Transcultural Nursing

The third millennium is challenging nurses and other health care professionals to think and act with a global perspective as they may encounter and assist people from virtually every place in the world today. Indeed, our world has become conceptually smaller yet more complex and diverse as nurses assist people from many different cultures with their concerns, beliefs, values, and lifeways. In the mid 1950s I anticipated this marked cultural diversity and the trend toward globalization and realized the need for the new field of transcultural nursing worldwide.[1,2] Since then transcultural concepts, principles, and research-based knowledge have helped many nurses to function in our present world of transcultural diversity in nursing and health. Accordingly, globalization, transculturalism, transcultural nursing, culturally congruent care, and related ideas are becoming meaningful to nurses and other health care providers as they serve the culturally different. This has been a rather slow evolution, but it has been encouraging to see diverse cultures respond to nurses who understand and help them appropriately. Major challenges exist in educating nurses and health care professionals worldwide to work together to make transcultural health care meaningful and beneficial. Learning about

different cultures and understanding ways to help them appropriately is not an easy endeavor as it requires entering the world of the people, learning from them, and using knowledge that fits the client's cultural expectations and needs. Achieving this goal can bring many satisfactions to the provider and benefits to the client.

With transcultural nursing and the trend toward globalization of health care, nurses are challenged to learn about different cultures locally and worldwide in this century. The increased number of immigrants, refugees, and other people from many different cultures has made transcultural nursing imperative for nurses today and in the future. The increased use of cybernetics and modern electronic modes of communication and transportation has brought people worldwide almost instantly in close contact with one another. These changes and many others are challenging nurses and other health personnel in transcultural health care services with a global perspective.

Amid these globalization trends are great opportunities for nurses to learn about different and similar cultures and discover ways to help them with their special needs. Indeed, the central purpose and goal of transcultural nursing is focused on promoting and maintaining the cultural care needs of human beings. Nurses who are prepared in transcultural nursing know how to identify and provide for cultures. They learn ways to discover and provide safe and meaningful care to people of diverse cultures. Since nurses remain the largest health care providers worldwide, they have a unique opportunity to learn about cultural strangers and help them with their particular lifeways and in their environmental contexts. Essentially, transcultural nursing provides nurses a new way to learn about and provide culturally congruent and meaningful care to people in the world. It is a new and different pathway for most nurses from their traditional nursing orientations and modes of helping people. Today nurses must learn about and respect different cultures and their care needs in different life contexts to be transcultural nurses.

Nurses who have been involved in learning transcultural nursing through formal study see the tremendous importance of this unique field. It is changing their ways of thinking and working with diverse cultures with many satisfactions coming to them. These nurses recognize that the greatest challenge for nurses today and in the future is to learn how to care for different people of diverse cultures with compassion and understanding. They realize that nurses must function in a much broader world and that they need substantive transcultural nursing knowledge and skills to be competent and effective in human caring services. Transcultural nurses' thinking and actions need to be based on a body of humanistic and scientific knowledge about specific cultures with their values, beliefs, and caring patterns.

Since launching the field of transcultural nursing in the mid 1950s, I continue to hold that nursing must shift its focus and become transcultural nursing in philosophy, education, administration, research, consultation, and practice to survive and remain relevant to serve people of diverse cultures.[3,4] Transcultural nursing has become imperative as the area of study and practice for all professional nurses to fulfill their societal and global professional mandate today and in the future. Nurses as the direct care providers must be prepared to function with transcultural nursing knowledge and competencies to ensure beneficial outcomes to people of different cultures. For without such preparation in transcultural nursing, nurses will be greatly handicapped, disadvantaged, and culturally ignorant to help people of different lifeways, beliefs, and values. Such transcultural caring knowledge of different cultures was clearly missing in education and practice

prior to the advent of establishing and developing the discipline.[5] Nurses needed to know how to help cultures to prevent serious illness and maintain wellness within a cultural perspective. Transcultural caring knowledge and practices of diverse cultures were greatly needed at the midcentury and remain essential today. Nurses also needed to be aware of their own cultural background and how it could influence the client's care and relationships with other nurses and disciplines. Nurses also needed a theoretical and research framework to discover and understand cultures. Hence, in the mid 20th century transcultural nursing theory, research, and practices were much needed for these and other reasons soon to be discussed.

Today, transcultural nursing and the concept of globalization are heard worldwide. Globalization is a recurrent term being used by many people and businesses. One hears of global technologies, global communication systems, global economics, global politics, global transportation, global health care, global marketing, and many other global ideas and products. The globalization theme assumes one has worldwide perspectives, knowledge, and competencies when discussed as a service. However, there are often major gaps in knowledge and understanding of cultures and of the nature, uses, and practice related to globalization. Transcultural nursing and globalization have similar uses, but the former is a professional service and the latter is a concept. Nonetheless, globalization is important to help nurses expand their worldview and to think broadly about the idea of nurses functioning worldwide. The expansion of one's view to a much wider world than one's local or neighborhood view is essential to grasp transcultural nursing as a global and comparative field.

During the past four decades, transcultural nursing has been soundly established as an essential and formal area of study and practice.[6,7] It is a major field of study to pursue and has a rapidly growing body of transcultural knowledge to guide nurses in care giving. Specific transcultural nursing concepts, principles, and research findings are available to help nurses provide a new kind of health service, namely, care that is culturally congruent, meaningful, and beneficial to people. A wealth of knowledge with care modalities is the new paradigm and way to care for immigrants, refugees, and minorities of many other cultures from virtually every place in the world. Moreover, there are signs that transcultural nursing is slowly transforming health care systems and changing health care providers to think and act transculturally. Accordingly, consumers of diverse cultures are valuing the times when health care providers know how to talk, listen, and respond appropriately with them. It is, indeed, a cultural movement that continues to take hold worldwide. This movement offers new hope to both cultures and cultural providers.

The challenge, as well as the goal, is to prepare nurses to provide sensitive, safe, beneficial, and meaningful care to people of different cultures. It has been difficult, but yet one of the most significant and important developments in nursing and the health fields during the past century.[8,9] As nurses use transcultural nursing concepts, principles, theories, and research-based knowledge relevant to cultures, one can find evidence of client satisfaction, recovery, and healing. Nurses soon realize the importance of culturally based care that leads to understanding and helping clients of different cultural backgrounds. They learn about the client's specific cultural lifeways and ways to modify their traditional nursing practices to provide care that fits the client's needs. This learning has necessitated a new way to know and give care.

In recent years health disciplines such as medicine, social work, pharmacy, physical therapy, and others are gradually becoming interested in transcultural health care and discovering similar reasons to modify their practices. Therefore, as all health providers learn, value, and understand transcultural health care, one can predict even greater benefits in the future for clients and for provider satisfaction. With this trend, traditional medical nursing and other services will be transformed from largely *uniculturally* based health practices and systems to *multicultural* ones. It is important to keep in mind that transcultural nursing was the first professional discipline to establish culturally based care as a formal area of study and practice. Only recently have other health care professions begun to move in the direction of teaching and developing transcultural professional knowledge and practices.[10] So, as transcultural health care becomes fully recognized and valued by all health disciplines, there will be many benefits to consumers and seekers of health care services worldwide. Moreover, this cultural movement needs to move forward soon to prevent negative and harmful outcomes

to clients such as cultural clashes, cultural conflicts, stresses, and destructive practices.

It is encouraging that a small cadre of transcultural nurses took leadership steps to prepare nurses to discover and use culturally based knowledge and practices to change traditional nursing practices in the early 1960s. Since then its leaders and followers are continuing to discover new knowledge about human caring among cultures and to initiate changes in client care and health services. It has been through sound educational preparation of nurses that such different ways to help people have occurred. No longer can nurses use biased and superficial knowledge or rely on tourists' visits to foreign cultures to be a professionally transcultural nurse. Nor can nurses rely on being of a culture to know accurately and fully one's cultural heritage and use this knowledge safely with other cultures. Superficial knowledge about cultures and human caring can lead to unfavorable and non-beneficial outcomes. Indeed, cultural ignorance, tourists' biases, racism, and a host of other negative practices must be replaced with scientific and humanistic transcultural nursing care knowledge and practices. Thus learning about specific cultures and their care and health needs has been the new and important challenge for nurses as they discover a different way to know and help the culturally different with a global view.

In this chapter, basic definitions and the nature, scope, and importance of transcultural nursing are presented with important and interesting historical facts about the unique development of transcultural nursing over the past five decades. The rationale for this field of study and practice, as well as some of the challenges, barriers, and difficulties encountered, are discussed with a substantive body of knowledge and clinical competencies so that today nurses can move forward into this 21st century with confidence as they make transcultural nursing a global reality.

 ## Definition, Nature, Rationale, and Importance of Transcultural Nursing

Transcultural nursing has been defined as a formal area of study and practice focused on comparative human-care (caring) differences and similarities of the beliefs, values, and patterned lifeways of cultures to

provide culturally congruent, meaningful, and benefi-cial health care to people.[11,12] To understand this def-inition several important ideas are considered. First, transcultural nursing is a *legitimate* and *essential area of formal study* requiring in-depth pursuit of knowl-edge and skills to function effectively with individuals or groups of designated cultures. For human care to be meaningful and therapeutic, professional knowledge needs to fit with the cultural values, beliefs, and expec-tations of clients. If professional knowledge and skills fail to fit the client's values and lifeways, one can antic-ipate that the client will be uncooperative, noncompli-ant, and dissatisfied with nursing efforts. Clients from different cultures are generally quick to show signs of conflict, discontent, distrust, resentment, and general dissatisfaction with nurses who do not know how to provide culturally based care. Transcultural nursing is challenging but complex and requires nurses to study the client's culture care values, beliefs, and lifeways and then to identify how to incorporate nursing knowl-edge to best help the client and usually the family. Transcultural nursing is highly creative and requires knowledge of specific cultures and their care and health lifeways. Culture and care are usually so embedded in each other and closely linked with a client's beliefs and practices that they cannot be overlooked or neglected in the helping-healing process of transcultural nursing.[13]

Today and in the future, cultures have *the human rights* to have their cultural values, beliefs, and needs respected, understood, and appropriately used within any caring or curing process, and so this necessitates that nurses are educated about culture and care phe-nomena. In fact, it is a moral and ethical responsibility for nurses to be attentive to and respond appropriately to the client's cultural care and other needs.[14] This means nurses must study the ethical and moral aspects of the client's culture. Transcultural nursing has become in-creasingly important and a legitimate area of study so that nurses can become knowledgeable about cultures with their human rights and ethical considerations.

The constructs of culture and care are two ma-jor transcultural domains that require in-depth study of people to have *holding knowledge* to guide nurses' thinking, actions, or decisions. For without such knowl-edge, nurses can be ineffective and even danger-ous. Learning about cultures in the past and today is important, and it takes time to gain understanding of

clients. Nursing students soon discover that there is considerable knowledge about cultures and caring to be understood, and then they use this knowledge prac-ticing transcultural nursing. Such knowledge is consid-ered to be equally as important as nurses studying about the heart or how muscles function in the body. For in-deed, culture and caring have functions and patterns that are different and that greatly influence how human beings are living and functioning in their daily life. Cultures and caring are complex phenomena with di-verse meanings and comparative expressions that must be studied and fully understood. It is a moral and eth-ical responsibility for nurses to learn about different cultures and their patterns and needs if nurses are to function effectively in a world of cultural diversity.

It is of interest that in the early history of nursing and until the early 1950s the concepts of culture and care had not been systematically studied nor made ex-plicit as central to nursing.[15–18] Nursing education and practice still tends to place much emphasis on biomed-ical and pathological diseases and curing and on how to manage symptoms with largely a focus on the mind-body perspective. Cultural and care phenomena fac-tors are often largely invisible or taken for granted in the healing and well-being of clients. With the intro-duction of transcultural nursing in the mid 1950s, the meanings, expressions, and patterns of care from the client's cultural background or lifeways began to be systematically studied, emphasized, and valued.[19,20] Cultural and social structure factors, the ethnohistory of clients, folk care, worldview, and other critical and similar factors are becoming a major focus of nursing. With establishing transcultural nursing came a wealth of new knowledge and practices that opened the door to the importance of understanding people from differ-ent cultures. Formal instruction and clinical preparation with mentoring of students have become imperative to learn about culture and caring to make these areas an integral part of nursing and health care.

The *goal of transcultural nursing* has been to pre-pare a new generation of nurses who would be knowl-edgeable, sensitive, competent, and safe to care for people with different or similar lifeways, values, be-liefs, and practices in meaningful, explicit, and bene-ficial ways. It is largely this new generation of nurses who see the great need to be prepared in transcultural nursing along with other nurses who are actively trying to provide care to many new immigrants and migrants that they are trying to serve today. Many undergraduate and graduate nursing students today know they can no longer be ignorant of cultures and need to study and use transcultural nursing principles, concepts, research findings, theories, and practices to function in this intense multicultural world.[21] Some nursing service staff also are becoming aware of the need for transcultural nursing.[22]

Accordingly, nursing students expect their faculty to be knowledgeable and competent in transcultural nursing so they will be effectively guided to provide culturally congruent and safe care. In fact, students who become knowledgeable about transcultural nursing concepts, principles, and research-based knowledge become upset with faculty who are culturally ignorant. They often say, "We teach the faculty through our presentations and clinical practices." Hence, an intergenerational faculty-student knowledge gap exists in some institutions. It is, however, encouraging to know that, with a rather large body of transcultural nursing knowledge with a comparative global perspective, many nurses are using the ideas to care for people of diverse cultures. Indeed, teaching and learning of transcultural nursing has become an exciting and relevant new area for many nursing students today. Moreover, nursing students learn to expand greatly their worldview and knowledge base by taking elective courses in anthropology, sociology, music, art, and related fields to grasp a holistic comparative perspective of human beings. A truly holistic transcultural nursing perspective has become exciting to learn and use with diverse culture care. Students are encouraged to maintain an open mind and genuine interest in learning about cultures, human caring, and health. Thus the original goal of transcultural nursing remains today to provide culturally competent and meaningful care by learning about cultures and their special care needs.

In the definition of transcultural nursing there is an inherent expectation that students, faculty, and clinical staff need first to become aware of their own cultural biases and prejudices as they learn about cultures. Some nurses and students may have long-standing biases and prejudices about cultures that make it difficult for them to become effective transcultural nurses. These nurses require mentoring by transcultural nursing faculty and others who are knowledgeable and able to help nurses

deal with their cultural biases and other problems to be therapeutic with clients. Many cultural biases and prejudices are learned in one's own family or community. These prejudices can be offensive and hurtful to clients and their families. Such tendencies along with cultural myths, beliefs, or racial views about cultures can seriously limit the nurse's effectiveness with clients, families, or groups. Hence, the first important principle in transcultural nursing is to "*know thyself*" to be helpful to people of different cultures. It is also a principle to help one to learn anew about one's self through other cultures.[23] Self-discovery and changing the biases and negative values of nurses takes time and skilled mentoring from transcultural faculty and others in diverse nursing and life experiences. However, nurses can and do learn about their cultural and caring tendencies while studying in the field. In fact, students often talk about how valuable learning of themselves has been as they observe and cared for clients under qualified transcultural nurse mentors. Learning about one's own culture and others is a dynamic, essential, and very important part of transcultural nursing learning and practices.

Within the definition of transcultural nursing is the expectation that transcultural nursing faculty are qualified and responsible to help students discover themselves by using transcultural knowledge. Knowing how to use transcultural knowledge appropriately and meaningfully is an art and an important skill so that learners can make appropriate care decisions and actions with clients for beneficial care services. Transcultural nursing faculty, however, need to be prepared in the discipline to ensure quality-based teaching and guidance as they need to shift from traditional nursing knowledge to largely new and unfamiliar knowledge related to transcultural nursing. Having nursing faculty who are knowledgeable and competent to guide undergraduate and graduate students to become sensitive and competent transcultural nurse practitioners in hospitals and community agencies remains a critical need in many schools of nursing. It is of interest that students (especially master and doctoral nursing students) seek faculty who are prepared in the field before enrolling in transcultural courses. They also expect faculty to use a holistic perspective and not a narrow mind-body or disease-symptom management focus. Students want and expect faculty to help them discover culturally grounded knowledge and use it to improve care to cultures. Discovering care differences and commonalties among cultures and the way cultures keep well or become ill is an integral part of teaching and practicing transcultural nursing. Using historical data, art forms, and both material and nonmaterial data also helps students to learn how cultures live and survive over time.

From the above definition of transcultural nursing, one has to shift from largely a medical disease model and traditional nursing to incorporate major dimensions about cultures, caring, and health or illness patterns. Students also realize that while they have spent considerable time learning anatomy, physiology, biology, microbiology, chemistry, and other similar courses, they must now reconsider knowledge with a much broader perspective about human beings over time and in different geographic locations. Transcultural nursing, therefore, provides a different view of human beings through transcultural nursing research, which must be integrated into selected and appropriate professionally learned knowledge, as well as using ideas from anthropology, philosophy (secular and theological), and other humanity areas. Students learn to discover people as cultural beings who have culturally defined care needs and rights that are important. They also realize that a "little knowledge of cultures can be dangerous," and so they value in-depth knowledge to understand cultures. At the same time they are challenged to use any appropriate medical and nursing knowledge but within a transcultural nursing perspective. These features are part of knowing and becoming a transcultural nurse to serve those with culturally different needs and expectations.

A major feature in the *definition of transcultural nursing is the focus on comparative differences (diversities) and similarities (commonalties) among cultures in relation to humanistic care, health, wellness, illness, and healing patterns, beliefs, and values.*[24] The nature of transcultural nursing requires a *comparative focus* to know patterns, expressions, values, and lifeways within and between cultures. Discovering how and why cultures are alike or different with respect to care, health, illness, death, and other areas provides new insights to improve or advance transcultural nursing care practices. *Why* cultures have different patterns of caring and different ways of healing, keeping well, becoming ill, or dying is of critical importance to nurses and especially to transcultural nurses. Comparative cultural interpretations and explanations of cultural and care expressions and meanings provide a wealth of different knowledge from traditional nursing or medical knowledge. It also leads to different practices and benefits to clients.

In transcultural nursing, one gradually learns how to do comparative cultural care and health assessments with individuals, families, groups, institutions, and communities. From assessment data one discovers cultural variations with similarities and differences within and between cultures. Remaining alert to subtle and gross differences among clients from Western and non-Western cultures helps nurses to understand why cultures are different and to understand client explanations or reasons over time. By discovering cultural differences or similarities, the nurse learns how to preserve, accommodate, or deal with differences that are not beneficial to clients and that there may also be some shared commonalties among and between cultures. To treat all clients "just alike" is generally very problematic and fails to respect culture-care differences. The author's concept of "the all alike syndrome" fails to recognize cultural variations and comparative differences among clients that can lead to nontherapeutic outcomes.[25] For example, some Anglo-Americans nurses believe they must treat Russian immigrant children just like all American children without realizing that Russian children are different and have different pain responses and experiences than Anglo-American children. Children in Russia are taught to respond to pain in a stoic way and to accept much pain compared with most Anglo-American children who express pain, often loudly and want immediate attention with their cries and complaints. Russian children have been enculturated in their lifecycle to accept pain in a stoic and nonexpressive way rather than crying or seeking immediate attention for pain relief. Such strikingly different cultural expressions are important comparative differences if the nurse is to provide therapeutic or helpful care to Russian children. With comparative transcultural knowledge, nurses are alert to watch for such differences and to respond in appropriate ways.

With the comparative focus as a dominant feature of transcultural nursing, nurses become knowledgeable about *cultural variations*; recognize subtle, covert, and overt differences among clients, families, groups, and institutional systems; and make appropriate responses. By knowingly responding to cultural differences or variations, the nurse can provide sensitive, compassionate, and competent care that promotes healing and well-being and fits cultural needs and expectations. Lumping or stereotyping people into one fixed mold is not congruent with transcultural nursing as it does not take into account cultural variations. Recognizing transcultural comparative care knowledge with variations helps to maintain quality care practices. Transcultural nurses are taught to identify comparative cultural meanings, body gestures, symbols, values, beliefs, use of space, perceptions of events, and even historical accounts about past and current life experiences. Such data are extremely valuable to approach and work with clients. Learning how to discover transcultural differences and similarities in a knowing way with clients and groups is a fascinating experience as it helps to validate findings and leads to accuracy. At the same time, one learns to respect and appreciate cultural differences, variabilities, and shared cultural attributes as an important part of transcultural nursing using comparative knowledge as an art and skill that takes astute observations and the perfecting of one's analytical and assessment abilities.

The term "*culture-specific care*" was coined by me in the early 1960s to designate care that is tailor-made and fits specific cultures such as Italian, Jewish, and others in appropriate ways. For example, many cultures will vary in what they eat, what they do, and how they want to be cared for when they become ill, disabled, or are dying. The nurse can provide sensitive and specific cultural care by using the client's beliefs, values, and practices that fit their particular needs. Culture-specific is an important concept to focus on with a designated culture to prevent using the "all alike" nursing or standard medical treatment regimes. Currently, the concept is being used by health personnel as they learn how to provide specific health care practices and decisions tailored to clients' cultural needs and lifeways. When carried out, clients say they benefit from health services or treatments in meaningful and acceptable ways. Culture-specific care is the art of using culture-specific knowledge and making it fit with the clients' needs, values and desires for cultural and health care reasons. As a consequence, client satisfactions, quick recovery, or healing often occurs with culture-specific care, and they

are usually willing to cooperate and comply with nurses and other health care services or expectations.[26] Negative client views or being resistant to nursing care can often be traced to health care personnel who fail to use culture-specific care practices. Indeed, culture-specific care can make a great difference in how quickly clients will cooperate with staff when they see their values and beliefs are incorporated into their care. Culture-specific care is also an integral part of the theory of culture care as it supports the goal of providing culturally congruent, responsible, safe, and beneficial transcultural nursing care.[27] Many examples are presented throughout this book with the theory, research findings, and practices.

Another major feature embodied in the definition of transcultural nursing is that culture and care are *holistic constructs* that can lead to knowing, understanding and helping people in their fullest and most meaningful lifeways. Culture comes from the discipline of anthropology and has long been studied and used by anthropologists as the totality of material and nonmaterial features of a culture, including language, history, art, spiritual, kinship, and many other aspects.[28,29] While there are many definitions of culture, the author has defined *culture* in the 1960s as *the learned and shared beliefs, values, and lifeways of a designated or particular group that are generally transmitted intergenerationally and influence one's thinking and actions modes.*[30] This definition has become central to transcultural nursing and guides nurses to grasp the holistic dimensions of a culture, and it is broad enough to develop and serve the purposes of the discipline. Culture is a very powerful and comprehensive construct that influences and shapes the way people know their world, live, and develop patterns to make decisions relative to their lifeworld. Culture is known as the blueprint to guide human lifeways and actions and to predict patterns of behavior or functioning. Culture is so much an integral part of our way of living, doing, and making decisions that one seldom pauses to think about it as culture. Culture has many hidden and built-in directives as rules of behavior, beliefs, rituals, and moral-ethical decisions that give meaning and purpose to life. It is one of the broadest ways to think about human beings in their world and the larger world in which they live. Cultures influence how one lives or exists each day or night and over time. Cultures influence choices and actions in specific ways such as what one chooses to eat, the way one sleeps or prepares food, and even becomes ill or dies.

Anthropologists are the experts who have studied western and non-western cultures for over 100 years and have valuable research data about many cultures that transcultural nurses study as holding or background knowledge about cultures, but always with awareness that cultures change and are not static over time. Indeed it is important to emphasize that cultures are *dynamic and not static as they change in different ways over time and under different circumstances or conditions.* As the first professional graduate nurse anthropologist to focus on cultures and nursing, I deliberately chose and defined culture as above for the full development of transcultural nursing as a new and different discipline than anthropology and traditional nursing. I could envision a new field of study and practice that had not been developed, but would be the hallmark of transcultural nursing. Indeed, transcultural nursing is *not* the same as anthropology, psychology, or other fields as it has been developed and shaped with distinctive features that make it unique as a discipline and professional practice. It is transcultural nursing with its unique body of culture care knowledge and practices that can serve clients worldwide and in special ways.

Since the phenomenon of culture is so central and important to transcultural nursing, one needs to realize that all human beings are born, live, marry (or remain single), stay well, become ill, and die within a cultural frame of reference. An awareness of the significance of culture with its shared values, beliefs, and action modes makes one realize how important it is to clients whether well, ill, disabled, or dying. As one notes, I have used the term *holding knowledge* to refer to substantive background knowledge about a culture or other phenomena that serves as known knowledge on which to reflect on ideas or experiences. Holding knowledge about culture care values, beliefs, symbols, and material culture forms that are usually transmitted over time and can change are relatively patterned and stable and need to be recognized. As one studies particular cultures over time and in-depth, the lifeways become evident and can guide the nurse's decisions.

Verbal and nonverbal communications are essential in studying the cultural beliefs and lifeways of different people. The nurse can identify patterns of culture, patterns of communication, and patterns of care through communication modes. Identifying different cultural patterns of daily or nightly living is also an essential focus of culture and transcultural nursing. It is always so intriguing to observe why cultures select what they do and what they reject or avoid. For example, if a client rejects pork, it may be because he is an Arab Muslim and pork cannot be eaten according to the Koran. However, other clients may also reject eating pork, so one has to study further the reasons and patterns. In another situation, a Mexican client rejected drinking ice water on a hot day. The Anglo-American nurse found this behavior "peculiar," "strange" and "irrational" on a hot day. This Mexican client believes in their culture's folk hot-and-cold theory with the cultural rule not to drink ice water when it is hot as it can lead to illness. Identifying and understanding such cultural taboos, expressions, and patterns and their need to be respected and understood within each culture is necessary to give culture-specific care. Every culture generally has different values and patterns of expression that need to be identified and understood to provide transcultural nursing care.

Another major and important theme in the definition of transcultural nursing is the focus on *human care and caring expressions, values, patterns, symbols, and practices of cultures.* In establishing transcultural nursing as a researcher and clinical practitioner since the mid 1950s, the author has held firmly to her position that *human care is essential for health and well-being* and is the *essence and central major focus of nursing.*[31,32] I held that humanistic care also had therapeutic benefits in healing and well-being, but in those early days many nurses did not agree with me. Indeed, the phenomena of human care is desperately needed to be studied in-depth to understand it, especially in relation to how cultures know and use care. Prior to the 1950s, nurses had not studied care in-depth nor did they claim *care was the essence of nursing,* even though they linguistically used the words care and nursing care.[33] The meaning of human care was largely unknown and not valued by many nurses until care was pursued by transcultural nurses and later by a few nursing-care scholars interested in the phenomenon, such as myself (beginning in the late 1940s and into the 1950s and 1960s)[34,35], Gaut,[36] Bevis,[37] Watson,[38] and Ray.[39]

Both the nursing care scholars of the mid 1970s along with transcultural nurses opened an entirely different pathway of knowledge and practice.

The author defined *care* as those *assistive, supportive, enabling, and facilitative culturally based ways to help people in a compassionate, respectful, and appropriate way to improve a human condition or lifeway or to help people face illnesses, death, or disability.*[40,41] I also made these firm statements: *care is an essential human need; caring is nursing; caring is the heart and soul of nursing; caring is power; caring is healing; and caring is the distinctive feature that makes nursing what it is or should be as a profession and discipline.*[42] I also discovered that care was embedded in culture and had to be teased out through research. Slowly, care and caring became valued by more nurses. Today, care is being studied and used as central to many nursing curricula, research, and ways of practice. Care is also being realized to be closely linked to culture with meaning and relevance to consumers, which necessitates that nurses fully understand cultures under consideration and in diverse health care systems.[43] In conceptualizing care, I held that caring must exist for curing to occur in most human beings and that caring and curing have different meanings and therapeutic outcomes.[44]

The above definition of transcultural nursing, therefore, embodies a number of important ideas to be understood such as the following:

1. Care needs to be systematically studied to learn about human care (caring) in diverse and similar cultures in the world and environments.
2. Nurses need to be knowledgeable about their own cultural care heritage and of biases, beliefs, and prejudices to work effectively with clients.
3. Nurses need to use transculture-specific and comparative knowledge to guide caring practices for culturally congruent care.
4. A focus on cultural care competencies for diverse cultures and universals (commonalities) is essential.
5. Nurses should seek comprehensive, holistic, and comparative culture care phenomena.
6. Maintaining an open learning-discovery process about care and culture is imperative.
7. Nurses need creative ways to provide culturally congruent care practices.

To achieve these important dimensions of transcultural nursing, nurses should be well grounded in transcultural nursing knowledge to guide their thinking and actions. Fortunately, there is a wealth of available transcultural nursing knowledge and practice guides that can be used today in hospitals, clinics, and a variety of community health services to prevent unfavorable outcomes.

Most importantly, nurses need to learn how to do cultural care assessments, which have different emphasis from traditional physical and mental nursing assessments. They are discussed later in this book. Grounded in transcultural nursing, nurses are discovering and using some entirely new sources of knowledge and practice ways related to healing, health, and well-being about cultural accidents, illnesses, disabilities, and death rituals with practices. Learning how cultures have maintained or preserved their health and prevented illness is generally new knowledge to most nurses. If nurses trust and respect clients they will often discover "cultural secrets" and special knowledge about traditional healers and carers of cultures and their roles. Cultural secrets are seldom shared with health professionals unless one has gained client trust and has a genuine interest in the person. Focusing on different language expressions, caring practices, stories, and life experiences, transcultural nursing care is learned and is meaningful to guide care practices.

Today, one hears a lot about "travel nurses," "tourist nurses," and "exchange nurses," but generally these nurses have not been prepared in transcultural nursing. They often have limited knowledge to function with different cultures. There are also nurses in military service, religious missions, or in other overseas assignments, and they too often lack preparation in transcultural nursing and struggle to understand and help the culturally different. These nurses often tell of their cultural and travel experiences and how they managed to "get by" or failed to do so. Some recognize their prejudices, biases, and misinformation about cultures. Today, nurse educators and others offer "professional seminars" and overseas exchange programs without preparation in transcultural nursing, which has led to questionable and unsound cultural learnings. Assuming one knows "all about a foreign culture" and can teach comparative knowledge is questionable. Even being raised in a culture may not make one an expert or competent transcultural nurse. To be a transcultural educator or practitioner requires one to study and be prepared in the discipline like all other discipline expectations. One must learn important transcultural nursing concepts, principles, and practices to provide safe and sound care practices.

Finally and most importantly, the ultimate *goal* of transcultural nursing is to provide *culturally congruent and competent care.* This term was first coined by me in the early 1960s as part of the theory of Culture Care Diversity and Universality. *Culturally congruent care refers to the use of sensitive, creative, and meaningful care practices to fit with the general values, beliefs, and lifeways of clients for beneficial and satisfying health care, or to help them with difficult life situations, disabilities, or death.*[45] This definition and similarly derived ones are now being used today by other health disciplines because they see the urgent need for culturally competent care with minorities, immigrants, and others. Nurses and other health practitioners are struggling to learn about cultures and their care practices to obtain client cooperation and beneficial outcomes. It is imperative today to attain and maintain beneficial and quality-based care. Culturally congruent care should become an integral part of a nurse's thinking and decisions for family and individual care practices. Thus the above definition of transcultural nursing is packed with meaning that one needs to reflect on to grasp its full and important dimensions. The definition also incorporates the general purpose of transcultural nursing in discovering and using culturally based research care knowledge to promote healing and health or to deal with illnesses, life-threatening conditions, or death in beneficial ways with clients. Providing culturally competent, safe, and congruent care to people of diverse or similar cultures is the central and dominant goal of transcultural nursing and should be with all health care providers worldwide.

The Scope and Rationale of and the Factors Influencing Transcultural Nursing

As the world has become increasingly global and complex, several factors have made transcultural nursing imperative in education, research, practice, and consultation. Some of these important worldwide factors will be identified and briefly discussed. The following global factors have significantly influenced the need for transcultural nursing:[46–48]

1. The steady and marked increase in the migration of people worldwide, especially with immigrants, refugees, the displaced, and others moving to diverse geographic locations within or outside a culture, country, or territory.
2. The worldwide fluctuation in cultural populations varying in different countries such as the marked increased numbers of Hispanics moving into the United States in the last decade.
3. The rise in cultural identities with health consumers expecting that their cultural beliefs, values, and lifeways will be respected, understood, and appropriately responded to in health care.
4. The worldwide increase in the use of Western modern high technologies, cyberspace, and electronic communications and health technologies bringing communication and technologies close to people of diverse cultures.
5. Increased signs of cultural conflicts and clashes, wars and violent acts among and between different cultures and nations influencing the health, survival, or death of people of diverse cultures.
6. The marked increased number of nurses, physicians, and other health care providers working in many different places in the world with cultural strangers since World War II.
7. An increase in cultural legal defense suits resulting from serious cultural conflicts and problems in health care services showing cultural care and treatment conflicts, ignorance, imposition, and offensive practices by health care providers who are unprepared in transcultural health services.
8. The rise in women's and men's human rights among cultures regarding their needs for health care services and for staff to understand their cultural care needs and desired treatment modes.
9. A marked increase in ethical and moral cultural health care concerns with evident conflicts between the "cultures of life and death" (the *culture of life* supporting newborns, elderly, and

youth and the *culture of death* supporting euthanasia, abortions, genetic manipulations, cloning, and a host of other destructive biotechnological treatment modes found in some health systems).

10. A major shift in Western cultures from hospital-managed services to community-based consumer health care, which is intended for more direct care to cultural minorities, the poor, the homeless, and other neglected and vulnerable groups.

11. An increased use of complementary, "alternative," folk, or generic health care practices, medicines, treatments, and healing modalities for prevention, healing, health maintenance, cost control, and perceived better health outcomes.

12. Increased consumer demand from minorities and the "culturally different" for better access to professional cultural health care and treatments that fit their cultural expectations and values.

13. A growing gap between the cultures of the poor and homeless and the cultures of the rich, showing a need for social justice and equal human rights in health care.

14. An increase in violence worldwide, revealing evidence of violence among diverse cultures who have been oppressed, poor, or neglected.

15. A general increased awareness by people that we need to find ways to live together in the world with many diverse cultures for reasonable peace, harmony, and healthy living and survival modes.

These factors and others remain significant influencers of the need for transcultural nursing and health care worldwide. In addition, cultures have their own unique cultural concerns that influence their health, well-being, or death that they want health care providers to address. For these reasons and others, transcultural nursing is needed to meet many of these global health concerns and people needs. Let us now briefly consider some of these trends.

The first and major factor that has influenced transcultural nursing has been *the marked increase in immigration and the migration of people within and between countries worldwide.* While most countries have been established on an immigrant basis, the trend in the past several decades has been a marked increase with many

cultural migrants. Never before in the history of humankind has there been so many people moving in and out of virtually every place in the world. So, while migrations and migrants have always been characteristic of the human species in different lands, the number and frequency of migrations have markedly increased since World War II largely as a result of wars, famine, oppressive political and economic regimes, and religious persecution.[49] In addition to wars, politically oppressive conditions, and poverty, unexpected natural disasters such as hurricanes, tornadoes, and typhoons have been major reasons for migrations. Other reasons include human freedom and perceived new opportunities for employment with better living conditions or for survival, especially in the United States, known as a land of freedom and respect for human rights.

The collapse of the Iron Curtain in Eastern Europe, the fall of communism in the Soviet Union in 1989, the Persian Gulf War in the Middle East, and the oppressive political war conditions in China, South Africa (especially Sudan), and the Balkan region with killings and threats to lives have led to many migrations and refugee placements in freedom countries. For 200 years, immigrants and refugees have been a major reason for many people migrating to the United States, Australia, Canada, and other perceived freedom or "safe" places in the world, but the numbers and intense favor for migrations have increased markedly in recent years. Since World War II, many refugees have come to the United States from Cambodia, Bosnia, Middle East, Europe, South and East Africa, Vietnam, Ethiopia, Sudan, Russia, Israel, Iran, and China, as well as from several Southeast Asian and Pacific areas. Immigrants from many Latin American and Caribbean regions have increased in recent decades bringing many Spanish-speaking people to North America, South America, and Canada. Many migrants such as the Vietnamese refugees were critically ill, and nurses were expected to understand and help them. Unquestionably, migrants and refugees have been seeking and relocating in many foreign areas worldwide, which has led to the need for transcultural nursing and healthcare.

It is important to state that climatic and natural disasters such as droughts, floods, earthquakes, and hurricanes have also led to migration of often large numbers of people to safe lands and on short notice. The strong desire and urgent need for human survival for physical protection, justice, freedom, and economic and religious needs of people have been important reasons for migrations along with the hope of better living opportunities. As a consequence of these worldwide migrations, immigrations, and refugees, a great diversity of cultures can be found in most communities and countries today. Some cultures have arrived almost overnight, and nurses and other health care providers have been expected to communicate with understanding to help them. Such humanistic needs remain critical with moral and professional obligations to serve cultural strangers. Cultural shock and feelings of helplessness with a lack of confidence and limited understanding of the strangers have been apparent with some nurses and other health professionals. The need for transcultural nursing has been clearly apparent through educational and health service programs established to meet migrant needs, and yet there were virtually no educational programs nor health services until after transcultural nursing was launched and established in the early 1960s and developed in subsequent decades.

The second major factor that led to establishing transcultural nursing was *an implicit societal moral and professional expectation that nurses and other health care providers need to know, understand, respect, and respond appropriately to care for people of diverse cultures.* Slowly, this moral and ethical imperative has begun to be realized in different countries, but with different action and attitude responses. The societal mandate to provide knowledgeable understanding, respectful, and compassionate care and other health services for the culturally different was a critical and urgent need in most countries. The rise in cultural identity, human rights, and cultural justice expectations became evident among cultures, especially in the United States, Canada, Australia, and several other countries. Nurses and other health care providers needed to understand diverse cultures to care for them. The oppressed, neglected groups — the refugees, the poor, and the homeless from many other cultures — posed real problems to health personnel. Immigrants from different cultures had different values, beliefs, and expectations for health care, and they wanted to be understood with regard to their premigration cultural history, traumatic experiences, and many cultural conflicts in their old and new locations. Many migrants such as the Bosnians had experienced extensive cultural

pain to see their many family members and neighbors horribly killed before their eyes in war and oppressive regimes before migrating. For example, the Bosnians and Sudanese in the United States saw millions of their people killed, raped, and tortured in terrible ways and over time. Such traumatic experiences necessitated culture-specific care and human compassion by health care providers. It has been largely professional nurses in community and home contexts or in emergency clinics who have tried to care for many of these refugees. Many nurses experienced cultural shock and felt very hopeless and helpless to work effectively with these people. Yet they felt a professional and moral obligation to help them. Clearly, transcultural nursing knowledge and competencies are much needed to meet these migrant and other refugee needs for several decades.

The third factor and rationale for transcultural nursing was *the rapid increase in the use of high technologies in caring or curing with different responses and effects on clients of diverse cultures.*[50,51] With the tremendous increase in the use of a great variety of types of electronic equipment for modern assessment and communication modes such as the internet, digital computers, organ imaging machines, and many other health diagnostic and treatment machines came new concerns and reactions with clients of different cultures. Many immigrants and non-Western clients have experienced cultural shock, fear, and disbelief with such powerful technological machines. This response was especially evident with non-Western immigrants living in the United States, Canada, Europe, Australia, and other Western cultures where high technologies dominate health care services. Many strange technologies were used for diagnosis, treatment, communication, and in other areas with migrants from nontechnological cultures and with the poor and homeless. Some of the clients had great fears of being electrocuted or killed with powerful machines. Some Vietnamese feared their soul would be taken with the machines. Clients from poor and rural areas and from non-Western cultures were often suspicious and frightened of the technologies even with the nurses' or physicians' best explanations. Using high-technology equipment such as CAT scans for tumors and other x-rays were especially feared. Hearing the terms "radiation beams," "ultrasound test," and "imaging one's body" were frightening to many clients. The personal attention to the client was often missing as the machines "took over and controlled their bodies" and decisions. Accordingly, some clients rejected or declined high-tech treatments. The use of high technologies with different cultures showed different responses that necessitated nurses understand cultures *before* using high-tech equipment, explanations, and care practices. As I predicted in the 1970s, with increased use of high technologies, there would be a decrease in interpersonal relationships and communication leading to nontherapeutic outcomes.[52] This has been evident in the past two decades. Nurses need transcultural nursing to study negative and positive client outcomes and to maintain interpersonal relationships.

The fourth reason why transcultural nursing has been essential is related to *increased signs of cultural conflicts, cultural clashes, and cultural imposition practices between nurses and clients of diverse cultures.*[53,54] While nurses are expected to care for all clients encountered, this is most difficult without understanding cultural differences among clients. As nurses work with clients, there are inevitable differences between the client's and nurse's beliefs and values. Nurses caring for clients such as recent immigrants and refugees, who have experienced violence and killings resulting from cultural clashes and conflicts, pose major nursing challenges and difficulties. Many clients from Bosnia, Rwanda, Sudan, and other places in the world today have often been deeply hurt by violent acts of killing, rape, and torture. Such atrocities have been some of the worst in the past century among cultures of very different political, economic, and religious values. Cultural conflicts, violence, and killings are often what nurses are expected to understand and deal with in nurse-client and home-community contexts today. Only with transcultural knowledge, compassion, and understanding of these people's historical, political, religious, and other cultural areas can nurses work effectively with such tortured refugees, immigrants, and other traumatized migrants. Transcultural nursing concepts and principles and anthropological, cultural, political, social, and historical insights are important to care for people of such different cultures, especially where traditional hatred and killings have occurred over a long time between and within subcultures. There are also signs and acts of increased violence in homes, schools, local communities, and workplaces where many signs of cultural clashes, conflicts,

and violence are evident. In addition, there are juvenile, adult and drug gangs found in most countries with whom nurses are expected to work, as well as prisoners and others who violate the law. Psychiatric, psychological, and other explanations are often used to explain such behavior, but cultural factors related to history are essential to understand these gangs, prisoners, and groups. Unfortunately, cultural conflict explanations are often missing, and only mind-body explanations prevail. Nurses prepared in transcultural nursing, anthropology, law, and political justice are often in a good position to grasp the clients' world and make appropriate actions and decisions related to caring for them. For often intercultural domestic, public, and other arenas of interacting will help to show the sources of prejudices, racism, anger, and violence. Cultural taboos are also usually unknown to health care providers or underestimated. Cultural gender abuses that are often intergenerational and are patterned need to be understood. All too frequently, school teenage violence is related to cultural differences and serious gender conflicts. The *culture of violence* is with us and nurses need to understand some of the reasons for so much hatred among cultures. A transcultural caring holistic approach is much needed so nurses can grasp the bigger picture of humans related to cultural values, religion, and many other cultural factors influencing human responses in the home, workplace, schools, and communities. Such intercultural violence with cultural clashes will continue, and this is why transcultural nursing preparation and skills are essential. Already, this approach in the discipline is providing some very different insights to deal with traditionally labeled psychological and medical diseases.

A fifth factor influencing transcultural nursing has been *the marked increase in the number of nurses who travel and work in different places in the world.* Today, and more so in the future, nurses will be traveling worldwide and will be employed in many different or limitedly known cultures and geographic locations. This trend will markedly increase in the 21st century, but nurses will soon realize that they must be grounded in substantial transcultural research knowledge to live and function successfully in different cultures.[55,56] This trend was anticipated in the early 1950s when nurses began to travel abroad, some being in military or mission roles. These nurses needed transcultural nursing knowledge and skills along with earlier nurse leaders who ventured to foreign lands such as Florence Nightingale and others. Cultural ignorance and cultural stresses have been evident with the great need to understand the values, beliefs, and major features of cultures *before* going to a foreign country. It was important to give care and to use medications and treatments with the culturally different. Still today nurses are traveling to different countries for employment, out of curiosity, or for different experiences, and these nurses could benefit from transcultural nursing concepts, principles, and competency skills for safe and effective employment and relationships. However, nurses do not have to go to a foreign country for cultural experiences as there are many cultures within one's local or regional geographic area that can provide rich learning with transcultural nurse mentors. Learning how to assess care patterns, needs, and health practices of families and individuals of different cultures necessitates knowledge and skills found in transcultural nursing. It is then that one can predict effective outcomes in nursing care and client satisfactions.

Currently, nurses employed in foreign countries or with national cultures generally need to know the culture and speak some of the language. Otherwise, misinformation, misdiagnosis, and misunderstandings of cultures can occur. Language barriers remain a major and significant factor in becoming an effective caregiver for the culturally different. In the future, nurses will also need to speak several languages as they work in different world cultures. For language is the critical communication mode to know, respect, and obtain accurate information from others. Language skills enable the nurse to enter the world of the client and to discover what will be helpful to people. In a way the new knowledge of transcultural nursing also becomes like a new language essential to assess and to know how to help others.

As nurses work in distant lands or at home, they will be caring for cultural strangers. This can be stressful and threatening unless one has some *holding* or *background knowledge* of the clients' cultures. Moreover, cultural strangers can test nurses to see if they can be trusted and to see if they are genuinely sincere and will be safe and helpful to them. Functioning with cultural strangers such as people of the Sudan, Vietnam, Ethiopia, Old Order Amish, Jehovah's Witnesses, and others can lead to destructive or negative outcomes un-less one has some background knowledge of who these people are, their cultural values, and lifeways. Thus transcultural nursing is essential to work effectively and safely with clients of foreign or different cultures — a major reason to establish transcultural nursing.

The sixth factor that influenced establishing transcultural nursing was *anticipated legal defense suits against nurses resulting from cultural negligence, cultural ignorance, and cultural imposition practices in working with diverse cultures.*[55] I predicted that by the 21st century legal suits would occur with nurses and other health personnel as clients from different minority and majority cultures sought justice for their human rights, values, and desired health care. If nurses were not prepared to support what they did and why, they would be defenseless and unable to protect themselves with clients. To prevent cultural ignorance, neglect, and insults to clients of diverse cultures, transcultural nursing was greatly and urgently needed. In time, nurses will probably need additional courses on the rights and process of legal torts in different cultures. Unquestionably, our world is a litigious one, and people know how to get their rights or harm abated. Cultures that have long experienced violations of their rights, values, and norms are finding ways to seek cultural justice and some with huge monetary claims. When cultural rights are violated, cultures will respond today for justice. Presently, transcultural nurses in the United States have been called to testify at legal suits when cultures contend that their rights have been violated, neglected, or misrepresented. Cultures vary with their different legal sanctions, norms, and interpretations of what exists or what they believe occurred in health care situations. This may greatly differ from health professional views. With more immigrants and migrations worldwide one can predict there will be many more lawyers working with health personnel and administrators to handle culturally based defense suits.

A few examples of legal suits are offered to help students understand culturally based legal action.[59] A Laotian family living in the United States found their cultural values and beliefs were violated when a community nurse reported and insisted that a child with a cleft palate be admitted to a hospital for surgery to correct the defect. The Laotian family, however, strongly refused the surgery because of their cultural beliefs and religious ideas about the sacredness of the head and for other cultural reasons. A legal suit began after this large extended Laotian family raised funds to sue the hospital for doing the surgery without their extended family's full consent. The Laotian family held that the hospital violated their cultural beliefs because the cleft palate was viewed as a "gift from God" and their rights "to protect sacred head spirits." The family had been caring for the child and had no concerns. Moreover, they believed the child's palate would heal with their folk care practices. The Laotian family and large community pleaded their case to the judge and won.

Another example of legal action was with a Jehovah's Witness family who refused blood transfusions for their child. They strongly opposed their son having the transfusion because of their religious beliefs. They challenged the United States legal and medical system; however, they did not win their case. Today, other cultures in the United States with similar expectations are becoming alert to their cultural rights and will sue if health personnel fail to know and respect their cultural norms and beliefs. One can predict there will be many legal challenges with culturally based health services when clients' human rights and cultural norms and values are violated. It will therefore be imperative that nurses have transcultural nursing preparation with ethical and legal, culturally based insights to function and understand what constitutes a legal and cultural offense. Moreover, nurses will be called to testify or be witnesses for cultures and for health institutions or agencies in the future.

A seventh factor that led to the development of transcultural nursing as a discipline of study and practice was *the rise in gender and special groups issues and rights.* In recent decades, the feminist cultural movement has markedly increased so that women assert their rights, especially those related to leadership positions, unfair gender practices and other discrimination issues. Women's rights have been violated in nursing and health systems, and now women are speaking out to redress such concerns. Male groups and other special groups are also taking active leadership for their rights when they experience reverse discrimination, abuses, or have not had similar opportunities of women. Both women's and men's rights are being pursued in the Western world, but in some non-Western cultures, women are seeking ways to deal with male abuse and oppressive acts or practices that have long been traditionally destructive to them. For example, some Iranian women are seeking ways to select their spouses, to not wear chadors, to vote, to drive cars, and to seek health care for themselves and their children. In southern Africa, some women are trying to stop genital mutilation, and older women want more freedoms and less abuse from men. Changes in women's roles and their rights are becoming transculturally known and recognized. Men in several cultures are learning how to alter their patriarchal or autocratic roles and to be effective in child care and in shared domestic spouse activities. Children and teenagers are also witnessing and discussing gender and parental changes in many cultures worldwide. Such changes in women's and men's roles necessitate comparative historical, transcultural, and anthropological knowledge to be effective in the human-caring change processes.

Likewise in the health field, changes are needed transculturally as males alter their oppressive and often autocratic decision-making roles to accommodate women nurses who are capable of making health care decisions. However, these changes often show signs of cultural conflicts, stress, and pain with traditional and long-standing norms of behavior.[60] Such changes necessitate transcultural insights to understand and effectively make gender changes to support gender rights. Transcultural nursing, anthropology, and other social science research-based knowledge are imperative to understand, appreciate, and respect the fact that cultural differences related to gender changes, human rights, and other consequences occur with gender violence and cultural clashes.

Changing gender roles in non-Western and Western cultures necessitates a broad and open view about cultural differences and similarities with reasons why gender differences have existed over time. Moreover, to change gender roles in different contexts requires extensive knowledge of historical social-structure factors and cultural norms. Learning through transcultural nursing how best to support women's and men's traditional healing and care-giving roles in diverse cultures is also important to recognize and uphold. For example, Wenger's research with the Old Order Amish[61] and Leininger's work with the Gadsup[62] are good examples of gender role differences in cultures over time and how to work carefully with the people in making changes. Cultures have beliefs and ideas of what constitutes good or acceptable healthy family and community gender role changes and the potential consequences. Nurses learn about these ideas and beliefs in transcultural family counseling, specific cultural therapies, and lifecycle care processes. This requires focused study in transcultural nursing so that nurses can be truly therapeutic with different clients in Western and non-Western cultures. Hence another important reason why transcultural nursing was much needed.

The eighth factor that gave rise to transcultural nursing was *the growing trend to care with and for people whether well or ill in their familiar or particular living and working environments.* From an anthropological perspective, it became clear to me that health care services needed to become more community-based and regulated by consumers of different cultures in the future. Indeed, cultures and subcultures in different communities are the natural place for healing, maintaining well-being, or for dying. I envisioned that consumers will gradually take hold of their health care needs, rights, and services within their local and familiar communities in the 21st century and with health personnel as facilitators.[63] As health care becomes more *community-based and regulated*, nurses and other health personnel will need to know and understand cultures in their community contexts. Many traditional professional health institutions such as hospitals will markedly decrease in the future, being replaced by new kinds of community-based health services that will flourish and that health-invested consumers will largely control.

As a futurist, I envisioned that global health care models and practices will be shared and become patterned in cultural environmental areas such as health spas, natural exercise areas, and many different community-based services using modern technologies and interpersonal skills.[64] Health care will be transformed from the traditional patterns of the 20th century and will become transculturally sensitive to serve many people of diverse cultures with new kinds of prevention and health maintenance services. Serving the poor, politically oppressed, and underrepresented cultures who need health care must occur in community contexts that are familiar, acceptable, and with less costs. Managed care practices and many present forms of health care will be changed to some entirely new, transculturally focused, health care systems. Health personnel

will need to know much about local community cultural beliefs, values, and practices. Transcultural nursing and all areas of nursing will focus on functioning in transcultural community contexts and on becoming knowledgeable of diverse cultures living and working in these communities.

In light of the above eight global trends influencing the development of transcultural nursing, a major and critical need will be for more prepared transcultural nurses who can provide culturally congruent, safe, and meaningful care. This need will be fully evident in the 21st century, but there will be far too few nurses prepared in transcultural nursing to prevent serious culturally based illnesses, accidents, violence, famine, drug usage, poverty, and a host of other human conditions and needs. The third millennium will clearly be the era to focus on prevention and health maintenance and on reducing chronic illnesses, accidents, and disabilities with diverse cultures worldwide. Culturally based illnesses will become of heightened interest along with traditional healing practices. The holistic transcultural perspective will become a dominant theme and goal by the year 2015. While the biophysical and genetic engineering and other new treatment modes will exist along with modern high-tech equipment, there will be many cultures wanting to be treated and understood holistically with their values. Treating and caring for the whole human being as an integrated being will be expected. *Partnerships* between consumer and health professionals as coparticipants will be needed to ensure quality care and cultural human rights — all major changes.

In the early 1960s and 1970s, I had the opportunity to study the importance of village and local life and how extended families and communities maintained health and prevented cultural illnesses and unfavorable practices with several cultures. It was evident that Western nurses and physicians need to learn about non-Western health care in community contexts to understand *why* some cultures remain well and others become ill. We still need to study the strengths and positive healthy lifeways of cultures with a comparative transcultural focus. Such knowledge remains imperative today for transcultural health care providers and educators to maintain healthy lifeways.

Unquestionably, transculturally prepared and practicing nurses will be in great demand by the year

2015 as community-based cultural maintenance services for diverse cultures become recognized. Both transcultural nurse generalists and specialists in life-cycle areas and in prevention and health maintenance will be greatly needed to provide safe and competent care. It will be a great opportunity for nurses prepared in transcultural nursing to make health care culture specific, safe, and meaningful to consumers. Hence, for all these major reasons, transcultural nursing became of critical importance and a necessity for today and the future.

In considering the above reasons for establishing the transcultural nursing discipline, several questions can be raised for reflective consideration and discussion:

1. In what ways are dominant Western health practices helping to facilitate non-Western or minority cultures today with their desired health care goals?
2. How can nurses deal with their biases, prejudices and ignorance when working with many immigrants, refugees, and the culturally different?
3. What current factors limit nurses in providing care to cultural strangers, immigrants, poor, and underserved?
4. What nursing factors limit nurses in providing culturally based care today?
5. How can we best prepare nurses for current and future changes in a global world through transcultural nursing education and practices?

These questions and others are important to move transcultural nursing forward in study and practice. Many nurses realize the great need for transcultural nursing, but they need support and encouragement to pursue this goal.

Envisioning the Global Scope of Transcultural Nursing

It is often difficult for some nurses to envision transcultural nursing from a global perspective. However, a global or worldwide view of transcultural nursing becomes essential to help nurses see the *scope* of transcultural nursing in many places in the world. A global perspective of transcultural nursing helps to expand nurses' thinking worldwide and to envision how one might function in different places in the world in education, research, and practice. Unquestionably, as nurses think and act globally as professionals their endeavors to understand and serve people effectively worldwide could occur.

In the early 1950s, I wondered what would happen to nursing if there were no geographic boundaries as cultural barriers. Could nursing survive and grow if its members kept a narrow and local view of serving people? Also, as the world was changing and globalization became a reality, how could nurses expand their parochial and local views to a worldwide view? It was a world in which nurses would be functioning in the future. The above functions had implications for education, research, and practice to survive in a rapidly changing world.

To help nurses envision the scope of transcultural nursing, I developed the logo shown in Fig. 1.1, with the message "*Many Cultures One World*," and predicted: "That the culture care needs of people will be met by nurses prepared in transcultural nursing." This logo offered a new challenge and different vision for nurses to function as transcultural nurses in the future.

This logo has served as a cognitive image and philosophical guide to help nurses realize the large scope of transcultural nursing. It helps nurses to think globally with a moral obligation to serve human beings wherever necessary. It has been the official logo of the Transcultural Nursing Society since I launched this organization in 1974 as a worldwide one for all

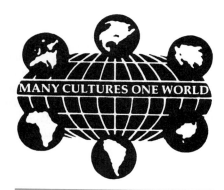

Figure 1.1
The global view of transcultural nursing.

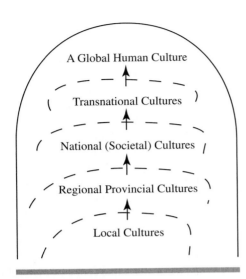

Figure 1.2
The scope of transcultural nursing.

nurses. The motto has helped nurses to think about many cultures in our global world of transcultural nursing, and as formal field of study and practice. [65] It continues to serve as the logo hallmark of transcultural nursing.

Still another visual aid to help nurses expand their worldview and the scope of the profession was developed as shown in Figure 1.2.

As one reflects on Figure 1.2, nurses may be working with specific cultures such as Mexican, African, Vietnamese, and others in a local geographic area. Usually, this is where nurses begin to develop their knowledge and skills by focusing on one culture using concepts, principles, and transcultural nursing knowledge. Later nurses are functioning in a regional or province area with several cultures such as in Australian, African, and Canadian provinces or in a region in the United States. This is more difficult and requires more comparative transcultural nursing knowledge. For example, a Canadian nurse was working with several Native American Cree families and also Portuguese families, which is a much larger geographic area of transcultural nursing responsibility. There are regional communities such as the Old Order Amish population in the United States. The transcultural nurse could be working with Aborigines in a regional area in Australia. Nurses in the United States often work in regional areas to care for Native Americans where the scope of practice is much larger than a specific tribal culture. Then there is the societal or national cultural scope, which is a very large area of responsibility for transcultural nurses. This may be government controlled or through private organizations or institutions. For example, Indian Health Services or national-specific cultural organizations function with many cultures within a society. Nurses in the United States, England, Canada, and elsewhere may be employed with cultures nationwide and practice transcultural nursing for a national organization. Currently, there are few transcultural nurses prepared and ready to function effectively and knowledgeably in regional and national programs. However, the interest and requests are being made and this will increase in the future. Most assuredly, nurses assuming the regional, national, and societal roles as transcultural specialists will be required to be well prepared in transcultural nursing through master and doctoral programs as the knowledge need and scope of responsibility are considerable.

It is important for nurses to envision the total scope of transcultural nursing to appreciate its potential to serve human beings worldwide. This scope goes *beyond international nursing*, which is much smaller in scope than global transcultural nursing. International nursing is usually between two cultures or countries such as the United States and Thailand. Transcultural nursing is the broadest and most encompassing scope that includes several cultures and requires comparative knowledge and skills of several cultures. Hence, the idea and scope of transcultural nursing reflects many cultures from a comparative worldview. Transcultural nursing is the largest perspective in scope as one maintains a focus on several interacting cultures in the world. In contrast, international (as the term implies) is between two cultures, not several. It is a limited and narrow focus and perspective. In the future, transcultural nurse experts and others will seek patterns and lifeways of people that are global and universal. When this occurs, many new discipline domains and practices will be established to help nurses move between many cultures with greater comparative knowledge, confidence, and competencies. Then the true and predicted essence of transcultural nursing will be worldwide, hopefully by the year 2030.

 ## Historical Development of Transcultural Nursing

The historical development of transcultural nursing is important, interesting, and unique as it evolved over the past five decades. As the founder and a central leader of transcultural nursing, I am able to share this lived experience firsthand along with the challenges and barriers. In fact, the evolution might best be portrayed as analogous to salmon trying to go upstream against strong waters, but struggling to reach their goal or homeland. This has been transcultural nursing and its struggles for several decades.

Some of the recurrent questions often posed to me are as follows:

1. What factors led you to establish transcultural nursing as an area of study, research, and practice?
2. What were your visions, dreams, and hopes for transcultural nursing that were needed and yet not recognized and developed as a formal area of study and practice?
3. What were some of the major hurdles or barriers you encountered to establish transcultural nursing through education, research, and practice?
4. What facilitated your endeavors as largely a lone explorer and leader to establish transcultural nursing worldwide?

These questions and many more continue to be of great interest to many nursing students and others since starting the field five decades ago. Because of space limitations, only major highlights can be presented in this chapter. This account will be told with the personal pronoun "I" to capture my direct experiences, challenges, and involvement through time.

It was in the mid 1950s while working as the first, graduate, child-psychiatric clinical nurse specialist in a psychiatric unit in the United States that I discovered major cultural differences among the children and parents.[66] I saw the need to address the fact that culture was the critical and major missing dimension of care. As I observed and tried to help the children from several different cultures, I experienced cultural shock and felt

helpless to respond to the children and their parents. Recognizing such major differences among the children and from my cultural Irish-German background, I knew changes had to be made. Culture was missing not only in nursing but in medicine and other health fields. Even though this treatment center was recognized as desired for mildly disturbed children, the cultural needs of African, Mexican, Jewish, German, and other culturally different were not being in met in 1950. These children were clearly different in their needs, responses and care expectations. Some children spoke different languages, some liked only certain foods, and some accepted or rejected medications and treatments in certain ways. They had different play patterns and different sleep rituals at bedtime. Some children were very talkative about their parents, others were silent, and still others were stoic. The Anglo-American children played aggressively, while the Mexican and Appalachian children played quietly. The Appalachian child carried a wooden stick and string and slept with it at night. Euro-Americans hugged stuffed animals at bedtime. When the Jewish parents came to visit their son, he clung to his mother for some time and talked a lot to her. The German child was independent as ever and remained "brave" when injured and seldom complained. Mexican parents were always asking if their child was lonely for the family.

Such gross differences in the daily life and with many other observations made me keenly aware of cultural differences among the children and parents. Nursing and medical staff seemed unaware of such cultural differences. I did not understand these children's behavior except from my narrow nursing and psychoanalytical view, which failed to explain what I saw and heard. I had recently completed a master's (graduate) degree program in psychiatric nursing and had worked as a nursing clinician and administrator for several years, but my nursing education (in the 1940s) had never prepared me for understanding cultural differences. I had heard that anthropology was focused on culture, and so I began reading anthropology books where available. A short time later, I pursued graduate education in cultural and social anthropology at the University of Washington.

While in the five-year anthropology program, I realized the wealth of rich and valuable knowledge about many different cultures. I became quite excited about how this knowledge could potentially help nurses and clients. I was, however, distressed that anthropological and related cultural information had not become part of nursing. I discovered there were no nursing books on transcultural care. There were no nursing theories or research literature specific to caring for clients of diverse cultures in the pre-1950 years. The more I studied anthropology literature, the more I could envision a close relationship between nursing and anthropology. I could see there were differences in philosophy, goals, and practice for nursing from anthropology. They were two different fields. While each discipline was different, there were some shared potential features that needed to be considered as I envisioned developing a new field of transcultural nursing. Some of these ideas have been presented in *Nursing and Anthropology: Two Worlds to Blend*.[67] It soon became clear to me that there was a critical need for the field of transcultural nursing.

Nurses needed to consider selected concepts and research from anthropology in reconceptualizing and developing the new field. In my first transcultural nursing book, *Nursing and Anthropology* (1970), I discussed the commonalities and differences between nursing and anthropology and the potential to support the a new field of transcultural nursing.[68] It was clear that anthropology was a social science field and transcultural nursing was a professional practice field with societal obligations to care for people. In 1978 I published the first book focused on and entitled *Transcultural Nursing Concepts, Theories & Practices*.[69] In this book, I identified basic concepts and principles and some theoretical ideas and practices for transcultural nurses. I emphasized that care was central to nursing and needed to be studied transculturally. This came from my basic direct experiences in nursing but not from nurse leaders. I also realized nursing needed to study cultural phenomena to make care meaningful and relevant to clients and practices. Nursing in the mid 1950s was deeply involved in learning about medical knowledge and practices and related knowledge areas such as microbiology, chemistry, anatomy, and physiology, but failed to realize the cultural and care dimensions. There were no courses focused specifically on culture and caring in United States nursing curricula. These were major areas still to be incorporated into nursing.

Since there was no emphasis on care and culture and no field of transcultural nursing, I began to carve out and develop the field anew. The philosophy, purposes, scope, and nature of the new field and potential discipline had to be established. There were no explicit theories or conceptual or practice models for transcultural nursing. It was mainly a one-woman leadership challenge. Florence Nightingale had not discussed and explicated care and culture even though she worked with Crimean soldiers and traveled.[70] It is of interest, however, that today (and 150 years later), there are some nurses proclaiming that Nightingale's focus was on care, yet it was never defined or made explicit by Nightingale.[71] This is a common tendency in the culture of nursing when new ideas become meaningful and popular; they are acclaimed to have always existed earlier.

My first challenge was to develop a body of transcultural nursing knowledge to teach and guide nurses into the new field. In the mid 1950s and from my clinical work and study in anthropology, I envisioned that by the year 2000 transcultural nursing would be imperative, but there was a critical need for research-based knowledge and practices for the field. As an Anglo-American Western nurse, I chose to study a non-Western culture and to rigorously study two different worlds for comparative knowledge. So, in the early 1960s for my PhD study I went to the Eastern Highlands of New Guinea to study people in two villages who had had limited contact with Western peoples. It was a non-Western and totally different culture than the United States. I observed and studied in-depth for nearly two years Gadsup lifeways in two remote non-technological and non-Western villages (Color Insert I). I lived day and night with the villagers while they observed me and I observed and learned much from them.[72,73]

During this intense and stimulating field study with dark-skinned Gadsups and no modern Western technologies or conveniences, I learned much as a white-skinned woman about their lifeways and world, which were in sharp contrast with my Anglo-American and early rural farm (and later urban) lifeways in middle America. My rural experiences in Nebraska, my Christian philosophy to know and respect God's people, and my experiences of living through a severe depression in the 1930s all helped me considerably to learn and survive in a largely unknown culture. I became immersed daily and nightly into the culture by joining in some of their activities. I adapted to the absence of modern facilities such as an indoor bathroom, electric lights, and piped-in water and to a very different environment and language for nearly two years. It challenged me in many ways and taught me a lot about myself and comparative American lifeways with the Gadsups.[74] The language was extremely complex and had to be studied and documented, but my openness to learn and listen to them was important. Reflections on general anthropological concepts and research of other non-Western cultures was helpful along with some of my nursing skills to remain with and listen to people. Every daily experience was almost a new one, which gave me enthusiasm for field study of strangers or limitedly known people.

While in New Guinea I became convinced that Western nurses would need transcultural and anthropological knowledge to function and survive and to care for the people of drastically different cultures. Western nurses had much to learn and study about non-Western cultures to be effective or therapeutic with clients of diverse cultures. Nurses needed substantive preparation in the concepts, principles, and available research data to help them to provide care in diverse cultures. Nursing texts and articles of their caring, health, and illnesses modes were practically nonexistent in non-Western cultures. So, on returning to the United States from New Guinea in the early 1960s, I began to develop transcultural nursing content and courses, but was baffled on how best to entice nurses into this new area of study and practice. Initially there were no nurses interested to support and help me, and there were no financial resources. So while I was eager to develop the field and realized the critical need, I found very few helpers and financial resources.

I soon realized that there were very few nurses who shared my interest, enthusiasm, or goals. In the 1960s, several nurse leaders told me, "We have too much to do and develop in the medical and nursing area; there is no interest nor time to think about other people or cultures. Besides we need to help our own people and take care of them at home in the USA." Another prominent nurse leader said, "Transcultural nursing will never be realized in nursing as nurses must become good medical, physical, and mental-health nurses dealing with diseases, symptoms, and medical treatments to survive. Learning about cultures is a waste of our time." Still another prominent nurse leader said, "Nurses will never change their practices for cultures and caring. Besides nursing is always the same wherever nurses work — there are no cultural differences." A nurse administrator said, "Your ideas are totally strange, foreign, and unacceptable to nurses. It will take years before nurses will ever value ideas about transcultural nursing practice to give care to specific cultures." An educator stated, "There is no room in the nursing curricula to study culture." Despite these negative statements and others in the 1960s and 1970s, I kept pursuing my goal with hopes to make transcultural nursing a reality someday and to make it worldwide.

It is also important to state that in pre-1960 days, health care emphasis was largely on the *mind* and *physical* needs of patients in Western cultures and on post World War innovations in medicine with new techniques and medicines. There was limited interest in non-Western cultures with their healing, curing, or caring practices. A few anthropologists were beginning to study medical disease conditions in non-Western cultures, but had no interest in caring phenomena. There was limited interest in studying the relationship of culture to care in Western or non-Western cultures. Despite these trends, I continued to introduce ideas about transcultural nursing and taught about "cultural differences that needed attention," "vulnerable cultures," "neglected cultures," "culturally congruent care," and "cultural imposition practices" within and outside the classroom. I took the philosophical position that if you valued and believed in something, you should persistently pursue it because someday it could become a reality. Interestingly, most anthropologists did not understand nursing and were far more interested in medicine and physicians' roles and their practices. A few exceptions were Margaret Mead, Lyle Saunders, and Esther Lucille Brown. However, with Saunders and Brown their interests were largely in medical and social science institutional practices. So they did not influence my work, and I never discussed ideas related to transcultural nursing and human caring with them. The relationship of nursing and anthropology remained strong with me.

In 1968 I established the Committee on Nursing and Anthropology within the Medical Anthropology Council and served as Chair for several years.[75] The purpose of this Committee was to exchange common ideas, research, and theories between the disciplines of nursing and anthropology. It was also to help nurses who I had encouraged to take anthropology courses to link ideas with the new field of transcultural nursing. It was seen as a temporary "stepping stone" for transcultural nursing. However, some nurses saw it only as anthropology and still do today. This organization exists today with few attendees and is focused largely on anthropology. In 1972 to 1974 I launched the Transcultural Nursing Society as the official organization for transcultural nursing. It has been very important to nurture and socialize practitioners, leaders, teachers, and researchers into transcultural nursing. Nurses without transcultural nursing, but with preparation in anthropology, remained in anthropology, and some have given limited leadership to the discipline of transcultural nursing. Several of these nurses became salaried employees in schools of nursing and taught mainly anthropological concepts with limited transcultural nursing research, concepts, and theories. Many graduate and undergraduate students prepared in transcultural nursing courses and programs have been outstanding leaders and advocates of transcultural nursing. These nurses quickly recognized the need in their clinical work and valued the concept of human caring within a cultural focus. Educating nearly 10,000 nurses over the past four decades has been essential to develop and educate nurses while promoting transcultural nursing worldwide.

After my first courses at the University of Colorado, I went to the University of Washington in Seattle as Dean and Professor of the School of Nursing and taught students at this institution on human caring from a transcultural perspective with field studies in the community. The first individual Ph.D. in Nursing with a focus on transcultural nursing was established from 1969 to 1975. In 1975 I was appointed Dean and Professor at the University of Utah (Salt Lake) and established the first master (M.S.N.) and doctoral (Ph.D.) programs focused specifically on transcultural nursing in the world. Several transcultural nurse leaders completed these programs along with students and faculty to support transcultural nursing conferences. In 1981 I went to Wayne State University (Detroit) and developed master (M.S.N.) and doctoral (Ph.D.) courses and programs in transcultural nursing. From 1981 to 1995 we had the largest program offerings in trans-

cultural nursing in the world at Wayne State University. Twenty-three Ph.D.s and approximately 30 master degree nurses were prepared as transcultural nurse specialists.[76] These were significant historical developments and breakthroughs to institutionalize programs in transcultural nursing with a cadre of nurses prepared in transcultural nursing. It has been encouraging to see other undergraduate and graduate transcultural nursing programs become established in the United States in the 1990s. Most assuredly, it has been the education of nurses into this new pathway of knowledge and practice that was the significant means to establish and maintain transcultural nursing.

In the late 1980s publications on "people of color" and "ethnic nurses of color" became popular with minority nurses in the United States. They had limited linkages to transcultural nursing and to anthropological research, concepts, or theories. Some articles led to misconceptions about relying on skin color and cultural diversity. Hiring minority nurses to teach cultural diversity without formal preparation or mentorship in transcultural nursing was also problematic. As a consequence, it thwarted knowledge development by some minority nurses to become effective teachers of transcultural nursing because many were placed in teaching roles without preparation in the discipline. Early affirmative-action programs helped in some schools of nursing to increase the numbers of minorities, but many were unable to teach and do research on Western and non-Western comparative aspects of cultures and about transcultural nursing. Today, many minorities are now enrolling in transcultural nursing graduate programs and are prepared to teach and do research in the discipline.

In tracing further the historical development of transcultural nursing education in the United States, Canada, and Europe, great variability existed with faculty, students, and curricula. As transcultural nurses endeavored to establish courses and get new content into nursing curricula, some repeated themes from nursing faculty were: "There is no room for courses in transcultural nursing in the curriculum," "We have gotten along without cultures since nursing began, and we know all about care/caring," "If we are to get jobs, we have to be competent medical practitioners," and "All cultures and care are alike for people." Many of these repeated statements were protective cliches. Some

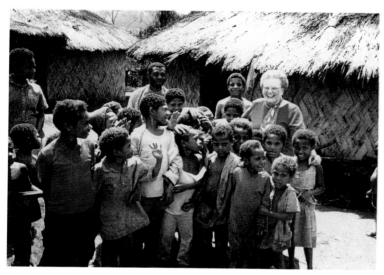

Gadsup children with Dr. Leininger in their New Guinea village.

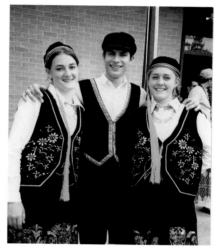

Greek teens in ceremonial dance attire.

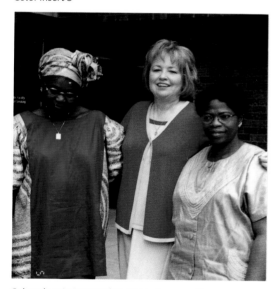

Cultural variations within and between cultures.

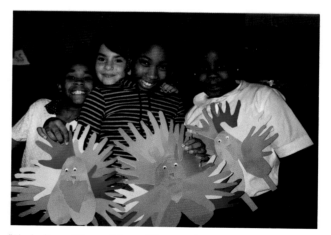

"Black-skinned" hues of three different cultures.

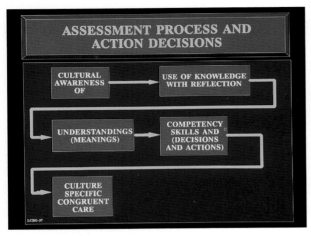

Cultural assessment process.

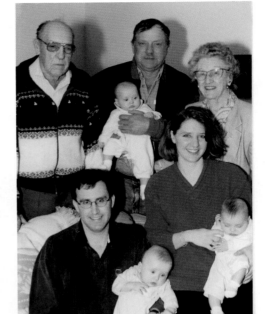

Four-generation family-care assessment.

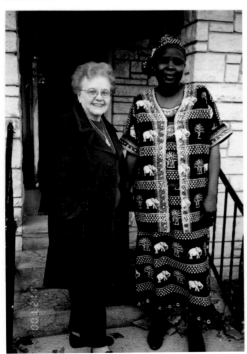

Dr. Leininger and Southern Sudanese refugee.

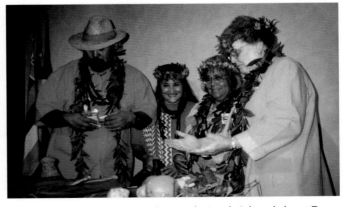

Polynesian traditional healers and carers sharing their knowledge at Transcultural Nursing Conference.

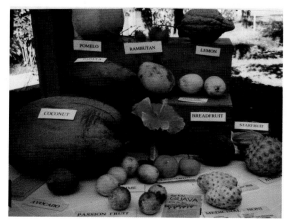

Pacific Island generic fruits and vegetables valued by indigenous people.

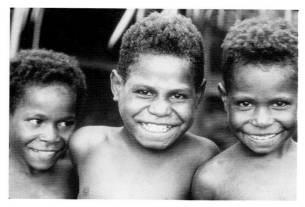

Three Gadsup children.

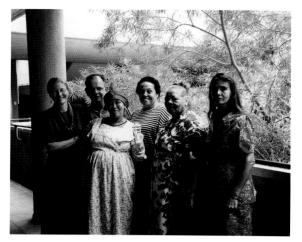

Drs. C. Leuning and L. Small (at left) with key Namibian informants.

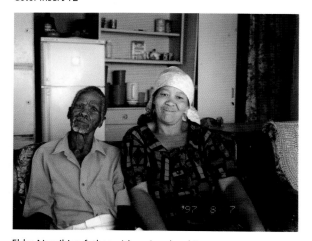

Elder Namibian father with caring daughter.

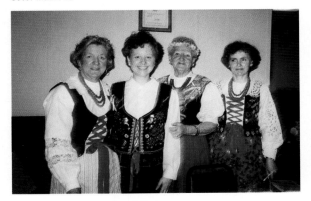

Polish American women in folk dresses.

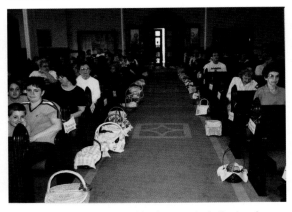

Blessing of Polish Easter food basket in a Catholic church.

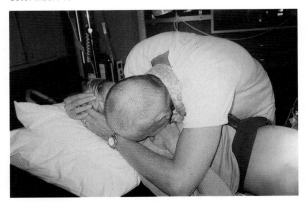

Physical presence as Comfort Care.

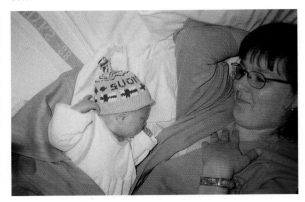

Trust as Protective Care.

faculty greatly feared teaching or dealing with cultures as this would lead to racial discrimination hassles. Most of all, faculty had no preparation in transcultural nursing, anthropology, or in-depth knowledge about caring in different cultures. Hence the dictum, "Stay away from it (cultures) but don't admit your real concerns."

Only a few schools of nursing worldwide had established undergraduate and graduate transcultural nursing courses by the late 1980s. The term "cultural diversity" was being used as popular culture by faculty, but seldom linked to care, health, or well-being with few exceptions. Accordingly, some schools labeled their courses "Cultural Diversity," "Culture and Health," or "Culture and Nursing" by early 1990s. A few progressive nursing schools had transcultural nursing courses and carried forth the philosophy, concepts, goals, and practices related to the discipline. At the University of Hawaii at Hilo, Dr. G. Kinney in the early 1990s established the first integrated undergraduate program focused totally on transcultural nursing throughout the curriculum.[77] Since then, other schools of nursing are beginning to follow this trend. Still today, however, nurse practitioner, advanced nurse specialists, and other nurse practitioners continue to have a heavy curricular emphasis on medical, psychologic, computor science, physical sciences, and many medical developments along with largely unicultural nursing foci. These are important, but must be linked to culture care.

Since the 1990s several United States hospitals, clinics, and community health agencies are beginning to introduce transcultural nursing concepts and research-based knowledge into their practices, but considerably more emphasis is needed. Staff nurses tend to treat "all clients alike" to prevent racial discrimination and other cultural conflicts and related problems. Clinical nursing staff, staff physicians, and other health personnel in the 1980s were sometimes avoiding some cultures because they were uncomfortable with different cultures. Some said they relied heavily on their "own common sense" and "home beliefs" about cultures. However, as more nurses became prepared in transcultural nursing, they were employed in schools of nursing and in a few hospitals and health agencies. These nurses demonstrated ways to work effectively with the culturally different. In some settings they dramatically transformed clinical practices with their com-

petencies and leadership. This led to increased requests for transcultural nurses to explain and help guide staff nurses and others to provide culturally satisfying and appropriate client care.[78]

Around 1988 certification of nurses was initiated as an important step to protect the public from unsafe cultural care practices. Consumers needed to be protected from nurses who were culturally ignorant and generally unsafe to care for clients of diverse cultures. It was also to prevent unethical and illegal care practices with consumers of different values and practices than those of professional health personnel. With the certification of nurses through the Transcultural Nursing Society, experts in the discipline were able to guide nurses to become culturally congruent and safe carers. Certification standards were established to promote cultural competencies and protect the public. By establishing the first certification in 1989 (by oral and written exams and a portfolio of evidence of competencies), the Transcultural Nursing Society became the first nursing organization to certify nurses *worldwide* for cultural care practices.[79] This was a major and important means to show the value of transcultural nursing education and practice and to protect clients. It also was a hallmark with certification and recertification to assure the public that nurses could provide culturally competent and safe care.

From 1990 to Present Era

There have been many significant developments to establish and maintain transcultural nursing since the mid 1950s, and the complete history is yet to be written. Today, transcultural nursing has become globally recognized as a legitimate and essential discipline with a growing body of knowledge for teaching, research, practice, and consultation. Transcultural nursing is not only recognized in most countries worldwide, but also in other health disciplines. In fact, medicine, dentistry, social work, and other professional disciplines have recently begun to use the term transcultural health and to develop educational programs.[80] It was, indeed, futuristic to launch transcultural nursing nearly five decades ago in anticipation of the present need to respect, serve, and provide competent care practices. Moreover, the concept of "culturally competent care" (that I coined in the 1960s) has now become a national goal in the United

States and in many health care systems and disciplines. The original predictive logo statement for transcultural nursing remains a central goal and challenge to many nurses; namely, *"That the cultural care needs of people in the world will be met by nurses prepared in transcultural nursing."*

Since the 1990s more nurses are valuing and recognizing the relevance of transcultural nursing in their practices and in education in many places in the world. Transcultural nurses are discovering different ways to teach, do research, and practice transcultural nursing with evidence indicators today. The discipline is slowly expanding nurses' worldviews, challenging their past unicultural and traditional ways, and providing fresh insights and rewards to be competent transcultural nurses. Most importantly, transcultural nursing is gradually transforming nursing education and health care systems and institutions by offering different kinds of transcultural health care services. Other current trends and developments in transcultural nursing are discussed in subsequent sections, especially as related to the evolutionary phases of transcultural nursing.

 ## Philosophical and Practical Views of Transcultural Nursing

Repeatedly, I am asked what philosophical and conceptual ideas led me to develop this discipline of transcultural nursing. While I have stated earlier my clinical and knowledge experiences that hastened me into action, some historical facts and conceptual ideas can be briefly highlighted.

After World War II and as a United States cadet nurse, I realized that all human beings and especially nurses were living in a large global world. Global interaction was bringing people into almost instant contact with strangers through rapid transportation, communication, and many new technologies within and outside health care systems. New medicines, treatments, and many new technological gadgets were evident. However, the missing dimension and the most critical was to understand, respect, and value people of diverse cultures being encountered with increasing frequency each day or night. Philosophically, professionally, and anthropologically, how could nurses and all health personnel learn about and respect cultural differences? How would nurses as the largest health care providers

learn about cultures and their caring needs and practices? What really happens when nurses care for cultural strangers? How do nurses discover, communicate, and understand their caring and health needs? Anthropological insights would help nurses but they needed to know and understand caring, health, and cultural professional needs of people. Many new immigrants entering a country overnight could baffle most nurses and health care providers. Philosophically, as a caring advocate, I was deeply concerned that technologies, the medical disease emphasis on mind-body practices, or professional task directives could obliterate human caring. Caring from spiritual, cultural, historical, environmental, and other perspectives would be lost. Cultural strangers with different values, language, and needs could be avoided, shunned, or patently neglected with the growing dominant and pervasive technologies in health systems. The nature of caring needed to be known and used with cultures. Modern technologies, robots, and a host of other nonpersonalized or nonhuman modalities could well negate or threaten care as the essence of nursing. Human caring within a cultural perspective was distinctive to nursing and needed to become fully known and used in practice.

With these perspectives, I also envisioned that transcultural nursing with a holistic perspective was much needed to help nurses function worldwide by the 21st century.[81,82] However, it was a shocking idea to think that nurses and health professionals were not prepared to care for clients from many different cultures in the world. Accordingly, nurses needed knowledge of cultures and their specific care needs, including substantive and in-depth knowledge about spiritual, kinship, political, economic, educational lifeways, language, folk practices, worldview, specific culture values, and historical aspects. Philosophically, nursing needed to shift drastically into a much broader worldview and knowledge base to guide nurses. Western and non-Western comparative knowledge needed to be studied, taught, and practiced. Anthropological knowledge along with humanities, philosophy, science, and moral-ethical academic preparation could greatly expand and enrich nurses' knowledge. Nurses, faculty, and nursing service organizations needed to value such a comprehensive cultural care educational and practice perspective while drawing on relevant existing medical and nursing knowledge appropriate to cultures.

Many nurses seemed committed to Florence Nightingale's emphasis on the patient's physical environment and health. These dimensions were not sufficient and failed to explicate human care/caring phenomena and to use cultural care knowledge.[83] Nightingale's British heritage and Victorian lifeways in Europe offered different insights of patient needs, and nursing. The International Council of Nursing (ICN) had been established as a nursing organization in the late 19th century, but its major focus was on establishing professional nursing standards and practices among nurse leaders largely from a Western nursing world view. This organization gave no emphasis to the idea of the *formal* educational preparation and focused research on different cultures to practice culturally based care.[84] Still today ICN's important role is to remain active to promote standards, practices, and norms of professional nursing organizations with selected membership. At the recent 100th anniversary of ICN (1999) my theoretical research paper was the first and only paper on transcultural nursing. My theoretical ideas and research findings could well transform ICN into transcultural nursing with a global care focus.[85]

Nurses in military and missionary services recognize the great need for transcultural nursing with their diverse cultural experiences. Many have told of their cultural shock experiences, cultural conflicts, fears, frustrations, and even threats to their lives in working with cultures they did not understand. Besides language needs, they have struggled to get cooperation and to understand the values and thinking of diverse cultures. The idea of being educated in transcultural nursing education was of much interest to them and *before* they went to foreign cultures. Many overseas nurses felt transcultural nursing was long overdue and imperative — and still today it is much needed.

At this point it is important to clarify why I philosophically and practically coined and used the term "transcultural nursing" rather than "medical anthropology" or "cross-cultural nursing." I saw the need to differentiate this new area of study from anthropology and to identify theoretical and research knowledge distinct to transcultural nursing. While anthropology has been a legitimate and recognized discipline with a focus on the study of diverse cultures (material and non-material) in different geographic places over great time periods, the purpose, nature, and professional aspects of transcultural nursing were quite different. *Transcultural nursing was a theoretical and practice discipline focused on comparative cultural care, health, well-being, and illness patterns in different environmental contexts and under different living conditions.*[86] Transcultural nursing was not primarily focused on medical mind-body symptoms, diseases, or pathologies, but rather on comparative human care and health to help people attain and maintain wellness, or to face death, disabilities, and dying within the client's cultural care values and lifeways. Medicine and medical anthropology were focused heavily on diseases, illness, and treatments rather than on care, health, or prevention of illnesses. From my anthropological and clinical field studies, it was caring and health phenomena that needed emphasis. Indeed, *transcultural nursing was not anthropology nor medical anthropology.* It had a different scientific and humanistic focus but related goals. It was a different field of study that required theoretical research and a professional body of *transcultural nursing knowledge and competencies.* Transcultural nursing was focused on comparative care and health phenomena with potentially different findings and benefits to human beings than other established disciplines. Some nurses had a narrow international focus without substantive cultural knowledge and practices. I saw the urgent need for holistic comparative-care research and theory for all future professional practices. I deliberately coined the term "*culture-specific care*" and "*holistic-particularistic care*" to support my conceptual and practice goals in the early 1960s and since. Hence, the philosophical, epistemic, and ontological basis for transcultural nursing as a discipline and profession were different from other fields for potential new knowledge and practices in nursing.

In conceptualizing transcultural nursing, I developed the Theory of Culture Care Diversity and Universality in the 1950s, which was conceptually broad in scope and yet culture-specific findings were essential for the new discipline of transcultural nursing. The goal of this theory was to discover transcultural nursing knowledge to provide *culturally congruent and responsible care.*[86] Discovering both universal and diverse transcultural care and health patterns worldwide was predicted to greatly generate a wealth of new knowledge and to provide both specific and general needs of cultures. The theory and the method were also conceptualized to focus primarily on informants' *emic* and *etic* knowledge and practices. The Culture Care theory is discussed by several experienced authors in this book to show definitive aspects of the theory and research findings.

Evolutionary Phases of Transcultural Nursing Knowledge and Uses

Students of transcultural nursing find it is helpful to envision the interesting phases that occurred with establishing transcultural nursing over the past five decades. Figure 1.3 shows the different evolutionary phases of transcultural nursing from the first phase of awareness to that of practicing transcultural nursing. These phases can be used to assess one's own progress in becoming a knowledgeable and competent transcultural nurse by studying each phase.[87]

In Phase I, the nurse is gaining cultural awareness and becoming sensitive to the needs of cultures. Cultural awareness or sensitivity is only the beginning phase to become transculturally competent. Sensitivity to another person, situation, or event is helpful, but the nurse must go further and gain confirmed cultural knowledge and understandings. Superficial awareness or opinions can be dangerous and often lead to misunderstandings and problems. The nurse enters Phase II to gain in-depth cultural knowledge, to use transcultural nursing concepts and principles, and to guide thinking and practices. The learner often needs a mentor in transcultural nursing to help see and reaffirm clients'

beliefs and expressions. The newcomer to this field needs a substantive course in transcultural nursing to discover differences and similarities and for accurate assessments. Transcultural nursing holding or reflective culture care knowledge of concepts, principles, and theories are powerful guides to assess what one observes, hears, and experiences while in Phase II of gaining in-depth knowledge and understandings. The theory of Culture Care is an important guide to discover the largely unknown about individuals and groups of a culture. For without theory, one cannot discover and explain phenomena in a systematic way and arrive at credible ideas and decisions.

In Phase III the nurse uses observations, experiences, and knowledge documented with clients to provide culturally competent care. This is the creative part of transcultural nursing to find ways to use client and professional knowledge for beneficial outcomes. The nurse documents and evaluates the outcomes when providing culturally based care and often with observations of others working with the client. The client's participation in the evaluation is very important and valued. In this last phase the nurse discovers the importance of using theory-based knowledge along with transcultural nursing concepts, principles, and available research findings to provide meaningful, safe, and beneficial care. It is in this third phase that the nurse assesses her (his) competencies and areas that need to be strengthened or modified. All three phases help the nurse to assess how one is becoming a knowledgeable, competent, and confident transcultural nurse.[88]

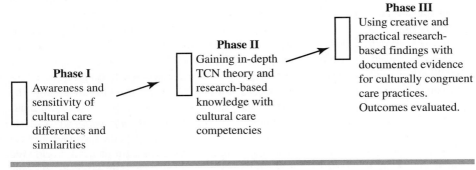

Figure 1.3
Evolutionary phases of transcultural nursing.

Glimpses of Transcultural Nursing Education

Ever since transcultural nursing began, it has been important to educate nurses to this new field to ensure that nurses become knowledgeable and understanding of transcultural nursing. This is in accord with nurse educators who value and uphold the importance of education to guide nurse's thinking and practices. In this section a general overview of transcultural nursing education today will be highlighted. At the outset, it is important to state that there are many countries in the world that are at different phases of learning about and developing transcultural nursing education. The statements below are largely based on the author's review of available literature and interviews and privileged visits to many schools of nursing and health agencies in the world over the past four decades (1960–2000). Only current glimpses of what is happening is offered with these summary statements.

First, transcultural nursing education and practice are generally known in most places in the world and many nurses see it as essential for practice. However, great variability exists in teaching, learning, and actual progress in different countries. Generally, nursing faculty recognize the need for nurses to be sensitive and knowledgeable and to have skills to care for clients who are culturally different, and so some transcultural nursing courses and programs are upheld. However, there are some faculty who contend, "Students know all about cultures" or "We have gotten along without such transcultural nursing in the past so why today." Yet, when students pose major cultural issues and conflicts, faculty begin to support transcultural nursing education.

Second, there are some places in the world in which formal transcultural nursing courses in educational instruction have been a reality for several decades, such as the United States, the birthplace of transcultural nursing. Courses are offered in Japan, Africa, Canada, Australia, Sweden, Finland, the Caribbean, Philippines, South America, and a few places in Europe. Some places offer course, modules, or units of instruction. Short-term workshops with or without credit are also available. In some countries it is only a plan yet to be realized. In other places there are related topics such as "culture and health" but no transcultural nursing or in-depth courses or programs.

Third, there are schools of nursing today that realize the great need for formal substantive courses and mentored field experiences but that have not been able to achieve these goals because of several factors:

1. Lack of prepared or qualified transcultural nursing faculty.
2. Noncommitted academic leaders and faculty or ambivalence about its importance.
3. The lack of funds or not using funds to support transcultural faculty and students because administrators are still wed to the medical mind-body emphasis.
4. The fear of not knowing how to handle racism, cultural clashes, biases, and ethnocentrism issues.
5. The lack of leadership and risk-taking abilities to initiate and establish transcultural nursing education alien in a region or area where transcultural nursing is greatly needed.[89]

Amid these hurdles and realities, there have been noteworthy and creative transcultural nurses who have successfully established courses and programs in schools and clinical practice settings. Most of these successful transcultural nurse leaders have been prepared through graduate programs in transcultural nursing. They are actively teaching and mentoring students, as well as conducting research and practicing in the field as time permits. They are also providing local, national, and transnational consultations. It is rewarding to see these leaders demonstrate how to change nursing education and practice into a dynamic transcultural nursing program to serve many multicultural groups in their area. For example, transcultural nursing courses or programs are offered in Minnesota, South Dakota, Michigan, Missouri, Colorado, Australia, Saudi Arabia, Hawaii, South Africa, Sweden, Finland, and Japan. This has required active leadership and firm commitments and persistence to initiate the offerings. The offerings have been welcomed by nursing students as a necessity and have given them a new career pathway. Some very creative teaching projects, research studies, and clinical innovations have been documented by undergraduate and graduate students prepared in transcultural nursing with many positive outcomes.[90–94]

While there are many positive developments and trends, there are areas to be strengthened and many more courses and programs are urgently needed in transcultural nursing. From a recent survey (2000) in the United States, approximately 48% of baccalaureate-degree nursing programs offer a unit of instruction or a course in transcultural nursing. There are only 20% of master's degree-bound nursing students receiving formal instruction in transcultural nursing and less than 2% of doctoral nursing students educated in the discipline.[95] Other reports generally support these findings.[96] Associate degree students are receiving instruction in transcultural nursing, but the data are not clear at this time. Master's degree students receive less preparation in transcultural nursing largely because of a heavy emphasis on preparing advanced nurse practitioners and primary care practitioners with a dominant medical-surgical, disease and symptom management or treatment emphasis. Preparation in clinical specialties such as cancer, gerontology, cardiovascular, and many other medical specialties continues to hold nurse practitioner interests. Unquestionably, nurse practitioners greatly need transcultural nursing research knowledge, basic concepts, principles, and theories to guide and provide care to individuals and families of diverse cultures.

As transcultural nursing with its standards, policies, and certification continue, all professional nurses will be expected to practice transcultural nursing worldwide by the year 2020. Recently, the United States government has recognized the need for such standards to support "Culturally Competent Care" (the term I coined in the early 1960s as part of my theory) to be promoted in health care and especially for practioners and minorities. Culturally competent care is an example of a cultural lag that finally took on relevance in the culturally diverse society of the United States. The concept is also being disseminated in other places in the world. However, to attain this goal transcultural education is imperative for health personnel and to address critical issues related to ethnocentrism, cultural biases, racism, and many other areas. Obtaining qualified faculty to educate health personnel and to mentor their work is another major need in the United States and worldwide to provide culturally congruent and safe care practices.

As educational and service exchanges occur among all health disciplines in this third millennium, there will be very great demands for transcultural health education, research, and practice and the need to evaluate the outcomes and problems. The current popular trend of educational foreign exchanges is a major issue because of so few health professionals prepared to teach and guide students in limitedly known and diverse cultures.[97] Major problems such as homicides, cultural shock, and cultural backlashes occur with such exchanges. While such educational exchanges are intended to be beneficial and are done in good faith, they can lead to less favorable and unanticipated outcomes largely resulting from transcultural nursing ignorance of the host cultures. Far more attention is critically needed to make them safe, beneficial, and effective.

In the United States and worldwide, graduate (master's and doctoral degree) students need in-depth transcultural nursing knowledge of and guidance in what strategies and ways can be most helpful to people in other cultures. Transcultural mentoring is much needed to help students understand the complex and diverse multifaceted issues related to cultures with their political, religious, economic, and cultural history lifeways and health care. Graduate students need to use theories and practices that *fit* cultures and not impose their desires and expectations onto a host culture. *Learning from the people* (the emic perspective) and reflecting on professional beneficial knowledge (the etic base) require serious study and mentoring with qualified transcultural nursing faculty and preceptors. Since transcultural nursing uses a more holistic comparative and broad knowledge base than traditional nursing or the mind-body medical model, this necessitates an open discovery mind with depth and breath of knowledge. As graduate students learn how to document the lifeways, patterns, values, and practices of cultures with a care and health focus, they discover some very different perspectives. Helping students to grasp the broad, comparative view and synthesize the knowledge for culture-specific care usually necessitates mentoring. Nurses prepared in transcultural nursing graduate programs can demonstrate differences to become culturally competent nurses and achieve desired professional goals. Conferences, workshops, short and long-term courses, and lectures have also been essential to maintain transcultural nursing education as cultures change and nurses have to deal with acculturation issues. Currently, there are many "cultural diversity" courses, books, and conferences, but many of these are generally not transcultural. They tend to be mainly anthropology and sociology focused on culture.[98–100] Graduate education programs in transcultural nursing remain needed in teaching, research, and practice. Undergraduate programs remain essential as background preparation for graduate education. A critical crisis remains in transcultural nursing education worldwide for qualified and prepared faculty and practitioners in transcultural nursing. Funds and programs or courses are needed to meet global and local cultural care needs of clients. It is anticipated that some needs will be met by modern electronic (internet) modalities, but content accuracy will be a major educational issue, as well as cultural privacy. Electronic courses, the internet, and other information labeled cultural diversity, ethnicity, culture, health and illness, medical anthropology, or multiculturalism are usually *not* transcultural nursing. They may be helpful as anthropology, sociology, or other non-nursing disciplines' courses, but the missing ingredient is usually transcultural nursing. Mentoring and guiding novices on the internet and modern cyber modes is a big challenge for the future.

Unquestionably, faculty prepared in transcultural nursing make a great difference in learning outcomes. Still today cultural minorities and nurses not prepared in transcultural nursing are teaching transcultural nursing. While faculty may be born into a culture, one should not assume these faculty are knowledgeable and competent in transcultural nursing. Some minority faculty may deny their cultural background for various reasons, but their cultural biases and acculturation factors may become evident and limit student learning. In general, one should never assume minority faculty or faculty of the *same* culture are the best or most competent to teach transcultural nursing. Contrary to Aleordi's view of the faculty of the same culture as "best or most effective" faculty, this position has not been found in transcultural nursing and is highly questionable.[101] Likewise using lay health aides as stated by Poss for teaching transcultural nursing because they speak the native language is also unacceptable and often dangerous with many problems.[102] Such unwise remedies deprive students of substantive and essential transcultural nursing needed to function competently with diverse cultures. Sometimes, speakers and interpreters of the same culture may try to impose what they feel is "politically correct and safe," but this may not accurately represent transcultural nursing content.

Currently, where there are nonprepared transcultural nursing faculty, there is a tendency to only teach about their local cultures and without comparative or global view of cultures. This practice also poses problems as students become handicapped to work effectively with immigrants and other cultures in the region or nation. There may also be faculty who emphasize only certain concepts as "cultural safety" as in New Zealand, but fail to see that this concept is already an integral part of transcultural nursing and the culture care theory.[103] There is also the practice of sending students to "foreign cultures to learn about and have special overseas experiences." Such "experiential experiences" with no transcultural nursing holding knowledge is educationally unsound and sometimes dangerous to clients and students. In other schools of nursing, students are to have "reflective encounters," but again with no prior or very limited preparation about the culture or country. Students often say "I reflected but often I had no holding knowledge to reflect upon, and so I rely upon my culture as I can't make sense out of the clients." Such practices appear questionable and educationally unsound.

There is also the current issue in academic settings of faculty without any preparation in transcultural nursing developing research and educational teaching projects to get available funds to deal with cultural problems, racism, and inadequate care practices. Again, such practices by faculty can lead to many problems and questionable results in interpretation of findings. So, while some progress has been made in transcultural nursing education, there are also problems that exist with the great need to prepare a new generation of transcultural nurses to give care in a multicultural health world. It is essential that faculty and students be prepared with and under the guidance of those who are well prepared, experienced, and educationally sound in transcultural nursing to prevent negative and destructive nursing educational outcomes and in client care. Although the demand is great for cultural care competencies, one must not yield to incompetent ways to meet a long-standing need worldwide.

General View of Transcultural Nursing Practices

While it is impossible to give an accurate picture of transcultural nursing practices locally, regionally, or worldwide because of great variability and different conditions and practitioners worldwide, some broad glimpses and general perspectives from literature, from the author's worldwide visits, and from direct observations and experiences with nurses are offered. The most encouraging recent development is that efforts are being directed toward valuing and providing culturally congruent, responsible, and meaningful care to clients of diverse cultures in many nursing and interdisciplinary places. The idea of "culturally congruent and responsible care" has linguistically taken hold as a desired goal to assist clients, but the full implementation in most places has not been realized except for places where transcultural nurses are persistent to maintain quality care outcomes. In the last decade in the United States, the idea of cultural competencies has spread to other health disciplines and to local, regional, and national health centers and institutes and is now of interest in medicine, social work, dentistry, and other health professions. It is most encouraging that all disciplines are involved.

Recently (1999), the Office of Minority Health of the US Department of Health and Human Services advocated cultural competence in health care with some national standards and outcomes.[104] Unfortunately, the focus was mainly on preventing "ethnic minority" discrimination in health care of a few cultures and failed to focus on all underrepresented cultures. The proposal also failed to draw on nearly five decades of transcultural nursing and health research-based knowledge, concepts, principles, and theories to guide health personnel to achieve culturally competent care. This was disappointing as it revealed interprofessional discrimination and failure to use and build on an available body of research and professional knowledge. Addressing only a few selected minority cultures rather than focusing on many immigrant and vulnerable cultures is important. Moreover, none of the transcultural nursing and other transcultural specialists' thinking and work were used. Such practices and projects need to be avoided by building upon existing knowledge and experts.

In recent decades, it has been encouraging to see transculturally prepared nurses functioning in hospitals, clinics, and community health agencies with highly positive feedback and outcomes.[105,106] These transcultural nurse generalists and specialists have been active to help immigrants, minorities, refugees, home-less, drug addicts, gangs, prisoners, and many neglected indigenous cultures such as Native Americans, Australian Aborigines and other groups receive quality cultural care. Undergraduate and graduate students who have had transcultural nursing preparation and received mentoring have been most helpful and warmly welcomed by cultures such as the Vietnamese, Sudanese, Russians, Somalis, and local native groups. It has been encouraging to see how transcultural nurse experts and generalists can work together in providing culturally congruent care. They have established several innovative transcultural nursing clinics since the early 1980s that are functioning well and valued by cultures.[107,108] Such leadership efforts in diverse settings and geographic locations worldwide are to be highly applauded and demonstrate hope for the future.

In selected health services and especially in new transculturally focused centers, graduate-prepared (master's, doctoral, and postdoctoral) transcultural nurse experts are providing counseling and therapy services to immigrants and refugees, as well as other kinds of transcultural nursing therapies related to mental health, maternal-child care, and elder care. Such encouraging directions are helping many neglected indigenous, homeless, drug dependent, and mentally ill to get the care they need. Many of these client concerns are derived from cultural stresses, conflicts, shock, pain, and offenses that violate cultural norms, values, and beliefs. In subsequent chapters, several excellent examples of these effective endeavors by transcultural nurses based on research and theory are found such as culture care to the homeless in Western USA (Peters chapter), care for Polish and American elderly (McFarland and Leininger chapter), and Arab Muslims (Luna chapter). Transcultural nurses are also working with cultures experiencing family violence as discussed in this book by Ehrmin with Africans and Euro-Americans, and giving focus to HIV/AIDS victims in Africa as presented in MacNeil's chapter. Transcultural nurses are studying and helping Mexican Americans as shown in Zoucha's chapter and many other groups within and outside health institutions such as hospitals and community agencies and in rural and urban locations.

These are all most encouraging signs that transcultural nursing can make a great difference in discovering cultural needs and providing quality of care that is different from past mainline nursing and health services. Culturally based caring practices are powerful for healing, well-being, and helping to face death and disabilities in meaningful and satisfying ways to clients and families. Much more effort is needed for nurses to apply or use such transcultural research-based knowledge in similar settings with clients of similar cultures.

Finally, there is an urgent and great need for the public through public media coverage to help people learn about the nature, focus, and ways transcultural nursing is practiced to help cultures. The public media needs to shift its focus from a heavy emphasis on medical discoveries of techniques, new gadgets, medicines, and treatments and to consider transcultural healing and curing modes that could be readily understood by many cultures. To date there has been very little emphasis made by television and other modern technologic modes to show some of the major breakthroughs by complementary folk and professional caring modes or the successful outcomes of transcultural nurses dealing with cultural conflicts, stresses, and cultural taboos or imposition practices. Worldwide media needs to give attention to transcultural health maintenance and to healing methods, especially through transcultural nursing skills with individuals, families, and institutions during this new century for beneficial outcomes.

◼ Some Myths and Misunderstandings

In any discipline or profession, there are always some myths and misunderstandings that need to be known and clarified. This is especially true in transcultural nursing. The following mythical statements or misunderstood beliefs are important to identify to prevent unfavorable consequences and help to summarize points made above:

1. There is the myth that "*if one uses common sense and has a smile*" *that this is all that is needed to care for cultures.* While "common sense" is always important and generally helpful, it is not always sufficient to help people with values and beliefs very different from the practitioner. A smile or opinion may not be helpful with some cultures, but in some cultures a smile may indicate distrust, manipulation, or to be on guard for a potential enemy.

2. There is the myth that "*one good, day-long conference or workshop is all that is needed to be a transcultural nurse.*" This myth fails to understand that transcultural nursing is complex and requires diligent and extensive study to be a knowledgeable and competent transcultural nurse.

3. There is the myth that "*any faculty can teach, conduct research, and guide students and staff to give culturally competent care.*" This myth and the practice of employing faculty and clinical staff without graduate preparation in transcultural nursing to teach and guide nurses is educationally unsound and leads to serious and unfavorable outcomes. For example, a Mexican nurse without preparation in transcultural nursing was employed to teach and mentor nursing students about "Hispanics" without awareness that there are many cultures with the Hispanic label such as Cuban, Haitian, and Caribbean cultures. This faculty member resigned after one semester as she began to realize she was not prepared to teach transcultural nursing and knew only her own recent experiences with Mexicans within one state in the United States.

4. There is the myth that a "*good medical and nursing psychophysical assessment with modern technologic equipment will tell you all you need to know today about any human beings.*" This is another false statement as the human is a cultural being in which culture is a powerful influencer of the wellness or illness, as well as caring modalities. Moreover, other factors have to be identified and validated with clients such as environment, life history patterns, genetic-family patterns, and others. Holistic culture care assessments are essential with cultures for beneficial practices.

5. There is the myth that "*all nurses need is to interact or experience different cultures, and they will know how to care for them.*" This is helpful but again insufficient to understand and work with cultures. Reflective experiences also need to be grounded in *holding knowledge* to make sense out of what one reflects on and understands. One may reflect on only one's own biases and home beliefs.

6. There is the myth that "*If nurses only had a 'cookbook' listing of all cultures with their values, practices, and beliefs, then nurses could provide culturally competent care.*" Such "cookbook fixes" are quite inadequate as the nurse needs to assess, study, and discuss with clients and determine acculturation extent and many other variability considerations. Cookbook recipes can lead to

stereotyping, which is counterproductive and not a desired practice in transcultural nursing as it fails to understand the individual and group dynamic expressions and lifeways of the clients.

7. There is the myth that *"transcultural nursing is the same as anthropology."* This is untrue as anthropology and transcultural nursing are two different disciplines, but they usually share some common interests and perspectives as discussed above.

8. There is the myth and misunderstanding that *"transcultural nursing, international nursing, and cross-cultural nursing are one and the same."* This is incorrect as each construct is defined differently with different goals, purposes, scope, and functions. As discussed earlier each construct must be well understood and used properly.

9. There is the myth that *"if the nurse uses the North American Nursing Diagnosis Association (NANDA) or the Iowa Classificatory repertoire that these tools will cover all cultures and the nurse will be able to identify and assess accurately the 'problem,' area of 'dysfunction,' or 'disease' and manage the client."*[109] This also is erroneous as NANDA and other nursing classificatory diagnostic tools woefully fail to identify, know, and classify accurately cultural and care phenomena due largely to lack of culture and care knowledge. These tools tend to be culturally biased and inaccurate about cultures, and are inadequate to use as an assessment and classification guide for cultures. The reader needs to study my writings on this critical and major movement, which started in the Western nursing cultures during the 1970s and has now spread to many nursing countries. Imposing axioms, diseases, or human conditions onto other cultures is questionable and often unethical, leading to serious problems with potentially destructive and inaccurate outcomes. Western diagnosis such as "needs parental alterations" may not be helpful to a culture where the nurse fails to understand parent lifeways and child guidance. Such cultural imposition practices must be avoided. There is the related myth that all mental and physical illnesses are alike or can be classified within Western categories. Again this is a myth or assumption to be avoided and seriously questioned as most physical and mental conditions have different expressions and meanings in different cultures. (See chapter on Mental Conditions and Cultures in this book.)

10. Last but not least, there is the myth that *"any nurse who travels to a foreign culture or works in a culture qualifies as a transcultural nurse."* Again this is a myth as transcultural nurses give evidence of knowledge and competencies to be a transcultural nurse. "Travel nurses" are generally not prepared in transcultural nursing and may be unsafe practioners with a culture.

These myths and others alert the reader to some major misconceptions, misinformation, and potentially non-beneficial outcomes. Nurses need to be alert to these myths and help to correct them, as well as others in the literature.[110]

 ## Summary of Facts about Transcultural Nursing

In this last section, the following summary points will be made to bring together some of the major points, themes, and facts presented in this chapter.

1. Transcultural nursing was envisioned in the early 1950s as a formal and essential area of study and practice by its founder, Madeleine Leininger. There was a critical, unrecognized and long-standing need in nursing and the health professions to appreciate and incorporate culture and care into nursing education, research, and practice. Accordingly, there was a critical need to develop transcultural nursing content and educate nurses in this new and essential field. Formal programs of education and research were greatly needed to care for many culturally different, neglected, and vulnerable cultures and subcultures. The founder prepared herself with a master's degree in nursing and a Ph.D. in cultural and social anthropology and did original field research to show the close relationship between two disciplines with different foci. One is a professional field (nursing) and the other a nonprofessional field (anthropology). Over the past five decades a body of transcultural nursing knowledge has been soundly developed and established as essential to nursing practice. Providing culturally congruent and comparative care has been a major contribution to humanity, nursing, and the health professions. Major transcultural nursing concepts, principles, theories, and research practices are beginning to guide nursing care practices with many cultures. Transcultural

nursing has been a new paradigm and new pathway to knowledge and practice that is stimulating nurses thinking and actions. It is considered by many as the most significant development in nursing in the 20th century and will be imperative in the 21st century.

2. The first transcultural nursing research study was done by Leininger in the early 1960s with the Gadsup of the Eastern Highlands of New Guinea. She did an ethnographic, ethnologic, and ethnonursing research study and also systematically examined her theory of Culture Care Diversity and Universality. The theory of Culture Care has become a major theory today to discover the close interrelationships of culture and caring to guide transcultural care practices.[111] The ethnonursing method (developed in the early 1960s) was the first nursing research method used to study nursing phenomena with a cultural care focus. The method was unique as it was designed to *fit* with the theory of Culture Care Diversity and Universality. Since then, Leininger has studied 15 other Western and non-Western cultures using the Culture Care theory and the ethnonursing research method. She wrote the first qualitative nursing research book in 1985 and encouraged other nurses to use qualitative research methods to study complex and covert care, health, and related nursing phenomena.[112] It was a major shift in nursing for nurses to use potentially 25 qualitative methods rather than relying so heavily on borrowed quantitative methods and instruments.

3. The theory of Culture Care Diversity and Universality is unique as it is focused on care and cultural factors to predict and explain (or arrive at) the health, well-being, illnesses, and other factors. It was one of the earliest (mid 1950) nursing humanistic and scientific theories with the goal to provide culturally congruent care.[113] The theory was slow to take hold because so few nurses were prepared in transcultural nursing and anthropology and caring phenomena to understand the purpose, goal, and meaning of the transcultural nursing theory. The theory is directed to discover both universal (common) and diverse culture care phenomena. It remains the only major theory for comparative culture care with both abstract and very practical practice features.

4. The first formal transcultural nursing courses and distant learning were initiated by Leininger in 1965 to 1969 at the School of Nursing at the University of Colorado (Denver). This was also the place where Leininger initiated the first Ph.D. Nurse-Scientist program with a focus on transcultural nursing and anthropological phenomena in doctoral education.

5. Leininger was Dean and Professor at the University of Washington (1969–1974), the first academic department to focus on transcultural nursing theory, research and practice. Dr. Beverly Horn was the first nurse to complete an individualized Ph.D. program with a focus on transcultural nursing in 1974. When the founder was then appointed Dean and Professor of Nursing at the University of Utah, she initiated the first master's (M.S.N.) and doctoral (Ph.D.) programs in transcultural nursing. Drs. Marilyn Ray, Joyceen Boyle, and Janice Morse were the first Ph.D. nurses prepared specifically in transcultural nursing. Since then, approximately 130 nurses have completed Ph.D.s in nursing with a focus on transcultural nursing within the United States and in a few other countries. There are approximately 70 nurses who have been prepared as anthropologists, but only 30 are functioning as transcultural nurses and several remaining with only anthropological interests.

6. The Committee on Nursing and Anthropology (CONAA) was launched in 1963 by Leininger to stimulate dialogue and to share common interests, theories, and research findings between nurses who were new anthropologists and with non-nurse anthropologists. It was envisioned as an important stepping stone to transcultural nursing. In 1973 the first transcultural nursing conference was held in Honolulu, Hawaii. In 1974 the Transcultural Nursing Society was established as the official worldwide organization for transcultural nursing.[113] The Society was developed to organize and enculturate nurses into transcultural nursing and to promote quality-based research, teaching, practice, and consultation in transcultural nursing worldwide. It was the first professional nursing organization to advance knowledge, research, and consultation in clinical transcultural nursing education and practice. (See Appendix 1-A for annual Conferences since 1974.) In late 2001, there are approximately 500 active members worldwide and many working with different regional chapters and transnationally. Annual and regional conventions are well attended. Through the Transcultural Nursing Society, certification was launched in 1989 to protect the public from unsafe transcultural care practices and for the public to recognize transcultural

nurse specialists who were knowledgeable and competent to practice culturally competent care.
7. Undergraduate, graduate, and continuing education courses and programs have been established in the United States and in several other countries. A summary of these current graduate transcultural nursing courses and programs are listed in Appendix 1-B.

- The first undergraduate and graduate transcultural nursing courses were offered in the School of Nursing at the University of Colorado (Denver) in 1965 to 1968 under Leininger.

- In 1978, the first doctoral (Ph.D.) and the first master's degree (M.S.N.) programs in transcultural nursing were established at the University of Utah by Leininger, but the program is no longer available (although much needed). As of late 2001, there were ten graduate programs offering courses, certificates, or master-doctoral programs in transcultural nursing.[114] Transcultural nurse specialists (graduate study) and generalists (undergraduate studies) are emphasized in the United States and in a few other countries. In 1982 Wayne State University College of Nursing (Detroit) initiated undergraduate studies and had the largest enrolled students in graduate (master, doctoral, and postdoctoral) studies in transcultural nursing with Leininger as Program Director. Other transcultural leaders are establishing programs in their countries.

- The Universities of California (Los Angeles and San Francisco) have offered a few graduate courses and mainly overseas exchange experiences focused on international nursing since around 1985, but offer no degree or in-depth study in transcultural nursing. Likewise, the University of Florida (Miami) initiated a few graduate courses focused on "Culture, Care, and Health" around 1988 under Dr. Lydia DeSantis, but these offerings are no longer available. The University of Washington has continued to offer cross-cultural nursing and anthropological courses under Dr. Noel Chrisman, a long-time anthropologist and College of Nursing instructor. Dr. Beverly Horn

guides students in community health and transcultural nursing care. Since 1990 several overseas schools of nursing have been offering graduate courses in transcultural nursing such as the Faculties of the University of Sydney and The Catholic University in Sidney, Australia, the University of Kuopio in Kuopio, Finland (graduate courses with administration focus), and others. New offerings focused on graduate study in transcultural nursing in the United States are at Duquesne University (Pittsburgh), the University of Southern Mississippi (Hattiesburg, Mississippi), Augsburg College (St. Paul, Minnesota), the University of Northern Colorado (Greeley), and Kean University in New Jersey. See Appendix 1-B. The University of Nebraska Medical Center (Omaha, NE) offers two short graduate seminars under Dr. Leininger each summer. Other educational institutions are offering continuing education conferences or units of instruction with an emphasis on transcultural nursing in Canada, Japan, Sweden, Australia, and Africa.

8. Publications in transcultural nursing have been extremely important to inform nurses and others about the field since the early 1960s. Many articles, book chapters, video tapes, and internet websites have been invaluable. It is estimated that there are over 1000 publications for nurses, students, and other disciplines to learn about transcultural nursing. This has been a significant development because prior to 1950 there were no books on transcultural nursing and virtually none on care and culture. The first book, *Nursing and Anthropology: Two Worlds to Blend* was written in the mid 1960s and published in 1970, which opened the door to transcultural nursing and with anthropology as an academic support area. Anthropology and nursing needed to come closer together, but had to be reconceptualized for the transcultural nursing discipline. The second book and the first substantive one entitled, *Transcultural Nursing*, was published in 1978 by Leininger. A book of anthropology readings for nurses entitled, *Readings in Transcultural Nursing*, was published by P. Brink.[115] Eight other transcultural nursing books

with caring focus were published by Leininger from 1979 through 1988. In 1985 M. Andrews and J. Boyle published and updated in 1999 a book, *Transcultural Concepts in Nursing*, which has been extremely helpful to advance undergraduate transcultural nursing education.[116] In 1995 Leininger's second edition of *Transcultural Nursing: Concepts, Theory, Research and Practices*[117] was published and contained practical experiences in transcultural nursing care. This current third edition shows the tremendous growth in transcultural nursing and the contributions of many nurses actively involved in teaching and research in transcultural nursing and practice. Other books as Geiger et al.[118] and Purnell et al.[119] are labeled transcultural nursing, but have limited focus on this subject but more on cultures.

Since 1995 the title "transcultural nursing" has become popular in nursing but not fully comprehended. As a result some nurses are publishing books and articles on this subject. Some publications are *not* reliable or accurate on transcultural nursing as a result of authors' limited knowledge but a desire to publish. In 1983 to 1985 I initiated plans for the *Journal of Transcultural Nursing* with the first issue published in 1989 and served as Editor. This *Journal* was a very significant development to let the world know about transcultural nursing. The second editor was Dr. Marilyn McFarland (1995–1999). Currently, Dr. Marilyn Douglas is the editor under Sage Publications (1999 to present time), which many contend has mainly a multidiscipline focus. A number of transcultural nursing films and video tapes have been prepared and have been excellent to help nurses, practitioners, and leaders to envision ways to help nurses understand and use transcultural nursing. A Leininger Collection of her books has been established at Madonna University since 1995 and of unpublished papers at Wayne State University.
9. Currently, there are approximately 300 graduate-prepared (master's and doctoral) transcultural nurse specialists and approximately 90 certified and recertified transcultural nurses (CTN). Although Leininger has taught many nurses (in conferences and courses) over the past five decades along with other faculty, still a critical shortage exists for more transcultural nurses as faculty members, practitioners, and administrators to meet needs for culturally competent, safe, and responsible care worldwide. Transcultural nurses with graduate preparation are especially in great demand in many schools of nursing and health settings to teach, conduct research, and mentor students in clinical practices. Employing unprepared nurses in transcultural nursing remains of deep concern to protect clients, students, administrators, and consultants from unsafe and nonbeneficial services.
10. Most encouraging and exciting is the recent establishment of the Worldwide Transcultural Nursing Society Office at Madonna University in the College of Nursing (Livonia, Michigan) in 2001. While a small office had been established at Madonna in 1985, the need for a larger office was evident for global and transnational services. The new office will serve nurses worldwide interested and involved in transcultural nursing for meetings and special conferences. Through the Society of Transcultural Nursing, an internet website has been established (www.tcns.org) to provide communication with nurses worldwide. These global facilities support the mission of transcultural nursing as a global discipline and profession in this new millennium and beyond.

In this chapter some definitive and highly relevant ideas and historical data on transcultural nursing have been presented. The intent was to give a broad and updated picture of the rapidly growing field of transcultural nursing in education, practice, and research progress since the second edition was published in 1995. The historical aspects with the evolutionary phases should be helpful to the readers to know and understand developments in the field since the beginning. This chapter was written by the founder and a central leader in transcultural nursing over nearly 50 years with many lived-through experiences. Many unique insights and documentary facts have been presented and especially facts, myths, and questions commonly asked by interested nurses and other disciplines. The chapters that follow build on and will expand to make meaningful many general ideas presented in this chapter with practical examples. This chapter was presented as the state of transcultural nursing and as a foundation to understand the focus, scope, nature, definitions, and other major ideas and facts in transcultural nursing from a global and historical perspective.

Appendix 1-A

Twenty-Five Years of Knowledge and Practice Development

Transcultural Nursing Society Annual Research Conferences (1974–2001)*

Compiled by Dr. M. Leininger, Founder of Transcultural Nursing

YEAR	LOCATION	CONFERENCE THEME	KEYNOTER(S)	CONFERENCE CHAIR(S)	PUBLICATION EDITOR/ YEAR
1974	Honolulu, Hawaii University of Hawaii	An Adventure in Transcultural Nursing Communication (First TCN Conference)	Dr. M. Leininger	L. Bermosk	Bermosk and Leininger, 1974
1975	Salt Lake City, Utah University of Utah	Transcultural Nursing Care of Infants and Children (First Transcultural Nursing Society Conference)	Dr. K. Kendall	M. Leininger	Leininger, 1977
1976	Salt Lake City, Utah University of Utah	Transcultural Nursing Care of the Elderly	Dr. L. Gunter	M. Leininger	Leininger, 1978
1977	Salt Lake City, Utah University of Utah	Transcultural Nursing of the Adolescent and Middle-Aged Client	Dr. M. Brown Dr. M. Friedman	M. Leininger	Leininger, 1979
1978	Snowbird, Utah University of Utah	Transcultural Nursing: Cultural Change of Ethics and Nursing Care Implications	Dr. P. Albers Dr. M. Higgins	M. Leininger	Leininger, 1979
1979	Snowbird, Utah University of Utah	Transcultural Nursing: Teaching, Practice, and Research	Dr. M. Leininger	M. Leininger	Leininger, 1980
1980	Snowbird, Utah University of Utah	Developing, Teaching, and Practicing Tr anscultural Nursing	Panel	M. Leininger	Leininger, 1981
1981	Seattle, Washington Mayflower Hotel	Focus of Transcultural Nursing: Arching Across all Domains of Practice	Dr. M. Leininger	M. Binn	C. and J. Uhl, 1982
1982	Atlanta, Georgia Hyatt Regency	A Transcultural Nursing Challenge: From Discovery to Action	Dr. J. Glittenberg	L. DeSantis	J. Uhl, 1983
1983	Scottsdale, Arizona	Application of Cultural Concepts to Nursing Care	Dr. A. Aamodt	B. Peterson V. Evaneshko	J. Uhl, 1984
1984	Boston, Massachusetts Copley Hotel	Cultural Challenges for Expanding Choices in Nursing Care	Dr. B. Horn	C. Carneiro	M. Carter, 1985
1985	San Diego, California	Transcultural Nursing: A Futuristic Field of Health Care	Dr. L. DeSantis	T. Cooper	M. Carter, 1986
1986	Chicago, Illinois	Transcultural Nursing: Knowledge, Synthesis, and Application	Dr. B. Horn	J. Scott	Selected papers published in 1987 (Carter, ed.)

YEAR	LOCATION	CONFERENCE THEME	KEYNOTER(S)	CONFERENCE CHAIR(S)	PUBLICATION EDITOR/ YEAR
1987	Miami, Florida	Transcultural Nursing in a Multicultural Society: Clinical Innovations and Applications	Dr. M. Dryer	L. DeSantis	M. Carter (Editor)
1988	Edmonton, Canada Fantasyland Hotel	Political, Economic, and Cultural Care Issues	Dr. M. Ray	J. Morse	M. Leininger and M. Carter (Editors) (First Jr. of TCN 1989)
1989	Maastricht, The Netherlands University of Maastricht	Transcultural Nursing and Migration	Dr. M. Leininger	G. Evers	Jr. of TCN (M. Leininger, Editor)
1990	Seattle, Washington Mayflower Hotel	Transcultural Nursing: Clinical Challenges in the 1990s	Dr. M. Muecke	M. McKenna	Jr. of TCN (M. Leininger, Editor)
1991	Detroit, Michigan Westin Hotel	Transcultural Nursing in Rural and Urban Contexts	Dr. A.F. Wenger	M. Leininger	Jr. of TCN (M. Leininger, Editor)
1992	Miami, Florida Hyatt Miami Regency	Retrospect and Prospect in Transcultural Nursing	D. Riff	L. DeSantis	Jr. of TCN (M. Leininger, Editor)
1993	Flagstaff, Arizona	Transcultural Nursing of Native Americans	Rita Harding	O. Still E. Geissler	Jr. of Transcultural Nursing (M. Leininger, Editor)
1994	Atlanta, Georgia Radisson Hotel	Transcultural Interfaces in Health and Care	Dr. J. Camphina-Bacote	F. Wenger	Jr. of TCN (M. Leininger, Editor)
1995	Kamuela, Hawaii Royal Waikeloan Hotel	Moving Transcultural Nursing into the 21st Century	Dr. M. Leininger	G. Kinney	Jr. of TCN (M. McFarland, Editor)
1996	St. Louis, Missouri Regal Riverfront	Health Issues in Migration: A Transcultural Nursing Perspective	Dr. M. Muecke	I. Kalnins	Jr. of TCN (M. McFarland, Editor)
1997	Kuopio, Finland University of Kuopio	Transcultural Nursing: Global Unifier of Care: Facing Diversity with Unity	Dr. M. Leininger Dr. C. Rohrbach	A. VonSmitten	Jr. of TCN (M. McFarland, Editor)
October 14–17, 1998	Secaucus, New Jersey Mayflower Hotel	Transforming Health Care with Policy Uses of Transcultural Nursing	Dr. J. MacNeil	D. Pacquiao	Jr. of TCN (M. McFarland, Editor)
October 6–9, 1999	Snowbird, Utah The Cliff Lodge	Visions of the Past, Dreams of the Future 25th Celebration 1974–1999	Dr. M. Leininger	R. Zoucha	Jr. of TCN (M. Douglas, Editor)
October 4–6, 2000	Goldcoast, Australia Legends Hotel	Leading into the New Millennium	Dr. M. Leininger Sally Gould Sally Ramsden	Steering Comm. E. Percival, A. Omeri and others	Jr. of TCN (M. Douglas, Editor)
October 10–13, 2001	Pittsburgh, Pennsylvania	Culturally Competent Care in Health Organizations	Dr. D. Satcher Dr. M. Leininger	R. Zoucha D. Pacquiao	Jr. of TCN (M. Douglas, Editor)

* Leininger, M., "Twenty-five Years of Knowledge and Practice: Development of the Transcultural Nursing Society," *Journal of Transcultural Nursing*, 1998, v. 9, no. 2, pp. 72, 73 (updated through 2001).

Appendix 1-B
Current Graduate Courses or Programs in Transcultural Nursing 2001–2002

United States

University of Nebraska Medical Center, College of Nursing (Omaha, Nebraska).

- Offers two short-term intensive graduate courses (2 credits each) at master's and post-master's levels on transcultural nursing and human caring.
- Courses may be taken for college credit or through continuing education.
- Dr. Madeleine Leininger, Founder of Transcultural Nursing, Professor.

University of Northern Colorado, School of Nursing (Greeley, Colorado).

- Offers graduate certificate program with transcultural nursing with field studies.
- Instructors: Diane Peters and others.

Kean University (Union City, New Jersey).

- Offers graduate courses in transcultural nursing through Transcultural Nursing Institute.
- Professor Dula Pacquiao.

Duquesne University, School of Nursing (Pittsburgh, Pennsylvania).

- Offers graduate courses in transcultural nursing, post-master's program with focus on transcultural nursing, and a Ph.D. in Nursing with a focus on transcultural nursing (online instruction).
- Associate Professor and Director Dr. Rick Zoucha.

Augsberg College, College of Nursing (St. Paul, Minnesota).

- Offers graduate courses in transcultural nursing.
- Instructor: Dr. Cheryl Leuning.

University of Southern Mississippi, School of Nursing (Hattiesburg, Mississippi).

- Offers a graduate course in transcultural nursing.
- Dr. S. Jones.

Nazareth University, Department of Nursing (Rochester, New York).

- Offers a graduate course in transcultural nursing.
- Professor Margaret Andrews.

Madonna University (Livonia, Michigan)

- Offers graduate transcultural nursing courses.
- Dr. McFarland; P. Shinkel.

Overseas

University of Sydney, Nursing Faculty, Graduate Nursing Faculty (Sydney, Australia).

- Graduate seminars in transcultural nursing.
- Instructor: Dr. Akram Omeri.

University of Kuopio, Nursing Faculty (Kuopio, Finland).

- Offers study in transcultural nursing.
- Faculty instructors.

NOTE: Several schools of nursing offer some cultural or transcultural nursing and research, but no full courses or programs over academic terms focused in-depth on transcultural nursing.

References

1. Leininger, M., *Transcultural Nursing: Concepts, Theories and Practices*, New York: John Wiley & Sons, 1978. (Reprinted Columbus, OH: Greyden Press, 1994.)
2. Leininger, M., *Nursing and Anthropology: Two Worlds to Blend*, New York: John Wiley & Sons, 1970. (Reprinted Columbus, OH: Greyden Press, 1994.)
3. Leininger, M., "Culture Concept and Its Relevance to Nursing," *The Journal of Nursing Education*, 1967, v. 6, no. 2, pp. 7–39.

4. Leininger, M., *Transcultural Nursing: Concepts, Theories, Research and Practice*, Blacklick, OH: McGraw-Hill College Custom Series, 1995.
5. Leininger, op. cit., 1978.
6. Leininger, op. cit., 1995.
7. Leininger, M., "Twenty-five Years of Knowledge and Practice: Development of the Transcultural Nursing Society," *Journal of Transcultural Nursing*, 1998, v. 9, no. 2, pp. 72, 73.
8. Leininger, M., "Transcultural Nursing: A Worldwide Necessity to Advance Nursing Knowledge and Practices," in *Current Issues in Nursing*, J. McCloskey and H. Grace, eds., 1990, pp. 534–541.
9. Leininger, M., "Multidisciplinary Transculturalism and Transcultural Nursing," *Journal of Transcultural Nursing*, 2000a, v. 11, no. 2, p. 147.
10. Leininger, op. cit., 1995.
11. Leininger, op. cit., 1978.
12. Leininger, op. cit., 1995.
13. Leininger, M., *Caring: An Essential Human Need*, Thorofare, NJ: Charles B. Slack, 1981. (Reprinted Detroit, MI: Wayne State University Press, 1988.)
14. Leininger, M., *Ethical and Moral Dimensions of Care*, Detroit, MI: Wayne State Press, 1990.
15. Leininger, op. cit., 1981.
16. Leininger, op. cit., 1967.
17. Leininger, M., "Caring: The Essence and Central Focus of Nursing," Research Foundation Report, 1977, v. 12, no. 1, pp. 2–14.
18. Leininger, M., "Care: A Central Focus of Nursing and Health Care Services," *Nursing and Health Care*, 1980, v. 1, no. 3, pp. 135–143.
19. Leininger, M., *Care: The Essence of Nursing and Health*, Thorofare, NJ: Charles B. Slack, 1988. (Reprinted Detroit: Wayne State University Press, 1990.)
20. Leininger, op. cit., 1977.
21. Leininger, M., "Transcultural Nursing Education: A Worldwide Imperative," *Nursing and Health Care*, 1994, v. 15, no. 5, pp. 254–257.
22. Leininger, op. cit., 1980.
23. Leininger, M., "Transcultural Nursing is Discovery of Self and the World of Others," *Journal of Transcultural Nursing*, v. II, no. 4, October 2000b, pp. 312–313.
24. Leininger, op. cit., 1995.
25. Ibid.
26. Leininger, op. cit., 1978.
27. Leininger, M., *Culture Care Diversity and Universality: A Theory of Nursing*, New York: National League for Nursing Press, 1991.
28. Leininger, op. cit., 1970.
29. Kottak, K.K., *Anthropology: The Exploration of Human Diversity*, 5th ed., New York: McGraw-Hill, 1991, pp. 36–43.
30. Leininger, M., "Transcultural Nursing: Development, Focus, Importance and Historical Development," in *Transcultural Nursing, Concepts, Theories, Research and Practices*, M. Leininger, ed., Blacklick, OH: McGraw-Hill College Custom Series, 1995, pp. 3–52.
31. Leininger, op. cit., 1970.
32. Leininger, op. cit., 1977.
33. Leininger, op. cit., 1980.
34. Leininger, op. cit., 1988.
35. Leininger, M., "Identifying Care Needs and How These Needs Can Be Met Through Psychiatric Nursing," *University of Cincinnati College of Nursing Publication*, 1955, pp. 8–12.
36. Gaut, D., "Conceptual Analysis of Caring Research Method," in *Caring: An Essential Human Need*, M. Leininger, ed., Thorofare, NJ: Charles B. Slack, 1981, pp. 17–24.
37. Bevis, E. M., "Caring: A Life Force," in *Caring: An Essential Human Need*, M. Leininger, ed., Thorofare, NJ: Charles B. Slack, 1981, pp. 49–59.
38. Watson, J., *Nursing: The Philosophy and Science of Caring*, Boston: Little, Brown and Co., 1979.
39. Ray, M. "A Philosophical Analysis of Caring Within Nursing," in *Caring: An Essential Human Need*, M. Leininger, Thorofare, NJ: Charles B. Slack, 1981, pp. 24–35.
40. Leininger, op. cit., 1981, pp. 9, 3–15.
41. Leininger, op. cit., 1991, p. 46.
42. Ibid, pp. 44–45.
43. Leininger, M., "Towards Conceptualizing Transcultural Health Care Systems: Concepts and a Model," in *Health Care Dimensions*, Philadelphia, PA: F.A. Davis Co., 1976.
44. Leininger, op. cit., 1991, p. 43.
45. Leininger, op. cit., 1995.
46. Ibid.
47. Leininger, op. cit., 1994.
48. Leininger, op. cit., 1990.
49. U.S. Migration Reports and World Bank Reports, Washington, D.C., 1970–1999.
50. Andrews, M. and J. Boyle, *Transcultural Concepts in Nursing Care*, 3rd ed., Philadelphia, PA: Lippincott Williams and Wilkins, 1999.

51. Leininger, op. cit., 1995.
52. Leininger, op. cit., 1978.
53. Ibid.
54. Leininger, op. cit., 1995.
55. Leininger, M., "Nursing Education Exchanges: Concerns and Benefits," *Journal of Transcultural Nursing*, 1998, vol. 9, no. 2, pp. 57–63.
56. Leininger, M., "Transcultural Nursing: Quo Vadis (Where Goeth the Field)," *Journal of Transcultural Nursing*, 1989b, v. 1, no. 1, pp. 33–45.
57. Leininger, M., "Becoming Aware of Types of Health Practitioners and Cultural Imposition," *Journal of Transcultural Nursing*, 1991, v. 2, no. 2, pp. 32–39.
58. Leininger, op. cit., 1990.
59. Leininger, op. cit., 1995.
60. Ibid.
61. Wenger, A.F., "Cultural Context, Health and Health Care Decision Making," *Journal of Transcultural Nursing*, 1995, v. 7, no. 1, pp. 3–14.
62. Leininger, M., "Gadsup of New Guinea: Child-rearing Ethnocare, Ethnohealth and Ethnonursing," in *Transcultural Nursing: Concepts, Theories, Research and Practices,* M. Leininger, ed., Blacklick, OH: McGraw-Hill College Custom Series, 1995, pp. 559–589.
63. Leininger, M., "Future Directions in Transcultural Nursing in the 21st Century," *International Nursing Review*, 1997, v. 44, no. 1, pp. 19–23.
64. Ibid.
65. Leininger, M., "Desktoppers from 1989 through June, 1998," *Journal of Transcultural Nursing.*
66. Leininger, op. cit., 1995.
67. Leininger, op. cit., 1970.
68. Ibid.
69. Leininger, op. cit., 1978.
70. Nightingale, F., *Notes on Nursing: What Is and Is Not*, London: Harrisons and Sons, 1859.
71. Dunphy, L., "Caring Actualized," in *Nursing Theories and Nursing Practice*, M. Parker, ed., 2001, pp. 31–54.
72. Leininger, op. cit., 1995.
73. Leininger, op. cit., 1970.
74. Leininger, op. cit., 1995.
75. Leininger, op. cit., 1995.
76. Leininger, M., *Annual Report, College of Nursing on Transcultural Nursing Program*, Detroit, MI: 1995.
77. Kinney, G., "Personal Communication," University of Hawaii, Hilo, 1995–2000.
78. Leininger, M., "Transcultural Nurse Specialists and Generalists," *New Practioners in Nursing,* 1989, v. 1, no.1, pp. 4–15.
79. Leininger, op. cit., 1995.
80. Leininger, op. cit., 1995.
81. Leininger, op. cit., 1978.
82. Leininger, M., "The Third Millennium and Transcultural Nursing," *Journal of Transcultural Nursing*, 2000, v. 11, no. 1, p. 69.
83. Leininger, M., "Reflections on Nightingale with a Focus on Human Care Theory and Leadership," in *200 Year Anniversary Edition of Nightingale's "Notes on Nursing,"* Philadelphia, PA: J.B. Lippincott Co., 1992, pp. 28–39.
84. Leininger, op. cit., 1995.
85. Leininger, M., "Reflections on the International Council of Nurses and the Transcultural Nursing Society in London 1999," *Journal of Transcultural Nursing*, 1999, v. 10, no. 4, p. 372.
86. Leininger, op. cit., 1991.
87. Leininger, op. cit., 1995.
88. Ibid.
89. Leininger, M., "Transcultural Nursing and Education: A Worldwide Imperative," *Nursing and Health Care*, 1994, v. 15, no. 5, pp. 254–257.
90. Leininger, op. cit., 1997.
91. Leininger, M., "Quality of Life from a Transcultural Nursing Perspective," *Nursing Science Quarterly*, 1993, v. 7, no. 1, pp. 22–28.
92. Leininger, M., "Transcultural Nursing: An Imperative for Nursing Practice," *Imprint*, November–December 1999, pp. 50–53.
93. Andrews and Boyle, op. cit., 1999.
94. Leininger, M., "Survey Report on Transcultural Nursing Programs," Omaha, NE, 2000. Unpublished.
95. Ibid.
96. Ryan, M. et al., "Transcultural Nursing Concepts and Experiences in Nursing Curricula," *Journal of Transcultural Nursing*, 2000, v. 11, no. 4, pp. 300–307.
97. Leininger, op. cit., 1998.
98. Spector, R., *Cultural Diversity in Health and Illness*, Norwalk, CT: Appleton and Lange, 1999.
99. Cavanaugh, K. and P. Kennedy, *Promoting Cultural Diversity: Strangers for Care Professionals*, Newbury Park, CA: Sage Publications, 1992.

100. Purnell, L. and B. Paulanka, *Transcultural Health Care*, St. Louis, MO: F. A. Davis Co., 1998.

101. Aleardi, M., "Must Patient and Nurse Share the Same Culture?" *Nursing Spectrum*, 1999, v. 8, no. 20, pp. 4–5.

102. Poss, J.E., "Providing Cultural Competent Care: Is there a Role for Health Promoters?" *Nursing Outlook*, 1999, v. 47, no. 1, pp. 30–35.

103. Williams, R., "Cultural Safety: What Does It Mean for Our Work Practice?" *Australian and New Zealand Journal of Public Health*, 1999, v. 23, no. 2, pp. 213–214.

104. United States Office of Health and Human Services, "Assuring Cultural Competence in Health Care: Recommendations for National Standards and an Outcome-Focused Research Agenda," *Federal Register*, 1999, v. 64, no. 24.

105. Leininger, op. cit., 1995.

106. Leininger, M., "Transcultural Nursing to Transform Nursing Education and Practice: 40 Years Image," *Journal of Nursing Scholarship*, 1997, v. 29, no. 4, pp. 341–349.

107. Leininger, op. cit., 1989.

108. Leininger, op. cit., 1995.

109. Leininger, M., "Issues, Questions and Concerns Related to the Nursing Dagnosis Cultural Movement for a Transcultural Nursing Perspective," *Journal of Transcultural Nursing*, 1990, v. 2, no. 1, pp. 23–32.

110. Leininger, M. "Strange Myths and Inaccurate Facts in Transcultural Nursing," *Journal of Transcultural Nursing*, 1992, v. 3, no. 2, pp. 39–40.

111. Leininger, op. cit., 1991.

112. Leininger, op. cit., 1985.

113. Leininger, M., "What is Transcultural Nursing and Culturally Competent Care?" *Journal of Transcultural Nursing*, 1999, v. 10, no. 1, p. 9.

114. Leininger, M. "Graduate Courses in Transcultural Nursing," unpublished study, 2001, Omaha, NE.

115. Brink, P., *Transcultural Nursing: A Book of Readings*, Englewood Cliffs, NJ: Prentice Hall, Inc., 1976.

116. Andrews and Boyle, op. cit., 1999.

117. Leininger, op. cit., 1995.

118. Geiger, J. and D.R. Hizer, *Transcultural Nursing: Assessment and Intervention*, 2nd ed., St. Louis, MO: Mosby Book Inc., 1995.

119. Purnell et al., op. cit., 1998.

CHAPTER 2

Essential Transcultural Nursing Care Concepts, Principles, Examples, and Policy Statements

Madeleine Leininger

Professional caring for people of diverse cultures, necessitates the use of transcultural concepts, principles, theoretical ideas and research findings to reflect upon and guide actions and decisions. LEININGER, 1978

Transcultural nursing is a growing and highly relevant area of study and practice today that has great relevance for nurses living and functioning in a multicultural world. This area of study and practice often leads to some entirely different ways of knowing and helping people of diverse cultures. With a transcultural focus, nurses think about differences and similarities among people regarding their special needs and concerns to develop different ways to assist clients. As nurses discover the client's particular cultural beliefs and values, they learn ways to provide sensitive, compassionate, and competent care that is beneficial and satisfying to the client. Gaining a deep appreciation for cultures with their commonalties and differences is one of several goals of transcultural nursing. At the same time, the nurse discovers many nursing insights about her own cultural background and how to use such knowledge appropriately with clients whether in a particular community, hospital, or other type of health care service. Transcultural nursing is an area that opens many new windows of knowledge and competency that have previously been unknown to nurses.

In this chapter, several essential transcultural nursing concepts will be defined and discussed along with specific examples to guide nursing practices as used in transcultural nursing. In addition, generic and professional nursing care are defined and explained as major concepts, showing the differences and similarities as they relate to the practice of transcultural nursing. In the last section several recurrent, clinical, transcultural nursing incidents with interpretations are presented to help nurses understand and envision the therapeutic nature of transcultural nursing. Several questions are raised so the reader can reflect on ideas regarding transcultural nursing and can thus provide nursing care that is culturally competent, safe, and congruent. Discovering the *whys* of each transcultural incident with the concepts helps the nurse to gain in-depth knowledge of a culture.

In this chapter consider that you are functioning or living with cultures largely unknown to you. You might envision yourself in a hospital assigned to care for a client who spoke a different language, was dressed differently, and acted in strange ways. You are baffled by what you see and hear, but eager to know how you could give good nursing care. How would you feel? What would you do? This is a transcultural nursing situation that many nurses face today in most hospitals, homes, and health services. The situations offered in this chapter challenge one to realize the critical need for transcultural nursing knowledge, principles, and skills to work with cultural strangers in therapeutic ways.

Major Concepts and Definitions in Transcultural Nursing

In the evolution and development of this field of study and practice, it is essential for nurses to understand the major concepts, constructs, theories, and principles of transcultural nursing. The term *construct* is used to indicate several concepts embedded in phenomena such as care or caring. *Concept* refers to a single idea, thought, or object. Transcultural nursing leaders have identified, studied, defined, and explicated a number of concepts and constructs so nurses can use the ideas in meaningful and appropriate ways. Such fundamental knowledge can assist nurses to communicate effectively with others and to avoid unfavorable conflicts or troublesome interactions. It is, therefore, essential that nursing students study the concepts and apply the ideas to real-life situations.

In Chapter 1 the general definition of transcultural nursing was presented, but let us reflect further on its essential features. *Transcultural nursing is a substantive area of study and practice focused on comparative cultural care (caring) values, beliefs, and practices of individuals or groups of similar or different cultures. Transcultural nursing's goal is to provide culture-specific and universal nursing care practices for the health and well-being of people or to help them face unfavorable human conditions, illness, or death in culturally meaningful ways.*[1,2] This definition of transcultural nursing has many important ideas such as the focus on discovering culture-care values, beliefs, and practices of specific cultures or subcultures to assist people with their daily health care needs. The comparative viewpoint is emphasized to identify differences and similarities among or between cultures. It is this comparative viewpoint that enables the nurse to identify culture-specific and commonalities of care of clients or groups. The major goal of transcultural nursing is to *tailor-make* nursing care to reasonably fit the client's culture-specific expectations and care needs for beneficial health care outcomes and to identify any universal or common care practices. Culturally congruent care becomes the desired and ultimate goal of transcultural nursing.

As one ponders further about transcultural nursing, the idea of human-care (caring) values, beliefs, and practices becomes a central focus for nurses to learn about and practice transcultural nursing. The author has declared since the late 1940s that *care is an essential human need and the essence of nursing* on which the profession should be focusing.[3,4] Nursing is a *caring profession and discipline* that directs nurses to discover and provide knowledgeable and skilled care to clients. I have defined *nursing as a learned, humanistic, and scientific profession and discipline focused on human care phenomena and caring activities in order to assist, support, and facilitate or enable individuals or groups to maintain or regain their health or well-being in culturally meaningful and beneficial ways, or to help individuals face handicaps or death.*[5] This definition reinforces the idea of care as the essence and fundamental focus of nursing and transcultural nursing.

Human Care as Essence of Nursing

In considering nursing as a caring profession and discipline, it is important to remember that nursing as a profession has a *societal mandate to serve people*. The professional nurse is challenged to serve others who need the assistance of a person prepared and qualified to respond to or who can anticipate the actual or covert care needs of people. Nurses are professional persons who are ultimately held responsible for and accountable to people in a particular society or culture to give *care* that will help people to regain and maintain their health and to prevent illnesses. Nurses, however, function best as professional persons when they know and understand different cultures in relation to their experiences, human conditions, and cultural care values and beliefs. Today all professional nurses need to be culturally prepared to be effective and beneficial to clients. Nursing as a culture also has culturally defined modes of functioning and being which may change over time with societal changes. However, as a discipline the culture of nursing expects that nurses will discover and use knowledge that is distinctive and explains and interprets nursing's focus and essence.[6] Most importantly, nursing as a discipline implies that there is a substantive body of knowledge to guide its members' thinking and actions. The discipline of nursing needs to focus more on care/caring to explain health and well-being in different or similar cultures. Care, health, and well-being are central to what nursing is or should be.[7] Transcultural nurses are contributing some new, unique, and significant knowledge to nursing with the comparative care focus and with ways to use this knowledge to serve people of a specific culture, or a society worldwide.

In a number of publications I have discussed human care and caring as the central, distinct, and dominant foci to explain, interpret, and predict nursing as a discipline and profession, and encourage the reader to study them.[8–13] *Human care*, a noun, refers to a specific *phenomenon* that is characterized to assist, support, or enable another human being or group to achieve one's desired goals or to obtain assistance with certain human needs. In contrast, *human caring* is focused on the *action aspect* or *activities* to provide service to other human beings. Differences in the meanings of care (noun) and caring (an action mode) are extremely important in understanding and practicing transcultural nursing caring as a professional art. More explicitly, I have defined care and caring as follows:[13]

> **Care** (noun) refers to an abstract or concrete phenomenon related to assisting, supporting, or enabling experiences or behaviors or for others with evidence for anticipated needs to ameliorate or improve a human condition or lifeway.

> **Caring** (gerund) refers to actions and activities directed toward assisting, supporting, or enabling another individual or group with evident or anticipated needs to ease, heal, or improve a human condition or lifeway or to face death or disability.

These definitions of care and caring with culture are the foundational constructs of transcultural nursing and characterize the nature and focus of the discipline. They guide nurses in discovering care knowledge and ways to provide direct care. Care is embedded in culture as an integral part of culture that challenges nurses to understand both care and culture together to practice transcultural nursing.

Culture and Nursing

Culture comes from the discipline of anthropology. Culture has been defined and used by anthropologists and other social scientists for over 100 years. The term culture, however, was limitedly used and was not valued and explicated in nursing until I raised awareness that culture was a crucial and major dimension of nursing in the mid 1950s. Gradually and by 1990, culture began to be discussed and used in a variety of ways with some questionable and imprecise uses. Definitions are important in any discipline, and thus these definitions were developed early for transcultural nursing:

> **Culture** refers to the learned, shared, and transmitted knowledge of values, beliefs, and lifeways of a particular group that are generally transmitted intergenerationally and influence thinking, decisions, and actions in patterned or in certain ways.[14,15]

> **Subculture** is closely related to culture, but refers to subgroups who deviate in certain ways from a dominant culture in values, beliefs, norms, moral codes, and ways of living with some distinctive features that characterize their unique lifeways.[15,16]

Other Features of Cultures

Both cultures and subcultures are developed by peoples or population aggregates over time with distinct values, beliefs, and lifeways. They are preserved and usually transmitted intergenerationally. A subculture is a smaller population group that establishes certain rules of conduct, values, and living styles that are different from a dominant or mainstream culture, and yet it has some features of the dominant culture. Subcultures have distinctive patterns of living with their own sets of rules, special living ways and practices that deviate from the dominant culture. For example, there are subcultures of the homeless, substance abused, elderly, abused women and children, chronically disabled, mentally ill, the retarded, deaf, AIDS victims, and often some religious sects and cults. There are also special political and social groups that do not follow the dominant culture. These subcultures closely identify with their own group's beliefs and values and hold themselves as different from dominant cultures such as Anglo-Americans, African-Americans, British, Hispanic, Brazilians, and other major cultures. Transcultural nurses are expected to study both cultures and subcultures as they have different care and health needs.

Culture is a major construct to understanding in transcultural nursing, and it is also a key construct in anthropology. However, it is bringing culture and care *together* that is providing new perspectives to understand and serve people of different lifeways. Culture has been studied and used in anthropology since the 19th century, and it continues to be central to anthropology as the learned and shared values, beliefs, and practices usually passed on intergenerationally. In transcultural nursing, culture and care are conceptualized as bound together to provide special insights valuable to nursing. *Culture care is a synthesized construct* that is the foundational basis to understanding and helping people of different cultures in transcultural nursing practices. Anthropologically speaking, culture is the broadest and most holistic and comprehensive view of people; yet one can focus on specific ideas and practices to understand people. It was this culturally based care that was woefully missing in nursing until transcultural nursing came into focus. Today, culturally grounded care/caring are now becoming valued and being studied in nursing.

There are other features of a culture that need to be understood and will be highlighted. *First*, culture reflects shared values, ideals, and meanings that are learned and that guide human thoughts, decisions, and actions. With shared cultural values and norms, individuals and groups tend to uphold the rules for living in a culture because it brings security, order, and expected behavior. Cultural values usually transcend individual values and are influenced by groups and symbols. Cultural beliefs, values, and norms (or rules of behavior) are learned from others and are not considered to be genetically or biologically transmitted. It is the cultural values and practices that have a powerful influence on others and become like ethical and moral standards with expected obligations and responsibilities.

Second, cultures have *manifest* (readily recognized) and *implicit* (covert and ideal) rules of behavior and expectations. Manifest cultural norms or rules of behavior are the obvious and readily known beliefs and expressions such as greeting another person by a handshake. Implicit and ideal values are usually covert rules that are difficult to see or understand. They have, however, important influences on decisions and actions such as nodding one's head as "yes" or "no" to accept or reject medications. Care is often implicit.

Third, human cultures have material items or symbols such as artifacts, objects, dress, and actions that have special meaning in a culture. In the United States, drinking Coke (or Pepsi) and music both are associated symbols of teenagers, whereas in New Guinea, carrying bows and arrows are teenage symbols of hunters. Cultures also have nonmaterial expressions, beliefs, and ideas such as having "good and bad spirits" to guide oneself in unknown lands. Nonmaterial cultural symbols such as certain hand gestures or words when wanting to be cared for are important. Material symbols as crosses and special relics may be used for healing and protection from illnesses. Human beings are unique for symbolic thinking and reasoning and use of material objects for various reasons. Nurses are expected to learn about material and nonmaterial forms and their functions in different cultures and how they can influence caring, healing, and well-being or sickness.

Fourth, cultures have traditional ceremonial practices such as religious rituals, food feasts, and other activities that are transmitted intergenerationally and reaffirm family or group ties and caring ways (Color Insert 2). Cultural rituals are also found in nursing and medicine and serve certain purposes. For example, nurses have the morning and evening chart report rituals to keep nurses informed and united on care goals. Physicians have the ritual of "grand rounds" in a hospital to share ideas about patients. Cultural groups such as the Vietnamese have healing rituals and protective care rituals when a child comes to a hospital. Such rituals usually have therapeutic value and need to be known and respected.

Fifth, cultures have their local or emic (insider's) views and knowledge about their culture that are extremely important for nurses to discover and understand for meaningful care practices. Emic ideas and beliefs are often viewed as "secrets" and may not be willingly shared with cultural strangers such as nurses or physicians unless the stranger is trusted. Transcultural nurses are expected to tease out emic data when trusting relationships have been established. It is *emic* (inside cultural) knowledge that nurses try to obtain from their clients. In contrast, *etic* (outsider's) knowledge, such as the nurse's professional ideas, may be very different from emic views and experiences. Both emic and etic knowledge are important to assess and guide nurses' thinking and decisions with clients.

These construct terms of emic and etic, which I introduced into nursing in the early 1960s, have been extremely valuable to nurses.[17]

Sixth, all human cultures have some intercultural variations between and within cultures. *Cultural variation is an important concept to keep in mind when studying individuals and different cultures.* For example, African-Americans and Italian-Americans show cultural variations in their daily lifeways regarding food choices, communication, dress, and response to illness and death. There are slight and great variations within and between cultures (Color Insert 3). However, one can usually, find some common patterns of expressions, and lifeways within each culture. In transcultural nursing, intercultural and intracultural variations are important to observe in your response to people in your care. Amid cultural variations, the nurse remains alert to common patterns of values, beliefs, and lifeways among and within cultures to guide care practices. Individual and group variability is always taken into consideration to prevent stereotyping or treating individuals in a rigid and fixed way.

Ethnicity is a related term that is often used as the same as culture, but it has a different meaning. Ethnicity refers to racial and often skin-color identity of particular groups related to specific and obvious features based on national origins. This concept tends to be used more frequently by sociologists and psychologists than by anthropologists or by transcultural nurses. Ethnicity also tends to be used by lay people and others in vague, diverse, and often superficial ways. Culture is a much more holistic and comprehensive term that goes beyond ethnicity and selected racial features or national origins of people. Culture deals with beliefs, values, and lifeways of human beings in addition to traditional and current origins. Ethnicity and culture cannot be used interchangeably as they have different meanings and uses. We, therefore, use culture as the holistic and in-depth meaningful term in transcultural nursing.

It is essential and very important to understand *cultural values* in transcultural nursing because values greatly influence human beliefs, actions, and lifeways of people. *Cultural value refers to the powerful internal and external directive forces that give meaning and order to the thinking, decisions, and actions of an individual or group.*[18] Discovering and understanding the

cultural values of a culture are essential in transcultural nursing because they are major indicators that influence what cultures do, how they act, and what one can expect of them. Understanding culture-specific values becomes important "holding" or reflection knowledge to consider in assisting a client. Such holding knowledge is always held in abeyance until one has seen, heard, or experienced the values, beliefs, expressions, or interpretations by informants. *Cultural values become guides to nursing actions and decisions.* Unfortunately, cultural values are usually not readily identified nor shared with strangers until a trusting relationship is evident. Some cultures may not want to share their values as they may fear rejection if their values are different from the nurse, the hospital, or clinic. However, some cultures are more open and ready to talk and share their values. For example, most Anglo-Americans value their independence, freedom of speech, privacy, and physical appearance and want to talk about or see these values respected. When these values are not respected or are threatened, Anglo clients often speak out. One may recall that when Anglo-American men were held hostage in Iran, these American hostages were reported to be very depressed and frustrated, and they became ill. Another example of cultural values are with Malawi people of Africa who greatly value their extended family and children and feel lost when they are not near them whether they are ill or well. The Old Order Amish also value community living and praying together to keep well. Other cultures have their cultural values to guide their lives in sickness and when well. These cultural values are the *powerful forces* to guide nurses' response in caring for people of diverse or similar cultures. Observing and actively listening to clients are the critical means for learning about cultural values in addition to having holding knowledge about cultures. Cultural values tend to be stable and do not readily change because they are well learned and give security to cultures. Accordingly, the transcultural nurse must remain sensitive to cultural values and should not try to change them unless desired by the client.

Western and non-Western cultures and values are also important for transcultural nurses to understand and respect. *Western* refers to those cultures that value and *use modern technologies and that are industrialized.* Western cultures are known for their emphasis on being efficient and using scientific equipment that makes them "progressive" or "modern." Western cultures are younger and also are more current in the development of civilization materials and other modern modes of living that are largely dependent on high technologies. Western cultures generally include the United States, Canada, Europe, Russia, South Korea, and related areas. In contrast, the term *non-Western (sometimes imprecisely called Eastern) cultures* refers to those cultures that have existed for thousands of years and have a long history of surviving and living with different philosophies of life. They have *traditional values and lifeways and rely less on modern technologies than Western cultures.* Non-Western cultures have a rich, traditional philosophy of life that is supported by symbols, beliefs, and different patterns of living and dying. Non-Western cultures would include China, South Africa, Indonesia, Vietnam, Papua, New Guinea, Egypt, Borneo, and the Caribbean. These cultures, with their thousands of years of living and surviving, often look to Western cultures as "inexperienced cultures moving rapidly with strange ways of living." Some non-Western cultures have been slow to become "Westernized" for many good reasons such as economic factors and very different cultural beliefs and values. Transcultural nurses are expected to assess, know, and work with both Western and non-Western cultures in effective and knowledge-based ways.

Culture shock is another key concept used in transcultural nursing that has been derived from anthropology. It refers to *an individual who is disoriented or unable to respond appropriately to another person or situation because the lifeways are so strange and unfamiliar.* It leaves one feeling helpless, hopeless, and confused. Nurses, clients, families, and researchers experience cultural shock in a variety of ways when they are unable to know what to say or how to act in a given situation that is truly shocking to them. Nurses may be shocked to relate to cultures so different from their own or to situations that are drastically different. For example, the nurse may be surprised to find an Anglo mother failing to respond to a crying child until the child does very destructive acts. Or the nurse who saw a Chinese client eating fish eye soup. Or when I first went to New Guinea and found no Western living conveniences such as running water and electricity in the homes and had to live in a bamboo hut with snakes. An Old Order Amish client who has never been in a hospital may experience culture shock when suddenly in an emergency room with masked nurses, electronic equipment, and bright lights and with everyone staring and talking about his injured body. The Amish live in a non-modern, rural community with virtually no technologies. Nurses who assist unknown immigrants and refugees also experience cultural shock when they find these clients live and act very differently in their daily lives. Culture shock greatly limits one's ability to function with strangers and in strange or unfamiliar settings. Feelings of helplessness, depression, and not knowing what to do is often experienced by nurses with cultural shock. One can overcome and prevent some cultural shock by studying and knowing something about the people of a certain culture and their lifeways in advance of working with them.

Uniculturalism and *multiculturalism* are two important but different concepts to be understood by nurses in transcultural nursing. *Uniculturalism (or monoculturalism) refers to the belief that one's universe is largely constituted, centered upon, and functions from a one-culture perspective that reflects excessive ethnocentrism. Multiculturalism refers to a perspective and reality that there are many different cultures and subcultures in the world that need to be recognized, valued, and understood for their differences and similarities.* Multiculturalism helps people to appreciate the many cultures in a changing world. This view is extremely essential in developing respect for the many cultures in the world.

Ethnocentrism is an important concept in transcultural nursing because it strongly influences one's thinking and action modes. *Ethnocentrism refers to the belief that one's own ways are the best, most superior, or preferred ways to act, believe, or behave.* Ethnocentrism is a universal phenomena in that most people tend to believe that their ways of living, believing, and acting are right, proper, and morally correct. However, excessive or strong ethnocentric attitudes can become a serious problem with others. When one holds too firmly to one's own beliefs, values, and standards and is unwilling to accommodate or consider someone else's views, problems occur. Learning to value, appreciate, and understand *why* other cultures do and act differently with their particular viewpoints is essential in transcultural nursing. For it is this knowledge and awareness of *other's views* that leads to creative ways to serve people and understand oneself. Beliefs that seem bizarre or strange may be common and important to one culture, but differ greatly with other cultures. Strong ethnocentric views that are acted on can be destructive or harmful to cultures. Modifying or changing one's own strong beliefs is often essential for an effective professional relationship with clients, staff, and systems. Rigid ethnocentrism can limit professional growth and success. It is often a major concern for nurses who want to practice effective transcultural nursing, because excessive ethnocentrism can lead to a host of cultural problems such as cultural clashes, stresses, and negative outcomes.

Many examples of rigid ethnocentrism can be identified in nursing. For example, there is the nurse who believes that there is only one way to make a hospital bed, give medicine, or feed a child or adult. Clients will often challenge such views and show other cultural ways to be effective. If a bed is made that does not allow for one's height or weight such as with a tall Danish client who wants plenty of room for his feet, he is uncomfortable. Or take the example of the nurse who is ethnocentric and is upset to learn that other cultures eat snakes, bugs, kidneys, and opossum as delicacies. Some nurses may be so ethnocentric that they constantly misinterpret what is said or done by clients. Rigid ethnocentric practices and attitudes by nurses generally lead to unfavorable client-care practices. Transcultural faculty mentoring is essential to assess and prevent strong ethnocentrism. Sometimes the problem continues because no one wants to deal with ethnocentric biases and practices. Of course, all humans have some degree of ethnocentrism, but it is the narrow, biased, and nonrespectful ones that cause difficulties.

Cultural bias is closely related to ethnocentrism. It *refers to a firm position or stance that one's own values and beliefs must govern the situation or decisions.* A culturally biased person usually fails to recognize their own biases and persists in making their biases known to others. They are rigid in their thinking and constantly get into problems working with diverse cultures. Strong cultural biases usually lead to open resistance and negative relationships with clients and staff.

Cultural relativism is well known in anthropology and is studied in nursing. It *refers to the position that cultures are so unique and must be evaluated, judged, and helped according to their own particular values and standards.*[19] Cultural relativism may be desired by some cultures for security and political reasons. Cultural relativists who take an extreme position that one culture should not be judged by the values and lifeways of another culture or that all cultures are completely unique will encounter difficulties accepting variabilities and universal truths. Cultural relativists who firmly uphold a practice of a particular culture will fight to protect cultural values. For example, a father fought against deformed-child legislation because he held that dealing with a child's handicap must be based on the particular community's resources and beliefs. This may be difficult to accept by professional nurses but was important to the community. Cultural relativism may have both beneficial and less beneficial outcomes. It is again how knowledgeable one becomes to interpret and understand cultures. Generally, strong relativism upholds that there are no universal norms, beliefs, or practices and that all is relative to each situation, event, or happening, which leads to religious problems. Transcultural nursing remains open to discover what is *particularistic* and *universal* as found in the philosophy of my theory of Culture Care Diversity and Universality. Transcultural nurses need to be aware of excessive cultural relativistic positions and how to deal with them in relation to health care, religious beliefs, and use of professional knowledge. Transcultural nurses need to understand and find the best ways to help people, but not relinquish their faith beliefs.

Cultural imposition refers to the tendency of an individual or group to impose their beliefs, values, and patterns of behavior on another culture for varied reasons.[20] In the mid 1950s, I coined this concept in transcultural nursing as I could see in clinical practices and in teaching that cultural imposition was evident. Many nurses and health care providers seemed unaware that they were imposing their own cultural beliefs, values, and professional ways onto the client's culture. *Cultural imposition remains a major serious and largely unrecognized problem in nursing as a result of cultural ignorance, blindness, ethnocentric tendencies, biases, racism, and other factors.* Cultural imposition can be found between professional staff and clients and especially when staff hold considerably more power, influence, and authority over clients. Clients of some cultures, especially non-Western and vulnerable cultures, often perceive that they have virtually no rights, power, or influence to deal with others such as nurses and physicians who are in authority or have special power roles. To get tasks or procedures done quickly, cultural imposition practices exist. Cultural imposition practices occur between nurses and clients when the nurse believes that only his or her ethnocentric views are right or the best for the client who may seem to have strange, bizarre, or nondesirable views. For example, the nurse insists that a Vietnamese client must eat hamburger and drink milk without regard to the client's lactose intolerance condition or dislike for hamburger. Or consider the nurse showing cultural imposition with a family's way of feeding their elderly mother by feeling it is "impractical" and "a waste of time." Many examples can be found in nursing and in nursing educational institutions. Cultural imposition practices can also be found with physicians and other staff using their professional authority, status and position. Use of power, authority, and superior attitude are evident with cultural imposition and leave the client feeling helpless, angry, and that "one must comply" to get care or service.

Cultural blindness is another term the author coined in the late 1950s to *refer to the inability of an individual to recognize or see one's own lifestyle, values, and modes of acting as those based largely on ethnocentric and baised tendencies*. It may seem strange to think that some people are so "blind" that they fail to see and understand their own as well as other ways of living, believing, doing, or valuing. For example, an Australian nurse was caring for an Arab-Muslim client who told the nurse several times that he would be gone from his room to say his prayers at certain times in the day and evening. The nurse would still come to give his medication at noon and failed to see and understand he was gone and praying at another place in the hospital. This nurse was "blind" to recognize and accept what the client did and had told her. She did not accommodate the Arab-Muslim's prayer time. Or consider the British nurse who believes "every baby should be bonded with his mother" even though the male baby is being bonded to his father for cultural reasons. The nurse with cultural blindness needs mentorship to help her become sensitive and responsive to other ideas and ways that are different and beneficial.

Cultural pain is a relatively new concept in health care that the author coined and discovered while caring for cultures who said they experienced "pain" because nurses and physicians failed to recognize their cultural discomforts or offenses.[21] Cultural pain *refers to suffering, discomfort, or being greatly offended by an individual or group who shows a great lack of sensitivity toward another's cultural experience*. Nurses are taught mainly about psychophysical pain, but seldom learn that cultural pain exists and may be extremely hurtful to cultures. Transcultural nurses are in a good position to identify cultural pain as they listen to and observe clients of different cultures. For example, if a client or nurse breaks a family cultural taboo, this may lead to crying and to feeling pain. Nurses can induce cultural pain by what is said or done to clients, a situation in which the comment or action is offensive and very hurtful. For example, the nurse made demeaning comments about a family's Native American healer. Sometimes comments about body size such as being so tall, dark-skinned, or overweight may lead to cultural pain. These comments may be deeply felt and offensive to clients of different cultures. Cultural pain goes beyond physical and psychological pain to hurtful cultural offenses.

It is important to also be aware that cultures respond to real physical and emotional pain differently. Some cultures are very sensitive to physical pain and may cry loudly such as with some Jewish and Italian clients. In contrast, Russian, Lithuanian, German, and Slovenian clients often remain stoic and withhold physical pain expressions in learned and controlled ways. Cultures that are stoic or remain silent with physical pain such as with injections, cuts, or smashed fingers are noted by transcultural nurses and medical anthropologists. Some cultures learn how to express stoicism with physical pain, and children are taught early of ways to ignore or not complain about physical injuries. Accepting pain may also be linked with religious beliefs to gain spiritual graces as *redemptive suffering* with Roman Catholics. In contrast, there are cultures that quickly and loudly respond to even the slightest pin prick, injury, or bodily discomfort. Transcultural nurses learn to be aware of how and why cultures vary with physical and cultural pain with children and adults.

Such holding knowledge helps nurses to respond appropriately to cultural pain differences in therapeutic and sensitive ways and to not assume everyone experiences physical, emotional, and cultural pain in the same way. It is especially important to go beyond psychophysical pain and include cultural pain as hurtful suffering resulting from cultural reasons. The important principle is that what constitutes pain for one culture or individual is largely culturally learned and patterned throughout the life cycle. Transcultural nurses are discovering new insights about pain meanings and expressions with appropriate care actions.

Bioculturalism refers to biological and physical expressions in different physical environments or contexts related to care, health, illness, and disabilities. Humans are born and live within biophysical environments that influence their health and illness factors. Genetic, biocultural, and physical facts influence each other in different ecologies and cultural environments. Glittenberg's chapter in this book provides current insights on the genome factor that has become an important new area of study. Her other writings are also important to study.[22] The author's study in 1960 on bioecological variability in two Gadsup villages was an early nursing and anthropology study focused on health care.[23] Nurses work with clients in their biophysical and cultural settings and need to give attention to these factors and how they can influence caring practices and use of biocultural resources. Remaining knowledgeable about many new human genetic and biomedical research findings is very important in transcultural nursing.

The concept of culture-bound illness and human conditions is another essential concept to understand in transcultural nursing. *Culture-bound refers to specific care, health, illness, and disease conditions that are particular, quite unique, and usually specific to a designated culture or geographical area.* For example, in the Eastern Highlands of Papua New Guinea, *kuru* was discovered as a culture-bound illness in the early 1960s while the author was doing a field study in the area.[24] It was a condition in which adult females died within approximately 9 months and largely related to biocultural, viral, and other factors, but unique to the Eastern Highlands New Guinea region.[25] In Malaysia, one finds the culture-bound phenomenon of *running amok* in which males have violent running sprees and attack animals,

people, or objects. *Voodoo death* is another culture-bound condition largely found in the Caribbean where death follows a curse from a powerful sorcerer. Anthropologists have studied these culture-bound conditions and others for many decades with findings revealing specifically defined cultural, local, or regional areas. Until discovered elsewhere in the world, they are referred to as culture-bound. Transcultural nurses learn to be alert to culture-bound expressions and conditions to identify those care needs that are unique to some cultures. Culture-bound phenomena are essentially new to nurses and many health professionals due to cultural ignorance.

Cultural Diversity, Universality, Racism, and Related Concepts

Recently, cultural diversity and universality are of great popular and professional interest but often with limited knowledge of the terms. *Cultural diversity refers to the variations and differences among and between cultural groups resulting from differences in lifeways, language, values, norms, and other cultural aspects.* Cultural diversity was one of the first concepts emphasized in transcultural nursing. This was because nurses seemed to ignore cultural differences and treated "all clients alike" as if from the same culture in the pre-1960 era, and some still do today. By identifying cultural differences among and between cultures, nurses gradually began to value such differences and to provide culture-specific care. However, from the beginning I wanted nurses to discover and respond appropriately to both the diverse and universal features of cultural beings. Both dimensions were common to consider and have been the major focus of my theory to arrive at culturally congruent care practices.[26] By taking account of cultural differences of individuals and groups, the transcultural nurse can prevent stereotyping or viewing all as alike. Treating and seeing clients in fixed cultural ways and ignoring cultural differences is not helpful to most clients. Cultural diversity also helps nurses to value differences and provide culture-specific care practices. In this book there are many examples of cultural diversity to be studied.

Cultural universals refer to the commonalities among human beings or humanity that reveal the similarities or dominant features of humans. Universality refers to the nature of a being or an object that is held as common or universally found in the world as part of humanity. Cultural universals are the opposite of cultural diversity. With universals one seeks to discover and understand *commonalities* but not absolute universals as this may never be found to exist in statistical or precise quantitative ways. The theory of Culture Care Diversity and Universality is focused on what is *universal* and *diverse* about human caring and within cultural perspectives. The purpose of the theory is to discover similarities and differences about care and culture and to explain the relationship and reasons for the findings.[27] Discovering commonalties and differences in lifeways, values, and rules among cultures is essential for nurses in our multicultural world. For it is both the commonalties and differences among cultures that keep nurses alert to humanistic care practices. With research findings on many cultures this would be of great significance and help to nurses in caring and healing practices.

Racism is a major word used in most public and professional settings. It has become a popular lay term that is used for various political, legal, and other ways but one that is very limitedly understood in relation to common human features. Racism is derived from the concept of race, and race is generally defined as a biological factor of a discrete group whose members share distinctive genetic, biological, and other factors from a common or claimed ancestor.[28] Race has become used and often viewed as discrimination of oppressed minorities or people of different skin color. The outward or phenotype appearance such as skin color is not adequate as culture and genetic features need to be included to understand race. Skin colors as "red," "black," and "yellow" are inadequate as there are many in-between colors (Color Insert 4). For example, Native Americans are not "red," "yellow" or "white," and yet they are often referred to as the "red race." Likewise, black skin has various hues and cannot describe only Africans as many cultures have dark to lighter hues of color such as Maori, Fijians, Southeast Indians, Native Australians, and others. These color references are only one aspect to understanding people. The biological, genetic, and holistic cultural aspects must be considered for accurate usage. The Fijians in the Pacific Islands belong to the Polynesian culture with dark skin color, and they dislike being called "African blacks" as they know they have different cultural history and lifeways. Skin colors are, therefore, *phenotypes* and are external appearances of people based largely on physical features. They are generally crude indicators of the people for one must understand the culture of the people and their lifeways. The concept of *genotype*, which refers to genetic factors that help establish the biological and genetic base of a race, also needs to be considered. Genetic features such as DNA are being actively pursued today to predict many exact features about people.

Kottak discusses the idea that people are often talking about social races rather than genetic or biological races in public discourse.[29] Social attitudes and perceived differences often preclude prejudices, discrimination, and labels of racism. Racism often denotes subordination and the oppressive use of authority over others such as minorities, refugees, women, and religious groups. The term "ethnic people of color" is still used in nursing practice and literature. This phrase is misleading and tends to be used by some "minority" nurses. It is seldom used in transcultural nursing because of its ambiguity and impreciseness and because it leads to misleading ideas and often negative views. Unfortunately, racism and "racial profiling" can lead to vicious labeling of people with unsupported accusations and especially between "white" and "black" groups worldwide. It also leads to overt violence, cultural backlash, and often prolonged alienation and legal suits between groups or individuals. In nursing, "racist" discrimination practices exist and need to be addressed to prevent harm to clients and to the persons involved. Marked interpersonal tensions, isolation, violence, and other destructive behavior can occur where racism prevails. All nurses and health professionals need to address racism and discrimination problems and to discover the sources, reasons, and various factors leading to or aggravating racism. Learning about cultural differences in values, beliefs, patterns, and lifeways and understanding the why of these differences is crucial. In addition, one needs to seek information about the roots of institutional racial beliefs, gender biases, disruptive behavior, and prolonged animosity between different cultures. Transcultal nurses prepared through graduate programs can be very helpful in dealing with these major concerns and problems worldwide with other health personnel.

Since the terms prejudice, discrimination, and stereotyping are closely related, but often not used correctly, the following definitions have been developed and used in transcultural nursing. *Prejudice refers to preconceived ideas, beliefs, or opinions about an individual, group, or culture that limit a full and accurate understanding of the individual, culture, gender, event, or situation. Discrimination refers to overt or covert ways of limiting opportunities, choices, or life experiences of others based on feelings or on racial biases. Stereotyping refers to classifying or placing people into a narrow, fixed view with rigid, or inflexible, "boxlike" characteristics.* Stereotyping is often a "quick fix" to classify people without understanding individual and group cultural differences. So when nurses stereotype clients, they usually fail to recognize the individual or group cultural variations and cultural understandings. Stereotyping is not sanctioned in transcultural nursing, and so the nurse must be mentored and guided to prevent this practice. Limited knowledge and understanding of cultures usually leads to stereotyping, discrimination, prejudices, racism, and biases with an attitude set.

Cultural backlash is another phenomenon that is important to understand in transcultural nursing. It *refers to negative feedback or unfavorable outcomes after nurses have been working or consulting with cultures (often overseas) for brief periods.* The host country being served by a nurse(s) from another country feels their efforts failed to help the people in meaningful or beneficial ways. As a result, the host country or agency expresses negative views and feelings to the consultant, practitioner, or home agency. This phenomena makes one aware of the importance of providing help that *fits the culture,* thus avoiding a cultural backlash. As a consequence of such a backlash, nurses on exchange visits or as consultants are not invited to return to the host culture. Cultural backlash usually occurs with nurses who have not been prepared in transcultural nursing, or it may occur because of political reasons and conflicts that suddenly occur in the host country.

Another related phenomenon that can occur in serving other countries or cultures, I call *cultural overidentification.* This refers to *nurses who become too involved, overly sympathetic, or too compassionate with the people, situation, or a human condition.* As a consequence, the nurse is unable to be helpful to the culture or individual, and nontherapeutic and inappropriate actions are evident. Sometimes, this occurs when nurses have deeply sympathetic, biased, and emotional feelings about a culture or situation such as with poverty stricken, homeless, abused, oppressed, or battered individuals. The nurse's beliefs, attitudes, and actions become ineffective and often labeled by the host culture as "too compassionate or too emotionally involved with us." The nurse needs to be aware of overidentification tendencies in transcultural services.

The Five Basic Interactional Phenomena

Nurses working in transcultural contexts need to be clear on five basic concepts, namely, *culture encounter, enculturation, acculturation, socialization,* and *assimilation.* These concepts come largely from anthropology and are essential in transcultural nursing.

1. *Culture encounter or contact refers to a situation in which a person from one culture meets or briefly interacts with a person from another culture.* With brief, casual encounters and exchange of ideas, one rarely adopts the values, beliefs, and lifeways of a cultural stranger. A nurse having brief encounters with people from another culture or a client seldom grasps and understands strangers and their cultural lifeways. Nor does one then become an "expert" or an authority about a culture. For example, nurses giving tours, making brief visits, or having encounters with people of different cultures seldom become "transcultural experts" of the cultures. The lack of in-depth knowledge or preparation prior to the encounter is usually evident. There are, however, nurses in the past and today who have had such brief encounters such as giving tours or traveling abroad without cultural background knowledge. Some publish, give lectures, and declare themselves as "cultural experts" of designated cultures. This often leads to "cultural backlash" and ethical problems when local cultures discover their culture was not presented accurately or understood following such brief encounters. This remains a serious problem today in nursing.

2. *Enculturation* is a very important phenomenon to understand in transcultural nursing. It refers to *the*

process by which one learns to take on or live by a particular culture with its specific values, beliefs, and practices. One can speak of a child becoming "enculturated" in learning how to become an Italian, Anglo-American, Amish, or whatever the parents or individual lives by or chooses. The child becomes enculturated when he or she shows acceptable behavior of the cultural values, beliefs, and actions. Nurses are also enculturated within the nursing profession by learning the norms (rules of behavior), values, and other expectations of the nursing culture. It is important that nursing students become enculturated into nursing values, norms, and lifeways to survive, function, and become professional nurses. Nurses become enculturated into local hospitals, community agencies, and other health services to accept and maintain practice expectations. Some clients may become enculturated to a hospital, especially if they stay in the institution over a long period of time such as with chronic illnesses or disabilities. However, not all children, clients, students, and nurses become enculturated into fully accepting the values, norms, and practices desired. One has to assess if one is enculturated to another lifeway.

3. *Acculturation* is closely related to enculturation but has some differences. *Acculturation refers to the process by which an individual or group from Culture A learns how to take on many (but not all) values, behaviors, norms, and lifeways of Culture B.* Acculturated individuals generally reflect that they have taken on or adopted the lifeways and values of another culture by their actions and other expressions. It is, however, interesting that an individual from Culture A may still retain and use some traditional values and practices from the old culture, but this does not interfere with taking on new culture norms. With acculturation, one generally becomes attracted to another culture for various reasons and almost unintentionally learns to take on the lifeways of the new culture in dress, talk, and daily living. This person or family becomes acculturated to the new culture. For example, a Vietnamese family came as refugees to the United States and initially retained their own traditional values, but after 10 years had become acculturated and took on Anglo-American

lifeways. It is interesting that many acculturated Vietnamese families tend to retain their traditional religious beliefs and kinship values and seldom relinquish them for Anglo-American lifeways. Economics, education, and technologies are more readily accepted and taken on or adopted. Actually, few cultures become fully or 100% acculturated to another lifeway. Instead, cultures are *selective* in *what they choose to change and retain.* When many values and lifeways of a different culture are evident, they are usually acculturated. It is important that transcultural nurses assess individuals or families to determine *if* they are living by traditional or new cultural values for quality care outcomes.

4. *Socialization* differs slightly from the above concepts. It refers *to the social process whereby an individual or group from a particular culture learns how to function within the larger society (or country), that is to know how to interact appropriately with others and how to survive, work, and live in relative harmony within a society.* For example, when the Chinese and Japanese people first came to the United States, they were eager to learn how to become a citizen of the United States. They learned about becoming a United States citizen and how to buy goods, interact, and communicate with Americans and others in the American society. Other immigrants in many countries who want to remain in the society realize they need to be socialized into it. They often refer to this as "taking on the new ways" or "living in x society." Socialization is different from acculturation because the goal of socialization is to learn how to adapt to and function in a large society with its dominant values, ethos, or national lifeways. It is not necessarily becoming acculturated to a particular local culture or another culture. It requires becoming an acceptable member of the dominant and larger society.

5. *Assimilation refers to the way an individual or group from one culture very selectively and usually intentionally selects certain features of another culture without necessarily taking on many or all attributes of lifeways that would declare one to be acculturated.* It is fascinating to see how

individuals and families select or choose what they want or will accept of another culture. Assimilation is different from becoming fully acculturated or enculturated to another culture. With assimilation, the individual generally may be attracted to certain features, values, material goods or lifeways of a culture, but *does not adopt the total lifeways of another culture*. For example, a Navaho nurse liked the specific way that Anglo-American nurses fed newborn infants so she adopted these particular attributes to feed Navaho children. The Navaho nurse did not like the way Anglo-American nurses handled the Navaho mother's placenta and the umbilical cord after delivery, and she did not assimilate the total Anglo-American infant-care practices. The Navaho nurse knew what was acceptable and not acceptable to her people. This Navaho nurse encouraged American nurses to use the traditional Navaho infant cradleboard in maternal care while caring for Navaho women for several cultural reasons such as the infant feeling more secure in the cradle and the use of the cradle naturally fits in the mother's hogan (home). The Anglo-American nurse assimilated this practice into her nursing and found it helpful, but she did not adopt all the Navaho maternal-child traditional care practices. The five above concepts are important to understand to assess, interpret, and work effectively with different cultures.

Culture Care: A Central Construct with Related Concepts

It was in the early 1960s when I developed the construct of culture care to be used as central to transcultural nursing knowledge and practices. A construct has many ideas embedded in it, whereas a concept has a single idea. *Culture care has been defined as the cognitively learned and transmitted professional and indigenous folk values, beliefs, and patterned lifeways that are used to assist, facilitate, or enable another individual or group to maintain their well-being or health or to improve a human condition or lifeway.*[30] This construct is central to transcultural nursing and to the theory of culture care, which is discussed in the theory chapter with examples and uses in other chapters.

Culture care is focused on discovering and learning about the meanings, patterns, and uses of care within cultures. Identifying patterns of care and their uses provides data that are beneficial to clients. Culture and care are tightly linked together and interdependent. Both are needed to know and help people of specific or several cultures. From studying culture care has come subtypes such as *protective care* from several cultures. For example, American Gypsies value and use *protective care* for their daily survival to remain well and prevent illness. To this culture protective care refers to being very watchful of strangers or outsiders who could harm or be noncaring to Gypsies. It is the Gypsy males who are active in maintaining protective care. *Comfort care* is another major idea discovered in some cultures that is essential for healing and well-being. Many additional new discoveries have been made, such as *touching care, reassurance care, filial care*, and others, such as culture-specific holistic constructs. These constructs have many embedded ideas that can guide nursing decisions and serve as a new way to practice nursing.[31,32] (For further use of culture-specific care constructs, see Chapter 3 and the 1991 Theory book).

The idea of *culture-specific care/caring* comes from culture care but refers to *very specific or particular ways to have care fit client's needs*. I coined this term in the mid 1960s to help nurses focus on and provide care that fits the client's specific cultural needs and lifeways. To be culturally helpful to clients, care needed to be tailor-made and used in specific ways so that the client could experience benefits in meaningful and therapeutic ways, such as *protective care* being used and maintained with Gypsies or *touching care* with many Anglo-American children. Care could be almost as specific as a pill to cultures if fully known, valued, and applied to human beings in nursing care practices.

The construct of *generalized culture care* was also coined and developed at the same time as culture-specific care. It refers to *commonly shared professional nursing care techniques, principles, and practices that are beneficial to several clients as a general and essential human care need*. Generalized culture care can be used in several cultures, such as the construct of *respectful care* discovered in several cultures. Generalized care tends to be valued by many cultures as a more common or even a universal care need. The nurse considers both *culture specific* and *generalized culture* care in practicing nursing. The nursing goal is to provide *culturally congruent nursing care, which is defined as those assistive, supportive, facilitative or enabling acts or decisions that include culture care values, beliefs, and lifeways to provide meaningful, beneficial and satisfying care for the health and well-being of people, or for those facing death or disabilities.* Culturally congruent care remains the central focus and goal of the theory of culture care and a desired outcome of transcultural nursing practices.

Cultural care conflict is another essential construct to understand, which occurs when nurses work with mainly unknown cultures. *Culture care conflict refers to signs of distress, concern, and nonhelpful nursing care practices that fail to meet a client's cultural expectations, beliefs, values, and lifeways.* It is also closely related to *culture care clashes* except that with culture care clashes *obvious and known situations arise that are tense and cause overt problems.* Both client and nurse are usually fully aware of culture care clashes, but may be less so with culture care conflicts. In both situations, the client is usually uncooperative, emotionally upset, and dissatisfied with the care offered. Cultural clashes can be frequently observed in clinical and community settings between staff and clients from diverse cultures.[33] For example, a Korean client refused nursing care and became resistant, angry, and uncooperative because the nurse was taking his blood, which was strongly against his beliefs. It meant losing his distinct identity when the blood was taken. The client was very upset because the nurse did not understand the Korean's culture. Another example is a Vietnamese mother whose values clashed with the nurse's cultural etic professional values regarding the mother instantly breast-feeding her newborn. The mother refused to breast-feed as she held there was insufficient time for her "real and natural breast milk" to come into the breast. The mother knew she could not nurse the baby on "false milk." Some clients remain silent and use a "conspiracy of silence" to show their dislike for nursing or medical care when it clashes with their cultural values and beliefs. To prevent such potential cultural clashes, the nurse needs to know the culture and the mother's reasons for being noncompliant, tense, and resistive.

Still another example of both cultural clashes and conflicts occurred when the Arab-Muslim mother was told by the nurse in a large children's hospital that she could not remain with her child at night. The Arab mother's response clashed with the nurse when she said, "I must stay with my child while in the hospital." The nurse refused the mother's stay so the Arab-Muslim mother took her child home and did not return. In this incident, the child was acutely ill, but it was the Arab-Muslim mother's *cultural responsibility* and *obligation* to remain with her child day and night while in the hospital. The Arab mother clashed with the nurse and found her cultural values were much in conflict with nursing and hospital rules. Culture care holding knowledge about the Arab mother was essential but lacking with the hospital staff.

Two closely related but different concepts to understand are *cultural exports* and *cultural imports*. *Cultural exports refers to the sending of ideas, techniques, material goods, or symbolic referents to another culture with the intention they will be valued and used to improve lifeways or to advance practices.* Likewise, *cultural imports refers to taking in or receiving ideas, techniques, material goods, or other items with the position they can be useful or helpful in this culture.* These two concepts are found in transcultural and in other areas of nursing as nurses are exporting and importing many ideas between cultures today such as nursing ideas, clinical-practice modes, curricula, equipment, books and journals, and other items and ideas. Sometimes these exports and imports are useful, but sometimes less useful as they fail to fit the values, beliefs, or care practices of the culture and become troublesome or dysfunctional to the people. Far more thought is needed about what is exported and imported between nursing cultures for beneficial or desired uses and to prevent unethical practices.

Culture time is another major transcultural nursing concept to understand. It refers to *the dominant orientation of an individual or group to different past, present, and the future periods that guides one's thinking and actions.* Cultures generally have their own concept and meaning of time that tends to differ among cultures and often with the time orientation of health professionals. For example, Anglo-Americans, British, and Australians tend to focus on the immediate and exact present or future times; whereas, Africans, Hispanics, Latin Americans, and Southeast Asians tend to focus more on past and an extended present time so that noon may mean from 11 a.m. to 1 or 2 p.m. In the United States, African-Americans talk about "BCT" (black colored time). This means it is their own culture time, which is usually later than Anglo-American's precise clock time. This means African-Americans may be late for appointments and will gauge their activities within *their* time orientation and not the professional nurses' time. Since Anglo-Americans tend to live and function by nearly precise clock time for appointments made and kept, cultural conflict and stresses occur with those two cultures that fail to conform to clock time. Nurses, physicians, and others become quite annoyed with clients who are late or cancel appointments at the last minute. Vietnamese, Chinese, and Koreans especially value past traditional time periods when they talk to health professionals. However, as these cultures and other become acculturated, they soon learn how important Anglo-American and other Western-oriented time is to function, make money, and other gains. Business and employment agencies, as well as professionals, expect precise clock time to be maintained. Precise Western time functioning is associated with money gains (or losses), high productivity, product gains or outputs, and keeping products and people moving through systems. Hence, clients of a different time concept often become annoyed, frustrated, and upset with precise Western time expectations. It is one of the common sources of great tension and conflicts between nurse and client.

There is another kind of time, called *social time*, in several cultures. *Social time refers to time for leisurely interactions and activities in which exact time is of less importance. Cyclic time* may be used to refer to *when certain activities occur each day, night, month, or during the year, and cultures regulate their activities as a cyclic rhythm of life.* For example, the Gadsups of New Guinea live by cyclic times as they regulate their daily and nightly activities by cycles of doing and living. Most villagers have had no watches or clocks, and so they regulate their concept of time by garden activities, picking coffee, eating, and hunting, which are all regulated by the sun, day-night activities, and sequential rhythm of community activities. Transcultural nurses and other nurses need to learn about different time orientations to function with different cultures, or if studying them. Health personnel need to understand culture time and try to accommodate such time differences to reduce anger, frustration, and noncompliant

responses. Being aware of culture time orientations facilitates establishing and maintaining favorable and trusting relationships with individuals, families, and others of different cultures.

Cultural space is an important concept to understand in transcultural nursing. It refers to *the variation of cultures in the use of body, visual, territorial, and interpersonal distance to others.* An awareness of how cultures use space and expect others to recognize their territory is essential to prevent conflict, feuds, and violence. To violate the use of another's space can lead to interpersonal stress, anger, and a host of problems. Hall, an anthropologist, found that in Western cultures there were three primary space dimensions, namely, 1) the intimate zone—zero to eighteen inches; 2) the personal zone—eighteen inches to three feet; and 3) the social or public zone—three to six feet.[34] The use of personal space was also studied by Watson, who found that Canadians, Americans, and British require the most personal space, whereas, Japanese, Arab-Muslims, Latin Americans, and Africans use less personal space.[35] Africans seemed to tolerate crowding in public spaces, but Japanese like more open living spaces. Germans and Scandinavians like lots of personal and environmental space.[36] Other ideas about time and personal and public space are relevant to understanding and interacting with cultures in providing therapuetic care.

Body touching between and among cultures varies and is often gender and culture related. Arab, South Vietnamese, and Papua New Guinea men touch each other in public places more frequently than women. Non-Western, traditionally oriented women seldom touch men in public places, but are usually comfortable to touch appropriately and selectively social friends, relatives, and familiars in their homes and nonpublic settings. Westerners often touch friends and relatives in their own ways when they meet them. In some cultures gender touching may not be acceptable and may be viewed as homosexual behavior. However, in several non-Western cultures such as Indonesia, Africa, and New Guinea touching and holding hands is usually not interpreted or viewed as homosexual behavior. *Age grade companionship* with touching is found acceptable in Africa and other cultures. There is much to be learned about cultural space and personal and public touching in different cultures and as it relates to transcultural nursing. Body touching as human caring is largely culturally defined and valued as important modes of communication and human expression and for healing and well-being.[37] The therapeutic value of touching as healing is known and used by nurses, but few nurses know about cultures and specific outcomes that go beyond American and Western nursing views.

Cultural context refers to the *totality of shared meanings and life experiences in particular social, cultural, and physical environments that influence attitudes, thinking, and patterns of living.* Cultural context was first discussed in nursing by the author in a 1970 publication as an important concept for nurses to understand.[38] Today, understanding the meanings and responses associated with cultural context is extremely important. Cultural context that includes the cultural values, social structure, and environmental factors provides a holistic and totality view of the client within an environmental setting. It is the cultural context that gives meaning to understand situations and clients and as a powerful guide for nursing actions or decisions.

The concepts of *high and low cultural contexts* are essential in transcultural nursing. *High cultural context refers to people being deeply involved, knowing each other and the situation, and sharing and respecting values and beliefs almost instantly.* In contrast, *low context culture refers to people having less commonly shared meanings of life experiences or values, making it difficult to quickly understand strangers.* With low context there is a tendency to change or allow meanings and situations to be altered and to be explicitly stated. Hall, an anthropologist, introduced the idea of high and low cultural context.[39] In 1991 Wenger used these concepts with the Old Order Amish. She discovered the meanings and practices of high and low context meanings with the theory of Culture Care that gave valuable insights about the people.[40] Nurses need to understand high or low contexts in nursing for communication and to discover theory factors as shown in the Sunrise Model, such as environment, cultural values, family, education, worldview, politics, and other holistic factors. Nurses focusing primarily on diseases, physical symptoms, or individual behavior will miss valuable information about cultural context and totality data.

Cultural care therapy refers to qualified, transcultural nurses who offer assistive, supportive, and facilitative healing reflections and practices to individuals who have experienced cultural pain, hurts, insults, offenses, and other related concerns. The need for cultural care therapy has become important because of our intense and changing transcultural world. Clients, nursing students, practitioners, and families often need transcultural nurses who understand these needs and help clients regain their cultural well-being or health. The transcultural care therapist is a certified graduate (master and doctoral) professional nurse who is well prepared in transcultural nursing to help cultural clients. The therapist uses a *holistic approach* to assess and reflect with the client on the client's worldview, social structure, gender, employment, lifestyle patterns, and related factors influencing or causing cultural hurts, insults, or other concerns. Active participation of the client is important to achieve beneficial healing outcomes. Transcultural care therapy is a relatively new specialty that is growing in need and importance. It is not the same as psychiatric or mental health nursing as the knowledge and action base is holistic (beyond mind-body) and uses in-depth culture care knowledge and practices.

In this section, several important constructs and concepts have been presented as essential and relevant to transcultural nursing. In the past several decades a wealth of new and valuable culture care knowledge has been discovered such as comfort care, nurturant care, continuity care, and respectful care from specific cultures.[41] The reader is encourage to study these care constructs in this book and in other publications to appreciate the richness of culture care, which had not been discovered until transcultural nurse researchers and the field came into reality.[42,43]

Generic (Lay and Folk) and Professional Care/Caring

In developing the transcultural nursing field two very important ideas were developed to identify different kinds of care, namely, *generic care* and *professional nursing care,* which were based largely on *emic* and *etic* care discoveries. These terms are crucial to help nurses realize care with different sources, meanings,

Table 2.1 Cultural Informants' Views of Comparative Generic and Professional Care/Cure

Generic *(Emic)* Care/Cure	Professional *(Etic)* Care/Cure
• Humanistically oriented	• Scientifically oriented
• People based with practical and familiar referents	• Clients to be acted on with unfamiliar techniques and strangers
• Holistic and integrated approach with focus on social relationship, language, and lifeways	• Fragmented and nonintegrated services with focusing on physical body and mind
• Focus is largely on caring	• Focus is largely on curing, diagnosis, and treatments
• Largely nontechnological using folk remedies and personal relationships	• Largely technological with many diagnostic tests and scientific treatments
• Focuses on prevention of illnesses, disability, & maintaining lifeways	• Focuses on treating diseases, disabilities, and pathologies
• Uses *high*-context communication modes	• Uses *low*-context communication modes
• Relies on traditional and familiar folk caring and healing	• Relies on biophysical and emotional factors to be assessed and treated

and expressions to be used in people care. *Generic care (caring) refers to culturally learned and transmitted lay, indigenous (traditional), and largely emic folk knowledge and skills used by cultures.* In contrast, *professional (nursing) care (caring) refers to formally and cognitively learned etic knowledge and practice skills that have been taught and used by faculty and clinical services to provide professional care.* Generic care is derived originally and still today from *emic* or within the culture. Professional care is derived *etically* from largely outside specific cultures from professional and institutional sources. Both have been identified to provide assistive, supportive, and facilitative care for the health and well-being of people or to help people face death or disabilities.[44,45] During the past five decades, these two kinds of care have been studied by transcultural nurse researchers worldwide to discover new insights about human care of diverse cultures. The terms were coined and developed by the author to discover if differences and similarities exist among and between cultures from the viewpoint of the cultures—*emic* (insider's view) and *etic* (outsider's view). Generic or indigenous emic care had not been studied in-depth or used in nursing until transcultural nurses introduced the ideas in the 1960s. Professional nursing ideas and skills were mainly used but not generic care knowledge and practices. Accordingly, I predicted that such

differences in care could lead to different outcomes in quality of care rendered. With a focus on comparative generic (folk) and professional care, a wealth of new knowledge has been forthcoming with major contrasts with the two kinds of care. Table 2.1 presents some major differences between generic (emic) folk and professional (etic) data from cultural informants. These differences and many others presented in this book and in Chapter 5 are findings that merit urgent consideration by nurse professionals to provide culturally congruent, safe, and responsible care. Both generic (emic) and professional (etic) care need to be explicitly taught, further researched, and brought into care practices for the therapeutic healing and satisfying care of clients of diverse and similar cultures.

Transcultural Nursing Care Principles and Study Examples

In this next section some essential transcultural nursing principles are presented and followed with cultural study examples. It is important to remember that principles serve as reflective guides for transcultural nurses' thinking, decisions, and actions. These principles of transcultural nursing have become the "holding knowledge" to guide students, faculty, practitioners, administrators, and consultants in their thinking and deliberations with people of different cultures. So in studying each principle, think about the meanings and relevance as one cares for or about human beings who may be like or different from you or others and need to be respected and understood. It is these important principles that serve as a sound basis for guiding one toward beneficial nursing care practices or interactions. The following transcultural nursing care principles are guides to reflective thinking and lead to culturally congruent care.[46-49]

1. Human caring with a transcultural care focus is essential for the health, healing, and well-being of individuals, families, groups, and institutions.
2. Every culture has specific beliefs, values, and patterns of caring and healing that need to be discovered, understood, and used in the care of people of diverse or similar cultures.
3. Transcultural nursing knowledge and competencies are imperative to provide meaningful, congruent, safe, and beneficial health care practices.
4. It is a human right that cultures have their cultural care values, beliefs, and practices respected and thoughtfully incorporated into nursing and health services.
5. Culturally based care and health beliefs and health practices vary in Western and non-Western cultures and can change over time.
6. Comparative cultural care experiences, meanings, values, and patterns of culture care are fundamental sources of transcultural nursing knowledge to guide nursing decisions.
7. Generic (emic, folk, lay) and professional (etic) care knowledge and practices often have different knowledge and experience bases that need to be assessed and understood before using the information in client care.
8. Holistic and comprehensive knowledge in transcultural nursing necessitates understanding *emic* and *etic* perspectives related to worldview, language, ethnohistory, kinship, religion (spirituality), technologies, economic and political factors, and specific cultural values, beliefs, and practices bearing upon care, illness, and well-being.

9. Different modes of learning, living, and transmitting culture care and health through the lifecycle are major foci of transcultural nursing education, research, and practice.
10. Transcultural nursing necessitates an understanding of one's self, one's culture, and one's ways of entering a different culture and helping others.
11. Transcultural nursing theory, research, and practice is interested in both universals (or commonalities) and differences to generate new knowledge and to provide beneficial humanistic and scientific care practices.
12. Transcultural nursing actions or decisions are based largely on research care and health knowledge derived from in-depth study of cultures and the use of this knowledge in professional caring.
13. It is the culture care lifecycle patterns, values, and practices of cultures that are valuable means to help sustain or maintain the health and well-being of people, or deal with other human conditions.
14. Transcultural nursing necessitates coparticipation of client and nurse for effective transcultural decisions, practices and outcomes.
15. Transcultural nursing uses culture care theories to generate new knowledge and then to disseminate, use, and evaluate outcomes in practice.
16. Observations, participation, and reflection are essential modalities to discover and respond to clients of diverse and similar cultures with their care needs and expectations.
17. Verbal and nonverbal language with its meanings and symbols are important to know, understand, and arrive at culturally congruent and therapeutic care outcomes.
18. Transcultural nurses respect human rights and are alert to unethical practices, cultural taboos, and illegal cultural actions or decisions.
19. Understanding the cultural context of the client is essential to assess and respond appropriately to clients and their holistic health care needs and concerns.
20. Culture-care therapy may be needed for people who have been deeply hurt, insulted, or dehumanized because of cultural ignorance and noncaring modes.

Clinical Study Examples in Transcultural Nursing

In this section some reality nursing incidents between nurses and clients, or between nurses and other health personnel, are presented to gain fresh insights and reflect on the nature of transcultural nursing. You are also asked to consider specific concepts, constructs, and principles that have already been presented as situations and questions cited. These examples have been taken from real-life experiences, observations, stories, and recorded events in different cultures. As you read these transcultural study situations, you are asked to reflect on the following questions:

1. What do you think is occurring in this situation?
2. What transcultural nursing concepts, principles, and research findings would help the nurse respond to this incident in a culturally sensitive, responsible, and competent way?
3. What signs are evident that the nurse(s) and other health personnel failed to respond appropriately to this transcultural situation?
4. What would explain this situation from a transcultural nursing perspective?
5. What did you learn from these study examples that helped you value and understand transcultural nursing?

Clinical Example: Vietnamese Child

A Vietnamese child was hit by a car on the street and was brought to a general hospital emergency room. Six family members rushed into the emergency unit and hovered over the child's head. The Vietnamese elders quickly rushed to their child and placed a white cloth on his head. The family members cried loudly and were very upset. The emergency room nurses and physician were stunned with the extended family's behavior. They were baffled why so many family members came and why they persisted to be with the child and covering the child's head immediately. Unfortunately, the child died and the family members grieved very loudly and kept their hands on the child. The nurses and physician felt helpless and uncomfortable with the whole situation. Later a transcultural nurse specialist discussed the Vietnamese culture and the parents' behavior with the staff. Two major ideas were emphasized: 1) The extended family were expected to be present as an obligation and to cover the child's head with a white cloth because this is an important cultural belief and act. Covering the head is a sacred symbol and act with Vietnamese. 2) The white cloth was used to protect the spirits in the child's head, which are powerful and sacred forces affecting the child's and his well-being. Other cultural factors were discussed showing the need for "holding knowledge" to respond appropriately and to anticipate care to the Vietnamese child. How could this situation have been handled in a culturally congruent nursing way?

Clinical Example: African-American Woman

An African-American woman from a southern United States rural area was wearing a cord with knots around her abdomen when admitted for the delivery of her child. The delivery nurse said, "You need to remove this string as it is dirty and unnecessary." The nurse removed the cord without the client's consent and was putting it in a garbage container. The client, however, grabbed the cord and put it back on her abdomen saying, "I need this (cord) to have a safe delivery." After the mother was given the anesthesia, the nurse removed the knotted cord and destroyed it. Unfortunately, the infant died during the delivery, and the grieved woman attributed the death of her child to the fact that the nurse "took her cord and killed the child." When the woman left the hospital she was very upset and kept saying, "You killed my baby and destroyed my cord—I lost them both." The nursing staff did not understand why this dirty cord with knots was so important to this African woman. Staff cultural ignorance and hurtful actions were evident. How would a transcultural nurse have handled this situation to meet the mother's cultural and health needs?

Clinical Example: Chinese Man

A recent Chinese immigrant had major bladder surgery. He was told by the nursing staff to "force fluids." The client did not understand the "forced fluid" order. He refused to drink the glasses of cold water from the big pitcher left on his bedside table. Each time the nursing staff entered the client's room, they reminded him that he needed to force fluids and drink many glasses of water. They threatened that his physician would order intravenous fluids if he did not drink more water. He still refused to drink the cold water on his bedside. The staff said he was "uncooperative," "strange," and a "noncompliant" client. When the client's daughter came to see him she told the nursing staff that he would drink hot herbal tea but not cold water. Finally, the nurses gave him the hot tea and he drank several cups. The nurses did not understand why the hot tea was culturally acceptable and why he had refused to drink tap water. A transcultural nurse came to explain the clinical "hot and cold" theory of the Chinese and its importance in nursing care. What other cultural factors and principles in this nursing situation were evident that needed to be addressed?

Clinical Example: Navaho Mother

A Navaho mother gave birth to a baby girl in a large urban hospital. The nurses assisting with the delivery put the placenta and umbilical cord in a delivery pan and had the nursing assistant dispose of it. When the Navaho mother got ready to leave the hospital she asked for the placenta and umbilical cord. She learned that the nursing staff had destroyed it. The Navaho mother and her family were very upset and were shocked that the nursing staff did not understand the significance of the umbilical cord and that it should have been saved for the mother. To the nurses this woman's request was a very strange one as, "No other patients would want a bloody placenta and cord to take home, and no one had ever requested the placenta to take home." The Navaho mother and her kinsmen cried as they left the hospital and said, "We have no hope for our child. We must not return again to this hospital." What happened here and what concepts and principles were violated by nurses?

Clinical Example: Chinese, Italian, and Philippine Clients

An evening nurse was caring for traditionally oriented Chinese, Italian, and Philippine clients who had surgery that day. She observed that the Italian client frequently requested pain medication, which she gave to him. The Philippine and Chinese clients remained silent and asked for no pain medications. The nurse asked these clients if they were having pain and wanted the medication that the physician had ordered "per the request of the patient." The Chinese client, who had had major surgery, firmly refused the medication. The nurse "knew he had pain" and again offered him some pain medication. The Chinese client again refused pain medication and became angry saying, "I don't need anything." The nurse acknowledged his wishes. When the physician came, he noticed the client had received no pain medications. He ordered that these clients have a pain medication immediately. The Chinese and Philippine clients again firmly refused the physician's order. The latter said, "I don't take pain medicines as I know how to handle pain." The physician told the nurse to give a small dose to the client despite the client's protest, which she did. Interestingly, the Italian client who frequently called for pain medication never seemed relieved of pain. The Philippine client did not ask the nurse for pain medication, but he said to the nurse, "It is Bahala na (God's will) and I can bear the pain Jesus gives me." The nurse talked to the Philippine client and said, "I hear you, but God wants you to have some medication to ease your pain." The Philippine client finally but reluctantly accepted the nurse's expectation because nurses are "professionals with authority." The nurses did not understand why there were so many pain differences with the Italian, Philippine, and Chinese clients. Later, they learned that "God's will" and stoicism were some cultural values that guided the Philippine and Chinese clients' beliefs and decisions. The Italian client who cried for pain medication got medication immediately from the nurses. Cultural variabilities among the clients of different cultures were baffling to nurses on this critical care unit. None of the nurses had preparation in transcultural nursing and failed to provide culturally based care. What ethical and care principles were violated? Why did the physicians' pain orders not work with these cultures?

Clinical Example: Mexican-American Woman

A Mexican-American client had an appointment at 2:00 p.m. with a nurse and a physician for a "big lump in her abdomen and complaints of pain." At 2:00 p.m., the client did not appear at the office. The nurse and physician were upset and said, "If she comes, she will have to make another appointment as we cannot see her later or whenever she arrives." At 4:00 p.m., the client came to the office and was told, "You missed your appointment. We cannot take you and you will need to make another appointment." The client was upset as she attempted to explain that she could not find a relative to care for her three small children and she had to wait for someone to bring her to the clinic. She told how their car did not run well and was out of gas and that she had also lost the clinic address. These explanations did not seem to help the staff and she had to make another appointment. The client became upset and said, "I am in great pain and I hope I will still be alive if I return next time. I knew I should have gone to our local healer—they understand me." The physician appeared and gave the client a lecture saying. "Time is money for us, and you need to be on time." This Mexican-American client went home very upset and crying. She never returned to the clinic. What happened to this client and her concerns and needs? How might you have handled this situation using transcultural nursing principles and concepts?

Clinical Example: Fijian Man

A client from the Fiji Islands was admitted to an American hospital in Hawaii for diagnostic testing and a CAT scan. This Fijian man had never been in a large modern hospital nor in Hawaii. He was apprehensive about the many new things he and his family saw as they entered the city and the large public hospital. Nevertheless, he was urged to get the tests and CAT scan done quickly because of a possible brain tumor. As his extended family members remained in the waiting room, the client went into a room for tests without any family members with him. The family members in the waiting room were very anxious and requested to be with him. A hospital nurse told the family members, "It is against hospital rules for you to be with the client when the tests are given. We cannot change the rules for you." They were told to read the magazines on the table in the reception room. They were too anxious to read, and they also found the magazines were in English and not their language.

In the meantime, this client entered a room to have a CAT scan with two technologists and a nurse. They explained the machine to the client in scientific terms pointing to parts of the huge machine. However, the client was obviously anxious and his English was inadequate to share his feelings. He said, "It looks too big for me." He was told that the staff would put him inside the CAT scan and close the lid. Then they told him that they would "take slicing pictures or sections of different parts of your brain. The machine does everything. Just remain quiet and cooperate." The client was placed in the chamber, but he was terrified. He remained stoic and tried to show that he was a brave man with a fighting spirit, but inside he believed the machine would kill him. He envisioned that they would "slice" his brain and that it was a "death machine." After a few minutes, he called for his family members, but they were gone. The nurse kept saying to him, "It will take only a few more minutes, and you will be finished." The words did not satisfy him and he interpreted this to mean that he would soon be killed. He insisted on getting out of the machine. The "CAT scan" made him very worried, and it frightened him for a "cat" to have such power as it was a negative symbol in his culture. The whole experience was terrifying for him. He and the family left the hospital. He went back to Fiji and returned to his folk healers. Interestingly, he was apparently healed later by the local folk healers in his familiar environment and with his family present. He often tells others about his experience of going to a "strange country, a strange big city, and being with strange people who almost killed me." This is another example to show that transcultural understanding was urgently needed and especially with using a powerful and large high-tech machine. How would you have handled this situation?

Clinical Example: Arab Muslim Man

An Anglo-American senior baccalaureate nursing student was assigned to care for an acutely ill, dying client who had recently come from the Middle East. Unfortunately, the student had no courses or preparation in transcultural nursing, but was told by the head nurse to "care for a newly admitted client who spoke another language." When the student entered the client's room, she found eight people around the male client's bed. She asked all of the visitors to leave the room as she was to give "morning care to him." The visitors refused to leave the room and continued to talk to the client. The nursing student returned to the head nurse expressing her frustration as not being able to "get those visitors who speak a strange language to leave the room." The head nurse told her to return to the room and "to be firm." However, this time when she came into the room, the visitors had moved the bed so it faced an east window. The visitors, whom she realized later were close relatives, were praying loudly and calling for "Allah." The student became more upset and felt it was impossible to care for the client. She firmly told the relatives that, "This bed has to be returned to its proper place as it is a hospital regulation." One relative who spoke some English said, "It must be in this place to pray to Allah." The nursing student did not know who Allah was and tried to clarify this with the male relative, but she thought the explanation was strange. The student then returned to the head nurse and emphatically refused to give any care. She said, "It is impossible to give (him) care." Later in the day, the student learned that the client had died and that he was an Arab Muslim. This incident baffled her because the situation was so bizarre and the client with all the family was so different from Anglo-American clients she had cared for in the past. She felt so incompetent and unsuccessful in her nursing care. The "why" of the Arab Muslim behavior was never understood by the nurses and other Anglo-American health personnel. Later, when this critical incident was discussed in a transcultural nursing course, the student was so surprised about what had occurred with her and how she should have handled the situation. She said, "I did not understand this client and his culture." And to the faculty she said, "Why was I cheated in my nursing program without knowledge of these different cultures we are expected to care for in nursing?" The faculty explained they never had transcultural nursing and never thought students would need it today. This clinical incident makes students very eager to enroll in courses in transcultural nursing and to learn a new body of knowledge. Later this student became a transcultural nurse expert through graduate study, and nursing had some totally new meanings and goals for her.

Policy and Standard Statements to Guide Transcultural Nursing Practices

With the development of transcultural nursing as an important and legitimate professional discipline has come the need for policy statements and standards to guide transcultural nursing practices. Such statements serve several important functions.[50]

1. Serving as an explicit guide with standards to provide and evaluate quality-based transcultural nursing by educators, practitioners, consultants, and researchers
2. Providing some commonly shared policy and standard statements to maintain culture care competencies and beneficial transcultural nursing practices
3. Serving to provide standards to guide transcultural nursing decisions, actions, and practices
4. Providing some explicit philosophical position of values, beliefs, and standards held by transcultural nursing experts
5. Providing a policy document for use by public officials such as legislators, the public, and others interested in knowing and understanding transcultural nursing in relation to consumer care services.

Policy statements are *directive guides for action and decision making to maintain, protect, and ensure quality-based consumer services*. Webster's general definition is that policy refers to "a method of action selected to guide or determine present and future decisions."[51] *Standards* are criteria to *guide policies*. Transcultural nurses know that while cultures are relatively stable over time still they can change. Nonetheless, it is important to find some general guidelines to initiate and maintain standards and policies for safe, meaningful, and effective care practices. The statements offered here are some commonly shared and desired guides to generally support the common good or welfare of clients from diverse and similar cultures, as well as subcultures worldwide. They are offered to help nurses reflect on and arrive at culturally congruent and appropriate decisions and actions in the best interest and safety of human beings.

The following policy statements with implicit standards have been formulated from Leininger's extensive study and leadership work in transcultural nursing with many diverse cultures over the past 45 years and from other transcultural nursing experts with general endorsement by the Trustees of the Transcultural Nursing Society.[52] In addition, many participants in our preconference seminars at the annual meetings of the Transcultural Nursing Society have contributed to and shared their viewpoints as standards to uphold transcultural nursing practices.[53] These policies and standards support the phiiosophical and epistemics of transcultural nursing along with established concepts, principles, ethical considerations, and research theory–based knowledge and practices. It is important that the reader consider these policies as *directive guides* to establish, improve, maintain, protect, and evaluate practices related to culturally congruent, meaningful, and beneficial care of people of diverse or similar cultures. They have been formulated by the author with input from the Trustee document.[54]

1. Consumers of health care have a right to have their culture-care values, norms, and practices respected, understood, and used by nurses and other health care providers.
2. Immigrants, refugees, oppressed individuals and groups, the poor, the homeless, the vulnerable groups, "minorities" (under-represented groups), and subcultures have a right to have their cultural and general health care needs understood and responded to in ways that are meaningful, helpful, and congruent with their beliefs, values, and past-present life considerations.
3. Transcultural nursing needs to be grounded in *emic* (culture-centered) and *etic* (professional) humanistic and scientific research and theory-based knowledge to ensure culturally competent, congruent, safe and responsible care to cultures.
4. Transcultural philosophy and epistemic findings hold that care, health, illness, and dying are embedded in culture-care values, beliefs, and normative lifeways of cultures and subcultures, which are essential to know and explicitly used to guide transcultural nursing decisions and actions for beneficial outcomes.
5. Transcultural care *diversities* (differences) and *universalities* (commonalties) exist within and among cultures and necessitate that nurses discover their meanings and uses for culturally based care to guide nurses' decisions with clients and in different institutions, or in different contexts.

6. Effective and beneficial policies for consumers of diverse or similar cultures necessitates that policy makers are aware of their prejudices, biases, racial stance, and ethnocentric tendencies in providing respected and ethically sound policies and practices.
7. Transcultural nursing policies and standards require comprehensive knowledge of cultural consumers to prevent narrow and partial perspectives of culturally based people care.
8. Since transcultural care is culturally constituted and rooted in the peoples' generic (emic or, local, folk, indigenous, or insiders') knowledge and appropriate professional (etic) knowledge, it is imperative that effectively cultural policies reflect research-based data to attain culturally congruent care practices.
9. Ethical and moral transcultural knowledge, as well as human right principles, must be incorporated or given full consideration for culturally based health care policies.
10. Transcultural health care policies need to be supported by theoretical and research-based knowledge to sustain sound policy decisions and actions, especially for consultation practices.
11. Transcultural health care policies and standards need to consider the community and institutional context in which policies are used and evaluated over time.
12. The users of transcultural health and nursing care policies must be considered in light of those who are knowledgeable and skilled to use them with cultures.
13. National, regional, and local community hospitals, clinics, or other types of health care organizations should be grounded in transcultural or relevant anthropological insights to ensure sensitive, appropriate, effective, and culturally congruent health care practices.
14. Nursing faculty, administrators (academic and clinical), practitioners, researchers and consultants who use and evaluate transcultural policies and standards should be prepared in transcultural nursing to intelligently and wisely use them.
15. Transcultural nursing expert leadership and/or mentors are usually needed to guide government

officials, practitioners, academic and clinical administrators, faculty, researchers, consultants, minorities, and others who are unprepared in transcultural nursing or transculturalism.

16. Financial support is essential to initiate, maintain, and evaluate policy and standard outcomes.

◼ Summary

In this chapter a number of very important and fundamental transcultural nursing concepts, philosophical views, definitions, constructs, principles, clinical examples, standards and policies were presented with questions. The content in this chapter is essential to grasp the nature, scope, and important reasons why transcultural nursing was established and is needed today. Understanding the comparative nature of transcultural nursing and why nurses need to know and understand the differences between generic (emic) and professional (etic) care were discussed. The many real-life transcultural care examples should help the reader to identify transcultural situations and phenomena related to cultural conflicts, ignorance, blindness, cultural imposition, and other concepts and principles. The fascinating and unique history of transcultural nursing with the many reasons the discipline needed to come into nursing are crucial to understand the field. In the last section, specific transcultural nursing principles, study examples, and standard policy statements were presented as guides toward attaining and maintaining culturally competent and responsible care practices worldwide. In general, the content presented in this chapter is extremely important to understand the nature, goals, and purposes of transcultural nursing and as background for the rich information presented in subsequent chapters.

◼ References

1. Leininger, M., "Transcultural Nursing: A New and Scientific Subfield of Study in Nursing," in *Transcultural Nursing: Concepts, Theories and Practices,* M. Leininger, ed., New York, NY: John Wiley & Sons, 1978, pp. 8–12. (Reprinted Columbus, OH: Greyden Press, 1994.)

2. Leininger, M., *Transcultural Nursing: Concepts, Theories, Research and Practice,* Blacklick, OH: McGraw-Hill College Custom Series, 1995.

3. Leininger, M., *Caring: An Essential Human Need,* Thorofare, NJ: Charles B. Slack, 1981. (Reprinted Detroit: Wayne State University Press, 1991.)

4. Leininger, M., *Care: The Essence of Nursing and Health,* Detroit, MI: Wayne State University Press, 1988a. (Reprinted Detroit, MI: Wayne State University Press, 1990.)

5. Leininger, M., *Transcultural Nursing: Concepts, Theories and Practices,* New York, NY: John Wiley & Sons, 1978. (Reprinted Columbus, OH: Greyden Press, 1994.)

6. Leininger, M., "Care: A Central Focus of Nursing and Health Care Services," *Nursing and Health Care,* 1980, v. 1, no. 3, pp. 135–143.

7. Leininger, op. cit., 1995.

8. Leininger, op. cit., 1981.

9. Leininger, op. cit., 1988a.

10. Leininger, M., *Care Discovery and Uses in Clinical and Community Nursing,* Detroit: Wayne State Press, 1988b.

11. Gaut, D. and M. Leininger, *Caring: The Compassionate Healer,* New York, NY: New York Press, 1991.

12. Leininger, M., *Ethical and Moral Dimensions of Care,* Detroit: Wayne State University Press, 1990.

13. Leininger, M., *Culture Care Diversity and Universality: A Theory of Nursing,* New York, NY: National League for Nursing Press, 1991, p. 46.

14. Leininger, op. cit., 1995, pp. 9–10.

15. Leininger, op. cit., 1978, p. 491.

16. Ibid. p. 113.

17. Leininger, op. cit., 1995.

18. Ibid. p. 490.

19. Haviland, W., *Cultural Anthropology,* 7th ed., Orlando, FL: Harcourt Brace Jovanovich College Publishers, 1993, pp. 32–35.

20. Leininger, M., "Becoming Aware of Types of Health Practitioners and Cultural Impositions," *Journal of Transcultural Nursing,* 1991, v. 2, no. 2, pp. 32–39.

21. Leininger, M., "Understanding Cultural Pain for Improved Health Care," *Journal of Transcultural Nursing,* 1997, v. 9, no. 1, pp. 32–35.

22. Moore, L., P. Van Arsdale, J. Glittenberg, and R. Aldrich, *The Biocultural Bases of Health,* Prospect Heights, IL: Waveland Press, 1980.

23. Leininger, M., "Ecological Behavior Variability: Cognitive Images and Sociocultural Expressions in Two Gadsup Villages," Unpublished Document, Seattle, WA: University of Washington, 1996.

24. Leininger, op. cit., 1978.
25. Kottak, P., *Anthropology: The Exploration of Human Diversity*, New York, NY: McGraw-Hill Inc., 1991.
26. Leininger, M., *Culture Care Diversity and Universality: A Theory of Nursing*, New York: National League for Nursing Press, 1991.
27. Ibid.
28. Kottak, op. cit., 1991, p. 69.
29. Ibid.
30. Leininger, op. cit., 1991, p. 47.
31. Ibid. pp. 33–49.
32. Leininger, op. cit., 1988.
33. Leininger, M., "The Significance of Cultural Concepts in Nursing, "*Journal of Transcultural Nursing*, 1990, v. 2, no. 1, pp. 52–59.
34. Hall, E.T., *The Silent Language*. Westport, CT: Greenwood Press, 1996.
35. Watson, O.M., *Proxemic Behavior: A Cross-Cultural Study*, The Hague: Mouton de Gruyter, 1980.
36. Hall, op. cit., 1996.
37. Leininger, M., "Selected Care Findings of Diverse Cultures Using Culture Care Theory and Ethnomethods," in *Culture Care Diversity and Universality: A Theory of Nursing*, M. Leininger, ed., New York: National League for Nursing Press, 1991.
38. Leininger, M., *Nursing and Anthropology: Two Worlds to Blend*, New York, NY: John Wiley & Sons, 1970.
39. Hall, E.T., *Beyond Culture*, New York, NY: Anchor Press, 1976.
40. Wenger, A.F., "The Culture Care Theory and Old Order Amish," in *Culture Care Diversity and Universality: A Theory of Nursing*, M. Leininger, ed., New York: National League for Nursing Press, 1991, pp. 147–178.
41. Leininger, M., "Special Research Report: Dominant Cultural Care (emic) Meanings and Practice Findings from Leininger's Theory," *Journal of Transcultural Nursing*, 1998, v. 9, no. 2, pp. 45–49.
42. Leininger, op. cit., 1991, pp. 343–371, 359, 374, 376.
43. Leininger, op. cit., 1994, pp. 79–80.
44. Ibid.
45. Leininger, op. cit., 1991, p. 38.
46. Leininger, op. cit., 1995.
47. Andrews, M. and J. Boyle, *Transcultural Concepts in Nursing*, 2nd ed., Philadelphia: Lippincott, 1999.
48. Leininger, M., *Ethical and Moral Dimensions of Care*, Detroit, Wayne State University Press, 1990.
49. Leininger, M., op. cit., 1988.
50. Leininger, M., op. cit., 1995.
51. *Merriam-Webster Dictionary*, Springfield, MA: Merriam-Webster, Inc., 1994, p. 703.
52. Trustees of the Transcultural Nursing Society, "Policy Statements to Guide Transcultural Nursing Standards and Practices," *Journal of Transcultural Nursing*, 1998, v. 9, no. 2, pp. 75–77.
53. Horn, B. and M. Leininger, Preconference Seminars at Annual Transcultural Nursing Society Conferences, unpublished reports, Omaha, NE, 1988–1998.
54. Trustees of the Transcultural Nursing Society, op. cit., 1998, pp. 75–77 (also 2001 Certification Committee Standards).

PART I. The Theory of Culture Care and the Ethnonursing Research Method

Madeleine Leininger

Theories with appropriate research methods are the gateway to new or reaffirmed knowledge and practice. LEININGER, 1998

Theories and the use of appropriate research methods are creative ways to discover, explain, and interpret findings of largely unknown or vaguely known phenomena or human conditions. The discovery of new insights or the reaffirmation of knowledge about many life situations related to keeping people well or to relieving human suffering, illness, or other unfavorable conditions is highly important to nurses and other health care professionals. Theories are essential to guide and explain human discoveries, and so the Culture Care theory with the ethnonursing research method was developed with this goal in mind. In this chapter the theory of Culture Care and the ethnonursing research method will be presented in Part I, followed by selected research findings from the theory and method presented in Part II.

 ## Theory of Culture Care: Vision, Hurdles, and Creative Actions

During the past five decades, the theory of Culture Care Diversity and Universality has been developed to establish and advance the discipline of nursing and improve the quality of health care to cultures. The theory was one of the earliest nursing theories and the only theory focused explicitly on human care and cultural relationships. The theory was conceptualized as comprehensive, holistic, and different from traditional orientations of nursing. The identity, meaning, and expressions of care/caring in diverse cultures and subcultures needed to be discovered, explained, and understood for a multicultural world. Initially in the 1960s, the theory was slow to be recognized and valued because it was so "foreign and different" to many nurses. Gradually, the theory became meaningful and today is one of the most relevant and important theories to obtain knowledge and help nurses and others care for people of diverse cultures. Currently, the theory is in great demand and viewed by many nurses and practitioners as essential for quality health care and to help specific cultures receive meaningful care. Likewise the ethnonursing method is being used to discover some of the most covert and embedded culture and care phenomena.

In this first part, an overview with a brief history of the theory of Culture Care Diversity and Universality by the theorist is presented, which is followed by the ethnonursing research method and selected research findings from the theory. The first book on the theory, entitled *Culture Care Diversity and Universality: A Theory of Nursing*, was published in 1991 and remains the definitive theory.[1] However a few refinements, clarifications, and new ideas are presented here to update and reaffirm the theory. Most significantly, this book has twenty-four guest transcultural nurse experts who share their findings with the use of the theory, the ethnonursing research method, and ways to provide culturally based care to Western and non-Western cultures.

The reader is encouraged to read these chapters and other publications where the theory has been presented with the ethnonursing research method and findings. It is estimated there are over 600 publications today showing the use of the theory, the Sunrise Model, and scientific research findings. The *Journal of Transcultural Nursing* has some excellent refereed examples of using the theory that were conducted by transcultural nurse researchers and experts.

A Brief History on Developing the Theory

The initial idea to develop a nursing theory about human caring with a focus on cultural differences and similarities began in the late 1940s while caring for patients (as they were called in those early days) in a general hospital. This was before high technologies dominated hospitals and the workday of nurses' and physicians' time and activities. World War II had ended, but only a few technologies and medicines had entered the daily life of nurses. Nurses were expected to know and spend time caring for patients and families. As a consequence, I frequently heard patients say to nurses, "It is your nursing care that helped me get well"; "You took good care of me and now I am well"; "Your care was more helpful than the physician's quick drop-in to see me." These comments and others made me aware of the importance of human caring and healing. However, giving "good care or nursing care" was a cliché limitedly understood in terms of the mutual meaning to the patient and the nurse. Unquestionably, the term "care" was important in nurse-patient relationships, but care and caring had not been systematically studied, taught, or researched in the pre-1950 history of nursing. It was largely unknown but a linguistic cliché and practice goal. I found care was of great clinical and intellectual interest to me, but wondered why nurses used care and caring and failed to study and explain care with explicit meanings, uses, and documented evidence to patients and nurses in both the classroom and clinical areas. It became an even greater mystery to me while caring for people of diverse cultures, such as Italians, Jewish, German, Africans, and many others in the hospital and in homes. The care responses and needs of clients were different, but faculty, clinical staff, and nursing literature were of limited help to me and especially with cultures. Granted, I held care was important to human

beings, but the cultural care differences had not been studied nor available in the literature in the 1940s.

In the mid 1950s I experienced a great need to understand care phenomena and meanings while functioning as a graduate child psychiatric nurse in a child guidance residence in the midwestern United States.[2] As the first, clinical, child psychiatric nurse specialist and therapist, I was attempting to help children from several different cultures, namely, Appalachian, German, Jewish, and Euro-Americans.[3] I was baffled about *caring* for these children of different cultures who openly expressed differences in the way they wanted to be cared for during the day and night. I had received no educational preparation in my undergraduate and graduate programs about cultures. I was seriously handicapped to respond to these children's needs. This was a cultural shock as I was not able to help the children of different cultures. I soon took steps to remedy the situation by pursuing graduate (Ph.D) study in anthropology and doing field research study in a non-Western culture for nearly two years. This opened my eyes, ears, and desire to establish a new field I called transcultural nursing to remedy a critical and major need in nursing.

While studying culture and social anthropology, I remained focused on human care and its relevance to theory and transcultural nursing.[4,5] From the pre-1950 literature I found that the term "nursing care" was used by nurses, but care phenomena was not defined and explicated. Likewise, care with cultures was also not studied by anthropologists. Care was awaiting full study within nursing and transculturally. Indeed, care was a linguistic cliché in nursing with the meaning to nurses and clients with therapeutic practices and outcomes largely unknown in nursing textbooks and general usage. There were virtually no articles, research studies, or nursing courses explicitly focused on care or caring phenomena with different cultures.[6,7] It appeared to me that two of the most powerful constructs, namely *culture and care*, were missing in nursing theory and research and woefully neglected in clinical practices. I found no nursing research studies or theories focused explicitly on the relationship of culture to care. It was evident that both care and culture were taken for granted, were ignored, or were the invisible and unknown phenomena in nursing in the pre-1950s. There were nurses, however, who had encountered cultures, but had not studied them in systematic or scholarly ways. Interestingly, there were no graduate nurses prepared in graduate cultural and social anthropology courses or programs even though the discipline of anthropology was over 100 years old and had been available to nurses to study in universities. Nor were anthropology courses required or recommended in nursing curricula. Instead, many medical pathology, physical, chemistry, and psychology courses were major requirements in most nursing programs that reflected a strong medical and pathologic disease focus.

Recognizing these midcentury realities about culture and care as two potentially major and important domains to be fully studied and incorporated into nursing, I began to take steps to remedy the situation. I made bold proclamations that *care was the essence of nursing and a dominant, central, and unifying focus in nursing* that needed to be fully studied to explain and advance the discipline and profession of nursing.[8-10] Theoretical hunches were needed to explain and show the therapeutic benefits of care phenomena such as compassion, nurturance, protection, comfort, and other care expressions with their meanings and specific uses with cultures. I believed that humanistic care was *essential for human growth, survival, and health*, but varied between and within cultures.[11] The study and use of specific cultural care knowledge was much needed to prevent illnesses, promote healing, maintain health, and be of general help in recovery from illness. I also held that culture and care were *holistic* phenomena with powerful meanings within cultures. Culture and care also had *patterns* that had to be identified, used, and studied over time with cultures.

Culture was the learned, adaptive, shared ways of people with identifiable patterns, symbols, and material and nonmaterial data. Anthropologically, all human beings are born, live, and die within a culture. Culture had biological, physical, spiritual, and historical features for nurses to know and understand in health, illness, or other human conditions.[12] Theoretically, culture and care needed to be closely interfaced, synthesized, and brought into meaningful relationships for the new field of transcultural nursing. There were selected concepts that needed to bring figuratively two worlds together for transcultural care to occur. Bonding cultural and care as "culture care" I held that I could bring some entirely new insights and knowl-

edge into nursing to care for people of diverse cultures. I further predicted that the worldview, social structure, historical, language uses, and environmental factors could offer powerful explanatory knowledge to understand culture care phenomena. In addition, the arts, humanities, and other knowledge areas could offer meaningful care to cultures.[13] These broad, holistic, and yet specific knowledge areas were important for the new field of transcultural nursing and nursing in general.

The idea of discovering what is *universal* and *diverse* about human care worldwide also intrigued me as a sound basis to establish global, and ultimately transcultural, nursing practices. I predicted that such knowledge was imperative by the year 2020 or earlier for nurses to care for people of different cultures. The *universality of culture care* was based on the philosophical belief that all human beings needed care to survive, grow, get well, and be human. Care was a commonality among cultures. The *diversity of culture care* was based on the belief that human beings were born, raised, and showed differences or variabilities from universal or common care features. Nurses need to discover these individual and group differences and respond to such variabilities. Treating all cultures alike in care was of concern to me and could lead to nontherapeutic or destructive outcomes. I speculated that both *universal and diversity laws of culture care* could be established for the scientific and humanistic dimensions of transcultural nursing as the new field of nursing for the future.

Most importantly, I held that nursing theories and knowledge development must be greatly expanded and holistic from past and present local and Western views. Transculturally, there are many different ways of knowing that go beyond empirical, personal, aesthetic, or ethical nursing theories. Cultures influence and shape ways of knowing and explaining that may be religious (spiritual), materialistic, technological, experiential, and culture-value based theories. It remains the challenge for transcultural theorists and researchers to remain open to different ways of knowing and especially what is diverse or universal about culture care and other related knowledge areas. This was an essentially new theoretical, philosophical, and epistemic perspective to prepare transcultural nurses' need to discover Western and non-Western transcultural care knowledge.

Hurdles and Challenges Related to the Theory

Before the theory of Culture Care would be accepted and take on meaning within nursing and as a new discipline, however, there were several challenging hurdles that had to be faced. These hurdles are helpful to understand in developing this new field, using a different theory in nursing and different approach to nursing practice.

The *first* major hurdle to understand the theory of Culture Care was to help *nurses shift their thinking and mode of practice from being so wed to the medical model with physician expectations and medical treatment regimes* that was clearly evident in the 1960s and 1970s to an emphasis on *a discipline of nursing with human caring and transcultural caring knowledge and practices*. For in the post World War II period, nurses were deeply involved with medical ideas and performing medical tasks to treat and cure diseases. Many new treatments were brought into hospitals after the War, and nurses struggled to keep abreast of these new medical symptoms, treatments, procedures, and practices. Some creative nursing innovations and practices were evident, but there was limited time, money, and support to make them fully known and used. The study of caring phenomena of diverse cultures remained limitedly known, studied, and of interest to most nurses.

A *second* major hurdle to face was that *there were no formal, explicit, or specific nursing theories in the pre-1950s* except for a few conceptual notions. Peplau's philosophy supported her ideas of therapeutic nurse-patient relationships in psychiatric nursing.[14] This major contribution was not developed as a theory until the 1990s when I assisted a doctoral student with this effort. Nursing theories needed to be developed and valued to guide and advance nursing science and care practices. In the late 1950s, I encouraged nurses to hold nursing's first conferences on nursing science, which was a new challenge for many nurses as the word theory was generally viewed as "ivory tower stuff." Many nurses and physicians could not see the usefulness of nursing theories as nurses were "doers and practical" and were mainly expected to carry out physicians' orders in keeping with the old culture of nursing.[15] Physicians greatly feared that if nurses pursued academic study about theories and did research, they would lose their "handmaidens." So, developing and using theories in nursing was a major hurdle to deal with in developing and promoting my theory in the 1960s and 1970s.

Third, to establish the theory of Culture Care Diversity and Universality, another major hurdle was *to encourage nurses to study cultures and care phenomena to understand and use the theory appropriately*. Since there were very few professional nurses prepared in anthropology to study cultures, there was limited knowledge about cultures and the potential contribution of culture to nursing and caring. Courses in sociology and psychology had different focuses and seldom provided in-depth specific knowledge of cultures with anthropological theory-research perspectives. As the first Ph.D. graduate nurse prepared in cultural anthropology, I encourage many nurses to study anthropology as an excellent foundation to transcultural nursing. I wrote the first book, *Nursing and Anthropology: Two Worlds to Blend*, to show reciprocal potential contributions of anthropology to nursing and the reverse.[16] Gradually, several nurses began to take anthropology courses in the 1970s; these nurses were intrigued with culture. They needed to incorporate care into nursing. *Care was missing in anthropology as culture was in nursing*. A few nurses became leaders in education, research and clinical practices in transcultural nursing, but several remained in anthropology and were lost to nursing. In 1968 I launched the Committee on Nursing and Anthropology (CONA) to help nurse anthropologists bridge, critique, and build transcultural nursing perspectives as they dialogued with anthropologists.

The *fourth* major hurdle was *to establish undergraduate and graduate courses to prepare nurses in transcultural nursing theory*. Graduate courses and programs were much needed to prepare nurses as competent teachers, researchers, and clinicians in transcultural nursing. Still today, it is a major challenge to establish courses and programs in transcultural nursing within different university schools of nursing. Almost single-handedly I established four programs in transcultural nursing and many courses with field experiences so nurses were prepared in the new discipline. By the mid 1980s, transcultural nursing courses and programs had been established in several universities with a research-theory focus. Gradually, the Culture Care theory began to be meaningful and used as a guide for transcultural nursing research, teaching, assessments, and patient care. Through academic study nurses soon realized the importance of transcultural nursing in caring for many recent immigrants, refugees, and cultural strangers who were seeking health care from nurses. Indeed, community nurses were often working directly with new immigrants from Vietnam, Southeast Asia, and other countries. They urgently needed transcultural concepts, principles, and theoretical ideas to help them. The need for transcultural nursing education and practices far exceeded the limited financial and personal resources for nurse preparation and practice. As a consequence, cultural clashes, conflicts, racism, and other unfavorable practices became evident in health care settings where there were no formal educational preparation and faculty in transcultural nursing. In England, Africa, Europe, and other places the need was clearly evident in client care services. In the United States, the birthplace of transcultural nursing in the 1950s, some schools of nursing slowly began to value transcultural nursing so that by the 1990s several graduate and undergraduate courses and programs were established. A major hurdle, however, remained with the critical need for prepared faculty and more academic courses in transcultural nursing to teach and guide students.

A *fifth* major hurdle was *getting nurses to value and practice human care and caring and from a transcultural focus in educational programs and in practices.* There were many nurses who had difficulty accepting care and caring as the essence and central focus of nursing and transcultural nursing.[17,18] There were United States nursing leaders who strongly objected to human care as the essence of nursing as they held that care was "too feminine," "too soft," and would "never be acceptable to consumers, nurses, and physicians as it had limited relevance and could not be studied and measured." Instead, these United States nurse leaders began to promote *health, nursing, person, and environment* as the major foci of nursing and the central concepts of the metaparadigm of nursing.[19] Still today, in some schools these four concepts are used, taught, and written about with care and culture blatantly absent. Gradually, care has gained use by nursing students and worldwide nursing literature. This change was largely brought on by a small group of nurse scholars that I encouraged and spearheaded to focus on care phenomena in 1978. This Conference Care group later became the International Association of Human Caring. These care scholars

such as Gaut, Ray, Bevis, Watson, Horn, Leininger, and others studied and demonstrated the importance and therapeutic values of humanistic and scientific care in healing and well-being.[20–24] Nurses from the Transcultural Nursing Society also became very active studying care with a transcultural nursing focus.[25] Care as the essence of nursing is gradually changing nurses' views to value care within a transcultural perspective.

Transcultural knowledge has shown that some cultures do not focus on the person but focus on family or groups. For example, Eastern and Latin American cultures value and focus on families, groups and communities as central to their caring lifeways and beliefs. Moreover, one cannot declare nursing as central to nursing as it is unacceptable to use the same term to explain nursing. The concept of care in my theory of Culture Care showed the power and relevance of care in nursing when known and studied with a culture care perspective. Thus the four earlier metaparadigm concepts were questioned, but some nurses and schools still hold to them because of lack of transcultural knowledge about care and cultures. Most encouraging, and through persistent education in transcultural nursing, culture and care are today being valued more and studied in teaching, research, and in several clinical practices. This major change from 1965 until 2001 has occurred with transcultural nursing care being the major focus that is now known and used in nursing. It is as if care "has always been there" by some nurses who were unaware of the great difficulties to bring care into transcultural nursing and as a major focus of nursing in early years.

A *sixth* major hurdle, before the theory of Culture Care and transcultural nursing could be understood, valued, and studied, was related to the fact that nurse scholars prior to 1965 were relying *heavily on quantitative research methods as the only means for "scientific knowledge" and methods acceptable to science, medicine, and nursing as a discipline.* Diverse qualitative research methods had been limitedly studied, known, and used in nursing in the pre-1970s except for few descriptive narratives and surveys. While in doctoral study, I learned about diverse qualitative methods in anthropology, philosophy, and the humanities. I learned about ethnographic and ethnological qualitative methods and did the first studies in nursing with these methods in the early 1960s in a non-Western culture.[26] I also developed and used a new method I called *ethnonursing*, which was designed to focus explicitly on transcultural and related nursing phenomena. I used this method with the Culture Care theory in the 1960s in studying the New Guineans in the Eastern Highlands. This was the first nursing research method developed in nursing.[27] After teaching and conducting qualitative research studies with many nursing students for 15 years, I published the *first nursing research book in 1985*, entitled *Qualitative Research Methods in Nursing*.[28] These steps were major hurdles to help nurses discover embedded and complex care and culture phenomena in different contexts as quantitative methods were inadequate to tease out enormously rich, valuable, and largely unknown data for nursing and for the new body of transcultural nursing knowledge. I encouraged nurses, through my teaching and research, to use and value qualitative research and especially the research on the ethnonursing method with "enablers" where the method and the theory systematically fit with each other to get meaningful and accurate data. Cultural informants liked this ethnonursing research method, and nurses saw new hope as they had been borrowing methods, models, theories, and instruments from non-nursing fields that often failed to discover full meanings and explain nursing phenomena. Gradually, diverse qualitative research methods took hold in schools of nursing in the United States by the mid 1980s along with the ethnonursing method. There are some nurse anthropologists who still remain wed to ethnography and are not using the ethnonursing and other promising qualitative methods. Valuing and learning to use qualitative methods was a major change in nursing and worldwide. These methods are generating some entirely new scientific discoveries about nursing, but especially in transcultural nursing that go beyond empiricism. The culture of nursing often is reluctant to use entirely new methods and different ways to know and establish a new order of functioning such as using the ethnonursing method and transcultural nursing. These historical hurdles are important to realize and appreciate as transcultural nursing was developed, taught, and shaped into a new world of nursing and people care.

Purpose and Goal of the Theory

The central purpose of the theory of Culture Care was to discover, document, interpret, explain, and even predict some of the multiple factors influencing care from an *emic* (inside the culture) and an *etic* (outside the culture) view as related to culturally based care. With the ethnonursing research method and theory, the researcher was challenged to discover the similarities and diversities about human care in different cultures. The theory was predicted to help guide the nurse researcher to discover new meanings, patterns, expressions, and practices related to culture care that influenced the health and well-being of cultures or to assist them to face death or disabilities. Ultimately, the goal was to establish a body of transcultural nursing knowledge for current practices and for future generations of nurses in a global world.[29]

The goal of the theory was stated to provide *culturally congruent care* that would contribute to the health or well-being of people or to help them face disabilities, dying, or death using the three proposed modes of nursing care actions and decisions.[30] In the discovery process, both similarities (commonalities) and diversities (differences) would be identified with specific modalities to provide culturally congruent care related to the desired goal of health or well-being. The term culturally congruent care was first coined by me in the 1960s as the goal of the theory of Culture Care, which is now used but not always recognized by others as coming from me.

Philosophical Beliefs, Assumptions, and Hunches with the Culture Care Theory

In developing the theory, several philosophical ideas, assumptions, and beliefs are important to state. Philosophically, I believed that human beings were essentially good with caring attributes as created by God. I believed that diverse cultures were created for a purpose, but our challenge as nurses is to discover, respect, understand, and help cultures as needed with a caring ethos and with other health professionals. Philosophically, I held that the nursing profession had a moral and ethical responsibility to discover, know, and use culturally based caring modalities as one of our unique and distinct contributions to humanity. Our transcultural nursing challenge was to ultimately discover worldwide, comparative, culture care phenomena using the theory to develop humanistic and scientific culture care knowledge for practice.

Research findings from the theory were predicted to support a body of transcultural nursing research knowledge for the discipline of transcultural nursing. The theory findings would provide epistemic data for providing meaningful and appropriate decisions and actions for culturally congruent, safe, and responsible care to people of diverse cultures. Through current and future studies of many cultures in the world over an extended period of years, ultimately, there would be an identifiable body of *universal* and *diversity* knowledge that nurses would know and could be used among nurses worldwide. Such fundamental scientific and humanistic discipline knowledge would offer different ways of knowing and practicing nursing. It would go beyond current empirical and physical evidence-based knowledge to new kinds of therapeutic practices. Focusing on culturally based care was an ambitious and futuristic goal for a distinct, unique, and unifying hallmark of nursing and transcultural nursing. Traditional nursing needed to shift to global transcultural nursing in the immediate future to serve people in meaningful ways. Nurses needed to be grounded in transcultural nursing and not just have a unicultural focus. This philosophical stance was a very futuristic and visionary idea in the 1950s for nurses to function in a global world. More importantly and philosophically, nurses needed to greatly expand their worldview and to know how to care for many different cultures worldwide. Nursing was far too local, national, and parochial in the midcentury and needed a theory to expand its research, knowledge, and practice focus. The Culture Care theory was developed to remedy this concern.

To reach these philosophical ideals and practical goals, nurses had to expand their worldview to a multicultural one for studying immigrants, minorities, poor, wealthy, oppressed, homeless, disabled, and many more cultures and subcultures. To do this, nurse leaders needed to be prepared in transcultural nursing through substantive and rigorous graduate programs. They needed to demonstrate competencies to function with individuals, extended families, groups, clans, subcultures (elderly, drug abusers, etc.), communities, and in institutions with diverse cultures. Nurses in the mid 20th century needed a breadth and depth of transcul-

tural nursing knowledge to guide and substantiate their actions and decisions. However, shifting nurses from the medical model of mastering medical symptoms, diagnoses, and treatment of pathological diseases to a transcultural holistic caring profession focused on care maintenance, wellness, and prevention of illness was a major hurdle and challenge. Teaching nurses how cultures have prevented illnesses and maintained holistic healthy lifeways over time and intergenerationally was difficult and complex. At the same time, nurses would use relevant and appropriate knowledge from nursing, medicine, anthropology, the humanities, and other fields that might be appropriately incorporated into transcultural nursing caring practices.

Anthropologically, I had learned from my field studies that Western diseases and illnesses were often very different from non-Western cultures, and so a comparative knowledge base was essential in transcultural nursing. From my clinical professional nursing experiences, I believed that consumers of diverse cultures needed and expected nurses to be respectful, compassionate, and humanistic in their caring practices. How to redirect nurses into a caring ethos with different cultures in culture-specific ways would be essential in transcultural nursing, and the theory should guide this discovery. Moreover, I was concerned that nurses were fast becoming technologists and masters of sundry tasks with limited caring practices. Discovering and developing culturally based caring knowledge and competencies related to care phenomena such as respect, comfort, being present, offering protection, reassurance, compassion, and many other caring modalities needed to be rigorously studied in-depth with cultures under transcultural nurse mentors. Establishing ways to fit caring with the client's cultural values, beliefs, and expectations was needed. Cultural caring constructs should become valued as linked to cultures and benefits. There was also the continued challenge to change nurses' image from "technicians," "extensions of the physician," "mini docs," "physician's handmaidens," and "shot givers" to sensitive and competent transcultural caring nurses who could make therapeutic caring decisions for people of diverse and similar cultures. All of these philosophical beliefs, goals, hunches, and patterns of thinking and planning led me to the theoretical tenets and assumptions of the theory of Culture Care Diversity and Universality.

Theoretical Tenets and Specific Hunches

In conceptualizing the theory, the *first* major and central theoretical tenet was that *care diversities (differences) and universalities (commonalties) existed among and between cultures in the world*; however, their meanings and uses had to be discovered to establish a body of transcultural nursing knowledge.[31] It was predicted that diverse and similar care concepts, forms, meanings, expressions, and patterns existed with cultures, but were largely unknown to nurses and others. The discovery of this wealth of potentially rich knowledge would guide and provide new knowledge for nurses and better care to cultures.

A *second* major theoretical tenet was that the *worldview, social structure factors such as religion, economics, education, technology, politics, kinship (social), ethnohistory, environment, language, and generic and professional care factors would greatly influence cultural care meanings, expressions, and patterns in different cultures*. These factors also needed to be discovered for holistic and meaningful care to people as these dimensions had been woefully missing in nursing assessments, theories, and care practices. They were predicted to be powerful influencers to know and understand culturally based care for individuals, families, and groups and to function in health institutions. Moreover, these dimensional factors needed to be discovered *directly* with cultural informants from emic data as influencing (not casual) factors related to the health, well-being, illness, and death. Discovery of these dimensions with *generic* (folk, lay and naturalistic) *care* was predicted to be different from *professional care* practices in which the latter could lead to cultural clashes, racism, cultural imposition, and other nontherapeutic outcomes. Generic care was limitedly known in nursing and, if known, was not used in culture-specific ways. Cultural conflicts and gaps between professional and generic care were predicted to be of major concern for therapeutic culturally congruent care.

The *third* major theoretical tenet conceptualized and incorporated within the theory were the *three major care actions and decisions to arrive at culturally congruent care for the general health and well-being of clients or to help them face death or disabilities*. These three theoretical practice modes that had to be discovered with clients (informants) and used in care were as follows: 1) *culture care preservation and/or maintenance*, 2) *culture care accommodation and/or negotiation*, and 3) *culture care restructuring and/or repatterning*.[32] To arrive at these appropriate modes in client care, the researcher draws on findings that had been generated from social structure, generic and professional practices, and other influencing factors while studying culturally based care for individuals, families, and groups. Then the researcher with cultural informants (or in assessment care practices) discusses the best ways to provide *culturally congruent and beneficial care modalities*. The three modes might all be used, but maybe only one modality is used. The transcultural nurse researcher creatively identifies with clients (as coparticipants in decision making) the most appropriate, beneficial, safe, and meaningful ways that fit the client's (family) values, beliefs, and lifeways. These three theoretical modalities were a highly creative and new way for nurses to give care and to shift from symptom, disease, and medical treatment management modalities to culturally based caring. Thus the Culture Care theory had both an abstract intellectual discovery focus and a focus on discovering daily and nightly living ways of cultures. Obtaining grounded culturally based data was a powerful guide for the three modes. Already, the research findings from the three modes of action and decision have been extremely beneficial to clients of diverse or similar cultures to meet their specific needs, values, and expectations in professionally responsible and safe ways. The three transcultural care actions are viewed by many nurses as "refreshingly different" from present-day nursing practices. They are a valuable means to incorporate holistic culture-care findings with specific care needs that fit the client's culture and are often not included in symptom management practices. The three modes of action and decision, however, require highly creative thinking and explicit use of both *emic* and *etic* findings derived from the culture. Dominant culture-care constructs such as "being present," "protective care," "filial care," and many others become major foci to guide care practices using appropriate knowledge sources. Again, carefully selected medical, nursing, and other knowledge sources as genetics and humanities may be used only if appropriate and safe. The reader is encouraged to study care constructs already discovered and discussed in this book and others with specific cultures.[33]

In conceptualizing the theory, the Sunrise Model was developed to guide nurses like a visual and cognitive map to remain sensitive to multiple factors influencing culture care outcomes. The Sunrise Model is *not* the theory per se but a guide or enabler to consider multiple factors related to the major theoretical tenets to be studied and to the theory premises. After four decades, the Sunrise Model has been heralded by many nurses as most helpful in discovering holistic and particularistic aspects bearing on human care in diverse cultures. The Sunrise Model will be explained shortly.

Assumptive Premises of the Theory

Several assumptive theoretical premises (like givens) were formulated to support the theorist's position, tenets, and hunches. They are the following:[34,35]

1. Care is the essence of nursing and a distinct, dominant, central, and unifying focus.
2. Culturally based care (caring) is essential for well-being, health, growth, and survival and to face handicaps or death.
3. Culturally based care is the most comprehensive and holistic means to know, explain, interpret, and predict nursing care phenomena and to guide nursing decisions and actions.
4. Transcultural nursing is a humanistic and scientific care discipline and profession with the central purpose to serve individuals, groups, communities, societies, and institutions.
5. Culturally based caring is essential to curing and healing, for there can be no curing without caring, but caring can exist without curing.
6. Culture-care concepts, meanings, expressions, patterns, processes, and structural forms of care vary transculturally with diversities (differences) and some universalities (commonalities).
7. Every human culture has generic (lay, folk, or indigenous) care knowledge and practices and usually professional care knowledge and practices, which vary transculturally and individually.
8. Culture-care values, beliefs, and practices are influenced by and tend to be embedded in the worldview, language, philosophy, religion (and spirituality), kinship, social, political, legal, educational, economic, technological, ethnohistorical, and environmental context of cultures.
9. Beneficial, healthy, and satisfying culturally based care influences the health and well-being of individuals, families, groups, and communities within their environmental context.
10. Culturally congruent and beneficial nursing care can only occur when care values, expressions, or patterns are known and used explicitly for appropriate, safe, and meaningful care.
11. Culture-care differences and similarities exist between professional and client-generic care in human cultures worldwide.
12. Cultural conflicts, cultural imposition practices, cultural stresses, and cultural pain reflect the lack of culture-care knowledge to provide culturally congruent, responsible, safe, and sensitive care.
13. The ethnonursing qualitative research method provides an important means to accurately discover and interpret *emic* and *etic* embedded, complex, and diverse culture-care data.

The *universality of care* reveals the common nature of human beings and humanity, whereas *diversity of care* reveals the variability and selected, unique features of human beings.

■ Sunrise Model: A Conceptual Research Enabler

The Sunrise Model (Fig. 3.1) was developed as a conceptual holistic research guide or enabler to tease out the multiple theoretical factors.[36] The Model shows different factors or components that need to be systematically studied with the theory. It serves as a cognitive guide to tease out culture care phenomena from a holistic perspective of multiple factors that can potentially influence care and the well-being of people. Again, the model is not the theory *per se*, but depicts factors that need to be studied in relation to the theory tenets and the specific domain of inquiry under study. The model is different from Fawcett's (1989) and other nurse theorists' concepts of models as it serves different purposes within the qualitative paradigm and the Culture Care Theory and the method.[37] Misunderstandings and inaccurate perceptions and analysis statements on this

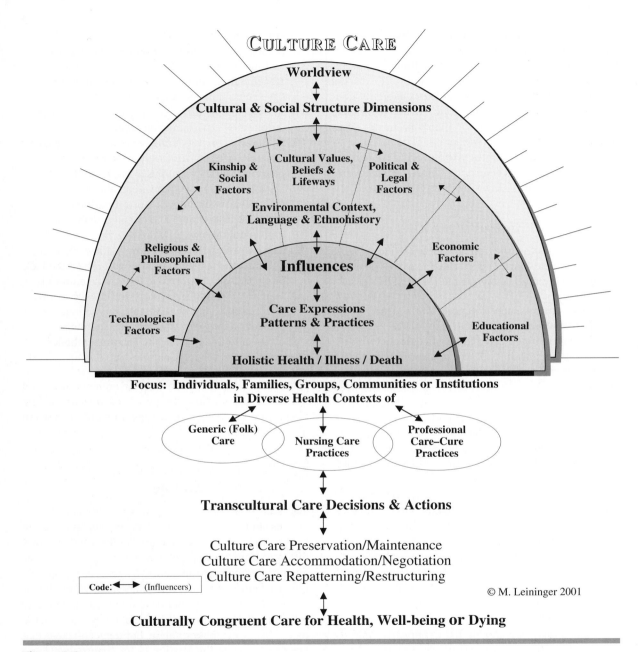

Figure 3.1
Leininger's Sunrise Model to depict the Theory of Cultural Care Diversity and Universality.

theory require critique for accurate use of the theory as with Bruni, Fawcett, and others.[38] It is important to always use the theorists' definitive statements and philosophical focus.

The Sunrise Model had some minor revisions from 1955 to 1985 to refine it in relation to the theory and the multiple holistic factors that could influence culture care. The model shows potential influencers (not causes) that might explain care phenomena related to historical, cultural, social structure, worldview, environmental, and other factors. It is important to understand that gender, age, class, race, historical, and other features are usually embedded or related to social structure factors such as religion, kinship, politics, and economics; cultural values are found linked to sex, age, etc. For example, gender, age, and race data are generally *embedded* in family ties, politics, and specific cultural norms and practices. In some families caring decisions and certain actions are related to male and female roles and often over generations. Likewise, biophysical, emotional, genetic, medical, nursing, and other factors may bear on generic and professional health or illness care. Hence, gender, class, age, and race factors are found in their natural cultural places and have to be discovered by the researcher in their familiar or natural cultural contexts.

In using the theory of Culture Care, nurses benefit from a broad, liberal-arts university preparation to identify and understand holistic dimensions such as social structure factors, ethnohistory, genetics, religion, spiritually, ethics, language uses, environment, politics, family structures, arts, and other ideas reflected in the Sunrise Model, *all as influencers or potential influencers of human care*. With the Sunrise Model, a truly holistic and comprehensive picture can be discovered to reflect the totality of knowing people in their lifeworld or culture.

As researchers use the Model, they will discover many hidden, obvious, and unexpected factors influencing care meanings, patterns, symbols, and practices in different cultures. "*Let the sun shine and rise*" figuratively means to have nurses open their minds to informants to discover many different factors influencing care in their culture with their meanings and the ways they influence the health and well-being of people. The Sunrise Model greatly expands the worldview and minds of researchers to look for obvious or covert embedded knowledge to obtain an accurate and comprehensive picture of influencers on care, health, illness, and dying or disabilities in cultures and goes beyond traditional mind-body-spirit holism views.

How to Use the Sunrise Model

As researchers use the Sunrise Model, they make choices about whether they will be studying stated individuals, groups, families, communities, or institutions in relation to culture care and their domain of inquiry. For newcomers to the theory, it is wise to begin with individuals and then gradually master studying families, groups, communities, and institutions, which are more complex. The researcher needs to remain focused on the theory tenets and the domain of inquiry under study (the latter varies with each researcher). One can begin the discovery process with the theory in the upper or lower part of the Sunrise Model according to the researcher's interests, knowledge, and competencies and the informant's interests. Some researchers are more comfortable focusing first on professional and generic care; whereas researchers prepared in graduate transcultural nursing programs and in anthropology often want to focus initially on the worldview, social structure factors, and other areas in the upper part of the Model. There is, however, *no set or rigid approach where one begins in using the Model*, for flexibility and choice is offered. However, the researcher is expected to explore generally *all dimensions or components in the Model* with the particular domain being studied to obtain a holistic, comprehensive, and accurate database. The researcher keeps in mind all aspects depicted in the Model, including generic and professional care and the three potential modes of action and decision. For example, a researcher may study a *domain of inquiry* (DOI) such as *Culture Care of Greek Mothers and Infants in the Hospital* and may wish to start with the kinship and cultural values and then focus later on the professional and generic care patterns in relation to the Greek history and environmental context. Cultural informants often have their interests of what they want to talk about first and last, and so the researcher tries to move with the informants' interests and comfortableness as much as possible to get in-depth data.

As the researcher probes for care meanings, beliefs, values, and practices in relation to social structure, environment, and other factors with the informants, one remains alert to the different areas in the model and thinks of the commonalties among informants whether studying individuals, families, or groups. For example, studying the religious and care beliefs of Arab Muslims generally requires a focus on their religious beliefs and cultural value lifeways of the family or group to discover their culture care. The researcher gently teases out religious data and remains cognizant to age, gender, and change factors influencing care. Physical, emotional, and other related knowledge that the informants share are important with their specific meanings and expressions, and suggested action care patterns are important. Generally, a full picture of the life of individuals (or family) becomes apparent if one remains genuinely interested and patient with informants while using the Sunrise Enabler.

At all times the researcher is careful to withhold any judgments and one's professional nursing etic knowledge, but instead focuses on discovering emic knowledge from informants. Teasing out embedded or concealed care practices with the client's meanings requires active listening, patience, and confirming what one hears and sees. Listening to how care is linked with and explained with kinship, religion, economics, politics, cultural values and beliefs, and other general factors in the Sunrise Model are essential to discover. Clients like to tell their story and are often pleased the nurse remains interested in their world of telling and knowing. Discovered meanings and practices about care are usually embedded or tucked into the social structure factors, cultural beliefs, language, and environment. This is why care phenomena has been limitedly known from clients, as it requires an in-depth and broad discovery of the client's world and experiences, including generic home care and what has influenced their care practices. Care practice discoveries such as protective care, supportive care, care as presence, care as respect, and care as family love have been identified using the theory and Sunrise Model.[39] Obtaining informants' *emic* knowledge first is important before reflecting on *etic* professional knowledge. Carefully and sensitive teasing out care meanings, expressions, and practices from informants with the Sunrise Model is generally most informative and rewarding to the researcher and informants.

As one continues with the use of the Sunrise Model, the researcher or assessor focuses on the three theoretical modes of culture-care actions and decisions that might be appropriate, congruent, satisfying, safe, and beneficial to people being studied or assessed. Since the theory has both abstract and practical features, the nurse needs to consider professional nursing knowledge with generic data. There is, however, a purposeful *built-in action* means to identify and confirm data with informants related to the three modes in order that congruent and meaningful nursing actions and decisions are identified. The three nursing modes of action or decision that the nurse researcher examines in the Model with informants are as follows: 1) *culture care preservation/maintenance*; 2) *culture care accomodation/negotiations*; and 3) *culture care repatterning/restructuring*.[40] The researcher and the informant can decide together appropriate care actions and decisions, which often leads to accepting the care offered. These modes, whether one or all, need to reasonably fit with informants' cultural lifeways and may need to include some beneficial professional suggestions that may be of benefit to the client(s). Again, the care action and decision data come from data obtained from the upper and lower parts of the Sunrise Model, all providing a wealth of rich and meaningful data to guide certain care actions and decisions. A coparticipant involvement approach is used with informants so that the client and professional use their knowledge and desires for culturally congruent care with the specific three action modes.

In general, the Sunrise Model is an invaluable guide to discover new knowledge or to confirm knowledge of cultural informants. Often nurses say, "The Sunrise Model became imprinted on my mind to alert me to many factors that had never explored been in nursing"; "The Model really helped me to get a holistic view of cultures and not just nursing diagnoses, symptoms, diseases, and medical views"; "The Model greatly expanded my view of what needs to be considered in nursing to reach out and help people of diverse cultures"; "After using this Model, I can see that fragmented, partial, and narrow views of clients often are used in nursing and medicine rather than the whole picture to arrive at a health care plan. I keep in mind to value clients' abilities to tell their story and to share their care knowledge and practices with my use of the Sunrise Model." Another nurse said, "I always use the Sunrise Model to do my culturological health care assessment to arrive at the comprehensive picture or holistic and effective care practices." These statements attest to the many users of the Model, which continues to reflect daily uses. Nursing students are very adept and skilled in using the Sunrise Model as it makes them understand the "whole person or family."

During the past four decades the theory with the Sunrise Model has led to a wealth of largely unknown care and health knowledge to provide culturally congruent care to individuals, families, and groups and for health institutions, which is the goal of the theory. The three modes of action and decision are specific ways to practice transcultural nursing and creative care and to back the decisions with hard data. Such findings have been major breakthroughs to explicate culturally based holistic care phenomena for the first time in nursing's history and to use this knowledge for new care practices. It is important to state that the *nursing intervention concept* (commonly used in nursing) is generally *not* used in transcultural nursing as it is often viewed by clients as "only professionals know best," when they often do not know clients' cultural care views and needs. The coparticipation concept is valued by most cultures. "*Patient problems*" is another phrase often used in nursing, but seldom used in transcultural nursing as the problem may not be that of the client but often the nurse's problem. Such traditional linguistic nursing sayings are often troublesome to clients of different cultures and can lead to cultural resistance and noncompliant responses when used with the theory and enablers. The reader will see how authors in this book have used the theory with the Sunrise Model with many cultures and different domains of inquiry areas. It is also used to do culture-care assessments, which are discussed later.

◼ Orientational Theory Definitions

With the qualitative paradigm, *orientational definitions* are generally used rather than *operational ones* as found in quantitative-oriented theories and methods. The following definitions are used with the Culture Care theory as a guide to discover culture care phenomena:[41]

1. **Human Care/Caring** refers to the abstract and manifest phenomena with expressions of assistive, supportive, enabling, and facilitating ways to help self or others with evident or anticipated needs to improve health, a human condition, or a lifeway or to face disabilities or dying.

2. **Culture** refers to patterned lifeways, values, beliefs, norms, symbols, and practices of individuals, groups, or institutions that are learned, shared, and usually transmitted intergenerationally over time.

3. **Culture Care** refers to the synthesized and culturally constituted assistive, supportive, and facilitative caring acts toward self or others focused on evident or anticipated needs for the client's health or well-being or to face disabilities, death, or other human conditions.

4. **Culture Care Diversity** refers to cultural variabilities or differences in care beliefs, meanings, patterns, values, symbols, and lifeways within and between cultures and human beings.

5. **Culture Care Universality** refers to commonalties or similar culturally based care meanings ("truths"), patterns, values, symbols, and lifeways reflecting care as a universal humanity.

6. **Worldview** refers to the way an individual or group looks out on and understands their world about them as a value, stance, picture, or perspective about life or the world.

7. **Cultural and Social Structure Dimensions** refers to the dynamic, holistic, and interrelated patterns of structured features of a culture (or subculture), including religion (or spirituality), kinship (social), political (legal), economic, education, technology, cultural values, philosophy, history, and language.

8. **Environmental Context** refers to the totality of an environment (physical, geographic, and sociocultural), situation, or event with related experiences that give interpretative meanings to guide human expressions and decisions with reference to a particular environment or situation.

9. **Ethnohistory** refers to the sequence of facts, events, or developments over time as known,

witnessed, or documented about a designated people of a culture.

10. **Emic** refers to the local, indigenous, or insider's views and values about a phenomenon.

11. **Etic** refers to the outsider's or more universal views and values about a phenomenon.

12. **Health** refers to a state of well-being or restorative state that is culturally constituted, defined, valued, and practiced by individuals or groups that enables them to function in their daily lives.

13. **Transcultural Nursing** refers to a formal area of humanistic and scientific knowledge and practices focused on holistic culture care (caring) phenomena and competencies to assist individuals or groups to maintain or regain their health (or well-being) and to deal with disabilities, dying, or other human conditions in culturally congruent and beneficial ways.

14. **Culture Care Preservation and/or Maintenance** refers to those assistive, supportive, facilitative, or enabling professional actions and decisions that help people of a particular culture to retain and/or maintain meaningful care values and lifeways for their well-being, to recover from illness, or to deal with handicaps or dying.

15. **Culture Care Accommodation and/or Negotiation** refers to those assistive, supportive, facilitative, or enabling creative professional actions and decisions that help people of a designated culture (or subculture) to adapt to or to negotiate with others for meaningful, beneficial, and congruent health outcomes.

16. **Culture Care Repatterning and/or Restructuring** refers to the assistive, supportive, facilitative, or enabling professional actions and decisions that help clients reorder, change, or modify their lifeways for new, different, and beneficial health care outcomes.

17. **Culturally Competent Nursing Care** refers to the explicit use of culturally based care and health knowledge in sensitive, creative, and meaningful ways to fit the general lifeways and needs of individuals or groups for beneficial and meaningful health and well-being or to face illness, disabilities, or death.

These orientational definitions allow informants and practitioners to discover care, health, and illness conditions within a cultural perspective. The above definitions facilitate emic and etic data discoveries from informants in naturalistic ways and in accord with the theory of Culture Care. Some social-structure definitions are found in the primary theory book, which the reader may wish to review.[42]

From the above philosophy, purpose, goal, major tenets, assumptions, and definitions of the theory of Culture Care, the nurse moves forward to systematically discover care and health outcomes. It is important to state here that other health and educational disciplines are using the theory and the method, but with slight modifications to fit *their discipline focus*. In fact some physicians, dentists, social workers, hospital and university administrators, and those of other disciplines are using the theory with the Sunrise Model and Enablers to obtain holistic, comprehensive, and specific areas of understanding of human beings, groups, and institutions in diverse cultures and contexts.

Some Unique Theory Features

The theory of Culture Care Diversity and Universality has several distinct features different from other nursing theories of which a few will be briefly highlighted. *First*, it is the only theory that is explicitly focused on discovering holistic and comprehensive culture care. *Second*, it is a theory that can be used in Western and non-Western cultures because of the inclusion of multiple holistic factors universally found in cultures. *Third*, it is the only theory focused on examining comprehensive factors influencing human care such as the worldview, social structure factors, language, generic and professional care, ethnohistory, and environmental context. *Fourth*, the theory has both abstract and practice dimensions that can be systematically examined to arrive at culturally congruent care outcomes. *Fifth*, the ethnonursing research method was the first nursing research method designed to fit a theory. *Sixth*, the theory is one of the oldest theories in nursing explicitly focused on culture and care of diverse cultures. *Seventh*, the theory is unique as it has three theoretical practice modalities to arrive at culturally congruent care decisions and actions to support well-being, health, and other specific care patterns. *Eighth*, the theory is designed to ultimately discover care—what is *diverse* and what is *universal* related to care and health with emic and etic multiple factors. *Ninth*, the theory has a *comparative focus* to identify different or contrastive transcultural nursing care practices, but with specific care constructs and their meanings to tailor-make care practices. *Tenth*, the theory with the ethnonursing method has Enablers designed to tease out in-depth informant emic data, and these Enablers can also be used for cultural health care assessments. *Eleventh*, the theory can generate new knowledge in nursing and health care to arrive at *culturally congruent, safe, and responsible care*. The term, *culturally congruent care*, coined by the theorist as the goal of the theory in the 1960s, is now being used worldwide by health and social science disciplines. *Twelfth*, the *ethnonursing research method with Enablers* is unique to obtain in-depth naturalistic qualitative data and to focus less on the use of scales and instruments that are often impersonal, offensive, and ambiguous to cultural informants.

It is also important to state that the Culture Care theorist does not endorse or value classifications of nursing theories as *low, middle range*, or *grand theories* as these often are reductionistic modes of analysis that fail to preserve holistic and natural qualitative data of cultures. Reducing data to numbers or statistical outcomes fails to meet qualitative criteria. Nor is this theory a *grand theory* as there may be small domains studied and discovered. Instead, the theorist has developed the four Phases of Quantitative Analysis, which have been tested and used in many cultures the past five decades. The analysis leads to grounded limited findings from cultural informants who provide emic data, but it can provide major "truths" or large data outcomes. The criteria for qualitative studies is used to arrive at credible informant truths and does not need to use quantitative criteria for a qualitative research study. It is also important to note that the theory and method are *not relativistic* as universal attributes and explanations are sought that transcend relativism. Most importantly, the goal of the theory is not for relativity, but seeks universal "truths" about many cultures. Let us turn to the ethnonursing research method to see how it fits with the theory as it is an original and unique research method in nursing and health care.

 ## Overview of the Ethnonursing Research Method: Major Features and the Enablers

The ethnonursing research method was specifically designed by the theorist to facilitate the discovery of data focused on the theory of Culture Care Diversity and Universality. The term *ethnonursing* was coined and developed by the theorist in the mid 1960s.[43–45] *Ethnonursing refers to a qualitative nursing research method focused on naturalistic, open discovery and largely inductive (emic) modes to document, describe, explain, and interpret informants' worldview, meanings, symbols, and life experiences as they bear on actual or potential nursing care phenomena.*[46] The ethnonursing method is a naturalistic (largely emic focused) and open inquiry mode to discover the informant's world of knowing and experiencing life. The research method is designed to focus on emic and etic knowledge and practices related to care, health, well-being, illness, lifecycle experiences, dying, disabilities, prevention modes, and other actual or potential areas of interest to nurses and transcultural nursing phenomena. The method facilitates the discovery of care and health knowledge related to areas such as worldview, social structure factors, ethnohistory, environmental factors, and other additional areas of the informant's cultural lifeworld.

There are several major features and reasons why the ethnonursing research method was developed with the theory of Culture Care. It was evident in the 1960s that nurses were heavily borrowing from other disciplines for research tools, scales, and instruments to quantify or reduce nursing phenomena to almost meaningless findings that limited nurses to discover caring and other data related to nursing insights and practices. Nurses were not developing methods or aids appropriate to studying nursing phenomena, but instead were using research methods, tools, scales, and statistical formulas from other disciplines. This was of deep concern to me as we were missing meaningful and in-depth nursing knowledge. Moreover, some quantitative methods and findings seemed highly questionable to discover meanings and to get accurate culture-care interpretations. Often, quantitative researchers were "lumping and dumping" findings together and even "population groups" so that specific cultures were omitted or obscured in the findings. Indeed, it was difficult to obtain findings of specific cultures and especially any full, in-depth, meaningful data with quantitative reductionistic and empirical research methods. *A priori* hypotheses with limited discovery of the cultural lifeways of people, the scientific method, and the manipulation and control of specific variables reigned, but *unknown "whole" cultures in context* were limited except for a few brief descriptions. Truths about a culture were questionable, vague, and partial knowledge with the quantitative borrowed methods and instruments as they were not designed to discover in-depth human care, health, ethnohistory, and values of cultures and lifeways.

Realizing these major shortcomings in the early 1960s about quantitative research methods, I took a bold and different step in nursing by developing the ethnonursing research method within the qualitative paradigm to fit my theory. This was a major new approach in nursing and different from the other borrowing practices of nurse researchers. After 20 years of studying nearly 25 different qualitative methods, I wrote the first qualitative nursing research book to guide nurses to use a different paradigm and a different method to discover nursing phenomena.[47] My philosophy and intent was for nurses to develop research methods that fit or were meaningful to their theories to get credible and full data and to not rely totally on reductionistic modes of testing and data outcomes for nursing phenomena. The idea of having nursing research methods fit or be congruent with nursing to discover complex, hidden, and covert nursing phenomena was important as related to care and health and in diverse cultures. It was essentially a new breakthrough approach. Still today, many nurse researchers continue to use borrowed research methods from nonnursing disciplines and quantitative instruments to test their theories.

The purposes of the ethnonursing research method were as follows:

1. To discover largely unknown or vaguely known complex nursing phenomena bearing on care, well-being, health, and related cultural knowledge
2. To facilitate the researcher to enter the people's emic (insider's) cultural world and learn from them first-hand of their beliefs, values, experiences, and lifeworld about human care and health

3. To gain in-depth knowledge about the care meanings, expressions, symbols, metaphors, and daily night-and-day factors influencing health and well-being as depicted in the Sunrise Model
4. To use standard and new Enablers to tease out covert or embedded care and nursing knowledge related to the Culture Care theory with both emic and etic data
5. To use a rigorous, detailed, and systematic method of qualitative data analysis that would preserve naturalistic cultural and contextual data related to the theory
6. To use qualitative criteria (not quantitative) for accurate, meaningful, and credible analysis of findings
7. To identify the strengths and limitations of the ethnonursing method in advancing transcultural nursing science knowledge and outcomes.[48]

The ethnonursing purposes seemed urgently needed in nursing but especially to establish a body of transcultural nursing knowledge to guide culture care practices. The ethnonursing research method was different from ethnographies as the latter was focused on broad cultural areas, which often failed to tap in-depth nursing care phenomena and perspectives.[49] Over the past several decades I have found that the ethnonursing research method is fully adequate to replace ethnographies and to get to the heart of nurses' research interests.

Qualitative and Quantitative Paradigms and Methods

To understand the ethnonursing qualitative research method, it is important to define and highlight below the major differences between the qualitative and quantitative research paradigms and their purposes:[50–53]

The purpose of qualitative paradigmatic research is to discover the essences, patterns, symbols, attributes, and meanings of human and related phenomena under study with informants in their natural or familiar environments.[54] Subjective, objective, philosophical cultural, historical, spiritual, gender, ethical values, life experiences, and other perspectives are studied with appropriate qualitative methods. These methods are used to obtain accurate meanings and holistic and related informant data within familiar and naturalistic environments, lifeworlds, cultures, or community contexts. With qualitative research, there is no controlling of informant ideas or manipulating variables by the researcher. Instead, informants are encouraged to share their ideas in their naturalistic ways with stories, life histories, and what they know and have experienced in their lifeworld. The emic or insider's world of information is the focus, but attention to etic or outsider's views are of interest. The researcher tries to hold her/his views in abeyance and without prejudgement of ideas expressed. The goal is to obtain qualitative in-depth findings of the domain under study.

In contrast, quantitative paradigmatic research uses a priori discrete variables and specific research hypotheses with statistical tools and methods to obtain measurable statistical data from preselected subjects in accord with reduced, statistical and measurable outcomes. The researcher is expected to carefully control, manipulate, and test selected a priori *variables with the scientific method of specific hypotheses.*[55] The purpose of the quantitative research paradigm is to obtain very precise measurements and to establish specific causal relationships among the variables. With this research approach, it is almost impossible to obtain and measure covert cultural care data and other largely unknown phenomena of importance to nursing, including cultural health, healing modes, meanings, expressions, and other related areas. Quantitative methods and goals are the opposite of qualitative methods as the purposes and views about ways of knowing are very different. Discovering in-depth and natural caring and healing practices, beliefs, and values of diverse and similar cultures is essential with the ethnonursing qualitative method to obtain credible transcultural nursing knowledge. From the author's many research studies in non-Western and Western cultures along with other research studies mentored over the past five decades it has been found that qualitative research is imperative to grasp the people's beliefs and lifeways.[56] Moreover, many immigrants and other cultures dislike being studied as "subjects," "cases," and "objects" in controlled or manipulated ways. Cultures like to tell their story, life histories, and experiences naturally from *their* ways of knowing, which are often counter to experimental and controlled ways of sharing by cultural informants.[57]

In general, qualitative and quantitative paradigms have different philosophies, purposes, goals, methods, and desired outcomes, and so they should *not* be viewed as the same and used in the same ways. Recognizing this reality, the two research paradigms and methods should *not be mixed* as it violates the philosophy, purposes, and integrity of each paradigm and leads to questionable outcomes.[58] Still today, some nurse researchers and others are mixing and using both qualitative and quantitative methods "to be sure" or "to get better findings." Such practices seriously violate the integrity and philosophical purpose of each paradigm. This is an important principle that needs to be understood and valued by researchers to obtain accurate and credible data in studying human beings. It is also important to realize that one does not have to add or mix many methods within the qualitative paradigm unless the researcher has good reasons and can justify using multiple methods. Most importantly, the researcher must know each qualitative method being used and analyze them fully with stated purposes. Qualitative research methods and findings can *stand alone* to study and explain findings, and quantitative methods with statistical treatments are not necessary or appropriate to justify qualitative studies. The ethnonursing qualitative research method was thoughtfully developed after studying the purposes and uses of both research paradigms.[59]

Although there are a number of different kinds of qualitative research methods, one chooses the method that fits the research area (domain) and theory, such as using ethnonursing research to fit the Culture Care theory. However, it is important that nurse researchers become aware of many different and distinct qualitative research methods to choose from, such as these (listed from the oldest to the most recent):[60]

1. Philosophical inquiry (oldest)
2. Ethnography (mini and maxi types)
3. Ethnology and ethnohistory
4. Phenomenology (German and French methods)
5. Hermeneutics
6. Life histories (autobiographic and biographic)
7. Ethnoscience
8. Daily diaries, narratives, and story telling
9. Historical (synchronic and diachronic types)
10. Audiovisual
11. Metaphoric inquiry
12. Ethnonursing
13. Symbolic interaction
14. Grounded theory
15. Action research
16. Critical social theory

17. Feminist theory
18. Constructionist
19. Deconstructionist
20. Focused groups (several different approaches)
21. A few others such as holographic and virtual reality methods

Each of these qualitative methods are different, but have some common philosophical attributes and characteristics that fit within the general purposes and goals of the qualitative research paradigm. Philosophical inquiry is largely based on reasoning and argumentative stances; however, the other methods are different and need to be throughly studied by the researcher *before* selecting and using the method and mode of analysis so they can be used properly to obtain credible findings based on the particular method used. It should be noted that some "grounded" methods use statistical or measurable techniques, and so they do not fit with the true philosophical purposes and attributes of the qualitative paradigm. Most qualitative studies use "grounded" or emic raw data; hence, it may not be unique to the grounded theory method. In the United States and a few other countries, nurses are using phenomenological (German and French) methods. More and more nurses knowledgeable about ethnonursing are using it with both "mini and maxi" studies (the terms I identified in the 1970s) for undergraduate and graduate nursing students which relates to the scope and domain under study. Again, it is important to state that with the ethnonursing method, one does not need ethnography and other borrowed nonnursing methods to tap nursing phenomena as ethnonursing is comprehensive and complete to study specific and diverse domains. To date, approximately 300 ethnonursing research studies have been done with mini or maxi methods.[61]

Criteria for the Qualitative Paradigmatic Studies

It has been interesting that in the past there has been a strong tendency for nurse researchers to use quantitative criteria for qualitative investigations. This is a questionable practice as it violates the philosophical basis and purpose of each paradigm leading to errors, inaccurate interpretations, and spurious qualitative findings.[62] Realizing this problem and that too few nurses were educated in qualitative methods in the 1960s and 1970s (and even today), I did an intensive and extensive literature study in the 1960s and identified specific qualitative criteria for qualitative studies over the past four decades. This was a critical and long overdue need in nursing and with other disciplines. Many researchers had believed that only quantitative criteria such as validity, reliability, and statistical criteria for any investigation were essential to have their research accepted by other colleagues. Qualitative criteria were much needed to substantiate and accurately interpret qualitative findings among nearly 25 different qualitative methods, including the ethnonursing research method. I, therefore, identified six major criteria that have since been defined and used for several decades and generally supported by Lincoln and Guba (educational researchers) and others today.[63] They are as follows:[64,65]

1. **Credibility** refers to direct sources of evidence or information from the people within their environmental contexts of their "*truths*" held firmly as believable to them.
2. **Confirmability** refers to documented verbatim statements and direct observational evidence from informants, situations, and other people who firmly and knowingly confirm and substantiate the data or findings.
3. **Meaning In-Context** refers to understandable and meaningful findings that are known and held relevant to the people within their familiar and natural living environmental contexts and the culture. (Note: This was not an explicit criteria of Lincoln and Guba, but deemed important for all qualitative studies by Leininger.)
4. **Recurrent Patterning** refers to documented evidence of repeated patterns, themes, and acts over time reflecting consistency in lifeways or patterned behaviors.
5. **Saturation** refers to in-depth information of all that is or can be known by the informants about phenomena related to a domain of inquiry under study.
6. **Transferability** refers to whether the findings from a completed study have similar (not necessarily identical) meanings and relevance to be transferred to another similar situation, context, or culture.

These criteria are studied before beginning a qualitative investigation such as an ethnonursing study. They are specifically, thoughtfully, and discerningly used with qualitative data to arrive at accurate interpretations and credible findings. These criteria are documented during the study and rechecked in the final analysis as one uses the Leininger Phases of Quantitative Data Analysis.[66] Some descriptive numbers (non-statistical) can be used to document patterns of use, directional foci, or patterned frequencies. The criteria are identified and documented while collecting data. The reader is encouraged to read other studies to understand the uses of qualitative criteria for accuracy from the beginning to the end of the research. The qualitative researcher needs to remain cognizant that the goal of qualitative studies is *not to produce generalizations*, but rather to document, understand, and substantiate the meanings, attributes, patterns, symbols, metaphors, and other data features related to the domain of inquiry under study drawing heavily on informant data. The researcher will find it is most rewarding to use these qualitative criteria as they confirm and reaffirm findings in process from the informants and in the final analysis and interpretation of findings. They are the scientific evidence with documentation.

 ## Enablers to Facilitate In-depth Discoveries

To tap the peoples' (or informants') world of knowing, the author developed several *enablers* (term coined by the author beginning in the 1960s) to tease out data bearing on culture care, health, and related nursing phenomena. Different enablers were developed to discover specific data related to the theory tenets and for in-depth data of overt, covert, unknown, or ambiguous nursing phenomena. Enablers sharply contrast with mechanistic devices such as *tools, scales, measurement instruments*, and other impersonal *objective distancing tools* generally used in quantitative studies. These tools are often viewed as unnatural and frightening to cultural informants, especially to minorities, refugees, immigrants, homeless, poor, elderly, oppressed, and other vulnerable groups, as well as to cultures in general. Accordingly, several Enablers were developed by the author as part of the ethnonursing method. They are as follows:

1. *Leininger's Observation-Participation-Reflection Enabler* (Fig. 3.2)
2. *Leininger's Stranger to Trusted Friend Enabler* (Fig. 3.3)

3. *Sunrise Model Enabler* (see Fig. 3.1) presented earlier as a cognitive visualization aid to see the totality of phenomena or dimensions under study
4. *Specific Domain of Inquiry Enabler* (this is always developed by the researcher doing the study)
5. *Leininger's Acculturation Enabler*[67]

Examples of using these Enablers and their uses can be found in this book and many publications where the ethnonursing method has been used. (See references at end of the chapter.) Each will be explained below.

The ethnonursing researcher often uses most (if not all) of the Enablers except for perhaps the Acculturation Enabler depending on the focus of the study. Enablers are used as a guide to gently tease out in-depth informant ideas and obvious facts related to a specific domain of inquiry under studied. With Enablers, informants are encouraged to talk out their ideas; tell stories; describe life experiences; share pictures, tapes, and any materials they feel comfortable sharing related to the areas being discussed. The researcher remains alert to the informant's accounts and is an active and genuine listener with informants. One always *moves with the informant's line of thinking or flow of ideas* so that one enters and learns from the informant. The researcher unobtrusively uses each Enabler as a guide to uncover specific knowledge areas related to the domain of inquiry, but does not give the Enabler to the informant to use. Throughout the use of the Enablers, the ethnonursing researcher pays attention to one's own responses, feelings, actions, and reactions reflecting on actual or possible influences of the researcher on the informant(s). Remaining in a nonintrusive role is desired, always sitting with the informant in a visiting style of relating to them and others. Let us briefly highlight these Enablers next.

The *Observation-Participation-Reflection Enabler*

This Enabler (see Fig. 3.2) is regularly used as a most helpful and essential guide to enable the researcher to enter and remain with informants in the familiar or natural cultural context while one is observing and doing the study. With this Enabler, the researcher moves from an observer and listener role to gradually a participant and reflector role with the informant(s) or with phenomena under study. The researcher moves in slowly and politely after seeking permission to be with the informant. The gradual entry helps the researcher to first observe what is occurring naturally in the environment and with the people. It helps to maintain the idea to enter naturally and with less emphasis on the researcher. Observing before, during, and after contacts is important with this Enabler. Observing the whole or total situation and remaining an active listener is important. Identifying symbols, documenting facts and historical events, and reflecting on reactions and interactions with one another are all essential to obtain comprehensive ethnonursing data. Gradually, the researcher moves into center visibility but maintains a more passive than active doing role. When this occurs, one begins to feel and experience the actual shared lifeways of the people and become part of the on-going situation and interaction. At all times the researcher encourages informants to explain and interpret what is being observed, done, or experienced.

With this Enabler, the researcher studies day and night experiences or events. They are clarified with the informants and with the researcher respecting and valuing what is shared or explained. The researcher remains an active observer, listener, and reflector as crucial to the ethnonursing research method while focusing on the domain of inquiry. The researcher learns how to use long silence-listening periods with cultural informants and how to respect and document gender status, especially with the elderly and children. Remaining patient and keeping focused on what is being said or not discussed is essential to get full data with meaningful, sequential, and authentic data. Documenting specific and unusual events, cultural care offenses, taboos, and activities that are acceptable and nonacceptable

is important. Past and present stories, incidents, and historical events about care giving and receiving are important sources of information. Throughout the use of this Enabler, the researcher remains alert to the Culture Care theory tenets and especially to what are the data diversities (variabilities) and commonalties. The ethnonurse researcher also reflects on transcultural nursing concepts, principles, definitions, and reflective holding knowledge about the culture to grasp what one observes and hears. One avoids labeling, social profiling, or stereotyping as unacceptable in transcultural nursing. Transcultural nursing research mentors will watch for these tendencies and discuss such behavioral tendencies with the researcher. A daily journal or field log is used to record what one observes, hears, and experiences with the Enabler. This Enabler is also most valuable to doing cultural assessments related to care and health practices. It should be noted that the *OPR Enabler* is quite different from the traditional participant-observation method used in anthropology in that the process is *reversed* and a new reflection phase has been added. In addition, the OPR Enabler has explicit expectations to guide the researcher in each phase of this Enabler, which is different from the PO in anthropology.

Leininger's Stranger to Trusted Friend Enabler

This Enabler (see Fig. 3.3) has been enormously helpful as the researcher enters and remains with informants as strangers in unfamiliar environments. If the researcher has been functioning in the culture earlier or is from the

Leininger's Ethnonursing Observation—Participation—Reflection Enabler			
Phases	1	2	3	4
Focus	Primarily Observation and Active Listening (no active participation)	Primarily Observation with Limited Participation	Primarily Participation with Continued Observations	Primarily Reflection and Reconfirmation of Findings with Informants

Figure 3.2
Leininger's ethnonursing Observation--Participation--Reflection Enabler.

culture, it still is very helpful. Looking anew at informants' ideas and responses, and not assuming "*one knows all about them and their culture*," remains extremely important in ethnonursing. With this Enabler, the nurse can learn much about oneself and the people under study with this guide. The goal with this guide is to become a *trusted friend* as one moves from the left side of the Enabler (distrusted friend) to the right side of the Enabler to become a trusted friend. Different attitudes, behaviors, and expectations can be identified with this Enabler as the researcher moves from a stranger to a trusted friend. (See Fig. 3.3.) The nurse

researcher can become a trusted friend as it is essential to be trusted for honest, credible, and in-depth data from informants. The author has found from several of her studies and from others using this Enabler that when informants considered the researcher to be a trusted friend, the findings have markedly increased the credibility and accuracy of the informant data. When one is a trusted friend, informants will generally share more openly their secrets and other insights than when one is a distrusted researcher. This is different philosophy from the quantitative researcher who tries to keep "subjects" at a distance and avoids being a friend.

The purpose of this Enabler is to facilitate the researcher (or it can be used by a clinician) to move from mainly a distrusted stranger to a trusted friend in order to obtain authentic, credible, and dependable data (or establish favorable relationships as a clinician). The user assesses oneself by reflecting on the indicators while moving from stranger to trusted friend. These are dynamic indicators from cultures.

Indicators of Stranger (Largely etic or outsider's views)	Dates Noted	Indicators of a Trusted Friend (Largely emic or insider's views)	Dates Noted
Active to protect self and others. They *are gate-keepers* and guard against outside intrusions. Suspicious and questioning.		Less active to protect self. More trusting of researchers (their *gate-keeping is down or less*). Less suspicious and less questioning of researcher.	
Actively watch and are attentive to what researcher does and says. Limited signs of trusting the researcher or stranger.		Less watching the researcher's words and actions. More signs of trusting and accepting a new friend.	
Skeptical about the researcher's motives and work. May question how findings will be used by the researcher or stranger.		Less questioning of the researcher's motives, work and behavior. Signs of working with and helping the researcher as a friend.	
Reluctant to share cultural secrets and views as private knowledge. Protective of local lifeways, values, and beliefs. Dislikes probing by the researcher or strangers.		Willing to share cultural secrets and private world information and experiences. Offers mostly local views, values, and interpretations spontaneously or without probes.	
Uncomfortable to become friend or to confide in stranger. May come late, be absent, and withdraw at times from researcher.		Signs of being comfortable and enjoying friendship—a sharing relationship. Gives presence, is on time, and gives evidence of being a genuine "true" friend.	
Tends to offer inaccurate data. Modifies *truths* to protect self, family, community, and cultural lifeways. Emic values, beliefs, and practices are not shared spontaneously.		Wants research *truths* to be accurate regarding beliefs, people, values, and lifeways. Explains and interprets emic ideas so researcher has accurate data of the culture and informant.	

Figure 3.3
Leininger's Stranger--to--Trusted--Friend Enabler.

The *process of moving from becoming a stranger to a trusted friend takes time and keen sensitivity while showing a genuine interest in the informants* and respecting their ideas, beliefs, responses, and cultural ideas. This Enabler is used early and throughout the research period to assess one's relationship with the informant to get accurate data.[68] It is also valuable for culturalogical assessments. By focusing on studying the attributes in the right and left parts of the Enabler, one can gauge and assess progress moving from distrusted to trusted researcher (or nurse clinician). This Enabler has been essential and a standard, required guide with the ethnonursing method. The author first developed this Enabler in the 1960s with the first transcultural nursing research study in the Eastern Highlands of New Guinea. It has proven to be enormously helpful to nurses working in any culture, but especially non-Western and unknown cultures. It also helps to obtain a wealth of *emic* and *etic* cultural data, including other cultural detailed information about the informants and their beliefs, values, and lifeways while learning about oneself as a researcher and stranger.

Domain of Inquiry Enabler (DOI)

The ethnonurse researcher develops a special *Domain of Inquiry Enabler* (DOI) that is specific to the researcher's interests and focused on the domain of study. For example, a Domain of Inquiry (DOI) might be stated as: "*Haitian Families and Care Meanings and Practices.*" Or another DOI would be "*Political Care Meanings of Czech Immigrants.*" This is a succinct tailor-made statement focused directly and specifically on culture care and health phenomenon. Questions or ideas can be stated as related to the domain to cover ideas with DOI. Several excellent examples of these special DOI Enablers are found in several research studies by transcultural nurses in this book and in the references listed at the end of Part II of this chapter.

Leininger's Acculturation Health Care Assessment Enabler

Another important enabler that is often used is the *Acculturation Health Care Assessment Enabler*. In studying any culture it is important to assess the extent of acculturation of the informants whether *more traditionally or non-traditionally oriented in their values,*

beliefs, and general lifeways. This enabler is presented in Chapter 4, Appendix B. It is most frequently used in doing culturalogical assessments, but is also used with ethnonursing research studies.

Sunrise Model Enabler

The *Sunrise Model Enabler* (see Fig. 3.1) has already been discussed earlier in this chapter. This Enabler remains one of the most valuable comprehensive guides for researchers to tease out data related to multiple factors influencing care and health outcomes and to remain cognizant of holistic lifeways to examine with the Culture Care theory.

 ## Guide to Using the Ethnonursing Research Method

In studying any theory it is important to understand and use an appropriate research method to collect and analyze data. The author's ethnonursing method is a very systematic and rigorous method to ensure a sound study. In this section an overview of the ethnonursing research method is presented, but the reader is encouraged to study further the method by reading completed research studies in this book and in other publications such as O'Neil's.[69] The first step in using the ethnonursing research method is to clearly and succinctly *state the domain of inquiry* (DOI) being studied by the researcher. The DOI is the major focus of the research, which is focused on culture care phenomena with the major theory tenets fully in mind. All key words stated in the DOI are thoughtfully selected as they are studied in-depth and comprehensively with the informants. For example, some stated domains of inquiry (DOI) might be: 1) *Culture care meanings, expressions, and patterns of elderly Old Order Amish*; 2) *Culture care meanings and practices of Chinese children living in a rural community*; or 3) *Afro-British teenagers and their cultural needs in an urban context.* You will note that they are brief DOIs, but *every word is fully the responsibility of the researcher* to discover all aspects of the DOI such as meanings, expressions, and patterns of X culture. Superficial knowledge is inadequate and would fail to be a sound ethnonursing research investigation.

Research problems are seldom stated as found in quantitative studies as the researcher's interest or concern may not be a problem to the people, but rather the researcher's problem or interest. Usually, a few research questions can be stated after the DOI to be sure that every idea in the domain is broken down and fully studied. These questions would be guides and do not have to be analyzed separately at the end of the study. Instead, the DOI data are fully analyzed. Additional questions may be raised while conducting the study. Some suggested examples of questions that might follow the domain of inquiry statement are: "Culture care meanings, expressions, and patterns of caring with Japanese families" followed by 1) What is the *meaning of care* (caring) to Japanese families? 2) What are the *caring expressions or overt action modes* with Japanese families? 3) What *specific care patterns* can be identified with Japanese families? 4) Which modes of action or decisions with the Culture Care Theory seem most appropriate to provide culturally congruent care to Japanese families? These questions are examples to help the researcher focus on the domain of inquiry in specific ways.

After clearly stating the domain of inquiry and identifying a few research questions, the researcher then develops her/his Enabler (DOI) related to the specific domain of inquiry under study. This may be developed further after preliminary visits with the people being studied. The theoretical hunches by the researcher and those bearing on the Culture Care theory are the focus throughout the study. In addition, the researcher should use other enablers such as the *Observation-Participation-Reflection Enabler* and the *Stranger-Friend Enabler* as an integral part of the ethnonursing research method. The *Acculturation Enabler* is often used to assess the extent of cultural changes with immigrants, refugees, and other groups.

The sequential steps for the ethnonursing method are summarized below to guide the researcher:[70]

1. Fully review literature related to the domain of inquiry under study and other close studies to the DOI. Identify how these studies are similar to or different from your investigation (including qualitative and quantitative studies relate to the DOI).
2. State the researcher's theoretical interests and assumptive premises about studying the domain of inquiry in relation to Culture Care theory. The

theory always serves as the overall focus with the DOI to refute or substantiate the theory.
3. State the orientational definitions (not operational ones) to clarify your terms being used. Some of the theorist's stated Culture Care definitions above may be used or modified to fit the researcher's DOI.
4. Clearly state the purpose(s) and goal(s) of the study and identify the potential relevance or significance of this study to advance transcultural nursing or related nursing knowledge and practice areas. It is well to discuss your research ideas and DOI with a transcultural nursing research mentor to ensure a clear domain, theoretical ideas, scope of the study, and research plans.
5. The researcher then selects informants usually after a preliminary visit where the study is to occur. *Key* and *general* informants are thoughtfully and purposefully selected after identifying potential ones for the study. Keep in mind that the *key informants* are studied *in-depth*, while the *general informants* are studied for reflection and for representations in the wider community. After selecting key and general informants with selection criteria and explaining the study, obtain informed consent of the key and general informants at the beginning of the study and also while the study is in process. The informants' willingness to participate with potential benefits are discussed, as well as the fact that the informants are free to withdraw anytime from the study. Consent from institutions or community agencies is usually necessary in most places to protect informants and institutional rights.
6. Use *Stranger-Friend Enabler* (Fig. 3.3), the *Observation-Participation-Reflection Enabler* (Fig. 3.2), and the *Sunrise Model* (Fig. 3.1) from the beginning to the end of the study. Frequently assess your own attitude, communication (including nonverbal) modes, gender, and any other factors that may influence informant responses. An experienced transcultural nursing mentor is highly encouraged to confer with the researcher or provide insights especially with nurses new to the method.

Throughout the study, the ethnonurse researcher keeps in mind that the key informants are to provide in-depth knowledge about the DOI focused on culture care phenomena. Generally, three to four 1- to 2-hour sessions are held with key informants as one focuses on the DOI and the six qualitative criteria. In contrast, the researcher spends approximately 1- or 2-hour sessions (30 minutes) with the general informants because they provide only *general ideas* about the DOI.[71] For a *maxi* ethnonursing study, usually 12 to 15 *key informants* are selected and approximately 20 to 25 *general informants* are needed. For a *mini* study (often done before a maxi study) about one-half the number of key and general informants is used, that is, 6 to 8 key and 10 general informants. The mini or smaller study helps considerably to gain skills and confidence in doing a large or maxi study. Often, baccalaureate and master nursing students do mini studies, whereas doctoral students are expected to do maxi investigations. These numbers for informants of maxi and mini studies have been found reliable to reach saturation and to meet other qualitative criteria based on nearly five decades of many studies with many nursing students and transcultural nurse research experts.

It is the responsibility of the principal investigator to regularly and systematically document all observations and work throughout the study. The researcher maintains a field journal log or may use an electronic mini hand computer to process data immediately after each session. Small note pads are used while talking with and observing informants or situations. Nonverbal and verbal observations and participatory experiences along with the researcher's reflections are documented. It is important for the researcher to record one's feelings, views, and responses, which are usually on a dated and separate log. Codes are used to protect identification of the informants and institutions, which are kept confidential and in locked files. Periodically, the researcher may need to clarify with informants the purposes or intent of the study so that no misunderstandings occur and to respond to their questions. Again, informants may withdraw without retribution or pressure at any time and must be thanked for their participation. Interestingly, very few withdrawals have occurred with ethnonursing studies as informants usually like the method and are eager to share their (emic) cultural stories and views, as well as past experiences with professional staff care practices.

During the study, the researcher tries to maintain a nonobtrusive or nondominating position when observing, talking to, or participating with people. Maintaining a genuine interest and becoming immersed in the culture are important. Learning with "new ears and eyes" about the people and their culture care bring many knowledge rewards. Time is needed to maintain a daily log, to reflect on what has occurred, and to plan ahead. Historical documents, pictures, and other documents from informants are important and part of the ethnonursing collected data to be studied. Descriptions of environmental context and special language statements need to be dated and recorded. Today, many types of hand computers and other voice aids are available to process data, which should be done immediately after each visit to get an accurate account and to prevent memory lapses. If a tape recorder is used and pictures taken, permissions are necessary from the informants. Permission for taking pictures or doing videotapes is with cultures and countries, but generally informant's rights are protected. Some cultures say their word is better than a written document and refuse written forms, such as the Old Order Amish. Computer field and research data need to be respected and protected by the researcher.

How long one spends doing an ethnonursing study depends on the domain of inquiry and if the study is a maxi (big) or mini (small) study. The research criteria need to support and substantiate the domain of inquiry throughout the ethnonursing study. Evidence from the six criteria are used to guide the researcher and to substantiate the qualitative study. Evidence for the six criteria are imperative, namely, 1) credibility, 2) confirmability, 3) recurrent patterning, 4) meaning incontext, 5) saturation, and 6) transferability as defined earlier. The *transferability* criterion is considered at the end of the study and requires very thoughtful consideration by the researcher to determine if the results are transferable to a *similar* context. The six criteria should be used to document different contexts and findings while collecting and analyzing data daily, rather than waiting until the end of the study. Informants with *emic* and *etic* views are also studied for comparative transcultural findings and in relation to particular environmental contexts, ethnohistorical data, gender, age, and language uses. During the study it is especially important for key informants to confirm, refute, or reconfirm findings with the researcher so that an accurate and truthful account is forthcoming. The researcher's personal and professional etic views should always be documented and studied for biases and racism and for differences, similarities, conflicts, and other factors related to interpretation of what one sees or hears. Remember the key informants are interviewed and studied *first*, and then the general informants near the end of the study to check out cultural representation of the findings. To reduce transcultural nurse biases and prejudices, considerable time is spent in transcultural nursing courses to deal with such realistic concerns under experienced transcultural nurse mentors.

 ## Phases of Ethnonursing Data Analysis

To facilitate a systematic data analysis, the author has developed the Phases of Ethnonursing Qualitative Data Analysis (see Fig. 3.4) and confirmed its importance

with approximately 100 studies over four decades.[72–74] The four phases provide a systematic data analysis when thoughtfully used. The Leininger Templin Thompson (LTT) Qualitative Software Data Program (or a similar one today) can be used to process a large amount of grounded raw qualitative ethnonursing data.[75] Data from key and general informants with all interviews, observations, ethnohistory data, social structure factors, generic and professional data, and other data are computer processed, coded, and classified for final analysis at each phase of analysis with final themes. All qualitative data are preserved in the researcher's data bank. Thus a large amount of data are analyzed and preserved for different uses by the researcher.

The *first two phases* of data analysis (see Fig. 3.4) include recording of all grounded data along with specific code indicators. The *third and fourth phases* of data analysis require that the researcher identify recurrent patterns (third phase) and themes (fourth phase).

Fourth Phase
Major Themes, Research Findings, Theoretical Formulations, and Recommendations
This is the highest phase of data analysis, synthesis, and interpretation. It requires synthesis of thinking, configurations, analysis, interpreting findings, and creative formulations from data of the previous phases. The researcher's task is to abstract and present major themes, research findings, recommendations, and sometimes theoretical formulations.

Third Phase
Pattern and Contextual Analysis
Data are scrutinized to discover saturated ideas and recurrent patterns of similar or different meanings, expressions, structural forms, interpretations, or explanations of data related to the domain of inquiry. Data are examined to show patterning with respect to meanings in-context and along with further credibility and confirmation of findings.

Second Phase
Identification and Categorization of Descriptors and Components
Data are coded and classified as related to the domain of inquiry and sometimes the questions. Emic and etic descriptors are studied within context for similarities and differences. Recurrent components are studied for their meanings.

First Phase
Collecting, Describing, and Documenting Raw Data (with Field Journal or Computer)
Researcher collects, describes, records, and begins to collect data related to the purposes, domain of inquiry, or questions under study. This phase includes: recording interview data from key and general informants; making observations and having participatory experiences; identifying contextual meanings; making preliminary interpretations; identifying symbols; and recording data related to the phenomena under study, from an emic focus, but attentive to etic data. Data from the condensed and full field journal is processed directly into the computer, coded by hand.

Figure 3.4
Leininger's phases of ethnonursing qualitative data analysis.

In the *fourth phase*, the researcher not only thoughtfully analyzes the themes, but arrives at synthesized formulations of the findings derived from the previous data from the other three phases. The fourth phase requires the researcher to do creative reflections and abstract thinking to synthesize the findings into dominant care themes related to the DOI and theory tenets. It is this phase that requires the highest level of abstraction and critical thinking by the researcher to arrive at succinct, accurate, and usually powerful explanatory themes from the mass of rich data processed. The researcher rechecks and does audits trails of all analysis themes to be sure they are substantiated with grounded evidence and credibility from the raw data of the informants. These themes are clearly stated as major dominant ones to guide nurses in providing culturally congruent and relevant care for cultures as the ultimate goal of the theory is to lead to health and well-being or assist in dying.

Transcultural nursing research mentors who are experienced with the ethnonursing method can be of great help to facilitate the researcher's thinking on the major themes for high or powerful levels of formulations for meaningful analysis themes. The ethnonursing researcher who has collected the data from informants (and not technicians or unprepared researchers) becomes the key person to analyze the findings for credibility and accuracy. The unique feature of the ethnonursing research method is that the findings are firmly grounded with the cultural informants, having both emic and etic findings. The researcher may share her/his own responses, special views, and immersion experiences that reflect her/his immersion in a special section or that are used as honest experiences with the culture and informants. The researcher's narratives and on-going extensive experiences over time are always of interest to readers to grasp the nature of interactive transcultural research process. Comparative perspectives of diversities and similarities with emic and etic findings among informants are important to document. Special experiences of the researcher, informants, and community participants are important to reveal humanistic findings as shown in several chapters by different authors in this book and elsewhere.[76]

In the final check of the Phases of Ethnonursing Analysis for Qualitative Data, the researcher rechecks the final themes to be sure the data supports them from the raw data (Phase 1) to the final step (Phase 4). Such a rigorous and systematic analysis shows the reader how the data were substantiated and how the themes and the conclusions were reached. The term *substantiation of findings* is used for reporting ethnonursing and other qualitative results rather than verification or generalization as the latter are used with quantitative research studies.

After completing the study, a summary of major findings are shared first with interested informants and then prepared for presentations and for publication. These are essential for ethnonursing research as informants are usually interested in findings and should be aware of them before they are publicly presented or published. It also provides time to thank the informants for their contribution to professional knowledge and practices. The informant summary can be a brief report and given near the research site.

The final step is writing and publishing the study as soon as feasible so nurses and others can benefit from the findings and recommendations. The final report should state whether the theory and the domain of inquiry have been substantiated or refuted with substantive evidence. In addition, the researchers discuss in published works how the study findings with the three modes of action or decision are used to provide culturally congruent nursing care in practical ways.[77,78] Both culturally diverse and universal findings are reported with the theory and ethnonursing research findings. Reflections, suggestions, and recommendations are offered rather than limitations. Reflections are presented on ways to strengthen ethnonursing research and to share satisfactions or challenges in the conduct of the investigation.

Summary

This chapter has presented an overview of the theory of Culture Care Diversity and Universality with the ethnonursing research method. In addition, general features of qualitative research methods contrasted with quantitative and with the use of qualitative criteria were used to support the use of the ethnonursing method. The general features of the theory and method were discussed to show the close and important relationship of theory and method for meaningful and congruent outcomes. This first part will help the reader to grasp the use of the theory and method as used by several authors in this book with 25 specific culture care studies by transcultural nurse experts. This chapter provides a bridge to Part II of this chapter to understand the many active researchers pursuing transcultural nursing research over the past five decades.

It is most encouraging to see so many nurses using the theory and method today worldwide to discover crucial and long overdue knowledge to help nurses function in our transcultural world. The researchers' enthusiasm with many positive feedback reports are most encouraging to receive, especially those of diverse cultures. Many users repeatedly say, "This theory is the most holistic, comprehensive, and reality-based one in nursing and the health disciplines"; "The theory and method are extremely important to help us practice nursing"; "The theory fits our desired way of functioning as nurses for we work with clients in many different settings"; "I am so pleased with the broad, holistic, and comprehensive theoretical features to expand my nursing perspective and yet tap highly particularistic data to guide my care with specific cultures. My practice of nursing is greatly changing, and it has been the theory research findings that has helped me the most in nursing"; and "This theory is timely and has come of age and is so relevant to nursing; we have long needed it to prevent racism and ethnocentrism." In general the theory of Culture Care with the ethnonursing research method has been probably the most significant breakthrough in nursing and will have even greater impact in this 21st century to improve culture care practices.

■ References

1. Leininger, M., *Culture Care Diversity and Universality: A Theory of Nursing*, New York, NY: National League for Nursing Press, 1991.
2. Leininger, M., *Transcultural Nursing: Theories, Concepts, Practices*, New York, NY: John Wiley & Sons, 1978.
3. Leininger, M., *Transcultural Nursing: Concepts, Theories, Research and Practice*, Blacklick, OH: McGraw-Hill College Custom Series, 1995.
4. Leininger, M., *Caring: An Essential Human Need*, Thorofare, NJ: Charles B. Slack, 1981. (Reprinted Detroit, MI: Wayne State University Press, 1988.)
5. Leininger, M., *Care: The Essence of Nursing and Health*, Detroit, MI: Wayne State University Press, 1988.
6. Leininger, op. cit., 1991, pp. 5–58.
7. Ibid.
8. Ibid.
9. Leininger, op. cit., 1988.
10. Leininger, M., "Caring, The Essence and Central Focus of Nursing," in *Nursing Research Foundation Report*, 1977, v. 12, no. 1, pp. 2–14.
11. Leininger, M., *Nursing and Anthropology: Two Worlds to Blend*, New York, NY: John Wiley & Sons, 1970.
12. Leininger, M., "The Culture Concept and Its Relevance to Nursing," *The Journal of Nursing Education*, 1967, v. 6, no. 2, pp. 27–39.
13. Leininger, M., "Transcultural Nursing: A Scientific and Humanistic Care Discipline," *Journal of Transcultural Nursing*, Jan.–June 1997a, v. 8, no. 2, pp. 54–55.
14. Peplau, H., *Interpersonal Relations in Nursing: A Conceptual Frame of Reference of Psychiatric Nursing*, New York, NY: G.P. Putnam and Sons, 1952.
15. Leininger, op. cit., 1970.
16. Ibid.
17. Leininger, op. cit., 1981.
18. Leininger, op. cit., 1988.
19. Fawcett, J., "The Metaparadigm in Nursing: Present Status and Future Refinements," *Image: The Journal of Nursing Scholarship*, 1984, v. 16, no. 3, pp. 84–87.
20. Leininger, op. cit., 1988.
21. Leininger, op. cit., 1991.
22. Gaut, D., "Conceptual Analysis of Caring," in *Caring: An Essential Human Need*, M. Leininger, Ed., Thorofare, NJ: Charles B. Slack, 1981. (Reprinted Detroit, MI: Wayne State University Press, 1988.)
23. Watson, J., *Nursing: The Philosophy of Science Care*, Boston, MA: Little, Brown and Co., 1979.
24. Ray, M., "Philosophical Analysis of Care," in *Caring: An Essential Human Need*, M. Leininger, ed., Thorofare, NJ: Charles B. Slack, 1981, pp. 23–37. (Reprinted Detroit, MI: Wayne State University Press, 1988.)
25. Leininger, M., "Culture Care Theory: The Comparative Global Theory to Advance Human Care Nursing Knowledge and Practice," in *A Global Agenda for Caring*, D. Gaut, ed., New York, NY: National League for Nursing Press, 1993, pp. 3–19.
26. Leininger, op. cit., 1978.
27. Leininger, M., "Ethnonursing: A Research Method with Enablers to Study the Theory of Culture Care," in *The Theory of Culture Care Diversity and Universality*, New York, NY: NLN Press, 1991, pp. 73–117.

28. Leininger, M., *Qualitative Research Methods in Nursing*, Orlando, FL: Grune & Stratton, Inc., 1985.
29. Leininger, op. cit., 1991, pp. 32–36.
30. Ibid, pp. 37–40.
31. Ibid, pp. 37–40.
32. Ibid, pp. 41–44.
33. Ibid, pp. 343–372.
34. Ibid, pp. 44–46.
35. Leininger, op. cit., 1995.
36. Leininger, op. cit., 1991, p. 43.
37. Fawcett, J., "Leininger's Theory of Culture Care Diversity and Universality," in *Analysis and Evaluation of Nursing Theories*, Philadelphia, PA: FA Davis, 1993, pp. 49–88 and "Faucett's Analysis and Evaluation of Contemporary Knowledges," *Nursing Models and Theory, 2000.* Philadelphia: F.A. Davis, pp. 511–548.
38. Leininger, M., "Response and Reflections on Bruni's Critique of Leininger's Theory," *Collegian,* 2001, v. 8, no. 1, pp. 37–38.
39. Leininger, op. cit., 1991, pp. 44–46.
40. Ibid, p. 43.
41. Ibid, pp. 48–50.
42. Ibid.
43. Ibid, pp. 73–119.
44. Leininger, M., "Ethnography and Ethnonursing: Models and Modes of Qualitative Analysis," in *Qualitative Research Methods in Nursing*, M. Leininger, ed., Orlando, FL: Grune & Stratton, Inc., 1985, pp. 33–72.
45. Leininger, M., "Ethnomethods: The Philosophic and Epistemic Basis to Explicate Transcultural Nursing Knowledge," *Journal of Transcultural Nursing*, 1990, v. 2, no. 1, pp. 254–257.
46. Ibid.
47. Leininger, M., "Ethnonursing: A Research Method with Enablers to Study the Theory of Culture," in *Culture Care Diversity and Universality: A Theory of Nursing*, New York: NLN Press, 1991, pp. 73–117.
48. Leininger, op. cit., pp. 73–80.
49. Morse, J., *Critical Issues in Qualitative Research Methods*, Thousand Oaks, CA: Sage Publishers, 1994.
50. Polit, D.F. & Hungler, B.P., *Nursing Research: Principles and Methods,* 5th ed., Philadelphia, PA: Lippincott, 1995.
51. Leininger, M., "Overview and Reflection on the Theory of Culture Care and the Ethnonursing Research Method," *Journal of Transcultural Nursing*, 1997b, v. 118, no. 2, pp. 32–53.
52. Leininger, op. cit., 1991, pp. 43–44.
53. Leininger, op. cit., 1985, pp. 12–24.
54. Leininger, op. cit., 1997b, pp. 73–90.
55. Ibid.
56. Leininger, M., "Ethnonursing Research Method: Essential to Discover and Advance Asian Nursing Knowledge," *Japanese Journal of Nursing Research*, 1997c, v. 30, no. 2, pp. 20–32.
57. Leininger, op. cit., 1985, 1995, 1997b.
58. Leininger, M., "Current Issues, Problems and Trends to Advance Qualitative Paradigmatic Research Methods for the Future," *Qualitative Health Research*, 1992, v. 12, no. 4, pp. 392–415.
59. Ibid.
60. Leininger, op. cit., 1997b.
61. Leininger, M., "Transcultural Nursing Research to Transform Nursing Education and Practice: 40 Years," *Image: Journal of Nursing Scholarship*, 1997c, v. 129, no. 4, pp. 341–347.
62. Leininger, op. cit., 1997c.
63. Lincoln, Y. and E. Guba, *Naturalistic Inquiry*, Newbury Park, CA: Sage Publications, 1985.
64. Leininger, op. cit., 1997b, pp. 44–45.
65. Leininger, op. cit., 1991, pp. 112–116.
66. Ibid, p. 95.
67. Ibid, pp. 90–104.
68. Ibid.
69. MacNeil, J., "Use of Culture Care Theory with Baganda Women as AIDS Caregivers," *Journal of Transcultural Nursing*, 1996, v. 7, no. 2, pp. 14–20.
70. Leininger, op. cit., 1991, p. 105.
71. Ibid, pp. 109–112.
72. Ibid, p. 95.
73. Leininger, op. cit., 1995.
74. *Journal of Transcultural Nursing*, Transcultural Nursing Society. Livonia, MI: Desktop Publishing, 1989–1999.
75. *Leininger, Templin, Thompson (LTT) Software.* Detroit, MI: Wayne State College of Nursing, 1988–2001.
76. Leininger, M., "Transcultural Nursing to Discovery of Self and the World of Others," *Journal of Transcultural Nursing*, October 2000, v. 11, no. 4, pp. 312–313.
77. Leininger, M., "Culture Care Theory: The Relevant Theory to Guide Functioning in a Multicultural World," in *Patterns of Nursing Theories in Practice,* M. Parker, ed., New York, NY: National League for Nursing Press, 1993, pp. 103–122.
78. McFarland, M., "Use of Culture Care Theory with Anglo and African American Elders in a Long-Term Care Setting," *Nursing Science Quarterly*, 1997, Fall Issue, pp. 940–951.

CHAPTER 3

PART II. Selected Research Findings from the Culture Care Theory

Marilyn R. McFarland

Over the past four decades approximately 300 known substantive transcultural nursing research studies have been done in Western and non-Western cultures. Many of these studies have been published in the *Journal of Transcultural Nursing*, the official publication of the Transcultural Nursing Society, but others have appeared in book chapters, special monographs, and related sources. Because of space limitations, only a few selected transcultural nursing studies and findings will be cited beginning in the early 1960s with others following until the year 2001. The reader is encouraged to read these studies to discover the use of the Culture Care Theory and the ethnonursing research method, along with the valuable findings to advance and substantiate transcultural nursing and to improve care in other health areas. Most of these studies are maxi-ethnonursing research studies with specific Western and non-Western cultures with approximately 12 to 15 key and 30 to 45 general informants. Only highlights are presented, and Appendixes 3-A and 3-B provide a partial list of additional research studies.

Early General Transcultural Nursing Studies

The first transcultural nursing study was with the Gadsup people of the Eastern Highlands of New Guinea in the early 1960s by Leininger which was approximately a 2-year in-depth study using ethnonursing and ethnographic research methods.[1–3] While many culture findings, beliefs, and values were discovered, the major care meanings and action modes of the Gadsup were explicated. Care meanings and actions

were as follows:

1. Nurturance (ways to help people grow) and survive
2. Surveillance nearby and at a distance (watchfulness)
3. Male protective modes
4. Ways to prevent illness and death
5. Use of touch as a caring modality.[4–6]

Kinship, politics, gender roles, cultural values, and other sociocultural factors were major influencers on care patterns, expressions, and lifeways. There were many other insightful findings discovered in this old non-Western, nontechnological culture that have been reaffirmed by Leininger with her return visits each decade since 1960. These findings affirm the tenacity of Culture Care values, beliefs, and lifeways as guides to transcultural nursing practices.[7] Most importantly, this first transcultural nursing study has inspired nurses to study cultures in-depth and over time for culture care patterns with the theory.

Another important transcultural nursing study conducted in an American urban hospital context with Philippine and Anglo-American nurses was done by Spangler in the late 1980s and reported in 1992. Findings from this early 8-month study revealed several diverse and two universal care themes and patterns that substantiated the theory of Culture Care. One of the many dominant care patterns demonstrated by Philippine American nurses in the hospital context was care as providing respect and physical comfort with therapeutic benefits and highly positive responses from clients. Philippine nurses showed competencies in using their generic traditional caregiving modes to provide smooth interpersonal relationships (or *pakikisama*) with clients, which prevented hurting patients' feelings and *saved face* as a dominant care value. Philippine nurses would avoid confrontational incidents and used *lambing* (playful coaxing or cajoling) when asking about or for an action or decision to be made with staff and clients.[8]

In contrast, Anglo-American staff nurses demonstrated a high regard for giving autonomous care or care that they controlled and gave independently to clients. These nurses were comfortable being assertive and confrontational in giving care that they valued, along with efforts to educate or teach clients. Anglo-American nurses showed signs of frustration when clients were noncompliant and when patients did not focus on initiating and maintaining self-care practices. Anglo-American nurses wanted patients to make decisions and choices that fit with professional (etic) nurse expectations and with what Anglo-American nurses believed "made sense to them." Being in control of the situation and "to be on top of things" was their way of caring and was very important to these Anglo-American hospital nurses. They drew on their professional (etic) knowledge "of what was taught to them" and were active in doing physical assessments. Anglo-American nurses demonstrated skills in mastery of situations, tasks (many technologies), and the use of "rational knowledge" as their action modalities of nursing care, but had limited knowledge about cultures and generic (emic) care knowledge. There were many culture care indicators of themes, patterns, and raw data from this study reflecting more diversities than universalities between Philippine and Anglo-American nurses. The only universal or common care theme for Philippine and Anglo-Americans was to work hard and to express frustration in different cultural ways about nursing situations or conditions. This remains an important comparative nursing staff institutional study of professional care meanings and practices between two nursing cultures within an urban United States hospital. Showing major differences, Philippine nurses used both generic and professional care practices, whereas Anglo-American nurses relied on only etic practices.[9]

Wenger's ethnonursing study of the Old Order Amish was the first transcultural nursing investigation to examine in-depth care meanings and action modes using the Culture Care theory.[10,11] Her in-depth emic findings of the Amish revealed that generic care had several dominant care meanings such as giving and accepting help generously and with humility from others. Care was very tightly embedded in the worldview and with social structure factors, especially religion, kinship, cultural values, and beliefs, and within their community-based daily modes of living. The use of technologies was counter to Old Order Amish cultural lifeways and was not seen nor generally desired as a care modality. The dominant core care meanings and action modes for the Old Order Amish were 1) providing anticipatory care (especially knowing about one another's cultural care needs); 2) practicing principled pragmatism (do what needs to be done with family and friends in traditional practical ways); and 3) being an active participant in daily community life activities that promote individuals, family, and community well-being. Care for the Old Order Amish was within high-context meaning, which meant care was readily known and understood by the Amish in their strongly oriented community lifeways. Culture care universals among the people were far more evident than diversities with signs of some intergenerational differences. Grandparents were highly respected and cared for by others in the Old Order Amish culture. This transcultural study was the first to discover the relevance and importance of culturally based care within the Amish community living context. It is the first study in nursing to show the meaning and practices of specific community caring modalities.[12]

Rosenbaum's transcultural nursing study of widows with the Culture Care theory was another first of its kind in that it was focused on care meanings and actions with Greek Canadians. The dominant care meanings and action modes were that care meant 1) being responsible for one's husband after death with the newly discovered construct by the researcher of "continuity care" for one's husband at the grave site; 2) showing active family protection for and concern about other Greek Canadians; and 3) demonstrating that caring means helping others in need and in daily life activities. The widow's spiritual belief in presence after her husband's death required comfort care, which was expected to be provided by nurses. The researcher discovered anew the construct of *cultural care continuity* with the use of the Culture Care theory, which meant that widows were expected to promote and maintain Greek Canadian health and well-being for both the living and the dead in special ways. Several additional, generic (emic), culturally based findings were discovered by Rosenbaum that can be studied with the three care action modes of the theory to maintain culture-specific health and prevent illness.[13]

In the late 1960s Leininger studied Mexican and Spanish American community care needs in a midwestern suburban community in the United States.[14] The Culture Care theory was used, which disclosed differences between the two cultures but also some similarities in religion, language, and kinship. In 1991 Stasiak and several graduate nursing students studied Mexican Americans with the Culture Care Theory in a large urban mid-Atlantic area of the United States. From these studies, several dominant cultural care (emic) meanings and action modes were discovered such as the following:

1. Filial love and respect for those in authority
2. Offering direct involvement as filial care with extended family members
3. Providing protective care by observing cultural taboos and using generic (folk) care by professional nurses and others
4. Being involved with other kin as "other care" rather than focusing on self-care
5. Accepting religious values and belief of God's will in caring, healing, and in death

See Table 3.2 for other care meanings and action findings. Religion, spiritual values, and extended kinship practices and knowing generic (folk) beliefs and caring actions were all held to be dominant and essential to provide culturally congruent care to Mexican Americans. Being attentive to different environmental contexts was also viewed as an important caring expectation for professional nurses who care for Mexican Americans.[15–17]

Stasiak was the first nurse researcher to discover *confidenza* or confidence as an important generic (emic) care construct for Mexican Americans. In his study he described confidence as trusting others and God as an essential goal for nurses in providing culture care accommodation practices. Stasiak's study revealed four major universal (emic) themes: 1) car-

ing is expressed through love of family and neighbor (filial love) and spiritual ties, including *compadrazgo* (fictive kin), and through invoking the power of God to heal by the use of prayer; 2) care means *todo o casi todo* or everything or almost everything, being with family, eating certain foods, and *bienestar* or well-being; 3) folk practices and rituals promote caring and healing among Mexican Americans; and 4) professional health care providers were seen by informants as an extension of God. The culture-specific and dominant care constructs were filial love, well-being, respect, confidence, and succorance—attention to direct assistance. These care constructs with cultural themes were held to be essential to provide culturally congruent nursing care using Leininger's three action modes. Nursing actions included: 1) culture care preservation of generic folk practices, use of Spanish, and use of religious signs, symbols, and maternal cultural goods with nursing care; 2) culture care accommodation actions, including earning confidence and respect that requires deference to family and community values; and 3) culture care accommodation and preservation of caring actions of folk and spiritual healers. A minimal restructuring of emic care practices was found, but professional nurses needed to incorporate generic care into professional practices for culturally congruent care.[18]

In 1998 Zoucha conducted an ethnonursing study to discover the experiences of Mexican Americans receiving professional nursing care.[19] The researcher, guided by the Culture Care Theory with the Sunrise Model, observed and interviewed Mexican Americans who were receiving nursing care from registered professional nurses in an outpatient surgical clinic context.[20,21] The researcher discovered that Mexican Americans preferred nurses who communicated with them in Spanish and that they expected and valued care expressions and practices that were personal, friendly, and respectful of family. Zoucha found that Mexican Americans preferred generic care and professional care to be combined for nursing care to be culturally congruent and appropriate. Nurses were also expected to earn the confidence of Mexican American clients when providing professional nursing care. The dominant culture care values of Mexican Americans discovered in this study were: confidence, attention, respect for client and family, concern, spending time, communicating in Spanish, and filial love.[22] This study substantiated the Culture Care theory and confirmed earlier Mexican American culture care findings of Stasiak and Leininger.[23–25]

Luna's study of Lebanese-Muslim immigrants was conceptualized with the Culture Care Theory and conducted during the early 1980s in a large metropolitan area of the midwestern United States. Her study covered a 3-year in-depth investigation of the culture in hospitals, clinics, and homes of the largest Islamic migrant group outside the Middle East.[26,27] Her interest in studying the Arab Muslim culture began before she entered her doctoral program in the 1980s and continued for several years. From her extensive in-depth study using the ethnonursing research method, she discovered several important findings: 1) gender role practices within the family and in religious and political activities were extremely important and could not be overlooked in Lebanese Muslim care; 2) generic care practices in the home and community contrasted sharply with hospital care in the United States and was limitedly known by hospital nurses and other staff; 3) professional hospital practices of Anglo-Americans with food uses, bonding of infants, and other professional practices reflected cultural imposition, stresses, conflict areas, and other noncaring practices for Lebanese Muslims. Luna's findings showed the critical need for transcultural nursing knowledge and skills to understand and work with Arab American Muslims in providing culturally congruent care. The three modes to provide culturally congruent care were clearly presented as guides to nursing practices. Findings from Luna's study identified specific gender role responsibilities for Lebanese Muslim males and females that should be maintained and preserved in both the home and hospital contexts. The positive culture care practices for men that should be preserved included surveillance, protection, and maintenance of the family. For Muslim women, educating the children and maintaining a family caring environment according to the precepts of Islam preserved culture care practices and values according to gender roles. Culture care accommodation and negotiation related to religious rituals needed to be provided as the nurse arranged for a place for the Muslim client to perform ritual purification before prayer. Providing a place for prayer and by making arrangements with the dietary department to provide nighttime meals for Muslim clients

who were fasting during Ramadan also needed culture care preservation practices. She recommended that if a cultural practice is potentially harmful to health, it is a legitimate area for cultural repatterning. She found that *Ko'hl*, a charcoal-like substance containing lead used in the Middle East as an eye cosmetic, was used by several informants on umbilical cords so that they would dry up quickly. Recent research has shown that the lead in Ko'hl is damaging to the growth and development of children, and so Luna recommended that cultural care repatterning for child eye care be established. The theory of Culture Care proved to be very essential to explicate highly covert Muslim culture care and health factors. The three care modalities were used for development of culturally congruent professional care practices and especially to incorporate several beneficial (emic) care practices into professional nursing. This early research has provided valuable cultural care findings that are used by many nurses today. Luna is currently practicing as a certified transcultural nurse specialist, teacher, researcher, and exemplar practitioner in an Arab Muslim hospital in the Middle East.[28,29]

Recently, in 1999, Wehbeh-Alamah conducted a 2-year ethnonursing study using the Culture Care Theory on the generic health care beliefs, expressions, and practices of Lebanese Muslim immigrants in two midwestern United States cities. Her findings (confirming many of Luna's findings from 1989) included the discovery of specific generic (emic) folk care diagnostic, preventative, and treatment beliefs, expressions, and practices used by Lebanese informants in a home context. Like Luna, Wehbeh-Alamah found that many generic care practices required culture care preservation/maintenance and culture care accommodation/negotiation in the home, as well as in the hospital. These generic care practices included providing for praying facing the east five times a day, having large numbers of visitors when ill in the hospital or at home, and eating only *Halal* meat (meat that has been processed in accordance with special Muslim guidelines). Gender care findings were similar to Luna's findings showing the persistence of many care patterns over time as predicted in Leininger's theory. However, the women in Wehbeh-Alamah's study believed the absence of extended family members in the United States had influenced men to assist them (wives, mothers, sisters) in the direct provision of care for family members. The researcher reported that acculturation had changed men's view of the act of providing care from the more traditional belief that the hands-on caring for the children, the elderly, and the sick belonged to women to the more contemporary belief in cooperation and participation on the part of Muslim men in direct care activities.[30]

Another important and timely transcultural nursing study was conducted by MacNeil in the early 1990s with Baganda people with AIDS in Uganda, Africa. The domain of inquiry was focused on the meanings, patterns, and expressions of Baganda women as AIDS caregivers. This in-depth ethnonursing field study guided by the Culture Care Theory covered approximately 2 years of observing and working directly with Baganda women. Several universal themes were identified and repeatedly documented with direct observations, participation with the women, and reflection analysis with the people. Some of the major universal theme discoveries were 1) culture care meant responsibility, love, and comfort measures derived from the Baganda kinship, religious, and cultural beliefs and values and from generic folk health care beliefs; 2) culture care meant survival to help secure a cultural future for the next generation through education and land claims; 3) culture care also meant to preserve and to continue being caring to others (especially kin), despite adversity and the tremendous burden of caring for AIDS victims over time; and 4) gender role differences were important, and caring for others after the death of a loved one were important. The universal care concepts of "being fully involved with" and offering presence and persistence in caregiving to others was evident. A few culturally diverse themes were identified among Baganda women such as the belief of making "the most out of life for the HIV-positive women." MacNeil's in-depth breakthrough research was the first non-Western (African) transcultural AIDS study to discover specific culture care (emic) knowledge to provide practical AIDS care for Bagandans. The complex ethnohistorical and social structure factors about the African culture with the Culture Care Theory and the Sunrise Model were extremely important to obtain comprehensive, convert, and accurate data for the domain of inquiry focused on AIDS care needs and values.[31]

Another in-depth and breakthrough transcultural doctoral study by Miller focused on the domain of inquiry regarding the American political context of professional (etic) and generic (emic) care patterns, expressions, and meanings of Czechoslovakian American immigrants living in one large urban midwestern United States city. Miller's findings not only substantiated the theory of Culture Care, but revealed the significant effect of politics for immigrants on the access and maintenance of culturally congruent health care in the American system, especially in hospitals. The United States health services' delivery system was discovered to have many differences for getting care for Czechoslovakian immigrants. Learning to be responsible for oneself was a dominant theme for Czechoslovakians in the United States, in addition to relying heavily on their generic (folk) care to survive for economic, political, and health reasons. Many cultural conflict situations arose for Czechoslovakian immigrants in getting health care in the United States, especially for young working parents. Care for children was highly valued by Czechoslovakian immigrants with action modes to actively seek and preserve and maintain child health care. Language, economics, politics, and technologies in United States hospitals were major influencers in accessing and receiving professional hospital care. Acculturation and generic care factors influenced the immigrants' recovery and the maintenance of care with professional nurses and physicians because of major intercultural care value differences. Learning about differences in cost, access to health services, and meanings and practices of health care were challenges for Czechoslovakian immigrants. There were many signs of "noncare" with nurses who did not understand the Czechoslovakian culture and generic care values. In general, Czechoslovakian immigrants found it was difficult to access the United States health care system. Hence, many Czechoslovakians spoke about "noncaring" when care and health services failed to fit the client's generic culture care values and political orientation.[32]

Life-Cycle Transcultural Nursing Studies

Transcultural nurses since the beginning have been interested in life-cycle, enculturation, and acculturation processes. This section presents brief summaries of selected studies focused on these processes.

In the area of parent and child nursing studies, several transcultural nursing studies have been conducted over the past four decades. Kendall, a nurse anthropologist and midwife, did an early life-cycle study in the late 1970s on maternal child care in an Iranian village with many important findings.[33] Horn did an in-depth research study of the Muckleshoot Native Americans using ethnography and ethnonursing research methods and found many important generic (emic) care findings for nurses to use in prenatal and postnatal care.[34] Bohay, using the Culture Care Theory, found that pregnancy and birth caring phenomena of the Ukrainians in the United States are deeply embedded in worldview, religion, and kinship expectations. Family care meanings for Ukrainians were care as obligations, care as presence with closeness, and care as helping others.[35,36] Finn did a phenomenological study of Euro-American birthing mothers in an American hospital context and discovered intracultural differences in the ways birthing women wanted personalized nursing care.[37]

Morgan conducted a study of pregnancy and childbirth practices with Hare Krishna devotees in the southern United States with a transcultural nursing focus. Her study showed that generic (folk) care beliefs and practices of the Hare Krishna were clearly evident and viewed as essential care that fit their religious, worldview, and cultural values and beliefs. More recently, Morgan, a certified transcultural nurse and an experienced nurse midwife, studied prenatal care of African American women in United States urban and rural contexts. From this ethnonursing study, four major themes were identified: 1) caring meant sharing; 2) caring was greatly influenced by social structure factors of kinship ties, spirituality, and economic factors to attain and maintain one's health and well-being; 3) professional prenatal care was seen by women as necessary and essential, but there were signs of distrust and noncaring by some professionals, especially physicians; and 4) generic traditional folk and life-cycle health beliefs and practices with indigenous health care providers were widely used by the women in both African American communities where available.[38,39]

Berry conducted an ethnonursing study on the expressions of the meanings of culturally congruent pre-natal care of Mexican American women in a large city in the western United States.[40] The study was conceptualized within the Culture Care Theory with the Sunrise Model.[41] The latter served as an important cognitive map to discover complex cultural components influencing prenatal care and caring. Berry discovered six universal prenatal care themes:

1. Generic (emic) prenatal care was identified as the protection of the mother and fetus, as transmitted (enculturated) intergenerationally over time by older Mexican American women, which was greatly influenced by generic (emic) life-cycle religion and family beliefs and practices.
2. Care was a family obligation for the provision of *filial* (family) *succorance*, sharing of self, and being with the childbearing mother.
3. Culturally sensitive care was viewed as respect for familial caring roles in relation to age and gender.
4. Childbearing Mexican American women described culturally competent care by professional nurses as concern for, professional knowledge, protection, being attentive to, and explaining.
5. Culturally congruent care was defined as the use of the Spanish language in caring interactions in diverse environmental contexts.
6. Professional prenatal care was valued by Mexican American women, but was influenced by legal, economic, and technological factors of the social structure.

The Culture Care Theory was essential to tease out complex and varied cultural values, beliefs, and practices of Mexican American women. It was extremely important to explicate the highly covert and largely unknown worldview, environmental context, social structure, language, life-cycle learning, and ethnohistory factors leading to the discovery of culturally congruent care for prenatal mothers. The informants affirmed that the intergenerationally learned life-cycle cultural values and practices were essential for delivery and care of healthy full-term infants. A follow-up study revealed that all key informants delivered healthy babies as their culture care values were upheld with the three modalities being respected and maintained. This supported the second assumptive premise of the Culture Care Theory that caring is essential for well-being and health—in this study caring was discovered to be essential for fetal development and a healthy birth.[42]

Ehrmin conducted an ethnonursing research study in the United States to discover expressions of violence with African and Euro-Americans intergenerationally, as well as cultural differences or commonalities with African and Euro-Americans life-cycle patterns. The focus was on violence intergenerationally and culture care practices that African and Euro-Americans used to reduce intergenerational conflicts to maintain peaceful and healthy lifeways. The broad, open, comprehensive, yet particularistic, in-depth Culture Care Theory was held as essential to identify complex and multiple factors such as the worldview, social structure, environmental context, and cultural care values and beliefs influencing intergenerational family violence. This study revealed the importance of nurses caring for clients experiencing difficulties with intergenerational life-cycle family violence within culturally congruent, meaningful, and safe ways. The Culture Care Theory was imperative to discover the comprehensive social structure factors regarding intergenerational family life-cycle violence within the African American and Euro-American cultures. This study further demonstrated the importance of transcultural nursing knowledge to reduce intergenerational violence and provide culturally congruent care. Ehrmin recommended a set of "Care Repatterning Guidelines" based largely on Leininger's major transcultural nursing concepts and principles and three modes of care to provide culturally congruent care. These guidelines are as follows:[43–45]

1. Take the time to learn specific cultural values, beliefs, and practices about care.
2. Communicate and maintain care modes to clients within culturally congruent, safe, and meaningful ways.
3. Negotiate, accommodate, and maintain cultural care values, beliefs, and practices that facilitate therapeutic caring.
4. Coordinate family and community referrals for clients to facilitate intergenerational caring values, beliefs, practices, and expressions of care.
5. Accommodate, preserve, and maintain healthy generic emic cultural care values, beliefs, and practices of clients.
6. Restructure lifeways that are noncaring or violent intergenerationally.
7. Empathize with clients and avoid judgmental nursing decisions and actions by providing culturally congruent care that leads to health and well-being.

A major transcultural ethnonursing study covering 2 years was conducted by McFarland starting in the late 1980s comparing Anglo- and African American groups living in a residence home for the elderly in one large midwestern United States city. The author's research was another in-depth emic and etic culture care investigation that revealed several significant findings and the importance of using Leininger's three caring modes for the elderly. The culturally congruent care findings were as follows: 1) Anglo- and African American elderly expect culture care preservation and maintenance of their preadmission generic (folk) care patterns; 2) doing for other residents (rather than a self-care focus) was a major care maintenance value for both cultures and was a dominant finding; 3) protective care was more important to African American than Anglo-American elders, but the nursing staff provided protective care and practiced culture care accommodation for both groups of elders such as accompanying them when they desired to go for walks in the surrounding inner-city neighborhood; and 4) African American nurses practiced culture care accommodation when they linked their etic care with generic emic care values and practices. Culture care maintenance/preservation and culture care accommodation/negotiation were new ways for nurses to provide culturally congruent and safe lifeway care practices for the elderly of both cultures. Based on the findings of this study, several institutional culture care policies were developed to guide professional elderly care.[46] This study substantiated many life-cycle care patterns that Leininger discovered in an early comparative study of African Americans and Anglo-Americans in two villages in the southern United States[47,48] and some African American life-cycle care patterns that Morgan discovered in her study related to childbirth practices in rural and urban areas of the United States.[49] The importance of obtaining life-cycle ethnohistories from informants and using them for generic care patterns was crucial for nurses to know.

Chiang's domain of inquiry was focused on care meanings and expressions of Taiwanese Americans in a large midwestern city in the United States.[50] The theory of Culture Care Diversity and Universality provided valuable guidance to discover the culture care values and beliefs of the Taiwanese with several Sunrise Enablers of the ethnonursing research method to tease out holistic, life-cycle, and acculturation data and specific culture care practice dimensions.[51] Five major universal themes were discovered from the analysis of this data:

1. Cultural care was reflected in the development of national and cultural identity.
2. Cultural care was reflected in the value of harmony and balance in daily life based on Taiwanese generic (emic) ethnohistory, social structure, and worldview to prevent illness and maintain well-being.
3. Culture care meant preserving generic (emic) traditional folk health care beliefs and practices and selectively using some Western health care practices for healthy outcomes.
4. Caring was an obligation for family members with different gender role responsibilities.
5. Caring was expressed as unconditional emotional, physical, and cultural life-cycle support for loved ones.

The tenets of the Culture Care Theory were substantiated showing both cultural universalities and diversities within Taiwanese culture largely based on acculturation factors. There were more universal patterns (similarities) than diversity findings from data. The ethnonursing research method was extremely important to uncover subtle and detailed differences between professional nursing and Taiwanese generic care and thus to provide culturally congruent care to acculturated Taiwanese Americans.[52]

Other Important Transcultural Nursing Investigations

George studied the culture care meanings, expressions, and experiences of the chronically mentally ill as a subculture living in alternative community settings in a midwestern United States city. The goal of the study was to discover knowledge to guide nurses in providing culturally congruent care for the chronically mentally ill in the community so that they could maintain or regain their health and well-being. This study clearly reaffirmed the importance of the theory of Culture Care Diversity and University to obtain subtle, complex, and covert data with the Enablers of the ethnonursing method. The findings suggested new approaches are needed in psychiatric/mental health nursing by incorporating transcultural care factors into nursing, which have been limitedly identified, valued, and understood. The care meanings and expressions related to mental health were embedded in the total fabric and patterns of living with the subculture of the chronically mentally ill. The findings of the study clearly showed that the worldview, cultural and social structure factors, and environmental context of the chronically mentally ill markedly influenced their care meanings, expressions, and experiences related to mental illness. There were three creative and recurrent care constructs discovered in the subculture as follows: 1) *Survival care* refers to the essential features of care that are needed to assist a chronically mentally ill person to live or make it through a period of time outside the mental institution in a given community and culture; 2) *Constructive care* refers to the recognition and use of clients' strengths and assets to maximize their health and well-being over time and to identify their strengths that are beneficial to chronically mentally ill individuals within the subculture and in the dominant culture; and 3) *Inclusive care* refers to assistive, supportive, and enabling actions that promote the participation of members of the subculture of the chronically mentally ill in the dominant culture. These new care constructs of knowledge need to be used by nurses with Leininger's three modes of action and decision to practice therapeutic transcultural mental health care with the chronically mentally ill living in an urban community.[53] This is another exemplar Culture Care study to discover new ways to understand and help the mentally ill in the United States.

Discovering the nature of moral caring of nurses as culturally constituted was Stitzlein's domain of inquiry with the Culture Care Theory. The goal of the study was the discovery of moral caring knowledge for use in nursing education, practice, and administration settings in the United States to promote morally congruent nursing care and professional satisfaction by documenting shared narratives of moral caring and nonmoral caring practice situations. Twelve nurse clinicians practicing in the United States, including African Americans, European Americans, and both males and females, participated in the open-ended, in-depth interview study from 1996 to 1998. The five dominant moral caring themes were discovered as follows:

1. Moral caring as nursing action emanating from personal and professional characteristics of the nurse and focused on a meaningful nurse-patient relationship
2. Family, religious, and philosophical (generic) and professional role modeling influences on the development of a definition and commitment to moral caring
3. Professional experiences of notable personal satisfaction, as well as intense moral distress and moral conflict
4. Economic, technological, political/legal, and human environmental influences on nurses' ability to give moral caring
5. Professional role satisfaction influence on the employment patterns

Three new care constructs were identified and are useful to nurses from this research, namely: 1) a need for a unified ethic of nurse caring; 2) the pursuit of professional care satisfaction; and 3) unresolved moral care distress.[54] The findings were congruent with the tenets of virtue ethics and confirmed Leininger's theoretical assumption that care is the essence of nursing, and they were supported by the researcher's speculation that moral caring is a virtue.[55] The complementarity of virtue ethics, obligation-based ethics, principle-based ethics, and a relational ethic of care were demonstrated. Social structure dimensions, especially generic and professional values and experiences, were powerful influencers on the moral caring practices of participants and showed the importance of Leininger's theory to tap these dimensions and the theoretical tenets and predictions from the Culture Care Theory.[56]

A number of other Culture Care Theory studies are in progress worldwide such as the study of youthful gang caring behaviors in juvenile detention centers[57] and others focused on Aborigines in Australia and native groups in the United States, Africa, Asia, and the Caribbean. The versatility, relevance, and meaning of the theory used worldwide is critical and imperative to advance transcultural nursing knowledge and practices in all areas of nursing. The reader is encouraged to read the full text of the studies summarized here to guide nursing actions and decisions.

Examples of Dominant Universal Culture Care Values, Meanings, and Actions of Selected Cultures (Emic Data)

During the past five decades approximately 100 Western and non-Western cultures have been studied by transcultural nurse experts. From these studies several recurrent and dominant universal culture care constructs have been identified and should be used to teach and guide practices and research to arrive at culturally congruent, meaningful, and responsible care. They are presented in priority of dominant rankings in meanings and actions of care transculturally and are as follows:[58]

1. Respect for/about
2. Concern for/about
3. Attention to (details)/in anticipation of
4. Helping/assisting or facilitative acts
5. Active listening
6. Presence (being physically there)
7. Understanding (beliefs, values, lifeways, and environmental context)
8. Connectedness
9. Protection (gender related)
10. Touching
11. Comfort measures

Examples from 22 studies reported in the Culture Care Theory book are shown in Tables 3.1 to 3.8, and are offered to show the specific cultural values and cultural meanings and actions of specific cultures.[59] The findings come from many culture care scholars, students, clinicians, and faculty and Leininger's work over five decades. They show the benefits of persistent studies to identify culture care phenomenon to be used

Table 3.1   Gadsup (Akuna) Eastern Highlands of New Guinea (non-Western Culture)*

Cultural Values	Culture Care Meaning and Action Modes

1. Egalitarianism
2. Marked sex role differences
3. Patriarchal descent recognized
4. Communal unity ("one vine/line")
5. Prevent social accusations (sorcery)
6. Maintain ancestor "life-essence" and obligations
7. Have "good women, children, pigs, and gardens"
	1. Surveillance (to prevent sorcery)
	  –nearby surveillance
	  –watch at a distance
	2. Protection (protective male caring)
	  –of Gadsups through life-cycle
	  –obeying cultural taboos and rules
	3. Nurturance
	  –ways to help people grow and survive
	  –know what they need (anticipate needs) through life-cycle
	  –eat safe foods
	4. Prevention (avoid breaking cultural taboos) to:
	  –prevent illness and death
	  –prevent intervillage fights and conflicts
	5. Touching

* This was the first transcultural care study by Leininger in two villages in the early 1960s with subsequent visits until 1992 (see chapter in this book). Emic data.

Table 3.2   North American (Indian) Culture*

Cultural Values	Culture Care Meaning and Action Modes
1. Harmony between land, people, and environment 2. Reciprocity with "Mother Earth" 3. Spiritual inspiration (spirit guidance) 4. Folk healers (Shamans) (The Circle and Four Directions) 5. Practice culture rituals and taboos 6. Rhythmicity of life with nature 7. Authority of tribal elders 8. Pride in cultural heritage and "Nations" 9. Respect and value for children	1. Establishing harmony between people and environment with reciprocity 2. Actively listening 3. Using periods of silence ("Great Spirit" guidance) 4. Rhythmic timing (nature, land, and people) in harmony 5. Respect for native folk healers, carers, and curers (Use of Circle) 6. Maintaining reciprocity (replenish what is taken from Mother Earth) 7. Preserving cultural rituals and taboos 8. Respect for elders and children

*These findings were collected by Leininger and other contributors in the United States and Canada during the past four decades. Cultural variations among all nations exist, but commonalities are evident as above emic data shows.

Table 3.3 Mexican American Culture*

Cultural Values	Culture Care Meaning and Action Modes
1. Extended family valued	1. Succorance (direct family aid)
2. Interdependence with kin and social activities	2. Involvement with extended family ("other care")
3. Patriarchal (machismo)	3. Filial love / loving
4. Exact time less valued	4. Respect for authority
5. High respect for authority and the elderly	5. Mother home care decision maker
6. Religion valued (many Roman Catholics)	6. Protective (external) care (male)
7. Native foods for well being	7. Acceptance of God's will
8. Traditional folk-care healers for folk illnesses	8. Use of folk-care practices
9. Belief in hot-cold theory	9. Healing with foods
	10. Touching

*These findings are from transcultural nurse studies (1970, 1990) and other studies in diverse regions in the United States. Middle and lower economic status. Emic data.

Table 3.4 Anglo-American Culture (mainly USA Middle and Upper Class)*

Cultural Values	Culture Care Meaning and Action Modes
1. Individualism—focus on a self-reliant person	1. Stress alleviation by:
2. Independence and freedom	−physical means
3. Competition and achievement	−emotional means
4. Materialism (things and money)	2. Personalized acts
5. Technology dependent	−doing special things
6. Instant time and actions	−giving individual attention
7. Youth and beauty	3. Self-reliance (individualism) by
8. Equal sex rights	−reliance on self
9. Leisure time highly valued possible	−self-care
10. Reliance on scientific facts and numbers	−independent
11. Less respect for authority and the elderly	−reliance on technologies
12. Generosity in time of crisis	4. Health instruction
	−teach us how 'to do' this self-care
	−give us the 'medical' facts

* Emic data from several transcultural nursing studies 1970–1995.

in transcultural nursing science and practices, which are much needed today. Granted, there was some variability within cultures and intergenerationally between individuals; however, the dominant care values and patterns became evident and were documented. Many can be identified in the research presented in this section and in this book. They are needed to serve as major guides for nurses to provide culturally competent care.

The reader is encouraged to read, study, and use the other 14 cited in the Culture Care Theory book such as the Vietnamese, Haitians, etc.[60]

Table 3.5   Philippine American Culture*

Cultural Values	Culture Care Meaning and Action Modes
1. Family unity and closeness 2. Respect for elder / authority 3. "Leave oneself to God" (*Bahala na*) 4. Obligations to sociocultural ties 5. Hot-cold beliefs 6. Use of folk foods and practices 7. Religion values (mainly Roman Catholic)	1. Maintain smooth relationships (*Pakisisama*) 2. Save face and self-esteem (*Amor propio*); (*Hiya* – avoid shame) 3. Respect for and deference to authority 4. Being quiet, privacy 5. Mutual reciprocity (*Utang Na Loob*) "the give and take" in relationships 6. Giving comfort to others 7. Tenderness 8. Being pleasant as possible

* These findings are from Philippines living in the United States for at least two decades and were collected by Leininger, Spangler, and other transcultural nurse researchers. Emic data.

Table 3.6   German American Culture*

Cultural Values	Culture Care Meaning and Action Modes
1. Industriousness and being hard workers 2. Maintain order and organization 3. Maintain religious beliefs 4. Stoicism 5. Keep environment and self clean 6. Cautiousness 7. Knowledge is power 8. Controlling self and others 9. Maintain rules and norms 10. Scientism with logic valued	1. Being orderly (orderliness) –things in "proper places" –right performance –being well organized 2. Being clean and neat 3. Direct helping to others –give explicit assistance –get into action 4. Watch details –follow rules –be punctual 5. Protecting others against harm and outsiders 6. Controlling self and others 7. Eating proper foods and getting rest and fresh air 8. Do not complain, "grin and bear it"

* Findings from urban and rural United States over the past four (4) decades by transcultural nurses. Similar values and care patterns also were observed and confirmed in Western Germany in past decades (1970–1990). Emic data.

Table 3.7 African American Culture*

Cultural Values	Culture Care Meanings and Action Modes
1. Family networks valued	1. Concern for my "brothers and sisters"
2. Religion valued (many are Baptists)	2. Being involved with
3. Interdependence with "Blacks"	3. Giving presence (physical)
4. Daily survival of poor	4. Family support and "get togethers"
5. Technology valued, e.g., radio, car, musical instruments	5. Touching appropriately
6. Folk (soul) foods	6. Reliance of folk home remedies
7. Folk healing modes	7. Rely on "Jesus to save us" with prayers
8. Music and physical activities	

* These findings were from Leininger's study of two southern USA villages (1980–1981) and from a study in two large northern urban cities (1982–1994) along with other studies by transcultural nurses. Middle and lower economic status. Emic data.

Table 3.8 Polish American Culture*

Cultural Values	Culture Care Meaning and Action Modes
1. Upholding Christian religious beliefs and practices ('pray')	1. Giving to others in need
2. Family and cultural solidarity (other-care)	2. Self-sacrificing for others and God
3. Frugality as way of life	3. Being actively concerned about
4. Political activity for justice	4. Working hard whatever one does
5. Hard work: 'Don't complain'	5. Christian love of others
6. Persistence: 'Don't give up'	6. Family concern for others
7. Maintain religious and special days	7. Eating Polish foods and folk care to stay well or recover from illness (including home remedies)
8. Value folk practices	

* These findings are from transcultural nursing studies with Midwest Polish Americans (primarily in Detroit and Chicago—two of the largest Polish settlements in the United States) by several transcultural nurses over the past decade. Emic data.

 ## The Internet and the Culture Care Theory Group

A Culture Care Theory Group has been formed to advance transcultural nursing and general nursing through the use of Leininger's Culture Care Diversity and Universality Theory in nursing practice, research, education, and consultation. This discussion group is open to all nurses worldwide who wish to have access to current news and developments related to the Culture Care Theory, methods, and research findings. An integral part of the Culture Care Theory Group is the use of the Internet. If you wish to join, send an e-mail to webmaster@tcns.org and request to be an online member of the Culture Care Theory Group (CCTG).

Appendix 3-A
Partial List of Users of the Culture Care Theory (Worldwide)

Author	Title
Anita Berry, PhD, RN	Mexican American Women's Expressions of the Meaning of Culturally Congruent Prenatal Care [*Journal of Transcultural Nursing.* 11(3) 2000]
Cynthia Cameron, PhD, RN	*An Ethnonursing Study of the Influence of Extended Caregiving on the Health of Elderly Anglo-Canadian Wives Caring for Physically Disabled Husbands* (PhD Dissertation, Wayne State University, Detroit, MI, USA – 1990)
Elizabeth Cameron-Traub, PhD, RN	*Conceptualizing Ethical, Moral, and Legal Dimensions of Transcultural Nursing within the Culture Care Theory* (In M. Leininger and M. McFarland (Eds.) *Transcultural Nursing* (3rd Edition) – in press 2001)
Lenny Chiang, PhD, RN	Taiwanese Americans Culture Care Meanings and Expressions (In M. Leininger & M. McFarland (Eds.) *Transcultural Nursing* (3rd Edition) – in press 2001)
Marguerite R. Curtis, PhD, RN	*Cultural Care by Private Practice APRNS in Community Contexts* (PhD Dissertation, Wayne State University, Detroit, MI, USA – 1997)
Joanne T. Ehrmin, PhD, RN	Culture Care: Meanings and Expressions of African American Women Residing in an Inner City Transitional Home for Substance Abuse (In M. Leininger & M. McFarland (Eds.) *Transcultural Nursing* (3rd Edition) – in press 2001)
Julianna Finn, PhD, RN	Culture Care of Euro-American Women during Childbirth: Applying Leininger's Theory for Transcultural Nursing Discoveries [*Journal of Transcultural Nursing,* 5(2) 1994]
Marie Gates, PhD, RN	Transcultural Comparison of Hospital and Hospice as Caring Environments for Dying Patients [*Journal of Transcultural Nursing,* 2(2) 1991]
Rauda Gelazis, PhD, RN	Lithuanian Americans and Culture Care (In M. Leininger & M. McFarland (Eds.) *Transcultural Nursing* (3rd Edition) – in press 2001)
Tamara George, PhD, RN	Defining Care in the Culture of the Chronically Mentally Ill Living in the Community [*Journal of Transcultural Nursing,* 11(2), 2000]
Barbara Higgins, PhD, RN	Puerto Rican Cultural Beliefs: Influence on Infant Feeding Practices in Western New York [*Journal of Transcultural Nursing,* 11(1) 2000]
Beverly Horn, PhD, RN	Transcultural Nursing and Child-Rearing of the Muckleshoots [In M. Leininger (Ed.) *Transcultural Nursing* (2nd Edition)]
Betty Horton, DNSc, RN	Nurse Anesthetists' Perspectives on Improving the Anesthesia Care of Culturally Diverse Patients [*Journal of Transcultural Nursing,* 9(2) 1998]
Judith Lamp, PhD, RN	Finnish Women in Birth: Culture Care Meanings and Practices (In M. Leininger & M. McFarland (Eds.) *Transcultural Nursing* (3rd Edition) – in press 2001)
Cheryl Leuning, PhD, RN (et. al.)	Elder Care in Urban Namibian Families: An Ethnonursing Study (In M. Leininger & M. McFarland (Eds.) *Transcultural Nursing* (3rd Edition) – in press 2001)
Linda Luna, PhD, RN	Care and Cultural Context of Lebanese Muslim Immigrants with Leininger's Theory. [*Journal of Transcultural Nursing,* 5(1), 1993]
Marilyn McFarland, PhD, RN	Use of Culture Care Theory with Anglo- and African American Elders in a Long-term Care Setting [*Nursing Science Quarterly,* fall issue 1997]
June Miller, PhD, RN	Politics and Care: A Study of Czech Americans within Leininger's Theory of Culture Care Diversity and Universality [*Journal of Transcultural Nursing,* 9(1) 1997]
Edith Morris, PhD, RN	*Culture Care Values, Meanings, Experiences of African American Adolescent Gang Members* (PhD Dissertation, Wayne State University, Detroit, MI, USA – 2001)
Akram Omeri, PhD, RN	Culture Care of Iranian Immigrants in New South Wales, Australia: Sharing Transcultural Nursing [*Journal of Transcultural Nursing,* 8(2) 1997]
Janet Rosenbaum, PhD, RN	Cultural Care of Older Greek Canadian Widows within Leininger's Theory of Culture Care [*Journal of Transcultural Nursing,* 2(1) 1990]
Zenaida Spangler, PhD, RN	Transcultural Nursing Care Values and Caregiving Practices of Philippine-American Nurses [*Journal of Transcultural Nursing,* 3(2) 1992]

(Cont.)

Appendix 3-A *(Cont.)*

Author	Title
Dorothy Stitzlein, PhD, RN	*The Phenomenon of Moral Care / Caring Conceptualized within Leininger's Theory of Culture Care Diversity and Universality* (PhD Dissertation, Wayne State University, Detroit, MI, USA – 1999)
Teresa Thompson, PhD, RN	*A Qualitative Investigation of Rehabilitation Nursing Care in an Inpatient Rehabilitation Unit Using Leininger's Theory* (PhD Dissertation, Wayne State University, Detroit, MI, USA – 1990)
VanderBrink, Yolande	*Transcultural Family Care at Home* (study using Leininger's Culture Care Theory to study family care of the Turkish/Dutch elderly from a care perspective, 2000, in Dutch).
Hiba Wehbeh-Alamah, MSN	*Generic Health Care Beliefs, Expressions, and Practices of Lebanese Muslims in two Urban US Communities: A Mini Ethnonursing Study Conceptualized within Leininger's Theory* (Master's Thesis, Saginaw Valley State University, University Center, MI, USA – 1999)
Anna Frances Wenger, PhD, RN	The Culture Care Theory and the Old Order Amish [In M. Leininger (Ed.) *Culture Care Diversity and Universality: A Theory of Nursing.* National League for Nursing Press, 1991]
Rick Zoucha, RN, DNSc, CS	The Experiences of Mexican Americans Receiving Professional Nursing Care: An Ethnonursing Study [*Journal of Transcultural Nursing*, 9(2) 1998]

(Prepared by M. Leininger, 2001)

Appendix 3-B
Dissertations on Transcultural Nursing Care Mentored
by Professor Leininger (*1988–2001*)

Author	Title
Edith Morris, PhD, RN (2001)	Culture Care Values, Meanings, Experiences of African American Adolescent Gang Members
Dorothy Stitzlein, PhD, RN (1999)	The Phenomenon of Moral Care / Caring Conceptualized within Leininger's Theory of Culture Care Diversity and Universality
Betty Horton, DNSc, RN (1998)	Culture Care by Private Practice APRNS in Community Contexts
Joanne T. Ehrmin, PhD, RN (1998)	Culture Care: Meanings and Expressions of African American Women Residing in an Inner City Transitional Home for Substance Abuse
Tamara George, PhD, RN (1998)	Meanings, Expressions, and Experiences of Care of Chronically Mentally Ill in a Day Treatment Center using Leininger's Culture Care Theory
Judith Lamp, PhD, RN (1998)	Generic and Professional Culture Care Meanings and Practices of Finnish Women in Birth within Leininger's Theory of Culture Care Diversity and Universality
Rick Zoucha, RN, DNSc, CS	The Experiences of Mexican Americans Receiving Professional Nursing Care: An Ethnonursing Study
Curtis, Marguerite R. (1997) PhD, RN	Cultural Care by Private Practice APRNS in Community Contexts
June Miller, PhD, RN (1996)	Politics and Care: A Study of Czech Americans within Leininger's Theory of Culture Care Diversity and Universality
Akram Omeri, PhD, RN (1996)	Transcultural Nursing Values, Beliefs, and Practices of Iranian Immigrants in New South Wales
Anita Berry, PhD, RN (1995)	Culture Care Expression, Meanings, and Experiences of Pregnant Mexican-American Women Within Leininger's Culture Care Theory
Marilyn McFarland, PhD, RN (1995)	Cultural Care of Anglo- and African American Elderly Residents within the Environmental Context of a Long-Term Care Institution
Rauda Gelazis, PhD, RN (1994)	Human, Care, and Well-Being of Lithuanian Americans: An Ethnonursing Study Using Leininger's Theory of Culture Care Diversity and Universality

(Cont.)

Appendix 3-B (*Cont.*)

Author	Title
Joan MacNeil, PhD, RN (1994)	Culture Care: Meanings, Patterns, and Expressions for Baganda Women as AIDS Caregivers within Leininger's Theory
Marjorie Morgan, PhD, RN (1994)	Prenatal Care of African American Women in Selected USA Urban and Rural Cultural Contexts Conceptualized within Leininger's Cultural Care
Julianna Finn, PhD, RN (1993)	Professional Nurse and Generic Care of Childbirthing Women Conceptualized within Leininger's Culture Care Theory and Using Colaizzi's Phenomenological Method
Zenaida Spangler, PhD, RN (1991)	Nursing Care Values and Caregiving Practices of Anglo-American and Philippine-American Nurses Conceptualized within Leininger's Theory
Teresa Thompson, PhD, RN (1990)	A Qualitative Investigation of Rehabilitation Nursing Care in an Inpatient Rehabilitation Unit Using Leininger's Theory
Cynthia Cameron, PhD, RN (1990)	An Ethnonursing Study of the Influence of Extended Caregiving on the Health of Elderly Anglo-Canadian Wives Caring for Physically Disabled Husbands
Janet Rosenbaum, PhD, RN (1990)	Cultural Care, Cultural Health, and Grief Phenomena Related to Older Greek Canadian Widows within Leininger's Theory of Culture Care
Linda Luna, PhD, RN (1989)	Care and Cultural Context of Lebanese Muslims in an Urban US Community: An Ethnographic and Ethnonursing Study Conceptualized within Leininger's Theory
Marie Gates, PhD, RN (1988)	Care and Cure Meanings, Experiences, and Orientations of Persons who are Dying in Hospital and Hospice Settings
Anna Frances Wenger, PhD, RN (1988)	The Phenomenon of Care in a High Context Culture: The Old Order Amish

This list has been prepared because of many requests for specific transcultural nursing doctoral studies mainly from Wayne State University (Michigan) as a major center producing transcultural nursing PhD investigations the past decade under Professor Madeleine Leininger.

References

1. Leininger, M., *Nursing and Anthropology: Two Worlds to Blend*, New York: John Wiley & Sons, 1970. (Reprinted in 1994 by Greyden Press, Columbus, OH.)
2. Leininger, M., *Transcultural Nursing: Concepts, Theories, Research, and Practice*, New York: John Wiley & Sons, 1978. (Reprinted 1994 by Greyden Press, Columbus, OH.)
3. Leininger, M., "Culture Care of the Gadsup Akuna of the Eastern Highlands of New Guinea," in *Culture Care Diversity and Universality: A Theory of Nursing*, M. Leininger, ed., New York: National League for Nursing Press, 1991a.
4. Leininger, M., op. cit., 1978.
5. Leininger, M., "The Theory of Culture Care Diversity and Universality," in *Culture Care Diversity and Universality: A Theory of Nursing*, M. Leininger, ed., New York: National League for Nursing Press, 1991b.
6. Leininger, M., "Ethnonursing: A Research Method with Enablers to Study the Theory of Culture Care," in *Culture Care Diversity and Universality: A Theory of Nursing*, M. Leininger, ed., New York: National League for Nursing Press, 1991c.
7. Leininger, M., "Gadsup of Papua New Guinea Revisited: A Three Decade View," *Journal of Transcultural Nursing*, v. 5, no. 1, 1993, pp. 21–29.
8. Spangler, Z., "Transcultural Nursing Care Values and Caregiving Practices of Philippine American Nurses," *Journal of Transcultural Nursing*, v. 3, no. 2, 1992, pp. 23–38.
9. Ibid.
10. Wenger, A.F., "The Culture Care Theory and the Old Order Amish," in *Culture Care Diversity and Universality: A Theory of Nursing*, M. Leininger, ed., New York: National League for Nursing Press, 1991.
11. Wenger, A.F., "Cultural Context, Health, and Health Care Decision Making," *Journal of Transcultural Nursing*, v. 7, no. 1, 1995, pp. 3–14.
12. Wenger, op. cit., 1991.
13. Rosenbaum, J., "Cultural Care of Older Greek Canadian Widows Within Leininger's Theory of

Culture Care," *Journal of Transcultural Nursing*, v. 2, no. 1, 1990, pp. 37–47.

14. Leininger, op. cit., 1970.

15. Ibid.

16. Leininger, op. cit., 1991b.

17. Stasiak, D., "Culture Care Theory with Mexican Americans in an Urban Context," in *Culture Care Diversity and Universality: A Theory of Nursing*, M. Leininger, ed., New York: National League for Nursing Press, 1991.

18. Ibid.

19. Zoucha, R., "The Experiences of Mexican Americans Receiving Professional Nursing Care: An Ethnonursing Study," *Journal of Transcultural Nursing*, v. 9, no. 2, 1998, pp. 33–34.

20. Leininger, op. cit., 1991b.

21. Leininger, op. cit., 1991c.

22. Zoucha, op. cit., 1998.

23. Leininger, op. cit., 1970.

24. Leininger, M., "Selected Culture Care Findings of Diverse Cultures Using Culture Care Theory and Ethnomethods," in *Culture Care Diversity and Universality: A Theory of Nursing*, M. Leininger, ed., New York: National League for Nursing Press, 1991d.

25. Stasiak, op. cit., 1991.

26. Luna, L., "Transcultural Nursing Care of Arab Muslims," *Journal of Transcultural Nursing*, v. 1, no. 1, 1989, pp. 22–23.

27. Luna, L., "Care and Cultural Context of Lebanese Muslim Immigrants with Leininger's Theory," *Journal of Transcultural Nursing*, v. 5, no. 2, 1994, pp. 12–20.

28. Luna, op. cit., 1989.

29. Luna, L., "Culturally Competent Health Care: A Challenge for Nurses in Saudi Arabia," *Journal of Transcultural Nursing*, v. 9, no. 2, 1998, pp. 8–14.

30. Wehbeh-Alamah, H., *Generic Health Care Beliefs, Expressions, and Practices of Lebanese Muslims in Two Urban US Communities: A Mini Ethnonursing Study Conceptualized Within Leininger's Theory*, unpublished master's thesis, Saginaw Valley State University, University Center, Michigan, 1999.

31. MacNeil, J., "Use of Culture Care Theory with Baganda Women as AIDS Caregivers," *Journal of Transcultural Nursing*, v. 7, no. 2, 1996, pp. 14–20.

32. Miller, J., "Politics and Care: A Study of Czech Americans with Leininger's Theory of Culture Care

Diversity and Universality," *Journal of Transcultural Nursing*, v. 9, no. 1, 1996, pp. 3–13.

33. Kendall, K., "Maternal and Child Care in an Iranian Village," *Journal of Transcultural Nursing*, v. 4, no. 1, 1992, pp. 29–36.

34. Horn, B., "Transcultural Nursing and Childrearing of the Muckleshoots," in *Transcultural Nursing: Concepts, Theories, Research, and Practice*, 2nd ed., M. Leininger, ed., Columbus, OH: McGraw-Hill College Custom Series, 1995.

35. Bohay, I., *Ethnonursing: A Study of Pregnancy and Childbirth in the Ukrainian Culture Within Leininger's Culture Care Theory*, unpublished master's thesis, Detroit, MI: Wayne State University, 1989.

36. Bohay, I., "Culture Care Meanings and Experiences of Pregnancy and Childbirth of Ukrainians," in *Culture Care Diversity and Universality: A Theory of Nursing*, M. Leininger, ed., New York: National League for Nursing Press, 1991.

37. Finn, J., "Culture Care of Euro-American Women During Childbirth: Applying Leininger's Theory for Transcultural Nursing Discoveries," *Journal of Transcultural Nursing*, v. 5, no. 2, 1994, pp. 25–31.

38. Morgan, M., "Pregnancy and Childbirth Beliefs and Practices of American Hare Krishna Devotees Within Transcultural Nursing," *Journal of Transcultural Nursing*, v. 4, no. 1, 1992, pp. 5–10.

39. Morgan, M., "Prenatal Care of African American Women in Selected USA Urban and Rural Cultural Contexts," *Journal of Transcultural Nursing*, v. 7, no. 2, 1996, pp. 3–9.

40. Berry, A., "Mexican American Women's Expressions of the Meaning of Culturally Congruent Prenatal Care," *Journal of Transcultural Nursing*, v. 10, no. 3, 1999, pp. 203–212.

41. Leininger, op. cit., 1991b.

42. Ibid.

43. Ehrmin, J., "Family Violence and Culture Care with African and Euro-American Cultures in the United States," in *Transcultural Nursing: Concepts, Theories, Research, and Practice*, 3rd ed., M. Leininger and M. McFarland, eds., Columbus, OH: McGraw-Hill College Custom Series, 2001.

44. Leininger, op. cit., 1978.

45. Leininger, M., *Transcultural Nursing: Concepts, Theories, Research, and Practice*, 2nd ed., Columbus, OH: McGraw-Hill College Custom Series, 1995.

46. McFarland, M., "Use of Culture Care Theory with Anglo- and African American Elders in a

Long-Term Care Setting," *Nursing Science Quarterly*, v. 10, no. 4, 1997, pp. 186–192.

47. Leininger, M., "Southern Rural Black and White American Lifeways with Focus on Care and Health Phenomena," in *Care: The Essence of Nursing and Health*, M. Leininger, ed., Thorofare, NJ: Charles B. Slack, 1984. (Reprinted 1990 by Wayne State University Press, Detroit).

48. Leininger, op. cit., 1991d.

49. Morgan, op. cit., 1996.

50. Chiang, L., "Taiwanese American(s) Culture Care Meanings and Experiences," in *Transcultural Nursing: Concepts, Theories, Research, and Practice*, 3rd ed., M. Leininger and M. McFarland, eds., Columbus, OH: McGraw-Hill College Custom Series, 2001.

51. Leininger, op. cit., 1991b.

52. Leininger, op. cit., 1991c.

53. George, T., "Defining Care in the Culture of the Chronically Mentally Ill Living in the Community," *Journal of Transcultural Nursing*, v. 11, no. 2, 2000, pp. 102–110.

54. Stitzlein, D., *The Phenomenon of Moral Care / Caring Conceptualized Within Leininger's Theory of Culture Care Diversity and Universality*, unpublished doctoral dissertation, Wayne State University, Detroit, Michigan, 1999.

55. Leininger, op. cit., 1991b.

56. Stitzlein, op. cit., 1999.

57. Morris, E., *Culture Care Values, Meanings, Experiences of African American Adolescent Gang Members*, unpublished doctoral dissertation, Wayne State University, Detroit, Michigan, 2001.

58. Leininger, M., "Special Research Report: Dominant Culture Care (Emic) Meanings and Practice Findings from Leininger's Theory," *Journal of Transcultural Nursing*, v. 9, no. 2, pp. 45–56.

59. Leininger, M., "Selected Culture Care Findings of Diverse Cultures Using Culture Care Theory and Ethnomethods," in *Culture Care Diversity and Universality: A Theory of Nursing*, M. Leininger, ed., New York: National League for Nursing Press, 1991e.

60. Ibid.

4

Culture Care Assessments for Congruent Competency Practices

Madeleine Leininger

To be culturally competent means to assess and understand culture, care, and health factors and use this knowledge in creative ways with people of diverse or similar lifeways. LEININGER, 1978

One of the greatest challenges for nurses is to discover how culturally based care factors can make a difference in providing meaningful, appropriate, and satisfying health care to those served. To achieve this goal, nurses need knowledge and skill to do culturalogical health care assessments. This means learning from people about their cultural care values, beliefs, and lifeways to understand their world, their needs, and the ways to provide professional practices. From accurate culturalogical care assessments nurses can greatly expand their understanding of people and discover ways to provide culturally competent, congruent, and responsible care practices.

The purpose of this chapter is to identify and discuss culturally based health care assessments with the goal to provide culture-specific meaningful care to people of different cultures. The author draws on transcultural nursing concepts and principles presented earlier and the theory of Culture Care Diversity and Universality with the Sunrise Model (Figure 3.1 in Chapter 3) and another circular version of the Model (Fig. 4.1 in this chapter) to guide nurses for culture care assessments. Either Sunrise Model has been used to discover holistic influencing factors related to arriving at quality care. The nurse keeps in mind the central goal of assessments to provide culturally congruent, specific, and meaningful care to individuals, families, special groups, or subcultures being served. To achieve this goal one enters the client's world to discover cultural knowledge that is often embedded within individual

and family values and lifeways. The Sunrise Model enables the nurse to discover what is valued, known, and practiced, as well as needs desired but not always attained. Both emic (client) and etic (outside) factors are discovered and used in culturally based assessments.

Environmental context factors and the use of principles presented in Chapter 2 are extremely important in doing any cultural care assessment with individuals families, groups, and institutions. Theoretical perspectives such as the Culture Care theory are kept in mind while using the Sunrise Model along with holding knowledge about the culture(s). Let us turn to the definitions, purposes, and characteristics of culturally based care assessments.

▪ Definition, Purposes, and Characteristics of Effective Cultural Assessments

Cultural care assessments refer to the systematic identification and documentation of culture care beliefs, meanings, values, symbols, and practices of individuals or groups within a holistic perspective, which includes the worldview, life experiences, environmental context, ethnohistory, language, and diverse social structure influences.[1] Culturally based care assessments are directed toward obtaining a holistic or comprehensive picture of informants with their particular factors that are meaningful and important to them. The *goal* of the assessment is to obtain a full and accurate account of

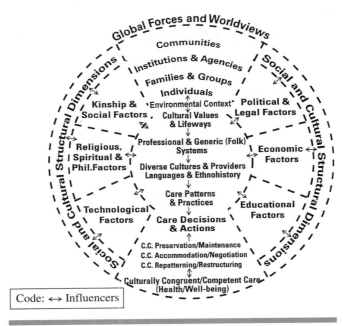

Figure 4.1

Another view of Leininger's Sunrise Model to generate culture competent/congruent care.

the client so that appropriate nursing care decisions can be made with the client for beneficial client health outcomes. The major focus of the assessment is to identify culture care beliefs, values, patterns, expressions, and meanings related to the client's needs for obtaining or maintaining health or to face acute or chronic illness, disabilities, or death.

Culturalogical assessments go beyond the traditional nursing assessments that focus on partial views as psychomotor, physiological, or mental conditions to that of holistic, cultural, environmental, ethnohistorical, and social structure factors, but still consider medical and nursing phenomena. While the traditional nursing areas are given attention, the nurse goes beyond these areas to tap holistic or totality living and functioning dimensions. Nurses are taught in transcultural nursing to use liberal arts and other broad areas of knowledge to get a realistic and accurate picture of people and their health needs or concerns.

The idea of culturally based care and health assessments began with my work in the early 1960s as

I drew on anthropological, cultural, and caring ideas from nursing.[1] It was not, however, until a core of nurses were prepared in transcultural nursing and in anthropology that these assessments were valued, understood, and used.[2] Today, culturalogical health care assessments are viewed as essential in nursing practice to provide accurate, meaningful, and congruent care to cultures. There are, however, some nursing schools and practice settings in which traditional psychomedical aspects are only emphasized in assessments or histories, and the cultural and care dimensions are clearly neglected or not recognized. Nurses prepared in transcultural nursing who use Culture Care theory with the Sunrise Model are especially skilled in doing culturalogical care assessments. These nurses know the great importance of a holistic assessment and can demonstrate the many benefits to clients, other nurses, and consumers.[3]

Today, 40 years later, there are now several models, views, and strategies for culturalogical assessments. Some definitions and models are very limited to small or partial areas of assessment. Other models focus primarily on psychophysiological and medical symptoms and diseases. Some use a few cultural factors and client behaviors or expressions and often use pieces of my assessment models and guidelines. For example, there are models such as Orque et al.,[4] Spector,[5] Parnell,[6] Campinha-Bacote,[7] Giger and Davidhizer,[8] and others. Most of these authors have drawn on my early writings and some from my theory of Culture Care, the Sunrise Model components, and related ideas with partial views. Several are not holistic and fall short to support a full cultural and care assessment. Several focus mostly on culture and not the cultural care aspects. Hence students, clinicians, and faculty always need to assess publications for their limitations and strengths before adopting them. Currently, my full or modified assessment remains the broadest and most holistic one with a specific theoretical perspective to assess outcomes for culturally congruent care. Dobson in 1991 provided a good summary of the different models and their particular focus.[9] Several models are now appearing in the literature, due to the demand for culturally competent care. They need to be thoughtfully assessed to ensure that comprehensive care and culture are fully considered, as well as a theoretical perspective, to guide the process and outcomes.

During the past four decades the author has identified several *purposes* of a culture care assessment. They are as follows:

1. To discover the client's culture care and health patterns and meanings in relation to the client's worldview, lifeways, cultural values, beliefs, practices, context, and social structure factors.
2. To obtain holistic culture care information as a sound basis for nursing care decisions and actions.
3. To discover specific culture care patterns, meanings, and values that can be used to make differential nursing decisions that fit the client's values and lifeways and to discover what professional knowledge can be helpful to the client.
4. To identify potential areas of cultural conflicts, clashes, and neglected areas resulting from emic and etic value differences between clients and professional health personnel.
5. To identify general and specific dominant themes and patterns that need to be known in context for culturally congruent care practices.
6. To identify comparative cultural care information among clients of different or similar cultures, which can be shared and used in clinical, teaching, and research practices.
7. To identify both similarities and differences among clients in providing quality care.
8. To use theoretical ideas and research approaches to interpret and explain practices for congruent care and new areas of transcultural nursing knowledge for discipline users.

Some nurses believe that the major purpose of a cultural assessment is to serve as a culture broker, but this is a limited view and may be a problematic goal. The concept of *culture broker* is derived from anthropology and refers to how one serves as a "mediator" or "broker" between two or more persons with different interests. In nursing one would be mediating between the client's cultural beliefs and values and the nurse's professional goals. While this concept has merit, however, the assessment goes beyond this role. Moreover, the nurse cannot be an effective culture broker or cultural mediator unless the nurse is very knowledgeable about the client's culture and diverse factors influencing the client's needs and lifeways. Health personnel with superficial, biased, or inaccurate views of a client's culture cannot function as effective culture brokers as limited knowledge often leads to many difficulties. For example, a Mexican nurse tried to serve as a culture broker for an Arab Muslim. She failed because she was unaware of the client's cultural background, values, and practices. She also had many biases and misconceptions about Arab Muslim people. To be an effective culture broker requires that the nurse knows general historical factors, as well as political, religious, kinship, and other social structure factors as depicted in the Sunrise Model. The culture broker who is prepared in transcultural nursing will use appropriate skills and holding knowledge to assess and be helpful to clients. Thus, it is very difficult to be a culture broker unless one understands the culture and if the client wants you to be a mediator. Instead, the nurse can serve as a care provider in different ways as discussed in the theory and in general mutually agreed on ways between client and nurse to avoid ethical problems and cultural imposition practices by nurses as cultural brokers. Few health personnel are effective cultural brokers today.

Culture care assessments are much needed today with the current trend that nurses are expected to make nursing diagnoses of clients' conditions such as those proposed by the North American Nursing Diagnoses Association (NANDA) and others, but most recently by the Iowa Classification System.[10,11] Through culturalogical assessment one frequently finds that nursing diagnostic labels and assessments are inadequate. Many diagnoses are derived from Western cultures and fail to fit non-Western cultures, minorities, or underrepresented cultures and subcultures. Diagnosing or labeling clients' behavior and needs in ways that are culturally inaccurate creates a host of ethical problems and often destructive outcomes. Most nursing diagnostic taxonomies or classificatory systems are heavily biomedically focused and fail to accurately include cultural and care knowledge. Diagnoses also fail to include accurate cultural language terms and specific emic cultural data. Gross cultural knowledge deficits exist with many classificatory schemes showing a lack of culture care knowledge and accurate assessments of clients from a specific culture.[12] For an accurate assessment, specific cultural terms and conditions need to be identified, understood, and correctly used to prevent serious misunderstandings and destructive practices. Moreover, some cultures do not have some Western medical diseases, symptoms, or explanations. Instead, these cultures may have unique kinds of human conditions that need to be assessed in *their cultural context* such as *susto* (magical fright), *evil eye*, and many other conditions. Many of these transcultural nursing problems and ethical issues have been discussed by the author in other sources.[13] In general, nurses must be grounded in transcultural nursing and other culture knowledge of Western and non-Western cultures before using global diagnostic labels to prevent grave problems with diagnostic labeling and a host of ethical, legal, moral, and other issues related to misdiagnosis and inappropriate treatment and care of clients of specific cultures. For example, a nursing diagnosis of "*Alterations Needed in Parenting*" with a Russian, Sioux, or Mexican child was a most questionable diagnosis and care plan as the nurse was ignorant of child-parenting practices, values, and lifeways of these cultures. Western nurses have exported such diagnostic systems to non-Western cultures, and tran-

scultural nurses are dealing today with these inappropriate exports. Thus, as the author has recommended since the early 1970s, such diagnostic and many culturally medical-bound labels should not be used until nurses are knowledgeable about cultures and transcultural nursing because of their potential destructive outcomes.

 ## Use of the Sunrise Model and Principles for a Culture Care Assessment

Instead of the focus on using the above diagnosis approach, let us turn to using the Sunrise Model as an extremely helpful and comprehensive guide for culture care assessments. In looking at Figure 4.1, the nurse can envision a total or holistic picture of many factors to be understood and assessed. Pharmacists, dental assistants, physicians, social workers, health anthropologists, and others in the health field have found that the Sunrise Model offers an excellent assessment guide to grasp the *totality* of the client's needs and lifeways. The Sunrise Model and Culture Care theory can be used with slight modifications by other disciplines according to their particular discipline interests and therapeutic goals. However, the nurse uses the Sunrise Model to assess the cultural care needs of individuals, families, groups, cultures, communities, and/or institutions in their naturalistic settings. The nurse keeps in mind the central focus of nursing regarding human care as the essence of nursing, but examines cultural factors to get full data and accurate meanings.[14] One can begin anywhere in the Sunrise Model according to one's focus, interest, or domain(s) of inquiry. For example, the nurse may see an urgent need to assess the kinship and technology uses along with generic folk practices seen as of concern to African mothers and their care needs during pregnancy. The nurse would start with these areas of the model, but ultimately needs to assess all factors in the model to get a comprehensive and accurate assessment.

The Sunrise Model serves as a guide to assess different holistic factors that tend to influence the clients' care and health. The major areas as seen in the model for assessment are worldview, environmental context, and social structure factors. The latter area includes the following:

1. Cultural values, beliefs, and practices.
2. Religious, philosophical, or spiritual beliefs.
3. Economic factors.
4. Educational beliefs.
5. Technology views.
6. Kinship and social ties.
7. Political and legal factors.

In addition, the nurse assesses generic (emic) folk and professional (etic) beliefs, practices, and experiences related to the client's cultural interpretations, experiences, and explanations with a caring focus. Ethnohistorical and environmental context factors also need to be assessed in general ways as they bear on care and health. The environmental context includes physical and social features, food resources, home conditions, and related factors.[15] Material cultural factors such as housing, land, water supplies, technologies used, and other factors are assessed to get a comprehensive picture of the client in his daily living environment. The nurse assesses these with a health care focus and draws on appropriate medical, nursing, liberal arts, and other knowledge relevant for professional care.

In using the Sunrise Enabler Model to obtain a holistic picture of the client(s), one should understand the different dimensions related to worldview, social structure, and all other domains of inquiry as offered in Appendix 4-A. Holding knowledge of these areas helps one to reflect on what one sees and hears. These areas such as ethnohistory and social structure factors are explored with the client. I have offered some communication "lead-ins" to tap gently the domains of inquiry to help nurses follow or enter the client's world. It is difficult for some clients to talk about these areas without nurses' understanding of them and some indirect suggestions, aids or examples. Thus the nurse is encouraged to study Appendix 4-A *before* using the Sunrise Model as background preparation for the assessment. The principles of doing the assessment (which follow soon) should also be studied in advance.

While doing the assessment, the nurse remains open to the client's ideas and leads. Granted, sizable amounts of data can be discovered with the Sunrise Model assessment. The nurse makes nonobtrusive brief notations which are later processed in full by diverse methods often using modern electronic data processing. The nurse seeks general knowledge of different dimensions such as folk and professional practices but also other areas. One remains a very active listener and observer of the client and context where the assessment occurs and constantly reflects on what *one sees, hears, and discovers* with very little interference in the flow of the client's ideas. The nurse reflects on the ideas with different dimensions on the model such as religion, kinship, and technologies and how they help to know care, health, or illness aspects. One must remain alert to special words or phrases used by the client as many may be special cultural terms and meanings. Nonverbal communication and use of space and language patterns (tone, style, body gestures) are also identified. Keeping an open mind and learning attitude is crucial to discover the client's ideas and not impose one's own views and interpretations. It is important to note subtle differences and commonalities about the client's ideas and views in relation to others in the culture for a later comparative view. With each assessment one can increase and perfect assessment skills and grasp comparative and highly individualistic needs.

Principles for Culturalogical Assessment

Since the nurse relies on general principles to guide the assessment for a comprehensive and holistic database, several principles will now be identified.[16,17] The *first principle is to show a genuine and sincere interest in the client as one listens to and learns from the client.* Respecting the client and being sincere and honest is crucial. The nurse tells the client of an interest to learn about cultural values, beliefs, and lifeways to provide good care. Showing genuine interest and respect are most important throughout the entire assessment.

The *second principle is to give attention to gender or class differences, communication modes (with special language terms), and interpersonal space.* The nurse gives attention to the gender or class roles and to styles of communicating and use of space. Physical appearance, gender, and class of the client are also observed and noted with this principle on culture and care aspects.

The *third principle is to study the Sunrise Model dimensions and Culture Care theory before doing the assessment to draw on and use different components of the Sunrise Model and their interrelationships.* A visual image and knowledge of the model serves as a road map and ascertains that all areas are considered for a holistic assessment. The nurse keeps alert to whatever the client wishes to share and explores ideas with focus on culture, care values, religion, kinship relationships, and other factors depicted in the model (Figs. 3.1 or 4.1).

A *fourth principle for an effective culture care assessment is that the nurse needs to remain fully aware of one's own cultural biases and prejudices.* As discussed earlier, nurse misconceptions, biases, prejudgments, and narrow views can greatly limit an accurate assessment. Some nurses have strong lifetime and negative views or prejudices about a culture that influence and distort what they see, hear, and interpret from clients.[18] Nurses from strikingly different cultures than the client may hold predetermined views about the culture that become evident in talking with the client and during the final assessment. Family and community biases are often related to cultural ignorance and blindness that limit reliable and accurate client data. The nurse's attitudes and viewpoints need to be assessed by oneself or a mentor often during client assessments. Currently, there is a belief in the culture of nursing that nurses from the client's culture are the best nurses to assess them. This may not be accurate because of nurses' own cultural blindness, strong ethnocentric tendencies, and sometimes being acculturated to an entirely different culture than the client's. Indeed, cultural blindness and cultural ignorance are two serious factors limiting effective nursing assessments and care practices. *Cultural blindness refers to the inability to know another culture because of cultural biases, attitudes, and prejudices.* Cultural blindness is generally related to strong ethnocentrism, cultural ignorance, and a lack of transcultural knowledge about a culture. Nurses may be acculturated to another culture and unable to see and know their own traditional and current culture. Or, if the person dislikes one's culture, they may not want to be identified with the culture and remain blind to it or deny it. Accordingly, health personnel need to assess their own cultural biases, prejudices, and other factors that limit accurate assessments. Transcultural

nursing mentors can be most helpful to deal with cultural blindness, biases, and myths about cultures and their own tendencies. Students in transcultural nursing are required to know and deal with their own cultural biases under a mentor's supervision. "Know thyself" remains critical and essential in transcultural nursing.

The *fifth principle to guide the nurse in doing a culturalogical assessment is to be aware that clients may belong to subcultures or special groups such as the homeless, AIDS and HIV infected, drug users, lesbians, gays, the deaf, and the mentally retarded, a knowledge of which is required to assess accurately.* These groups are often subcultures with particular cultural patterns, values, norms, and practices that fit with the criteria of a subculture. *Subcultures are small or large groups living in a dominate culture that retain certain values and beliefs that are different from the dominant culture.*[19] Subcultures show differences in their special ways of living that make them different in certain areas from the dominant culture and require attention to such subtleties as dress, actions, lifestyles, beliefs, and other areas. Often, these groups are labeled strange, odd, unacceptable, or questionable by the dominant culture. Gays, lesbians, the homeless, the retarded, the elderly, and others show patterns of living that are different yet unique. Nurses need to be aware of such subcultures in any society with their special features and health care needs. They must also be respected for their rights to be understood, heard, and assessed and to receive culturally congruent care that fits their lifeways.

While doing assessments, stereotyping of cultures is a transcultural nursing taboo and of concern. *Stereotyping refers to seeing people in rigid, fixed, or "cookbook" ways with prejudged views about them and their lifeways.* Nurses need to avoid stereotyping and profiling of people as it leads to the analogy of putting people "in a box and nailing it closed." Stereotyping and profiling people and cultures into tight molds limits individual variations and can be inaccurate and demeaning. There are many different role-playing exercises and games used in transcultural nursing to prevent stereotyping and prejudgements about cultures. Transcultural nurse mentors can help to deal with such long-standing prejudices. Practicing cultural care assessments in the classroom before working with clients is important to change attitudes and develop new skills and insights. In clinical settings transcultural nurse specialists are also helpful to staff nurses and interdisciplinary colleagues in identifying and dealing with stereotyping and other cultural discrimination and injustice practices.

The *sixth principle is that nurses need to know their own culture and areas of competencies along with their deficits to become culturally competent practitioners.* Nurses need to know their own cultural heritage, values, and lifeways as this influences assessment outcomes. This principle became especially evident to me when I first went to New Guinea. While I had some general ideas about my mother's Irish and my father's German American cultural values and roots, I discovered them more clearly as I studied the Gadsup and compared their lifeways with mine. Assessing a strange culture can make one keenly aware of one's own cultural differences and lifeway tendencies. Sometimes, nurses want to be like another culture and take on such lifeways and practices. Some may strongly deny one's own culture. Assessing a culture that is markedly different from one's own forces one to think anew, whereas a culture that is similar tends to make the nurse assume they "know all about the culture." Major differences between cultures can lead nurses to experience culture shock or to avoid learning about the people. The idea of knowing about a very different or strange culture I first learned from Margaret Mead in the 1950s; she always held that one learned and remembered more about a "new" or different culture than a familiar one. Accordingly, the shockingly different lifeways of the non-Western Gadsup in the 1960s with my American culture stimulated me to discover how they lived without technologies and Western comforts. Assessing sharp cultural differences and discovering why cultures are different or similar then leads to many new breakthroughs in knowledge and practices. Similarities within and between cultures is also important, but requires astute observations that are often subtle or not clearly overt.

The *seventh principle to guide the nurse in doing a cultural care assessment is to clarify and explain at the outset to the individual, family, or group the focus and purpose of the assessment, including times to visit with them about their health care beliefs and practices.* Since cultural assessments are quite different from "hands on" medical or physical assessments or psychosomatic exams, clients may wonder about them. The nurse should realize that assessments take more time and patience with clients and a broad knowledge base. Assessments in hospital settings often have to fit the busy hospital schedule. So the nurse has shorter times with the client, but arranges for several sessions. The nurse and the client need a reasonably quiet place so that disruptions will be minimal and that the client and nurse can talk about different areas in the Sunrise Model. Since a cultural care assessment may be a new experience for some clients, the nurse will often need to repeatedly clarify to the client and to others on the unit about the importance of the assessment to provide culturally competent care. Clients generally like the assessments as they value sharing ideas about their culture, family folk care, and practices, and hope that nurses will incorporate their ideas into their care.

The *eighth principle is to seek a holistic view of the client's world within his or her environmental context by focusing on familiar and multiple factors depicted in the Sunrise Model that influence care, illness, or wellbeing.* The Culture Care theory helps to explain and get a holistic or total client picture in their natural and familiar home or work environment. The nurse remains alert to use nursing, medical, and humanistic knowledge sources to understand the client in his or her environment. Traditional medical and nursing views that fail to include environmental, cultural, and other factors limit a holistic view. It may take time for some clients to focus on holistic culture care factors because they may be oriented to the medical diseases, symptoms, medications, and treatment modes. Encouraging clients to reflect on their cultural beliefs, values, and lifeways often stimulates them to renew their values with hopes that medicine, nursing, and others will incorporate their values into their health care. For example, an Arab Muslim woman from Saudi Arabia experienced severe cultural pain because she was very upset in the labor and delivery room with an American male physician delivering her baby. The female Arab client's values were counter to the Anglo-American male physician treatment modes especially touching and putting lights on her vagina and trying to deliver her baby. She became very upset and demanded a female physician who came to deliver the child. Today, many clients want culturally congruent care that is not offensive or counter to their cultural values and practices. Cultural assessments and education help to avoid these critical incidents. Many cultures, minorities, immigrants, and subcultures are becoming aware that *their* cultural practices should be respected such as the Armenian woman who said to the author, "I have long waited for this day, as I have been in this country for 20 years and never felt comfortable to talk about my cultural background, values, interests, and care expectations and now I can." Such statements and others reaffirm the need and benefits of culturalogically-based care and assessments and practices to fit people's needs.

The ninth principle is to remain an active listener and to discover the clients' emic *lifeways, beliefs, and values as well as* etic *professional ways, to fit client expectations and create a climate that is trusting so that the client feels it is safe and beneficial to share one's beliefs and lifeways.* Of course, some clients are more eager than others to share their beliefs and experiences such as Italians, Jews, Eastern Europeans, and Anglo-Americans. The way the client wants to be cared for or about is important, as well as preventing illnesses. Western clients are usually conditioned to recite medical symptoms, diseases, and medical treatments to health personnel which often makes it difficult to focus on their cultural lifeways, history, values, and beliefs. In contrast non-Western clients, I found from my research, view their family lifeways and folk caring practices of first importance.[20] Storytelling has long been valuable to non-Western and minority cultures, and only recently is this method or approach being emphasized by Western health care practitioners. Helping clients to be active sharers and participants in the assessment and to learn together about care and health patterns is a transcultural art and skill.

The tenth principle is to reflect on learned "transcultural holding knowledge" about the client's culture and research-based care and health knowledge available today. Using such culturally based knowledge and reflecting on what is being shared such as the evil eye, good and bad spirits, *susto* (fright), and many other cultural conditions with the care practices gives meaning and credibility to what is shared. Holding knowledge of such cultural conditions in advance helps the nurse to reflect upon and clarify the ideas directly with the client. Statements such as, "Tell me about *susto* or your condition," or "I would like to learn about your expe-

rience with your illness," or "Tell me about ways you care for your family." These are gateways for in-depth knowledge to understand what is being said and the meanings. Key cultural linguistic terms should be jotted down to be accurate and used in the assessment. Very few direct questions are used, but rather indirect and inquiry comments such as, "Could you tell me more about your experiences at home?" or "I would like to learn about your daily lifeways, your work, and your family." Reflections without cultural holding knowledge often leads to errors.

During the assessment the nurse remains alert to intergenerational differences and similarities within or between generations to discover changes in cultural values and practices influencing care practices over time. Intergenerational male and female role-taking differences are noted, especially in relation to human caring and health, along with social structure and historical factors influencing these changes. So, throughout the assessment, the nurse maintains a flexible and open attitude with a willingness *to listen and move with the client's* ideas and interpretations. Actually, there are no rigidly prescribed steps or prescribed technique for a culture assessment as it is a dynamic discovery and sensitive process to grasp the client's world about cultural meanings of care, health, sickness, and lifeways. *Moving with the client's thinking and interests and clarifying what is shared is an important principle.* If the above principles are understood, valued, and maintained, the nurse will obtain valuable insights and new data to make sound care decisions and actions appropriate for congruent care practices.

It is important to keep in mind that the nurse is not expected to cover fully and in detail all domains depicted in the Sunrise Model, but rather captures dominant themes and patterns from current and subsequent sessions with the client. It is wise to begin the assessment with comments such as, "I would like to learn about some of your ideas, experiences, and beliefs and about how you would like to be cared for or about while here." Or "I would like to learn about your cultural heritage or family roots to understand you and your care needs." Or "What would you like to share with me today about your lifeways." The first session is often in the hospital or clinic and is about 20 minutes in length but subsequent visits are usually longer, especially in the home. Allowing time between sessions for the client to think about ideas related to cultural beliefs, care, or health values with the nurse is important. During the early sessions, some clients may wonder if the nurse can be trusted and if the nurse is truly genuinely interested in the client's culture and may "test" the nurse on these areas. Distrust indicators usually reflect tension, caution, and sparse and inaccurate information. The nurse needs to use the *Stranger to Trusted Friend Enabler* (Fig. 3.3 in Chapter 3) to assess how to become a trusted friend with the client, group or family by using the indicators in the model.

Special Author Insights

From the author's 40 years of doing cultural care assessments, clients from non-Western cultures like to talk first about their family and their caring values and health beliefs, whereas those from Western cultures (particularly Anglo-Americans) like to talk initially about medical treatments, tests, medications, technologies, and their highly personal life and illness experiences. Transculturally, considerable variability exists among males and females worldwide in what they wish to share. The nurse holds in abeyance her experiences and views as this can lead to cultural imposition of ideas to please the nurse's interests. After each session the nurse always thanks the client or family in a sincere way and leaves the door open to bring forth new or reinforced ideas. If the client refuses a culturalogical assessment, the nurse respects such wishes. However, most clients find many benefits with the assessment and are eager to share their stories, beliefs, and lifeways as new modes of health care.

The real secret for an effective culturalogical care assessment is to remain an *active learner and reflector* of what the client has shared and what the client deems important. If the assessment is done in the client's home, the nurse has a wonderful opportunity to see firsthand the client's naturalistic environment and material culture items and often to meet family members or guests. Seeing the client's cultural context is extremely helpful, as well as talking with them about how they care for one another with their generic (emic) care practices and with local healers and curers. For example, a Mexican American woman wanted me to visit with her at the kitchen table and later to walk outside to see her many herbal plants (the generic folk herbs) that she

and her family used daily to "keep them well." She also introduced me to traditional healers and their roles and practices. Her home and garden were filled with folk herbs that have been used over time and intergenerationally for many different health conditions. They were taught healing ways from family elders, which reduced costs, and they seldom used professional hospital services. Other Mexicans in nearby homes came and told how they live and help one another and especially how children, elderly, and the dying are cared for. Within four visits much was learned about emic and etic care patterns with Mexican American families. Culture care preservation and maintenance were clearly and repeatedly noted and used.

It has also been interesting to note that negative experiences or stories are usually told at the end of the sessions along with valuable and "sacred cultural secrets," including those regarding generic local healers and cultural spiritualists and their practices. The reasons for this are to be sure one is trusted and will respect their cultural secrets and to be sure the nurse is a "genuinely trusted friend." If the assessment is done in the clinic or hospital, the sessions usually take more time as there are always many interruptions by other health personnel with medical regimes to be done. In addition, cultural secrets are often not revealed in the hospital as the clients fear that they will be recorded in the chart or that they will be demeaned by staff. Cultural minorities are often cautious to talk in hospitals and clinics about folk practices.

In general, culturalogical assessments are extremely valuable and essential for health care. I have found over the past five decades that culturalogical care assessments have not only been informative to get accurate and full data, but to grasp in-depth and accurate meanings of care, health, and life experiences of clients. One must however, be patient, persistent, and open to learn from others. Rich and meaningful data have been generated about care, health, well-being, illness consequences, and other areas with the Sunrise Model, the theory of Culture Care, and the Trusted-Friend Enabler. Such rich scientific data are often embedded in social structure factors such as family relationships, religion, politics, economics, and philosophy of life, which takes time to tease out gently and sensitively. These are scientific and credible data to be used with the three modes of the theory to arrive at culturally congruent and therapeutic health outcomes or for facing disabilities or death.[21] Indeed, cultural assessments must be congruent with the client's lifeways to be useable, beneficial, and acceptable to client's emic knowing world. Generic (emic) and professional (etic) knowledge should be integrated or blended together to provide *culturally congruent care* as discussed and shown in Chapter 5, Figure 5.1. The reader is encouraged to visit this synthesized Figure 5.1 to understand how cultural assessment emic data can or should be integrated with professional etic knowledge and practices to attain and maintain congruent care. Effective culturalogical assessments are the reality means to get into the clients' world and let them experience a sense of control and power with their ideas of what will be caring and beneficial to them within their cultural orientation and lifeways. There is nothing more valuable in health care than having good skills to do a holistic care assessment, and transcultural nurses have led the way to show how and why care assessments are beneficial to clients and rewarding to care providers.

 Transcultural Communication Modes

The challenge in doing culturalogical assessments today is understanding the many verbal and nonverbal modes of many diverse cultures. Transcultural communication has become extremely important for any assessment or to provide care to immigrants, refugees, and many indigenous people residing in a given country for short or long periods of time. Unfortunately, with some exceptions most USA nurses can speak only one language, and yet the nurse works more directly and often more continuously with clients than other health personnel. Understanding clients' verbal and nonverbal communication is imperative today in this multicultural world. Nurses should speak at least two languages today and in the future even more, and language learning should begin in grade schools and continue throughout the lifecycle. Nurse educators need to require language skills to care for clients of diverse cultures and to meet a critical need today for education, research, and consultation.

Nurses and health professions also need to learn about transcultural nonverbal communication for their meanings and especially when one cannot speak the client's language. Body language expressions are forms of communication and are culturally patterned. Facial expressions vary transculturally and need to be accurately interpreted. For example, most Anglo-Americans tend to maintain direct eye contact, whereas several Native Americans avoid direct eye contact as do Asians. Direct eye focus may be viewed as rude and a cultural taboo with some cultures. Moreover to "save face" in communicating with many non-Western cultures, direct eye contact by Westerners is often viewed as aggressive and threatening. Slapping Arab Muslims on the back is generally offensive and disrespectful. In Japan and in China one makes a deep bow of the head and body to greet and respect a guest or stranger from another culture. Shaking hands and showing broad smiles may be offensive in some cultures, yet often used by Anglo-Americans and Europeans. Crossing one's arms over one's chest is often viewed as a hostile act to non-Westerners, as well as crossing one's legs when talking to a stranger. These body languages are only a few important nonverbal communication expressions to learn and respect of cultures. Anthropologists such as Birdwhistell Hall and other linguistic scientists have studied different patterns of nonverbal communication and gesture language in many cultures over time.[22] Nurses need to use literature from scientists who have thoroughly studied and documented such findings and their meanings. Currently, some nurses are publishing books and articles on cross-cultural communications that lack accuracy or credibility because of the absence of in-depth language knowledge of cultures. Miscommunication of verbal and nonverbal expressions can lead to serious problems and destructive outcomes in client and family care.

In communicating with different cultures, there are many styles or patterned ways that people share their ideas. Figure 4.2 shows some common transcultural communication modes that nurses need to consider. These modes with the cultures are very helpful to illustrate different patterns of communication that one can anticipate in assessments and in caring processes. If aware of these differences, the nurse needs to be patient for a reply, especially with those cultures that communicate through extended families as with Mexicans and Southeast Asians or through several persons as with Europeans and Arabs. An awareness of these patterns is very useful in assessment and in daily care.

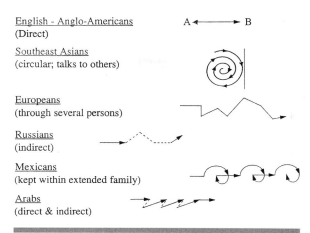

Figure 4.2
Transcultural communication modes.

However, there are other *patterns of communication* such as African Americans who like direct eye contact (often prolonged), speak with feeling and emotional gestures, and watch for times to speak. In contrast, Native Americans in the United States and Canada use an indirect look when speaking or listening, speak softly and slowly, use limited emotional gestures, like silent periods, and are seldom aggressive or interrupt others. As one reflects on Anglo-Americans, one finds (with individual variabilities) that they are very quick and direct to respond to whatever is being said; maintain eye contact while talking and listening; usually speak fast and loud; try to control the conversation; and use their hands, head, and body language as they state their "facts" or objective "scientific" evidence. This pattern of communication contrasts with traditional Vietnamese families that avoid eye contact when talking or listening to others (especially those viewed in high-status roles), speak softly and cautiously, and often delay giving any verbal answer or quick response using limited affective gestures. Since transcultural communication is focused on sending and receiving ideas or messages, these cultural differences are important to understand; however, one should always realize that cultural differences will exist in any cultures. Hence, this is why *patterns* are emphasized as they are more constant and consistent.

Much could be written about nonverbal communication and body expressions in different cultures.

Kinesics is the term that *refers to body movements' communication modes, which include posture, facial expressions (smile or anger), gestures, eye contact, and other body features.* Body expressions have different meanings transculturally as noted above with Asians and Anglo-Americans. Head, face, and hand movements are particularly important as nurses care for the culturally different. In New Guinea and with several other cultures nodding one's head up and down means "no" rather that yes. Shaking hands to greet others varies, but is a taboo in some cultures. Latin Americans shake hands firmly and actively for a period of time. With Asians and some Arab Muslims hand touching is a taboo. For Arab Moslems, shaking with the left hand is an obscenity as it is the unclean hand, while the right is "clean" and is used for food preparation and consumption. Hence, medicines should not be given to Arab Muslims in the left hand, but rather in the right hand. Japanese, Thai, Chinese, and other Asians generally bow their heads rather than shake hands as this has long been a cultural practice with deep respect and status significance.

Proxemics is another essential concept to understand in transcultural communication. *It refers to the use and perception of interpersonal or personal space in sociocultural interactions.*[23] In 1966 Hall identified and discussed the importance of proxemics and how cultures use space. For example, he found there were interpersonal distances or zones that were important. Americans liked personal space of 1/2 to 4 feet, social space of 4 to 13 feet, and public space (lectures and speeches) greater than 12 feet. In contrast, other cultures as Africans, Latin American, Indonesians, and French like closeness to relate to others. Personal space has major implications in doing an assessment and of where one stands or sits to talk to a client. Proxemics is very important in client care in the home, hospital, and other settings. Sitting behind a desk to interview or assess a client is often unacceptable for many non-Western immigrants, minorities, and strangers.

Finally, within the many areas of transcultural communication, a few pointers need to be given about the *use of interpreters to get accurate assessments.* Today, there are many articles and books about working with interpreters. It is important to study interpreter uses with researchers who have had direct working experiences in seeking health care information. From my experiences and other transcultural nurse experts, these interpreter points should be kept in mind:

1. Be sure the interpreter knows the client's cultural language and knows the culture.
2. Discuss in advance what you are doing in the assessment and its purposes to the client.
3. Insist on an exact interpretation from the client, not the interpreter's views of a desired response.
4. Write out terms in both languages to check when you are in doubt about the terms spoken or the interpreter's interpretation.
5. Try to get an interpreter of the relatively same age as younger clients, as children and teenagers may often communicate different intergenerational knowledge leading to errors in the data and different information.
6. Try to know a few words or phrases in the language being interpreted to occasionally check if the interpreter is sharing ideas accurately and completely (sometimes an interpreter may shorten or omit informant ideas for her or his personal reasons or comfortableness).
7. Always thank the interpreter afterward, and recheck ideas or observations that are unclear to you.

Central Goal and Steps to Provide Culturally Competent and Congruent Care

Goal

To provide respectful, meaningful, and competent care to people of diverse cultures that leads to health and well-being or to face death or disabilities of individuals or groups.

Ten Guideline Steps for Culturally Competent Congruent Care

1. Have holding knowledge of the individual or family culture being assessed from reliable literature and through transcultural nursing courses taught by qualified faculty.

2. Know your own cultural heritage, patterns, and biases and factors that may interfere with effective assessments and understanding the client.
3. Use a theory or theoretical perspective to guide your assessment such as the holistic Culture Care theory with use of the Sunrise Model and Enablers.
4. Know some common language phrases of the client to obtain accurate information and to work with qualified interpreters.
5. Show respect and a genuine interest in the informant and the culture while remaining an active learner, letting the informant tell his or her story, experiences, and ideas to you.
6. Be observant of the environmental context in which you are doing the assessment and document it.
7. As the client shares emic or etic data, reflect on and check the meanings with the client. (Be sure you get a holistic perspective as depicted in the Sunrise Model for a total and accurate picture of client/family needs and expectations.)
8. The client needs to be an active co-participant in the assessment to obtain credible and accurate data, especially with the Culture Care theory and the three modes of action and decision, and to provide culturally specific and congruent care.
9. Identify and then recheck specific and general cultural care values, beliefs, and needs related to generic (emic) and professional (etic) data for possibly integrated culturally congruent care.
10. Use the assessment findings in sensitive, knowing, creative, and meaningful ways with the client so that beneficial and satisfying outcomes are forthcoming. Do a follow-up with the client or family to document goal outcome(s).

From the outset, keep in mind the author's definition of *culturally competent and congruent care, that is, the use of culturally based care knowledge that is used in assistive, facilitative, sensitive, creative, safe, and meaningful ways to individuals or groups for beneficial and satisfying health and well-being or to face death, disabilities, or difficult human life conditions.*[24]

Color Insert 5 helps to envision the assessment process to arrive at culturally congruent actions and decisions. This figure should be kept in mind as one works with individuals and families or in community or institutional agencies.

Differences in individual and intergenerational assessments, as depicted in the four-generation assessment in Color Insert 6, make one realize that intergenerational assessments take more time, but can be very valuable to trace culture care, health, and illness patterns. The informants are encouraged to be active sharers for comparative generational perspectives. Families often say how much they learn from intergenerational family assessments.

Color Insert 7 shows a transcultural nurse visiting with a Southern Christian Sudanese client as a refugee living in the midwestern United States. The client wanted to wear her native attire to tell sad stories about her African country, family deaths, and how she became a refugee, leaving many of her extended kinsfolk in Sudan under terrible war conditions. The assessment took 20 hours (5 sessions) over 1 month at a refugee house. She always wore this same attire to make her feel "back home" as she talked about caring and noncaring, illnesses, family member killings, and the destruction of her home village. She looked forward to each visit and said they were most helpful to heal her sad experiences and memories.

An Alternative Short Assessment Guide

Another alternative assessment guide, which has been used with undergraduate and graduate students since 1985 and with nursing staff in short-term emergency and acute care centers, has been my *Short Culturalogical Assessment Guide* (Fig. 4.3).[25] This guide provides a brief and general assessment of the client, but does not usually provide in-depth holistic features as found with the Sunrise Model. It has, however, been very helpful to nurses functioning in an acute care or emergency setting where time and space constraints are very limiting. The assessment data offer general information to develop a quick nursing care plan or to make decisions about a client from a particular culture. The author often refers to this assessment guide as Model B to contrast it with the Sunrise Model (Model A). The nurse begins

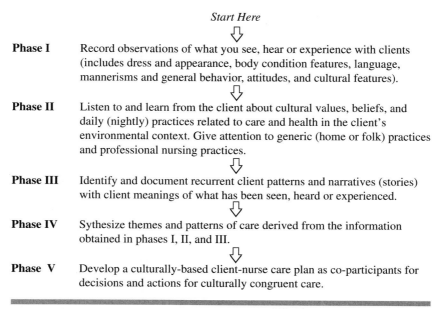

Figure 4.3
Leininger's short culturalogical assessment guide (Model B).

with Phase I and proceeds to Phase V to get an overall assessment of the client. Each phase has a clear focus and can be readily followed. One should indicate at the outset whether assessing an individual, small group, or family.

Caring Rituals Important to Assess

In doing culture care assessments there are special areas bearing on caring patterns and healing that provide valuable information. Practically all cultures have caring rituals that are sequenced activities people use to maintain wellness, prevent illness, ease dying, or regain health. *Generic (folk) caring rituals* are learned and used in the home, but they may be in demand in hospitals or clinics because they are held to be therapeutic and essential to clients. Generic folk caring rituals generally serve specific functions when used thoughtfully in the home or hospital. Nurses need to discover these particular rituals for their healing or other benefits with different cultures. Cultures have rituals in caring for one's skin, hair, and body and for gaining or losing weight. For example, Africans have very special rituals for their hair and to keep their skin healthy. Such rituals have cultural functions such as reassurance, security, protection, and feeling good. Rituals provide a sense of well-being through activities that need to be regularly performed each day or night. Professionals can learn these cultural rituals and develop ways that care rituals can be creatively used in transcultural practices with the client or family. Most rituals have healing attributes if one studies their benefits as learned from clients and from professional insights. Let us consider some types of caring rituals that nurses ought to know or be ready to learn:

1. *Eating Rituals*: All human beings have regular times and patterns of eating that are generally ritualized and expected to be respected. For example, in some cultures the people always wash their hands and put on clean clothes before eating, but the rituals and materials vary. Some traditional cultures still eat only in special attire because "our family has always done this" as the Japanese and some Southeast Asian cultures. Then there is the way the food is eaten, whether by fingers or tools. For example, the British

use their forks with prongs down, whereas Americans use forks with prongs upward. Chinese use chop sticks and other cultures use their fingers. Certain foods are ritually prepared and only eaten on special occasions. Arab Muslims eat no pork and drink no alcohol. Polish and Germans enjoy special sausage cooked in special ritualized ways for festive occasions. The nurse needs to know these rituals, culturally taboo foods, class or gender preferences, and especially ritually prepared cold and hot foods for clients when ill or well. The environmental setting and who eats and may pray together are important in several cultures. In several non-Western cultures women only eat after men have eaten the choicest foods. Children and teenagers have many rituals such as ways of eating an egg, fruit, or meat and drinking beverages. These rituals should be respected and facilitated in the hospital and can make a big difference in maintaining one's health. Poor and oppressed people eat food in many ways to survive.

2. *Daily and Nightly Ritual Care Activities*: It is always fascinating to observe the client's patterns of daily and nightly care rituals. What daily personal exercises are done each morning or evening are helpful to know. For example, traditional and many present-day Japanese maintain their early morning Tai Chi exercises for health and spiritual well-being. Americans now have many morning, noon, and evening running, walking, and other physical rituals to keep them well, to prevent heart illnesses, and to keep in good physical condition. Some cultures have praying rituals such as Arab-Muslims who pray five times a day using prayer rugs and beads and wash their hands and bodies before praying. Such ritual activities need to be respected, assessed, and understood for their meaning and contribution to cultural health or well-being. Nurses can often accommodate these expected ritual activities in the daily care plan and facilitate them if beneficial. Roman Catholics and other faith groups have prayer rituals for the sick and dying, which need to be respected and supported as priests, ministers, and family members carry out the religious rites with clients of diverse faiths. Assessing their effect on the clients' health is important.

3. *Sleep and Rest Ritual Patterns*: Cultures have patterns of sleep and rest that have usually been

established early in life and maintained throughout the lifecycle for their health maintenance. Children and elderly especially like and expect rituals of eating and sleeping. What are these rituals in different cultures, and how are they incorporated in nursing care practices? Nursing faculty and textbooks often fail to recognized cultural differences in eating, sleeping, and praying. If rituals are not known and used, how do they affect the well-being or lead to unfavorable client outcomes? Sleep and rest cultural patterns are especially important today in this busy and pressured world of tasks and activities. Such rituals are usually important to provide culturally congruent care for client health maintenance and preservation.

There are additional cultural rituals related to folk healing and caring that need to be learned from clients and studied for their uses in professional caring. Integrated generic and professional rituals are an important part of transcultural nursing care. Knowing and respecting generic emic healing rituals are being reestablished with many cultures, and nurses are expected to know these rituals and help the client use them. If rituals are nonbeneficial to the client, they need to be assessed and discussed with the client, family, and health care providers.

Lifecycle Rituals

Transcultural nurses and anthropologists have been studying lifecycle rituals in diverse cultures for many years to discover commonalties and differences related to healing and health. *Lifecycle rituals are especially crucial because they demonstrate patterns of caring for health, as well as illnesses and generic folk lifeways.* Life span rituals can help nurses know and value care from birth to old age if identified and respected. Hence, lifecycle rituals should be assessed and studied from birth and at special times as with marriage, death and specific illness, and wellness in cultures for their therapeutic or nontherapeutic outcomes. (See Chapter 10 for full lifecycle rituals.)

Some lifecycle cultural rituals are stressful, but most fit the culture and are held as essential and beneficial. One of the oldest theories about rituals comes from van Gennep in his classic study, *The Rites of Passage*, which was originally published in 1908.[26] Van

Gennep hypothesized that there were major phases of human rites of passage, which he identified as follows: 1) *a phase of separation,* 2) *a phase of transition, and* 3) *a phase of incorporation.* Persons experienced these phases in the lifecycle and when changing positions or statuses such as being separated from their past role and taking on a new role. One moves into the second phase as a transitional phase, but with uncertain role expectations. In the last phase, people learn to take on and incorporate a new role or position in the culture that gives them recognition or status such as being married, becoming a nurse, or becoming an elder or a prisoner. Rites of passage and rituals are extremely important to study in every culture as they are often unique and yet have some commonalities when used with the theory of Culture Care and with van Gennep's cultural perspectives.

Nurse and Hospital Rituals

Nurses and even the "tribes of nursing" have many rituals that are often not recognized nor assessed, and yet they exist in hospitals and other settings wherever nurses function or live.[27] There are nursing rituals of administering medications, giving baths, checking clients, and caring for acute and chronically ill clients. Some rituals appear more beneficial to nurses than to clients. Clients assess nursing "task rituals" and "good" caregivers. Nursing rituals such as morning reports and rounds with physicians tend to regulate the time when clients can expect to receive nursing care. New immigrants and cultural strangers may not know these rituals and receive less care. Some clients get very upset if nursing rituals related to food, medicine, and basic care needs are not explained or offered.

Periodically, nurses need to assess their own rituals for their caring benefits and values to clients of diverse cultures. Rituals can have favorable or less favorable caring and therapeutic features for clients. For several decades transcultural nurses have studied some nursing rituals and how congruent they are with client needs. Some nursing rituals may have limited benefits to clients, but may be more helpful to nurses as efficiency tasks and ritualized routines. Wolf's and Leininger's studies are a systematic discovery of hospital rituals to awaken nurses to their rituals and effects.[28-30] In addition, folk rituals and professional rituals need to be compared to prevent illnesses such as the folk evil eye (*mal ojo*) with nurses praising or envying a child, which can lead to cultural illness of the child. Nursing administration (academic and clinical) rituals also need assessment with students and consumers of different cultures for their beneficial and nonbeneficial features. Assessment of these rituals can often provide some entirely new insights about nursing practices and outcomes. For example, a Native American Sioux viewed hospital admission rituals as punishing, demeaning, and noncaring when the nurses failed to get the client's story and what actually happened on the Reservation. Nursing students often view administration and faculty rituals as having questionable value and mainly serving administrators more than students' and clients' needs.

Cultural factors related to rituals have meaning for clients in different cultural contexts such as the hospital. For example, in some cultures when individuals are separated from their extended family, they may feel abandoned at the hospital. In several cultures the ritual of admission often communicates to children and elderly clients that it is a place where they will die or be abandoned, and so they are very reluctant to go to the hospital except as a last resort. If the client dies in the hospital, the family usually goes into their immediate mourning or dying rituals at the hospital. Since the early 1970s transcultural nurses have been instrumental in establishing "mourning rooms" in hospitals for dying clients with their grieving rituals, especially for some Oceania, southeast Asians, and Native Americans. These mourning rooms have been most therapeutic and are now becoming part of the new hospital cultural context as another transcultural nursing contribution.

In general, cultural caring rituals of clients and nurses are powerful forces to know, understand, assess, and respectfully use. More and more nurses will be expected to incorporate generic rituals into client care for congruent and beneficial care. Comparative caring rituals of different cultures have greatly expanded transcultural nurses' knowledge for several decades. They are providing valuable new and specific care data to other nurses attentive to diversities and universalities using the Culture Care findings.[31,32] These transcultural care findings are used with the three modes of professional care, namely, culture care maintenance/preservation, culture care accommodation/negotiation, and cul-

ture care repatterning and restructuring.[33,34] These modalities are well demonstrated by several authors in subsequent chapters in this book to provide culturally competent and congruent care to clients in specific and therapeutic ways.[35] Staff nurses in other specialties need to study care rituals for their positive or less positive outcomes by using available scientific and humanistic transcultural nursing research findings. Chrisman has assessed and analyzed operating room rituals, which provides new insights and practice implications.[36] One must also remember that rituals can change over time, but usually slowly and partially because of their cultural security and consistency functions.

 ## Standards for Culturally Competent and Congruent Care

The standards below have been derived and modified from the *1998 Policy Statement to Guide Transcultural Nursing Standards and Practices*[37] and from *the Committee on Certification and Recertification of Transcultural Nursing Society 2001*.[38] They reflect the work of transcultural nurse experts in academic and clinical practice arenas. They began with Leininger's work in 1960 while establishing and leading the professional transcultural practices in education and service. It should be noted that other standards are rapidly coming on the market, but many of these fail to be transcultural nursing standards. They are often created by nurses not prepared in the transcultural field or by government officials pushing to proclaim their own standards. For example, a recent U.S. Federal document, with questionable statements and standards, was prepared for only a few minorities. The following transcultural nursing standards should be established, maintained, and upheld, as they have been developed by transcultural nurses knowledgeable and experienced in the field:

1. Consumers of diverse cultures have a right to have transcultural care standards used to protect and respect their generic (folk) values, beliefs, and practices and to have health personnel incorporate appropriate ways into professional practices.
2. Nurses assessing and providing care to diverse cultures or subcultures have a moral obligation to

be prepared in transcultural nursing to provide knowledgeable, sensitive, and research-based care to the culturally different.

3. Cultural assessments and practices need to demonstrate the use of transcultural nursing concepts, principles, theories, and research findings and competencies to ensure safe, congruent, and competent practices.

4. Nurses need to show sensitivity and ways to use cultural and care knowledge with competence for clients of diverse cultures.

5. Nurses as caregivers have an ethical, moral, professional obligation and responsibility to study, understand, and use relevant research-based transcultural care for safe, beneficial, and satisfying client or family outcomes.

6. Providing culturally competent and congruent care should reflect the caregiver's ability to assess and use culture-specific data without biases, prejudices, discrimination, or related negative outcomes.

7. Nurses caring for clients of diverse cultures should seek to provide holistic care that is comprehensive and takes into account the client's worldview and includes ethnohistory, religion (or spiritual), moral/ethical values, specific cultural care beliefs and values, kinship ties (sociocultural), economic, and political (legal) factors with references to their environmental living or working context.

8. Nurses practicing transcultural nursing give evidence in their actions and decisions of being able to deal with intercultural prejudices, biases, racism, and other expressions that are destructive or nonbeneficial to clients of diverse cultures.

9. Nurses demonstrating cultural competence and congruent care maintain an open, learning, flexible attitude and desire to expand their knowledge of diverse cultures and caring lifeways.

10. Nurses with transcultural competencies show evidence of being able to use local, regional, and national resources for beneficial care outcomes.

11. Nurses with transcultural competencies demonstrate leadership skills to work with other nurses and interdisciplinary colleagues who need

help to provide culturally safe and congruent client practices, thus preventing cultural imposition, cultural pain offenses, cultural conflicts, and many other negative and destructive outcomes.

12. Nurses with transcultural competencies are active to defend, uphold, and improve care to clients of diverse cultures and to share their research findings and competency experiences in public and professional arenas.

Other Enablers for Culturalogical Assessments

During the past several decades, two additional guides have been enormously helpful to nurses and other health practitioners in assessing clients' cultural care needs and behavior. They are the *Stranger-Friend Enabler*[40] and the *Acculturation Health Care Assessment Guide*.[41] These will be briefly highlighted.

The *Stranger-Friend Enabler*

This Enabler has been presented in Chapter 3 (Fig. 3.3) and is an integral part of obtaining accurate data for the Culture Care theory. The reader is directed to review this Enabler in Chapter 3. Now this same Enabler can be used with a different but related purpose to enter and effectively remain in the client's world when doing an assessment. It is a sensitive guide and barometer to indicate how nurses move from a stranger to a trusted friend to get accurate, in-depth, reliable, and trusted-friend data. If not a trusted friend, clients often give false and/or distorted data and are not always willing to share intimate and meaningful cultural knowledge and secrets. When signs of distrust exist, fear, doubt, and suspiciousness often prevail between assessor and assessee, and the data becomes questionable and sparse and may often be inaccurate. This Enabler helps the nurse move gradually and with criteria on becoming a trusted professional friend with the client. The nurse, therefore, needs to thoughtfully study this enabler before using it and then document what occurred as moved from stranger to friend. Cultural assessment labs for nurses are used today to increase competency skills and check interpretations with transcultural nurse specialists. As the nurse studies and uses the Stranger-Friend Enabler, self-awareness and interpersonal and intercultural factors can become known to the nurse. Considerable personal and professional growth has occurred with nurses and other health professionals who use this Enabler consistently and regularly. Indeed, one can also assess one's own progress of becoming a friend with other strangers with the Enabler that has been used for five decades in transcultural nursing with many reliable and scientific truths and benefits.

Acculturation Health Care Assessment Guide

This guide was developed and tested in several cultures since the early 1960s. It is shown in Appendix 4-B (at the end of this chapter). It has been one of the oldest and most continuous guides for assessing whether cultural clients are more traditionally or nontraditionally oriented to their cultures in diverse areas. Acculturation is a critical factor in assessments to determine whether a client takes on or adopts the lifeways of another culture. This dimension of assessment is important to obtain the dominant patterns of caring and health practices, whether one is dealing with a traditional or new lifeway. This influences nursing decisions and plans. This Acculturation Enabler was developed to obtain data with the ethnonursing method and the theory of Culture Care and has been used by several disciplines and health care providers to get credible, reliable, and meaningful assessment data about informants.[42,43]

The strength of this enabler is that one can obtain holistic assessments, especially when using it with the Culture Care theory and Sunrise Model. It offers a systematic assessment of the client (or family) of a particular culture with respect to worldview, social structure factors, language use, environmental context, appearance, generic and professional care practices, and other areas. The nurse assessor makes notations directly on Part I and uses this information in Part II to make a qualitative *summary profile* of the client regarding whether the person (or family) is more traditionally or nontraditionally oriented in cultural values, beliefs, and lifeways. These data are then used to develop guidelines or plans for nursing actions and deci-

sions with clients using the three modes of the theory, namely: 1) culture care maintenance/preservation; 2) culture care accommodation negotiation; and 3) culture care repatterning/restructuring. It is very important to document and describe the place where the assessment was done such as the home, hospital, or another setting because the context can greatly influence the responses and meanings. The enabler is not intended to be used by the client, but rather by the nurse who is responsible for the assessment and who uses the Culture Care theory with the Sunrise Model. This enabler is also used as a research guide for information to substantiate or refute theories related to the extent of acculturation, showing documentation of past or present lifeways. It provides more qualitative data indicators than quantitative data, but has been used with both data goals. Again, this enabler provides a holistic picture or profile of a cultural informant(s) as related to care, health, and special needs of clients of designated cultures. The nurse jots down general observations of the home, setting, person, and environment, as well as narrative information shared by the client. A more detailed summary account is generally prepared after the profile (B) is obtained.

 ## Important Summary Points for Effective Culture Care Assessments

In this chapter several principles, guidelines, models, and enablers have been presented to achieve culturally competent care assessments for quality care outcomes. The following summary points are important to keep in mind:

1. The Culture Care theory with the Sunrise Model serves as one of the best and most reliable guides to obtain a holistic view of an individual, family, or group and for institutional assessments of cultures. The worldview, social structure factors, ethnohistory, language uses, and environmental context are all essential areas to obtain a holistic and comprehensive picture with culture-specific information. Some areas will be of more interest than others in specific cultures and with the assessor. For example, Mexicans, Africans, Italians, and Arabs generally emphasize the

importance of extended family care. In contrast, Anglo-Americans emphasize individuals and their specific needs with a focus on costs, technologies, and legal and political factors of health care. The nurse actively listens to and observes the informants to enter their world and learn from them. Rather than a narrow mind-body pathophysiological or emotional symptom or disease focus, a broad and open view is maintained.

2. Throughout the assessment the nurse remains an active listener, learner, and reflector rather than a teacher or as a "know it all" medical specialist. The nurse refrains from using a lot of professional jargon or medical terms as this tends to suppress cultural data and prevents informants from sharing their ideas. If the informant inquires about professional knowledge, the nurse is obligated to share ideas but is careful not to practice cultural imposition or rigid ethnocentrism.

3. The nurse always keeps the assessment focused on the client's world of knowing (*the emic focus*) rather than on the nurse's views or professional (*the etic focus*) ideas about care, health, and lifeways. If the nurse is prone and eager to sell ideas or products to the client, this often leads to cultural conflicts and clashes and thwarts the client's participation and shared ideas.

4. The nurse always encourages the client or family to share their cultural care practices, including health values, beliefs, and lifeways and how they use them in daily life. Clients usually like to share their values and lifeways through stories, special life experiences, photographs, letters, or material cultural symbols such as talking about a "blue stone" or the "medicine bag" (of Native Americans) that promote or hinder healing and well-being in their culture. Clients like to share material items and nonmaterial ideas that have the most meaning for them in their life. Focusing on the meaning of clients' ideas to themselves during the assessment is extremely important. Some family members have diaries and videotapes to share their special life experiences, especially during a home assessment with the nurse. In the hospital such video and home artifacts are seldom used.

5. Throughout the assessment, the nurse asks very few direct questions, but instead uses indirect probing that focuses on areas of inquiry. Open-ended frames are used such as "Tell me about ____" or "I would like to have you to talk about yourself and your family" or "I need to learn more about the ways you care for children and elders." Encouraging the client to talk about their experiences is a good strategy. Also, it is important to clarify terms used as "comfort care." Eliciting ideas to help the nurses give "good care" is always welcome. The nurse tries to always use the client's words and frame of reference rather that those of the nurse. This preserves the client's world of knowing and understanding. This is a major approach today in developing culturally competent skills.

6. The nurse explores not only present-life experiences and values but also past historical events and future views related to the general assessment. These are discovered in relation to culture, care/caring, health, well-being, environmental context, and social structure domain factors influencing health or illness patterns.

7. The nurse identifies and appreciates that most clients are capable of explaining and interpreting *their* experiences related to care, health, illness, and maintaining wellness in their culture. Narratives, poems, cultural taboos, songs, pictures, and symbols have cultural meanings that the clients often may use to explain their ideas. The nurse should assume that she or he is not the expert interpreter and analyzer, but that the client is the knower. The nurse's etic (outsider's) views usually differ from the client's emic interpretations, so it is the responsibility of the nurse to hold back her or his ideas and interpretations. Knowledge of the language and being able to speak certain phrases or questions is critical to accurate assessments and interpretations. At the end of each assessment period (and there may be several), the nurse rechecks for accurate client interpretations and explanations.

8. Tapping the client's cultural secrets is done gently and sensitively. They are generally not shared unless the client believes that the nurse can be trusted, is genuinely interested in him or her and the culture, and can protect cultural secrets and viewpoints from being misinterpreted or used inappropriately. Some clients fear that their cultural ideas and experiences might be demeaned or devalued by outsiders. *Respect as caring* is practiced when doing assessments. Spiritual,

political, and legal ideas are usually guarded by clients and shared when trust is evident.

9. The client may want to wear traditional dress, adornments, or symbols for the assessment or bring items to tell "their story." The nurse respects and encourages this practice. Seeing the client in familiar dress and using certain material cultural items is valuable to learn the culture, health, caring, and healing modes as good talking cues.

10. Making the client or family comfortable and able to enjoy sharing ideas with the nurse is an important principle in assessments, so select settings that will help the client share ideas, including confidential and special secrets.

11. Throughout the assessment process, one seeks to assess if the information one hears, sees, or observes is accurate or credible to the client's lifeways. The family and other representatives of the culture may also confirm such knowledge with the informants. Individual and group variations always exist, and one must not generalize findings to other cultures.

12. The nurse remains appreciative of the client's willingness to share ideas by always thanking them after each session. Giving money or gifts for assessments is not generally practiced unless it is a research study. However, benefits (actual or potential) need to be discussed at the outset and at the end.

In general, a culturalogical care assessment is a very creative and dynamic discovery and learning process that brings forth valuable knowledge. It is often packed with surprises of information that are generally limitedly known to most nurses and health care providers about cultures. The Culture Care theory with the Sunrise Enabler and with other enablers presented in this chapter can make the journey an exciting and meaningful process with benefits to the client and rewarding experiences to the nurse or other health professionals.

Today, the phrase I coined in the 1960s, "culturally competent congruent care," has become popular and in demand worldwide with many researchers and other disciplines seeking it. Some are looking for "measurement tools," "instruments," and statistical data to be "scientific." However, it is the in-depth qualitative,

verbatim, and holistic data that will be most helpful to clients and nurses. Cultural care competencies are very difficult and imprecise to measure. Qualitative enablers are the most meaningful and rich data to obtain today and in the future. Moreover, the myth of what constitutes "science" is being challenged and slowly changing to value qualitative findings as one important type of science.[44] Very meaningful data has been forthcoming over the past four decades with this cultural care assessment process and with the theory and enablers. Today, many ideas, terms, models, and methods used by the author since the early 1960s are just beginning to be used, "diffused," and proclaimed by others, sometimes without full documentation of author source. Such unethical practices need to be abated and "to render honestly to authors their original work." Transcultural nurses have and continue to lead the way in making culturally competent and congruent care a reality with diverse cultures.

In sum, the reader has been presented with a theory and several principles, guidelines, models, and strategies to do a quality-based culturalogical care assessment. The purpose of this assessment was stated to obtain information to guide the nurse in providing culturally congruent and competent care to blend with the client's values, beliefs, and lifeways. Such emic and etic assessments are imperative to ensure quality care and to promote the health and well-being of diverse cultures. The Sunrise Model (derived from the theory of Culture Care) and other Culturalogical Assessment Guides and other Enablers were discussed. The Acculturation Enabler was presented to determine whether clients are more traditionally or nontraditionally oriented. Nurses prepared in transcultural nursing will find these aids meaningful and easy to use. Other disciplines will also find them helpful in making assessments. Assessment data are not only used for client care, but also for educational, consultation, and for research purposes. Nurses using the assessment data can greatly increase their ways of knowing clients, and it can become a most rewarding experience as they get a holistic view of cultures, as well as very specific and practical data.[45] Most importantly, nurses learn much about themselves that greatly expands their worldviews and gives them a deep appreciation for cultures and caring phenomena transculturally.

Appendix 4–A
Leininger's Suggested Inquiry Guide for Use with the Sunrise Model to Assess Culture Care and Health

Instructions: The purpose of this ethnonursing guide is to enter the world of the client and discover information to provide holistic, culture-specific care. Use broad and open inquiry modes rather than direct confrontational questions. Move with the client (or informant) to make the inquiry natural and familiar. These inquiry areas are examples for the inquiry and not exhaustive. Identify at the outset if assessing an individual, family, group, institution or community. (This inquiry guide focuses on the individual). Identify yourself and the purpose of the inquiry to the client, i.e., to learn from the client about his/her lifeway to provide nursing care that will be helpful or meaningful.

Domains of Inquiry: Suggested Inquiry Modes

1. Worldview — I would like to know how you see the world around you. Could you share with me your views of how you see things are for you?

2. Ethnohistory — In nursing we can benefit from learning about the client's cultural heritage, e.g., Korean, Philippine, etc. Could you tell me something about your cultural background? Where were you born and where have you been living in the recent past? Tell me about your parents and their origins. Have you and your parents lived in different geographic or environmental places? If so, tell me about your relocations and any special life events or experiences you recall that could be helpful to understand you and your needs. What languages do you speak? How would you like to be referred to by friends or strangers?

3. Kinship and Social Factors — I would like to hear about your family and/or close social friends and what they mean to you. How have your kin (relatives) or social friends influenced your life and especially your caring or healthy lifeways? Who are the caring or non-caring persons in your life? How has your family (or group) helped you to stay well or become ill? Do you view your family as a caring family? If not, what would make them more caring? Are there key family responsibilities to care for you or others when ill or well? (Explain.) In what ways would you like family members (or social friends) to care for you? How would you like nurses to care for you?

4. Cultural Values, Beliefs and Lifeways — In providing nursing care, your cultural values, beliefs, and lifeways are important for nurses to understand. Could you share with me what values and beliefs you would like nurses to know to help you regain or maintain your health? What specific beliefs or practices do you find most important for others to know to care for you? Give me some examples of "good caring" ways based on your care values and beliefs.

5. Religious/Spiritual/Philosophical Factors — When people become ill or anticipate problems, they often pray or use their religion or spiritual beliefs. In nursing we like to learn about how your religion has helped you in the past and can help you today. How do you think your beliefs and practices have helped you to care for yourself or others in keeping well or to regain health? How does religion help you heal or to face crisis, disabilities or even death? In what ways can religious healers and nurses care for you, your family or friends? What spiritual factors do we need to incorporate into your care?

6. Technological Factors — In your daily life are you greatly dependent upon "high-tech" modern appliances or equipment? What about in the hospital to examine or care for you? (Explain.)

	In what ways do you think technological factors help or hinder keeping you well? Do you consider yourself dependent upon modern technologies to remain healthy or get access to care? (Give some examples.)
7. Economic Factors	Today, one often hears "money means health or survival." What do you think of that statement? In what ways do you believe money influences your health and access to care or to obtain professional services? Do you find money is necessary to keep you well? If not, explain. How do you see the cost of hospital care versus home care cost practices? Optional: Who are the wage earners in your family? Do they earn enough to keep you well or help you if sick?
8. Political and Legal Factors	Our world seems full of ideas about politics and political actions that can influence your health. What are some of your views about politics and how you and others maintain your well-being? In your community or home what political or legal problems tend to influence your well-being or handicap your lifeways in being cared for by yourself or others? (Explain.)
9. Educational Factors	I would like to hear in what ways you believe education contributes to your staying well or becoming ill. What educational information, values or practices do you believe are important for nurses or others to care for you? Give examples. How has your education influenced you to stay well or become ill? How far did you go with formal education? Do you value education and health instruction? (Explain.)
10. Language and Communication Factors	Communicating with and understanding clients is important to meet care needs. How would you like to communicate your needs to nurses? What language(s) do you speak or understand? What barriers in language or communication influence receiving care or help from others. What verbal or nonverbal problems have you seen or experienced that influences caring patterns between you and the nursing staff? In what ways would you like people to communicate with you and why? Have you experienced any prejudice or racial problems through communication that nurses need to understand? What else would you like to tell me that would lead to good or effective communication practices with you?
11. Professional and Generic (folk or lay) Care Beliefs and Practices	What professional nursing care practices or attitudes do you believe have been or would be most helpful to your well-being within the hospital or at home? What home remedies, care practices or treatments do you value or expect from a cultural viewpoint? I would like to learn about your home healers or special healers in your community and how they help you. What does health, illness or wellness mean to you and your family or culture? What professional and/or folk practices make sense to you or are most helpful? Could you give some examples of healing or caring practices that come from your cultural group? What folk or professional practices and food preferences have contributed to your wellness? What foods are taboo or prohibited in your life or in your culture? In what ways have your past or current experiences in the hospital influenced your recovery or health? What other ideas should I know about what makes you well through good caring practices?
12. General and Specific Nursing Care Factors	In what ways would you like to be cared for in the hospital or home by nurses? What is the meaning of care to you or your culture? What do you see as the link between good nursing care and regaining or maintaining your health? Tell me about some of the barriers or facilitators to good nursing care. What values, beliefs or practices influence the ways you want nursing care? What stresses in the hospital or home need to be considered in your recovery or in staying well?

What else would you like to tell me about ways to care for you? What community resources have helped you get well and stay well? Give some examples of non-helpful care nursing practices. What environmental or home community factors should nurses be especially aware of to give care to you and your family? What cultural illnesses tend to occur in your culture? How do you manage pain and stress?(Clarify.) What else would you like to tell me so that you can receive what you believe is good nursing care? Give specific and general examples.

Appendix 4–B
Leininger's Acculturation Health Care Assessment Guide for Cultural Patterns Traditional and Non-Traditional Lifeways*

Name of Assessor _____ Date _____

Informants or Code No. _____ Sex _____ Age _____

Place or Context of Assessment _____

Directions: This guide provides a general qualitative profile or assessment of the traditional or non-traditional orientation of informants and their patterned lifeways. Health care influencers are assessed with respect to world-view, language, cultural values, kinship, religion, politics, technology, education, environment and related areas. This profile is primarily focused on emic (local) information to assess and guide health personnel in working with individuals and groups. The etic (or more universal view) may also be evident. In Part I, the user observes, records and assesses findings on the scale below from 1 to 5 with respect to traditionally or non-traditionally oriented lifeways. Numbers are plotted on the summary Part II to obtain a qualitative profile to guide decisions and actions. The user's brief guide is *not* designed to be a quantitative measurement guide, but rather a qualitative guide of information with respect to the above areas of informant knowledge as lifeway indicators.

....

Part I: Rating Criteria to Assess Traditionally and Non-Traditionally Patterned Cultural Lifeways or Orientations

	Mainly Traditional	Moderate	Average	Moderate	Mainly Non-Traditional	Rater Value
Rating Indicators:	1	2	3	4	5	No.

Culture Dimensions to Access Traditional on Non-Traditional Orientations

1. Language, communications and gestures (native or nonnative). Notations: _____
_____
_____

2. General environmental living context (symbols, material and nonmaterial signs). Specify: _____
_____
_____

3. Wearing apparel and physical appearance. Notations:_____
_____
_____

4. Technology being used in living environment. Notations:_____
_____
_____

5. Worldview (how person looks out upon the world). Notations: _____
_____
_____

6. Family lifeways (values, beliefs and norms). Notations:_____
_____
_____

7. General social interactions and kinship ties. Notations:_____
_____
_____

8. Patterned daily activities. Notations:_____
_____
_____

9. Religious and spiritual beliefs and values. Notations:_____
_____
_____

10. Economic factors (rough cost of living estimates and income). Notations:_____
_____
_____

11. Educational values or belief factors. Notations:_____
_____
_____

12. Political or legal influencers. Notations:_____
_____
_____

13. Food uses and nutritional values, beliefs, and taboos, Specify:_____
_____
_____

14. Folk (generic, lay or indigenous) health care-cure values, beliefs and practices. Specify:_____
_____
_____

15. Professional health care-cure values, beliefs and practices. Specify: _____
_____
_____

16. Care concepts or patterns that guide actions, i.e., concern for, support, presence, etc.: _____
_____
_____

17. Caring patterns and expressions:_____
_____
_____

18. Informants ways to:
   a) prevent illnesses:_____
   b) preserve or maintain wellness or health:_____
   c) care for self or others:_____
_____
_____

19. Other indicators to support more traditional or non-traditional lifeways including ethnohistorical and other factors._____
_____
_____

20. Other notations below_____
_____
_____

....

Part II: Acculturation Profile from Assessment Factors

Directions: Plot an X with the value numbers placed on this profile to discover the orientation or acculturation lifeways of the informant. The clustering of numbers will give information of traditional or non-traditional patterns with respect to the criteria.

Assessment:	Mainly Traditional 1	Moderate 2	Average 3	Moderate 4	Mainly Non-Traditional 5

Criteria:
1. Language and communication modes
2. Physical-social environment (and ecology)
3. Physical apparel appearance
4. Technologic factors
5. Worldview
6. Family lifeways
7. Social ties/kinship
8. Daily/nightly lifeways
9. Religious/spiritual orientation
10. Economic factors
11. Educational factors
12. Political and legal factors
13. Food uses/abuses
14. Folk (generic) care-cure
15. Professional care-cure expressions
16. Caring patterns
17. Curing patterns
18. Prevention/maintenance factors
19. Other indicators, i.e. ethnohistorical

Note: The assessor may total numbers to get a summary orientation profile. Use of these ratings with written notations provide a holistic qualitative profile. Detailed notations are important to substantiate the ratings in these areas.

*Note: This guide has been developed, refined, and used for four decades (since early 1960s) by Dr. Madeleine Leininger. It has been frequently in demand by anthropologists, transcultural nurses and others. It has been useful to obtain an informant's orientation to traditional or non-traditional lifeways. It provides qualitative indicators to meet credibility, confirmability, recurrency and reliability criteria for qualitative studies. This copyright guide may be used if the *full title* of the guide, recognition of *source* (M. Leininger), and *publication outlet (Journal of Transcultural Nursing)* are cited.[22] The author would also appreciate a letter to know who has used the guide, the focus and summary outcomes. Permission originally granted from Leininger, M., "Leininger's Acculturation Health Care Assessment Guide for Cultural Patterns in Traditional and Non-Traditional Lifeways, *Journal of Transcultural Nursing*, v. 2, no. 2, Winter, 1991, pp. 40–42.

▪ References

1. Leininger, M., "Culturalogical Assessment Domains for Nursing Practices," in *Transcultural Nursing Concepts, Theories and Practices*, M. Leininger, ed., New York: John Wiley & Sons, 1978, pp. 85–106.

2. Leininger, M., *Nursing and Anthropology: Two Worlds to Blend*, New York: John Wiley & Sons, 1970.

3. Leininger, M., *Transcultural Nursing: Concepts, Theories, Research and Practice*, Columbus, OH: McGraw Hill College Series, 1995.

4. Orque, M., B. Black, and L. Monroy, *Ethical Nursing Care*, St. Louis: The C. V. Mosby Co., 1983, pp. 55–74.

5. Spector, R., *Cultural Diversity in Health and Illness*, 5th ed., Upper Saddle River, NJ: Prentice Hall Health, 2000.

6. Parnell, L. and B. Paulanka, *Transulcultural Health Care, A Culturally Competent Approach*, Philadelphia, PA: F.A. Davis, 1998.

7. Campinha-Becote, J., *The Process of Cultural Competence: A Culturally Competent Model of Care*, 2nd ed, Wyoming, OH: TCN Care Associates, 1991.

8. Giger, J. and R. Davidhizar, *Transcultural Nursing: Assessment and Intervention*, 2nd ed., St. Louis: The C.V. Mosby Co., 1991.

9. Dobson, S., *Transcultural Nursing*, London: Scutari Press, 1991, pp. 41–138.

10. McFarland, G. and E. McFarlane, *Nursing Diagnosis and Intervention: Planning for Patient Care*, St. Louis: The C.V. Mosby Co., 1989.

11. Leininger, M., "Issues, Questions and Concerns Related to the Nursing Diagnosis Cultural Movement from a Transcultural Nursing Perspective," *Journal of Transcultural Nursing*, 1990a, v.2, no. 1, pp. 23–32.

12. Ibid.

13. Leininger, M., *Transcultural Nursing: Concepts, Themes, Research and Practice*, Columbus, OH: McGraw-Hill, 1995 pp. 115–143.

14. Leininger, M., *Care: The Essence of Nursing and Health*, Detroit: Wayne State University Press, 1988.

15. Leininger, M., *Cultural Care Diversity and Universality: A Theory of Nursing*, New York: National League for Nursing Press, 1991 pp. 1–64.

16. Ibid.

17. Leininger, M., "Transcultural Interviewing and Health Assessment," in *Mental Health Services: The Cross-Cultural Context*, Vol. 7, Pedersen et al., eds., Beverly Hills, CA: Sage Publications 1984, pp. 109–133.

18. Leininger, op. cit, 1995, pp. 65–66.

19. Leininger, op. cit, 1978, p. 113.

20. Leininger, op. cit, 1995.

21. Leininger, op. cit, 1991.

22. Hall, E. T., *Handbook for Proxemic Research*, Washington, DC: Society for the Ontology of Visual Communication, 1974.

23. Ibid.

24. Leininger, op. cit., 1991, p. 49.

25. Leininger, op. cit., 1995, p. 142.

26. Van Gennep, A., *The Rites of Passage*, London: Routledge & Kegan Paul, 1960.

27. Leininger, M., "The Tribes of Nursing in the USA Culture of Nursing," *Journal of Transcultural Nursing*; v. 6, no. 1 Summer 1994 (first published in 1980 in newspaper).

28. Ibid.

29. Wolf, Z.R., *Nurse's Work: The Sacred and Profane*, Philadelphia: University of Pennsylvania Press, 1990.

30. Leininger, M., *Care: Discovery and Uses in Clinical Community Nursing*, Detroit: Wayne State University Press, 1988.

31. Leininger, M., "Selected Culture Care Findings of Diverse Cultures Using Culture Care Theory and Ethnomethods," in *Culture Care Diversity and Universality: A Theory of Nursing*, New York: National League for Nursing Press, 1991, pp. 355–375.

32. Leininger, M., "Special Research Report: Dominant Culture Care (Emic) Meanings and Practice Findings from Leininger's Theory," *Journal of Transcultural Nursing*, 1998, v. 9, no. 2, pp. 45–48.

33. Leininger, M., *Cultural Care Diversity and Universality: A Theory of Nursing*, New York: National League for Nursing Press, 1991, pp. 1–64, 98–104.

34. Leininger, M., "What is Transcultural Nursing and Culturally Competent Care?" *Journal of Transcultural Nursing*, 1999, v. 10, no. 1, p. 9.

35. Leininger, M., "The Phenomenon of Caring: The Essence and Central Focus of Nursing," *Nursing Research Report*, American Nurse's Foundation, 1977, v. 12, no. 1, pp. 2–14.

36. Chrisman, N., "Cultural Shock in the Operating Room: Cultural Analysis in Transcultural Nursing," *Journal of Transcultural Nursing*, 1990, v. 1, no. 2, pp. 33–39.

37. Transcultural Nursing Board, "Policy Statements to Guide Transcultural Nursing Standards and Practices," *Journal of Transcultural Nursing*, 1998, v. 9, no. 2, pp. 75–77.

38. Leininger, M., ed., "Standards for Transcultural Nursing," unpublished draft for certification and recertification, Omaha, NE, 2001.

39. Ross, Houkje, "Office of Minority Health Publishers Final Standards for Cultural Linguistic Competence," in *Closing the Gap. Newsletter of the Office of Minority Health*, U. S. Dept. of Health and Human Services, February/March 2001, pp. 2–5, 10.

40. Leininger, op. cit., 1991, p. 82.

41. Leininger, M., "Leininger's Acculturation Health Care Assessment Tool for Cultural Patterns in Traditional and Non-Traditional Lifeways," *Journal of Transcultural Nursing*, 1991, v. 2, no. 2, pp. 40–42.

42. Leininger, op. cit., 1991, pp.

43. Leininger, M., "Overview and Reflection of the Theory of Cultural Care and the Ethnonursing Research Method," January to June 1997, v., no., pp. 32–51.

44. Leininger, M., "Types of Science and Transcultural Nursing Knowledge," *Journal of Transcultural Nursing*, October 2001, p. 330.

45. Leininger, M., "Transcultural Nursing: An Imperative Nursing Practice," *Imprint*, 1999, November–December, pp. 50–52, 60–61.

CHAPTER 5

PART I. Toward Integrative Generic and Professional Health Care

Madeleine Leininger

There remains extremely rich healing, caring and curing generic traditions of human beings from the distant past that are still limitedly known and await discovery for integration into today's modern professional health services. M. LEININGER

This chapter has two parts. Part I is written by the author, a nurse anthropologist, and Part II by a physician providing an ethical medical perspective of the major theme toward integrative generic and professional health care. This chapter is not intended to provide a comprehensive view of diverse kinds, uses, and techniques of generic healing modes and therapeutic outcomes. Instead, the purpose is to offer an overview about the rapid growing interest in generic traditional health and healing practices with reflections and comparisons with professional historical viewpoints, trends, and issues. Controversial issues related to the qualifications and efficacy of traditional roles of healers, carers, shamans, or medicine men in diverse cultures will not be discussed because of space limitations. Some of these areas can best be studied in the anthropological and other related science literature. The intent of this chapter is to provide some fresh insights of the nature, development, and importance of generic and professional care from a transcultural nursing perspective with the goal of facilitating integrative, culturally congruent care for people of diverse cultures. In Part II the author will provide some present-day perspectives of alternative medicine from a physician's viewpoint with ethical, professional, and research considerations. Hopefully, the reader will realize that transcultural nurses have a special interest in integrative humanistic, scientific, and generic-professional care and a unique role as direct care providers with special prepa-

ration to work with clients of diverse cultures in the world. However, before considering this reality, let us first consider why there is such a rapidly growing interest in generic (folk) or traditional health practices, especially in the Western world.

■ Fast Growing Western Interest in "Alternative" Health Practices

One of the fastest growing areas of interest and practice of Western health professionals is on traditional folk or indigenous medicines, healers, and naturalistic practices that have survived over thousands of years in non-Western cultures. While physicians have become interested in recent years, professional nurses who have worked closely with people in homes, hospitals, and community services have been interested to learn what cultures were using and why.[1,2] Transcultural nurses have stimulated nurses through education, practice, and research to learn about specific folk practices and how to incorporate them therapeutically into professional practices. Some nurses who work with immigrants such as the Vietnamese, Philippine, Chinese, Russian, and Cuban people have observed how families use folk practices in daily lives to maintain their well-being or to treat common ills. Some nurses traveling or working overseas have also become aware of folk or traditional health care practices in recent years.

Despite modern Western technologies and treatments, nurses, physicians, and pharmacists have been curious about how non-Western, traditionally oriented cultures heal and even "cure" clients with different herbs, rituals, and practices often at less cost and with some effective outcomes. When physicians saw or heard that transcultural nurses were using folk practices in the 1970s and 1980s, they often would demean the practices as superstitions and quackery.[3] Some physicians felt a loss of control and serious interference with scientific medicine largely because of a lack of knowledge about specific folk practices. Through graduate anthropological studies of non-Western and Western health and illness practices in the 1960s, I learned of their importance for transcultural nursing and general health care.

In the 1970s specific culture folk care practices were selectively and carefully used as part of transcultural nursing care. Physicians were not too interested except for a few who questioned such practices. At that time, physicians were greatly immersed in mind and body relationships and the use of new technologies. There was almost no interest in culturally and holistically based care related to healing and well-being. Nonetheless, transcultural nurses continued to explore the uses and caring practices with selected folk caring modalities. We were attentive to some potential dangers when folk modes were used with Western medicines and treatments, but remained interested in how cultures used familiar, inexpensive herbs and other folk healing and caring practices. Considerable folk caring and healing knowledge began to come into transcultural nursing in the 1970s, 1980s, and 1990s.[4,5]

As medical costs began to increase markedly in the 1990s, economically poor cultures had limited money for modern Western medical care and treatments. Furthermore, some traditional non-Western cultures feared surgical and medical Western interventions because of their beliefs in soul loss and the use of powerful Western medicines and treatments. Transcultural nurses continued to document these traditional cultural responses and were keenly aware of what clients preferred to use with their folk medicines and treatments. Protecting cultural practices was important while still discerning what would fit best with their cultural beliefs and be beneficial.

With the use of Culture Care theory, transcultural nurses became keenly aware of values and the importance of "holistic caring" and went beyond the medical focus on mind-body and partial care and cure. The holistic and totality view of cultures threw into relief the dynamic role of folk care healing practices as influenced by kinship, religion, specific culture values, and multiple other factors. Emic folk practices and their functions "made sense" as we took folk histories and studied the intergenerational use of these practices over time. Gradually, the holistic care and folk practices penetrated the thinking and practices of other nurses by the 1980s. Holistic care became a powerful means to shift some nursing dependence on medical diseases and symptoms to a broad transcultural professional and generic care focus. However, as managed care came into existence, holistic transcultural nursing care with a comprehensive focus became threatened. It was very difficult to maintain a client-centered emic folk and professional focus with a dominant emphasis on managed and limited care for cost reduction and early dismissal. Considerable efforts remain today to maintain the transcultural and holistic emic and etic nursing perspective in mainstream nursing and to reappraise managed care ideology and effects.

It is of interest that in the past two decades folk healing practices are being studied and recognized by more physicians and by other health disciplines and practitioners. The recent establishment of the National Center for Complementary and Alternative Medicine at the federal level in the United States is evidence of this rapidly growing movement. There remain, however, both doubters and supporters of the movement by physicians. The literature and practice evidence has dramatically increased in the last two decades on alternative medicine and naturalistic healing as presented in the works by Weil,[6,7] Pelletier,[8,9] and Chopra.[10] Currently, medical schools in the United States are now educating students in "alternative or complementary medicine" and some research is being conducted to document beneficial or less favorable outcomes. At the same time, many Americans are being attracted to naturalistic medicines such as herbs; vitamins; and diverse, traditional, cultural healing and curing practices. Large amounts of advertising money are being given today in the United States for "prescriptions for healthy living" by promoting dietary pills and foods as well as body-builders and exercise equipment. Books on alternative medicine of what is held to "work or not work" are available to the general public. Hopefully, in the 21st century, research and experiential data will clarify the beneficial or less beneficial outcomes.[11] Surveys continue showing the United States population relying quite heavily on alternative medicines or therapies and fewer patient visits to physicians.[12]

In this evolutionary development of folk practices, it should be clearly stated that anthropology, since its beginnings in the 19th century has led the way in the discovering, documenting, and interpreting of folk or traditional cultural healing and curing practices. Accordingly, health professionals prepared in anthropology, transcultural nursing, and medical anthropology have studied some of these past and present folk contributions to health care.[13] Anthropological literature has provided several research studies on traditional folk and professional health practices. There are some health professionals who have not discovered such research studies until very recently.

Amid these rapidly growing trends in the past decade have come many critical issues in the United States related to definitions of acceptable terms, ethical concerns, treatments, consumer and professional usage, and outcome indicators of beneficial and less beneficial uses of folk practices with professional regimes. Let us turn to definitions of concepts and uses of such terms from a transcultural nursing perspective.

 ## Definitions of Generic (Folk) and Professional Care

It was in the early 1960s when I began to realize the need for two major concepts in the development of the new field of transcultural nursing. There was evidence that the nursing profession was failing to study, teach, and integrate culture and human caring into nursing education and practice regarding folk or indigenous beliefs, values, and practices. Learning about and integrating cultural folk practices into nursing was meager, with doubts of its value or appreciation of folk healing, caring, and curing modalities. I, therefore, conceptualized and defined the terms *generic care* and *professional care* drawing from some anthropological

viewpoints for generic care and humanistic caring from nursing.[14] The need to explicate these two major perspectives was important to discover new knowledge and integrate findings into a new body of evolving transcultural nursing knowledge and practices.

I define *generic care* as *referring to the oldest or first folk, lay, naturalistic, and traditional cultural ways of assisting, helping, or facilitating the healing and caring process of human beings.*[15] The word generic refers to the original, root sources, the first or earliest knowledge sources. Anthropologically, humans lived and many survived in the world long before professions such as nursing, medicine, and other related fields came into existence. Human beings relied on what was natural biologically, but also on what was familiar to them interpersonally and spiritually within their total cultural ways of knowing and living in different environments. These early cultures had healers, carers, curers, medicines, rituals, and indigenous ways of dealing with daily common and recurrent life situations related to birth, living, and dying. Hence, the term generic seemed most appropriate to conceptualize and discover traditional ways of caring, healing, and curing in transcultural nursing, keeping the dominant focus on caring, health, illness, and well-being.

In the 1950s, Pike's linguistic terms *emic* and *etic* were of great interest to me to discover culture's inside (*emic*) knowledge and contrast it with outsider (*etic*) knowledge in transcultural nursing.[16] After conferring with Pike and getting his enthusiastic response, I introduced *emic* and *etic* into nursing in the 1960s with my teaching, research, and theory. Today, these concepts have now become part of professional discourse and use to discover embedded and overt phenomena.

The second major concept that was different from generic care was *professional care*. Professional care was defined as the *formally or informally taught, learned, and transmitted culturally based professional knowledge focused on human caring, healing, and wellness practices that are used to assist or facilitate well-being.*[17] Professional care and cure is often viewed as "scientific" knowledge about diagnosing, treating, caring for, or curing people. However, what constitutes scientific and humanistic professional, philosophic, and epistemic knowledge tends to vary in Western and non-Western cultures. Moreover, professional or modern nursing caring or curing is not as old as generic care, and yet the latter is important to many cultures, especially non-Western cultures. Professional care knowledge that is *culturally constituted, learned, and practiced* is a relatively new perspective and contrasts with generic care as defined above. I took the position that *both generic and professional care were crucial for professional nursing and needed to be rigorously studied and used appropriately.* These two constructs became an integral part of my theory of Culture Care in the early 1960s.[18] Today, transcultural nurses are using these definitions in research to discover major contrasts between these two types of care. (See Chapter 3.) From an epistemic viewpoint these two types of care are guiding many nurses to be aware of such expressions with people of diverse cultures in caring and curing processes. Generic and professional care must continue to be studied worldwide with focus on the dual relationships and their therapeutic values for human caring and well-being. In a way generic care is essentially new knowledge in nursing being promoted and taught by transcultural nurses and others knowledgeable of the phenomena.

The construct of *integrative care* was chosen as a desired outcome of generic and professional care when appropriately and meaningfully used in therapeutic practices. I have defined *integrative care to refer to safe, congruent, and creative ways of blending together holistic, generic, and professional care knowledge and practices so that the client experiences beneficial outcomes for well-being or to ameliorate a human condition or lifeway.* Integrative care is often the desired means to provide culturally congruent care and often the desired outcome generated through the theory of Culture Care. It is important to state, however, that sometimes in helping clients, there needs to be more emphasis on generic care than professional care modes. However, at other times, there may be more emphasis on professional care and very little on generic care. Such decisions require knowledge of both generic and professional practices along with consumer input. Most importantly, professional nurses have a societal and legal mandate to always inform and share relevant professional knowledge with clients and not neglect generic care knowledge to arrive at sound decisions. Currently, transcultural nursing promotes and practices

integrative care so that the client gets the better of the two worlds of knowing and therapies.

Presently, there are a number of different terms being used by different disciplines for lay, folk, or traditional healing practices. Terms such as "alternative," "complementary," "traditional," "non-Western," "lay," "folk remedies," "indigenous," "integrative," and "holistic" are being used, especially by health professionals and some consumers. Debate over the scientific and popular merit of these terms continues with confusion in usage and outcomes. Physicians tend to dominate in proclaiming and declaring what terms should prevail, but sometimes they may not be very knowledgeable about generic folk practices of different cultures and especially non-Western cultures. Transcultural nurses and anthropologists can serve as consultants with generic care based on their experiences with different cultures over time. Medical anthropologists can also be helpful, but sometimes they focus mainly on medicine and curing rituals. Transcultural nurses focus more on human caring, health, and well-being from an integrative and holistic perspective for reasons already stated.[19] Physicians and pharmacists tend to use "alternative medicine," and some use "complementary medicine." In general, there is a lack of consensual language usage and definitions, with the terms becoming politically and financially laden with some disciplines.

In studying and working with many cultures over the past five decades, I have discussed some of the linguistic terms with cultural informants. Most non-Western cultures disliked the use of the term "alternative" by professionals. They are quick to ask: "Alternative to what?" and say, "Our folk healing ways are *not* alternatives as they are basic and are the first and oldest ways to heal. They have been important to us for hundreds or even thousands of years."[20] Some traditional cultures reported that when the word "alternative" is used by physicians and nurses, it is insulting and demeaning to them, revealing a lack of appreciation and knowledge of their traditional practices. The majority of informants preferred the term "generic" as it conveyed the idea of the first healers with native (insider) views, which are often very different from professional views and practices. They also hoped that the idea of integrative care and cure would occur in the future. Traditional healers, carers, and curers were all concerned about demeaning or not respecting their practices, healers, rituals, and practices and the history of using native remedies over a long period. For these reasons and others transcultural nurses use the terms "generic," "integrative," or "holistic" care and encourage usage in others.

Reflecting further on the topic, I believe that the greatest potential benefit to consumers will be *blending generic and professional knowledge and practices together* when grounded in research-based knowledge of cultural data and caring. As B. Leininger emphasizes in Part II, rigorous and vigorous research must be forthcoming for alternative medicine. Most assuredly, biomedical and genetic factors will be important and need to be integrated. However, they may never adequately explain humanistic caring and healing related to social-structure, historical, language, and cultural values. These factors and others play an important part in providing truly integrative and culturally congruent care. It is also reasonable to predict that in the future dominant and specific culturally based caring and healing values and practices will be the powerful forces to explain and predict health maintenance and prevention for culturally diverse and similar cultures worldwide. The nature of human beings with generic (*emic*) and professional (*etic*) knowledge and practices are essential guides for wellness and especially to prevent illnesses, disabilities, chronic conditions, and destructive health acts. Integrative care that incorporates Western professional (etic) provider's knowledge with non-Western (emic) provider's remains an important goal for transcultural nursing practices in providing and maintaining culturally congruent care.

In Figure 5.1, the author shows a summary of the major differences between Western *etic* (column 1) and non-Western *emic* providers (column 2). These data are from cultural informants' viewpoints and assessments shared with the author over several decades. Understanding generic and professional care providers' viewpoints are extremely important in working toward the desired goal of integrative care that is culturally congruent care (column 3). The theory of Culture Care can be very helpful to health professionals in arriving at integrative and congruent care. Thus it is helpful to reflect on Figure 5.1 as one seeks to provide integrative care, keeping in mind both emic and etic perspectives. There

are additional chapters in this book and others from the past four decades that provide substantial information and findings with many cultures on generic and professional care outcomes. The reader is encouraged to study these sources.[21–26]

■ Transcultural Generic (Folk) Beliefs and Practices

With the growing interest in generic or traditional values, beliefs, rituals, and practices, nurses are challenged to study in depth such phenomena. There are many chapters in this book that will be helpful, as well as excellent books, articles, videos, and magazines on generic folk beliefs, foods, practices, and care-cure rituals. There are also sections in several transcultural nursing books and research articles about traditional generic or folk practices such as those in Andrews and Boyle's book with excellent clinical examples.[27] In contrast, Spector identifies many folk material items in different cultures, but, unfortunately, fails to discuss them within a transcultural nursing perspective or practices.[28] Some nurses unprepared in transcultural nursing or anthropology are now writing about folk practices with questionable interpretations and findings that need to be cautiously assessed and used. In this book are several chapters with excellent examples of generic folk healing and caring practices studied within the Culture Care theory. In addition, transcultural nurses have published several articles in the *Journal of Transcultural Nursing*. Higgins' article on Puerto Ricans is one of these research articles that show the influence of generic folk beliefs on infant feeding practices within the Culture Care theory along with some integrative practices.[29]

As transcultural nursing specialists or generalists, it is important to keep in mind that there are many different kinds of generic folk healers (including medicine women and men), care-takers (women and men), rituals, caring–curing strategies, beliefs, and symbolic material and nonmaterial ways of healing, along with different ways to integrate generic beliefs into professional practices. Keeping an open (discovering) mind along with active listening and documenting of what is seen, heard, and done helps the nurse to obtain accurate data. The transcultural principle of *learning from*

1. Western (Etic) Professional Providers Practices	2. Non-Western (Emic) Folk Provider Practices	3. Desired Attributes for Integrative Care
1. Relies mainly on etic biomedical knowledge of diseases, symptoms & practices.	1. Relies mainly on emic generic (folk) care healing, values & beliefs.	1. Desires trust and mutual respect in caring, healing, curing & well being.
2. Uses partial body-mind meanings, practices, & research findings.	2. Seeks holistic culturally-based meanings, beliefs & lifeways for healing.	2. Desires collaborative decision-making using the best of emic and etic practices.
3. Uses action-oriented modes & largely "scientific" medical facts but skeptical of folk practices.	3. Uses listening &watching about professional ideas and practices but often skeptical of them.	3. Seeks etic and emic care-cure practices that are congruent, safe and meaningful.
4. Defends etic professional knowledge & practices.	4. Uses and defends emic folk lifeways, values & experiences, especially in home context.	4. Seeks holistic care perspectives to ensure safe & congruent generic practices.
5. Relies heavily on medical, nursing, and other treatment modes as "scientific" and "the best".	5. Relies on folk healers & carers as safe, reliable & trustworthy.	5. Seeks beneficial care or healing practices that incorporate one's values, beliefs, and lifeways within their living environments.
6. Focuses on individual curing & symptom management relief for curing outcomes.	6. Focuses on caring modes & lifeway experiences in community context	6. Seeks competent, creative & compassionate practitioners.
↓	↓	↓
Professional Etic Care	**Generic Emic Care**	**Integrative Etic & Emic Congruent Care**

Figure 5.1

Comparative Western (etic) and non-Western (emic) cultural provider practices with desired integrative congruent care attributes.

others by listening to cultural informants and remaining nonauthoritative is strongly advised. Cultural healing and caring studies and obtaining life histories from carers and healers are valuable data sources. Families often like to share "their" foods, herbs, medicines, and practices if genuine interest and respect by nurses is evident. The use of Culture Care theory with the Sunrise Model of generic caring and healing is an excellent means to discover generic and professional care to provide culturally congruent care practices. (Color Inserts 8 and 9 show generic foods and transcultural healers sharing their knowledge with nurses.)

It is important to know there are many different types of ancient and current therapies, especially in non-Western cultures. Some of these generic procedures or therapies are diet, herbal, moxibustion, cupping, acupuncture, coining, massage and manipulation, dance, imagery, aerobic exercises, relaxation, breathing modes, energy, music, Reiki, spiritual meditation, sauna, and many others. Internal and external substances and amulets are used with these therapies in specific ways. There are also some generic folk therapies or practices that are already combined with medicines and nursing practices because the cultural uses were found to be beneficial. Indigenous cultures, however, may integrate several folk practices. For example, Oi Gong is an ancient exercise that integrates breathing, movement, and meditation. Hence, different cultures have different histories of their "favorites" or what they believe and have found through experiences to be the most efficacious to obtain certain results.

Transcultural nurses and others can learn about these different philosophies, schools of thought, and specific practices to understand and appreciate their usage over time. Many non-Western schools of thought and practice are very ancient such as Ayurvedic, which is India's ancient mode of naturalistic medicine and healing dating back to 3500 B.C. Hindu texts known as Vedas (meaning "science of life" from the Sanskrit Ayur) are very old traditions.[30] Ayurveda is claimed to be the oldest system of natural healing and the source for many other healing traditions. Some of these non-Western philosophies are being studied anew in Western contemporary health systems for their holistic and integrative practices in preserving and promoting optimal health or to help heal selected physical illnesses and chronic cultural conditions. Integrating generic spiritual aspects with exercises and with nutrition, sociocultural, and environmental factors are important in traditional and natural healing practices.

There are also Chinese and Tibetan philosophies with medicines and healing modes, naturopathy, homeopathy, chiropractic, reflexology and meditation, yoga, aroma, Rolfing, shiatsu, and many other therapies derived mainly from very ancient schools of thought. Recently, in Western professional institutions the focus has been to examine these therapies, medicines, and all natural food supplements for hard "scientific proofs" and repeated evidences. In the meantime, many lay people and professionals are using Eastern herbs, exercises, nutritional foods, and several traditional therapies from ancient schools of thought. Some are using them to regulate body weight, to prevent illnesses and diseases such as cancer and hypertension, and to promote and regulate healthy lifestyles. Nurses are using generic folk practices, and as they travel to many countries, they discover different and new uses of generic

care. All health professionals need to assess the costs, strengths, and limitations (or problems) with traditional medicines and treatments, as well as the effectiveness of these practices.

A groundswell of new ideas, practices, and discoveries from the traditional non-Western cultures has steadily increased in the professional world with nurses, physicians, social workers, pharmacists, and other disciplines. Some generic practices are entering professional health systems faster than anticipated, and nurses are often expected to know how to use them properly with professional medicines and care practices. Family members often bring some healing materials into health institutions and use them in their homes for healing or to "protect them" from perceived "dangerous" professional medicines, treatments, and practitioners.[31] Transcultural nurses, with knowledge of and experience in using both generic (folk) and professional practice care modes, should be called on to assess and help other nurses, physicians, and health providers in making decisions with consumers about the use of both of these modes. This can be an awesome professional responsibility with legal implications. However, as more health professionals are educated to use traditional generic practices with professional knowledge, the problems should decrease. The transcultural nurse is often asked to *protect clients* of non-Western cultures who are unfamiliar with Western medicines and treatments from being demeaned or shunned when using their folk remedies. Establishing mutual and genuine relationships between the health provider and the client or family is critical to promote and practice beneficial integrative care. A few examples of generic and professional situations with different cultures may help the reader to grasp the meaning and importance of ideas discussed above.

Examples of Generic (Folk) Care Practices and Professional Responses

There are many examples to show differences between traditional generic and professional care practices. The following clinical examples are offered with different cultures from data and real-life situations or observations by the author.

Vietnamese Child and Nurse Response Example

A community health nurse was asked to make a home visit to a traditionally oriented Vietnamese family, but especially to see a sick two-year-old child. When the nurse examined the child, she noted reddened welt areas by the spine and neck and some round reddened areas on the shoulders. She was very alarmed and immediately called the clinic physician to arrange for an x-ray of the child's spine. Since none of the family could speak English, the nurse assumed from her professional studies that it was a case of child abuse. The mother's nonverbal communication showed that she was upset that the nurse had called a physician. The mother kept shaking her head as if disapproving the nurse's actions. Unfortunately, this nurse had not been prepared in transcultural nursing and failed to recognize that Vietnamese family members use their traditional practice of cupping with warm glasses to promote healing of the child's cold or whatever was making her ill. The coin rubbing (Cao gio) was used near the spine and neck for similar reasons. The nurse was very concerned, but noted that the mother was affectionate to her sick child. The nurse felt helpless and left after she took the child's temperature and documented her observations. The Vietnamese believe that illness (or cold) needs to be drawn out of the body for healing to occur, hence, the generic practice of coining, rubbing, and cupping.

Chinese Immigrant and Nurse Example

A Chinese immigrant who had had major surgery was told by the nursing staff to "force fluids." The client refused to drink from the pitcher of water left on his bedside stand. The nurses and physicians threatened the client with intravenous fluids if he did not drink more fluids. The staff concluded that the client was uncooperative and noncompliant. When the client's daughter came to visit her father, she told the nursing staff that he would drink hot herbal tea, but not cold water. Herbal tea was culturally congruent based on the Chinese belief in the use of hot beverages for healing and well-being. The theory of hot and cold is major to understand along with the yin and yang beliefs. Many generic herbal teas are used daily by Chinese people and are viewed as healing. They expect teas to be used in caring for them while in the hospital.

Navajo Folk Birth Expectations Example

A Navajo woman gave birth to a child in a large urban hospital. After the birth, the nurses immediately disposed of the placenta and the child's umbilical cord. When the mother was ready to be discharged, she asked for her placenta and umbilical cord. She learned that the staff had destroyed these important human parts. The mother became very upset because she assumed the staff knew of the importance of the placenta and umbilical cord to the Navajo and to save them according to their tradition. The mother and her family left the hospital in great distress. Since the nurses were not educated about the Navajo culture and the importance of folk caring practice, they were ineffective to help the mother to preserve the child's future well-being. The mother performed some ritual ceremonies after she returned home to ease what happened to her and the child in the hospital. She also wanted to bury the placenta near the hogan and place a piece of the umbilical cord outside the hogan for the male infant. Cultural negligence by the nurses prevented the Navajo mother from completing the birth process and receiving culturally congruent generic care. Professional birthing practices failed to meet the client's needs and expectations.

Saudi Arabia Uses of Generic Substances Example

A transcultural nurse came into a hospital room in Saudi Arabia and found the mother placing a dark substance into the eye of her sick ten-month old child. The nurse was knowledgeable about kohl, which is used for cosmetic and eye conditions based on statements in the Koran (the holy book of Islam). This transcultural nurse discussed with the mother her reasons for using kohl. The mother said, "To make my child beautiful and to prevent diseases." The nurse helped the mother to understand that the kohl she was using contained lead sulfate as noted on the container. She advised the mother not to use the eye substance as it could lead to serious eye problems. The mother did not realize what was in the new medicine. She thanked the nurse for her caring advice and concerns. This is an example of professional care knowledge to a client and child to prevent an unfavorable potential consequence from a folk practice. It is an obligation of the nurse to inform clients when these situations arise and not to use a generic, traditional, and potentially harmful substance. However, the client ultimately has a right to make his (her) decision in many societies.

Southern African American and Pregnancy Example

When the author was working and studying in the southern United States with African American families, she found that several pregnant women craved clay dirt or ate laundry starch (Argo). The mothers said this tradition was "comforting" and that it helped "settle my stomach" and "build up my blood." The nurse recognized these cultural beliefs about generic cultural practices of consuming small amounts of clay. The pregnant mothers, however, feared there could be negative sanctions by the community health nurses after they saw mothers using clay dirt or Argo. One pregnant mother who ate the clay also had a string tied around their abdomen when she came to the hospital. The client quickly told the nurse that "it (the string) is for protecting my new baby." She also had a small scissors under her pillow "to cut the labor pains." The nurses practiced culture-care accommodation with the mothers and provided respectful caring and comfort. The mothers were willing to use modern professional nursing practices as long as their generic substances and practices were preserved. The mothers became trustful of nurses when they saw their beliefs and practices could be used as integrative generic and professional care practices.

Mexican Nurse and Abortion Example

Mary, a Mexican professional nurse midwife, was told by her supervisor to participate in a therapeutic abortion. Mary, a devout Roman Catholic, refused to participate in the abortion as this was against her religious beliefs. Her supervisor was most disturbed with Mary. She told her, "Other nurses accepted such assignments and that she had no other nurses available." The supervisor then said, "Well, you can set up the equipment, supplies, and the operating table for the abortion." Again, Mary refused this assignment and told the supervisor

"I will be aiding or helping in taking an innocent child's life and this is participating in murder." The supervisor was very angry, and later she threatened that she probably could not continue to employ her. Mary responded that she had a right to have her beliefs upheld and to practice professional nursing. In this situation great cultural conflict occurred between the supervisor and the nurse with caring for a client receiving an abortion. Mary also knew that the client was a Mexican American who did not want the abortion as promoted by a non-Catholic physician. Such religious conflicts and situations lead to noncongruent and unethical professional care practices. The nurse's generic (emic) values were in conflict with professional values of the supervisor.

 ## Summary Reflections and Challenges

In this section the doors have been open to encourage nurses to study in-depth and systemically generic care with diverse cultures and to reflect on their uses in professional care practices. Whether generic care and professional care can be appropriately used alone or integrated is a professional transcultural issue and responsibility to assess. During the past four decades, transcultural nurse researchers and practitioners have given leadership to the new doors of generic and professional care. They have also provided meanings and creative ways to apply the knowledge to care for people of diverse and similar cultures. The goal to integrate and appropriately blend or synthesize generic with professional care to provide congruent and safe care is important today and in the future. The study and identification of differences between generic and professional care remain essential to be an effective transcultural nurse practitioner. Generic care needs to be valued and nurtured for helpful relationships with clients of different cultures. Nurses prepared in transcultural nursing are expected to master knowledge of generic care comparable to nurses mastering cardiovascular knowledge. Cultures and generic care are complex phenomena requiring intensive study. Learning how to provide integrative holistic care requires a synthesis of both generic and professional care values and practices. Therefore, as transcultural nurses and other nurses move into the twenty-first century, they are challenged to practice integrative care or to justify generic (emic) or professional (etic) care when used alone. It is the philosophy of transcultural nursing to provide culturally competent caring practices that are safe, meaningful, and beneficial to people of diverse and similar cultures worldwide.

References

1. Leininger, M., *Transcultural Nursing: Concepts, Theories and Practices*, New York: John Wiley & Sons, 1978.
2. Leininger, M., *Nursing and Anthropology: Two Worlds to Blend*, New York: John Wiley & Sons, 1970 (Reprinted 1994 by Greyson Press, Columbia, Ohio).
3. Leininger, M., *Transcultural Nursing: Concepts, Theories, Research and Practice*, Columbus, OH: McGraw Hill, 1995.
4. Ibid.
5. Leininger, M., *Cultural Care Diversity and Universality: A Theory of Nursing*, New York: National League for Nursing Press, 1991.
6. Weil, A., "A New Look at Botanical Medicine," *Whole Earth Review*, Fall 1989, pp. 5–7.
7. Weil, A., *Natural Health, Natural Medicine*, Boston: Houghton Mifflin, 1995.
8. Pelletier, K., *Mind as Healer, Mind as Slayer: A Holistic Approach to Preventing Stress Disorders*, New York: Delta, 1992, Revised (First published in Fireside, W. 1977).
9. Pelletier, K., *The Best Alternative Medicine*, New York: Simon & Schuster, 2000.
10. Chopera, D. Ovantan, *Healing: Exploring the Frontiers of the Mind and Body Medicine*, New York: Bantam Books, 1989.
11. Pelletier, op. cit., 2000.
12. Eisenberg, D., et al., "Trends in Alternative Medicine Use in the United States," 1990–1997, *Journal of the American Medical Association*, v. 280, no. 18, pp. 1569–157, 1998.
13. Kottak, C., *Anthropology: The Exploration of Diversity*, New York: McGraw Hill, Inc., 1991.
14. Leininger, op. cit., 1991.
15. Ibid.
16. Pike, K., *Language in Relation to a Unified Theory of the Structure of Human Behavior*, Glendale, CA: Summer Institute Linguistics, 1954.
17. Leininger, op. cit., 1991, p. 48.
18. Ibid.
19. Leininger, op. cit., 1995.
20. Leininger, M., "Alternative to What?: Generic vs. Professional Caring, Treatments and Healing Modes," *Journal of Transcultural Nursing*, v. 19, no. 1, July to December, 1997, p. 37.
21. Leininger, op. cit., 1995, pp. 79–81.
22. Leininger, op. cit., 1970.
23. Leininger, op. cit., 1991.
24. Leininger, M., *Transcultural Nursing*, New York: Masson International Press, 1979.
25. Leininger, M., "Transcultural Nursing: Its Progress and Its Future," *Nursing and Healthcare*, September 1981, v. 2, no. 7, pp. 365–371.
26. Leininger, M., "Transcultural Nursing: A Scientific and Humanistic Care Discipline," *Journal of Transcultural Nursing*, v. 8, no. 2, January to June 1997, pp. 54–55.
27. Andrews, M. and J. Boyle, *Transcultural Concepts in Nursing Care*, 3rd ed., Philadelphia: Lippincott, 1999.
28. Spector, R., *Cultural Diversity in Health and Illness*, Upper Saddle River, NJ: Prentice Hall Health, 2000.
29. Higgins, B., "Puerto Rican Cultural Beliefs and Influence on Infant Feeding Practices in Western New York," *Journal of Transcultural Nursing*, v. 11, no. 1, January 2000, pp. 19–30.
30. Khare, R.S., "Dava, DaKar, and Dua: Anthropology of Practical Medicine in India," *Social Science Medicine*, v. 43, no. 5, 1996, pp. 837–848.
31. Leininger, op. cit., 1995.

CHAPTER 5

PART II. Ethics of Alternative Medicine: Primum Non Nocere

Bernard J. Leininger

Alternative medicine (AM) has enjoyed immense popularity in the past several decades as shown by the billions of dollars spent annually for herbal extracts, patent medicines, large doses of vitamins, special food supplements and forms of spiritual/mystical healing.

I will not attempt to define exactly what falls under the term AM, but for purposes here will arbitrarily designate AM as those therapies *outside the pale* of conventional medicine (CM). I fully realize the unfairness of such a sweeping generalization, particularly to conscientious practitioners of AM who have devoted a lifetime to study of natural remedies and some of the ancient healing arts of other cultures.

In modern society's quest for autonomy, people are eager to challenge what is perceived as the hegemony of medicine in matters of their personal health. Patients' ability to access instant, bona fide medical information backed with the latest scientific data through the electronic media endows them with a power previously reserved for the medical profession.

The incredible medical advances, fueled by scientific discoveries in technology, genomology, biotechnology and pharmaceuticals, resulting in costly, procedural-oriented care, have perhaps blurred the *art* of medicine—leaving, at least as perceived, a spiritual void in the healing process.

Morris' recent book, *Illness and Culture in the Post Modern Age*, describes society's current fascination with cultural and spiritual aspects of health, and rejection, in part, of the purely scientific (modern) approach.

Recently there has been an increasing number of medical conferences on the spiritual aspects of healing with sell-out audiences. In short, we are witnessing a groundswell of interest in things labeled *natural,* *organic, herbal, spiritual, mystical, non-invasive, and non-chemical.*

Needless to say, this movement has multiple facets. Many individuals with degrees related to AM have devoted years of study and research to advance the knowledge and practice of AM; health/nutritional gurus with varying degrees of training and information espouse beliefs with almost a messianic zeal. A rather large group might be said to fall into a *modern day fad* category that embraces *natural* and *organic* products as something good and safe for you.

Then we have the entrepreneurs who see *gold in them thar herbs*, aided and abetted by marketing on the Internet. Patent medicines, non-prescription drugs, vitamins, minerals, nutritional supplements and health aids have always contributed enormously to the bottom line of reputable pharmaceutical companies. Certainly a lot of money is being made by less-reputable purveyors with compelling advertisements of half-truths.

Suffice it to say, most of these items are being merchandised by incorporating the description *herbal, organic or natural* whenever feasible.

The 1994 Dietary Supplement Health and Education Act allows the sale of herbal remedies without manufacturers' having to prove their safety and effectiveness to the FDA. This Act was recently upheld by a federal judge in Utah who required the FDA to lift its ban on an imported cholesterol-reducing substance containing a natural form of lovastatin, a key chemical in Merck's Mevacor.

Even as the media reports cases of individuals suffering severe untoward toxic effects from the use of natural herbs and unregulated dietary supplements, this large industry netted over $5 billion last year in revenues on dietary supplements alone.

Prominent health-care institutions, responding to this growing popularity, and perhaps with an eye to the bottom line, are establishing departments of AM which would seem to open a Pandora's box of administrative conundrums. For example, by what criteria does one credential practitioners of AM? Will the Joint Commission on Accreditation of Healthcare Organizations (JCAHO) allow special concession for AM as in the legislation of the control of dietary supplements? And who will do the research and education on AM? Clearly, this is a quandary for CM with its lack of formal training in AM—vis a vis practitioners of AM with varying degrees of training in this medium of care. Who will be responsible for the quality of AM care in health-care institutions?

Physicians have been indirectly dealing with AM for the past decade through patients who, for the most part, have been reluctant to divulge their AM activities; and yet many of the compounds they have been taking are pharmaceutically active and difficult to quantify. This situation poses a moral and perhaps legal responsibility on physicians to be able to assess the effects of AM on patients' health, as well as its interaction with the treatments they may be prescribing.

Having posed this dilemma, it is perhaps fair to say that, much like hospice with its care of the dying and emphasis on pain management, AM is also coming to CM via the back door. Historically, CM, in its attempt to distance itself from origins steeped in witchcraft and therapeutic misventures (bloodletting, etc.) has scrupulously aligned itself on the side of science, even though much in the art of medicine has been, and still is, less than scientific. Hence the phobia of CM for anything that smacks of unorthodoxy by CM standards.

In a recent medical educational exchange trip to Cuba, we saw a rather large building that the Cuban government had designated as *a natural healing* center. It served both as a clinical facility for the community and as a required teaching rotation for the medi-cal students. Members of our group, particularly from the social sciences, were quite impressed. Witnessing "mud packs from a special pond" to treat osteoarthritis of the ankle, I remained very skeptical of the efficacies of such ministrations; but knowing how long it takes to effect changes in our medical school curricula, I was impressed by how quickly a totalitarian state responded to the perceived wants of its citizenry, as well how pervasive the interest is in AM.

In assessing the moral implications of AM, we might do well to go back to the Oath of Hippocrates and its tenet: Primum non nocere (first, do no harm). And while modern high-tech medicine renders this ancient dictum more or less an oxymoron and has been supplanted by "risk/benefit ratio," its historical context is important.

In the time of Hippocrates (circa 400 BC), the natural healing powers of the body were well appreciated, and honest practitioners realized that most of their ministrations were apt to interfere with that process; ergo, the hallowed dictum endured until modern medicine changed the balance of the risk/benefit ratio.

If much of AM allegedly is predicated on natural healing, then the excessive intake of vitamins and herbs with pharmacological activity, the reliance on faith healing, and use of unproven invasive or manipulative procedures—all these would interfere with the natural healing processes of the body and violate the concept that if we don't know the efficacy of the treatment—do no harm.

Morally, this is perhaps imposing a double standard and it's unfair to paint all forms of AM with a single broad brush; but medicine, it would seem, has an obligation to incorporate a discipline of research and education of AM into its educational institutions, and to evaluate with open minds the benefits and risks of these popular therapies—especially if carried out within its health-care institutions. But until we know more—primum non nocere.

6

The Biocultural Basis of Transcultural Nursing

Jody Glittenberg

Entering the 21st century, transcultural nursing has been active to solve health problems from local and global perspectives. Leininger's holistic Theory of Culture Care Diversity and Universality has provided one of the broadest and most promising theoretical frameworks for nursing and health-related disciplines and professions.[1-3] Nursing has been changed dramatically over the past three decades largely as the result of the creative and pioneering work by Leininger. This American Academy of Nursing living legend has been a leader to help nurses become more aware of the importance of transcultural nursing and nurses' responsibility in our culturally diverse world. How to practice culturally competent nursing care is as essential as giving good physical nursing care. In this chapter the author's ideas will build on the Leininger theory and model but with a focus on bioculturalism as discussed in work defining *bioculturalism as referring to how biological, physical, and different physical environments of diverse and similar cultures relate to care, health, illness, and disabilities.*[4] This definition is based on the work in *The Biocultural Basis of Health* authored by Moore, Van Arsdale, Glittenberg, and Aldrich.[5]

For transcultural nurses the interaction between biology (human bodies) and culture (human values, beliefs, and practices) is of great interest. How they interact for healthy and/or unhealthy outcomes is of professional interest. An example an of of an unhealthy outcome in some societies can be cited with present-day United States views that a "thin" female body is culturally highly valued as heard in the often-quoted statement, "You can never be too rich or too thin" — attributed to Wally Simpson, the Duchess of Windsor, in the 1940s. Practicing nurses know the negative outcomes of being "unhealthily" thin, especially for female teenagers, many of whom are anorexic or bulimic. In spite of news media constantly communicating how obese Americans are in the United States and that they are getting fatter, they continue to go to the nearest fast-food window and order burgers and fries, leaving the healthy vegetables and fruits untouched. Why such incongruent behaviors? This chapter will describe human behavior such as eating patterns within Leininger's broad theoretical framework that includes discovering transcultural health care by focusing on the worldview, social-structure factors (e.g., kinship, religion, and other factors), as well as historical, environmental, and language meanings to discover phenomena to arrive at culturally competent health care.[6]

Several important transcultural nursing textbooks such as Andrew and Boyle's book[7] describe giving competent biocultural nursing care by focusing on *individual* biological factors such as assessing skin color, hair texture, and other physical features. These approaches to care are very important; yet they lack an integrating framework that builds a synthesis of biology *with* culture. Transcultural nurses think more broadly about influencers of health problems and how to give culturally competent care within a biocultural ecosystem. Perhaps new research directions will emerge by using this approach in transcultural nursing, and more integrated solutions may be found for some perplexing nursing and health care problems.

The author's framework builds on how an *individual's* biology, culture, and caring modes are *part* of a whole human ecosystem. A human ecosystem is similar in concept to Leininger's holistic Sunrise Model as it incorporates multiple environmental factors in which humans are born, live, and die.[8,9] This ecological approach is understanding health at the societal level that affects large groups of people rather than just one individual or family. For instance, why do certain groups of people have a higher prevalence for some diseases — such as the Pima American Indians for non–insulin-dependent diabetes mellitus (NIDDM)? Historically, the pattern of increasing incidence of NIDDM throughout the Pima tribe, as well as other American Indian tribes, began to accelerate dramatically following the introduction of government commodity foods in the 1950s. Prior to this event the Pima had been accustomed to their high-protein diet based on food grown on their arid lands that required heavy physical labor to harvest these crops. However, when government high-carbohydrate-and-fat commodity foods became available as inexpensive or free food sources, the natives ate abundantly and did not do heavy physical labor to acquire such foods, then the Pima began to exhibit NIDDM. This is an example of the interaction of biology (diabetes) with culture (deficiency changes in diet).[10]

There are many other examples, such as why are some groups — such as poor women on welfare — kept from reproducing? Could eugenics still be a "policy" in the United States? Or, why are organ transplants an "ordinary" practice in the United States, while in some countries such as Germany there is an aversion to such practices?[11] Another example is that genetically altered sterile seeds are being sold to impoverished farmers throughout the world by large international agricultural corporations, thus keeping such farmers forever enslaved — needing to buy "new" seed for each planting. Does not this enslavement to technology affect health? Recently, anthropologists have become interested in researching such biocultural problems.[12–14] In nursing there is an increasing interest in environmental caring factors that influence health.[14,15] These environmental studies, with a transcultural nursing caring focus, point nurses into new areas of study. What biocultural knowledge do transcultural nurses need to study and use in their caring practices? It is important to understand the close relationship between biology/culture, caring modes, and health outcomes.

To aid in this discussion the human ecosystem model, as developed in *The Biocultural Basis of Health*[16], will be described. The human ecosystem operates within two subsystems: subsystem I, the macro-

level, and subsystem II, the individual or microlevel. Subsystem I, the macrolevel, is comprised of three environmental factors: 1) physical (e.g., climate, altitude, solar fields, earth movements, water, soil, etc.); 2) all living matter (e.g., fauna and flora, fertility of the land and people, etc.); and, 3) human-made environment (e.g., cultural rules, norms, meanings, practices, and social institutions such as family, education, religion, power and politics, economics, health, etc.). Two environmental factors at the macrolevel, physical and all living matter, are studied as factors that directly affect individuals. Transcultural nurses usually do not assess the specific effect atmospheric pressures have on clients, nor do they study the effects of climate changes on the health of people. However, dietary patterns of different cultural groups are assessed, and knowing what physiologic and caring adjustments may be necessary in accommodating new foods is important. Such interacting macrolevel physical factors and care patterns do affect the health or well-being of people.

Macrolevel Example: Physical Factor (an Earthquake) Interacting with Cultural Norms

The recent earthquakes in Turkey and Taiwan (June and September 1999) are an example of the interaction of macrolevel physical factors and cultural norms of people in those disasters. The media reported that in Turkey and Taiwan substantially more people died in poorly constructed buildings than in better constructed buildings — perhaps among the dead were people who lived in poverty. However, in the 1976 Guatemala earthquake Glittenberg discovered that the poor lived in thatched-roofed cane huts (a cultural pattern of housing) that simply collapsed during the earthquake, and very little loss of life occurred. Just a lot of dust fell as the light-weight cane roofs caved in, and the residents escaped with a few bumps and bruises. These huts were easily and quickly replaced and were very different from houses of wealthier people that were built with heavy brick and tiled roofs. In brick houses, Glittenberg discovered a pattern of differential loss of life among young mothers who huddled themselves (a cultural pattern) over their infants to save them, while their toddlers — the two year olds — remained unprotected. Unfortunately, many mothers and toddlers died from falling bricks, while the protected infants survived. Some fathers were crushed as they ran into the streets (a cultural pattern) to assess the damage.[17] This example illustrates a macrolevel biologic factor of small and frail bodies interacting with proscribed culture-care patterns of living that shaped mothers' and fathers' behaviors during a crisis. An earthquake is a macrolevel factor that illustrates the health outcome (a biologic survival of people) as the result of variation in the human-made environment (culture).

Macrolevel Example: Living Factor (Food Supply, ABO Blood Type, and Immune Systems)

Another example of a macrolevel "living" factor is the complex interaction between three factors: food supply, cultural dietary habits, and ABO blood type. It is hypothesized that when the immune system is in balance, it is considered to be healthy, but when the system is stressed and becomes imbalanced, it is said to be dis-eased. It is important for transcultural nurses to understand the potential effect of stressful *macrolevel* factors that can affect individual health by leading to an imbalanced immune system and subsequently to disease. An example of balance and imbalance in dietary habits resulting in potential dis-ease will be described.

Some diseases may be linked with blood type. Blood phenotype A, B, O, or AB is usually not considered an important factor affecting health — except when compatible blood type for transfusions is needed or during pregnancy for the mother and infant, then it is advantageous to have compatible Rh blood factors. In general, health care practitioners seldom ask, "What blood type are you?" Many people also do not know what type they are. From informal polls taken by the author, when people are asked about blood type, nearly 90% did not know their blood type. Anthropologists have long been interested in the ABO phenotype (the visible property of blood types) as a critical factor in human evolution, but patterns of distribution (i.e., patterns of clustering geographically) have been puzzling as they do not seem to follow any racial or ethnic lines.[18,19] For example, not "all" Norwegian Americans in one area will have the same ABO blood type nor will "all" Mexican Americans in that same area have the same type. Rather blood types are quite "mixed"

as a result of migrations from original birthplaces and intermarriages with people with other blood types. Certainly, diversity is not negative as human beings are biologically very diverse, and this biodiversity has contributed to the survival of the species.[20]

Snyder, an anthropologist, in the 1920s tried to classify people by blood type.[21] He found some patterns were associated with geographical distributions that *could* be associated with ethnic groups, but Snyder also found may strange groupings that were *not* aligned with ethnicity. For instance, he found that the majority of people in Korea, as well as the majority of people in parts of the Middle East, had the *same* blood type, yet they were from widely separated geographical areas.[22] Why did this occur? Another mystery that has intrigued some researchers is a possible association between blood type and disease. They have studied patterns of disease as linked with blood type (but *surely* not proven). For example, syphilis has been associated with type B or AB, gastric ulcer with type O, and cancer of the prostate with type A blood group.[23] D'Adamo has found *suggestive patterns* that type B people seem to have a higher incidence of bladder and kidney infections, as well as bladder cancer, and types A and O seem to be more predisposed to lymphoma, leukemia, and Hodgkin's Disease.[24] Questions have been raised about *why* these suggestive patterns exist, as there is no known theory to explain the pattern.

To explain some of these associations, D'Adamo[25] claims the ABO blood type is a genetic fingerprint that is more powerful in affecting individual health than other classifications of human populations. The D'Adamo *hypothesis* relates ABO blood types to an adaptive dietary process taking place over the past 10,000 to 15,000 years as human beings living in various geographical areas met their nutritional needs from the local fauna and flora. D'Adamo believes that the specific ABO phenotype of the people living in an ecological niche was compatible with the food supply available to them. Also he believes that negative effects on health can be noticed when people (like families and extended families) have migrated to different ecological niches where their familiar foods (nutrients) were not available, and they then had to survive on new and different fauna and flora to meet their nutritional needs. Although their blood types remained the same, the migrants' immune systems were/are under constant stress, and over time their bodies began/begin to show a variety of immune system–related disorders.[26] Through clinical studies D'Adamo has developed a framework of dietary needs for each blood type (recommending a return to the earlier, appropriate fauna and flora food supply). When these patterns of living are followed, D'Adamo claims, people become healthier individuals.

D'Adamo has written a best-selling book entitled, *Eat Right for Your Type*,[27] which is popular with lay people. To my knowledge the D'Adamo hypothesis has not been scientifically tested, but there are researchers from the Center for Integrated Medicine, College of Medicine, The University of Arizona, who are testing the D'Adamo hypothesis. In a graduate transcultural nursing course at the College of Nursing, The University of Arizona, in 1999, students investigated some of the D'Adamo ideas and found some suggestive support for his hypothesis. An evaluation of his work is not part of this chapter; however, the D'Adamo framework is an example of how to examine interacting factors in a macrosystem (fauna and flora and dietary needs) that may influence individuals' immune systems.

While the above example is suggestive, it presents many interesting questions for future research. Transcultural nurses using the theory of Culture Care with the Sunrise Model study social-structure, environmental, historical, and multiple factors related to food meanings and caring patterns. These broad, holistic, theoretical perspectives are crucial, especially when dietary changes are made during the acculturation process. The meanings of dietary norms and food uses need to be studied closely with physiologic adaptation to the food supply and the caring environment.[28]

By studying these two examples of environmental factors — physical and living — we can see how important it is to view macrolevel variables such as earthquakes and flora and fauna as important elements when unlocking the mysteries of adaptation. By using such principles we look not only at the individual human being or groups of people, but we also look for patterns of influence such as dietary patterns, change in climate, and change in water supply. Furthermore, we need to look at clusters of "trouble" in groups of people who have such disorders as arthritis, diabetes, chronic fatigue syndrome, and heart disease and ask questions: Why these people? Why at this time? Why not women? Why only some children? By asking such

questions transcultural nurses are *synthesizing biologic and cultural* factors in their search for answers. Such factors are important for transcultural nurses to consider in research, as well as in practice. In addition to looking at physical and living environmental factors, we shall now discuss the third macrolevel factor in the human ecosystem — the human-made environment (culture) — as important in shaping individual, as well as group, biocultural health.

 ## Some Important Human-Made Factors Within the Ecosystem

Within the ecosystem there are many examples of human-made factors (culture) that shape human health. In this chapter, only three categories of cultural factors will be discussed: mating, genetics, and biotechnology. How the ecosystem relates to transcultural nursing will be briefly summarized.

Mating as a Biocultural Adaptation

Mating is a complex adaptation of an individual's biologic need to procreate as is the cultural shaping that takes place within a common mating pool.[29] A mating pool is the group of individuals who usually associate together and who reproduce during the fertile time in their lives. Although a mating pool is not restricted to an ethnic group, closed ethnic groups can be viewed as a type of pool; for instance, cultural rules may prohibit inter-ethnic or interreligious marriages (i.e., mating), so that over many generations the mating group becomes more homogeneous in relationship to biologic diversity. For example, migration patterns of people looking for work or resource opportunities or, in contrast, the decimation of some groups such as in war or from natural disasters may result in loss of "ideal" mates for marriage. When this happens, new cultural rules must be developed and used regarding ideal marriages and mating. Thus we see that cultural rules (human-made environment) are dynamic and subject to change or adaptation.[30]

The Adaptive Link: Socialization of the Individual Within the Group The *adaptive link* between biology and culture is the individual *within* a group. For the infant, the individual, to survive and thrive (culturally and physically) he or she must be socialized into the group. Adequate socialization of an individual — the child — permits the group to survive both biologically and culturally. This assumption is important to remember for the sheer number of different cultures, about 5000 to 8000, in the world, into which an infant may be born.[31] Such immense diversity underscores how adaptive the human species really is, and it also points out how critical it is for infants/children to be socialized into their culture or group as shown with the Gadsup of the Eastern Highlands of New Guinea.[32] Norms and values that are taught prepare that child for survival and possible reproduction of their own children at an appropriate time in adult life. The adaptive link between biology and culture is the individual, and the shaping of the group is usually done within the family setting and often through care meanings and process. One of the best examples of biocultural shaping is that of choosing mates for passing on the culture and physical attributes of the family to the next generation.

Biocultural Shaping of the Family Through Transcultural Caring Process   Using Leininger's Culture Care theory, the kinship meanings become important as they link with physical, psychological, and cultural ideals that are usually shared by the family. Ideals are drawn from the larger culture of which the family is one part. In each culture, the physical and psychological image of an ideal male and female is transmitted and learned through the media, story, and myth. For example, having such characteristics as being "tall," "agile," "beautiful," "brave," "honest," "good mother," "good father" are reinforced as being ideal. The cultural norm takes shape also within the rules of religion, law, and economic and political structures of the dominant culture, although minority norms survive. These factors influence culture care norms, beliefs, values, and practices. Moreover, in kinship systems there exists a "preferred marriage" (i.e., mating), meaning that certain relationships within the extended family are maintained or avoided by means of cultural rules and norms. An example is that in some cultures "first cousin" marriages are prohibited by law, yet in other cultures this would be a preferred marriage. In most cultures there are extended family relationships that build alliances to protect the "in-group" through marrying within the group, known as endogamous

preferred marriages. Yet in other cultures to marry outside the group is preferred to establish, extend, or protect limited resources. Such preferred marriages are called *exogamous*. In anthropology, analysis of kinship systems is a starting point for understanding a cultural group, and a great deal has been written about the rules specific to marriage and mating.[33–36] Transcultural nurses also gain a fuller understanding of the biocultural structure of cultural groups by mapping kinship systems,[37] and then by linking the system to transcultural nursing phenomena related to care health, wellness, or illness.

For most of human history, the survival of offspring and ultimately the family unit has been very risky. In hunting-and-gathering and agricultural cultures, and even today in post-industrial times, women are able (without biotechnological intervention) to conceive and bring to full term only about six children during a lifetime of procreation.[38] In earlier times and in some environments fewer children survived. To sustain human populations, many rules for marriage or mating were shaped not only by cultural rules, but also by rules that would maximize physical reproduction capabilities. For example, a strong, healthy male would be able to provide physically for the family unit, and a female with sufficiently broad hips for a safe birthing and breasts for production of milk would likely provide the family with offspring for group survival. Choosing ideal mates was shaped by family guidance for productive mating. Even today, with biotechnological advances and in postindustrial economic systems, selection of ideal mates still is shaped through parents' or elders' advice. Advice can be given by parents to their soon-to-be mating offspring with statements such as "That girl (boy) would make a fine mother (or father), look at her or his parents." Or, "Would you really want your children to look like her or him?" "Marry him or her and you'll really have smart (or dumb) kids." Or, "It's better if you marry within your own religion, your own kind, etc." The shaping of preferred matings has a profound effect on the genetic pool of your ancestry and is greatly influenced by worldviews and social structures in different communities. It is the cultural norm for families to shape their kinship systems through pressing offspring to select future mates that complement the family system rather than a mate that would be detrimental to the family.

In today's world many changes are being made in family systems. For instance, in the past five decades in the United States (and in many other parts of the world) populations migrate rapidly, and family rules for shaping procreation of offspring change. Much more freedom is extended in making mating choices. Interreligion, interethnic marriages are far more common than in the past century, but they tend to occur in populations that have recently migrated rather than in populations that have remained stable.[38] Mating involves male and female individuals responding to a cultural pattern, as well as a biologic drive. There are few exceptions to this statement except for same-sex mating. Such couples are very rare, but with biotechnology, children can be conceived by a female couple or donor males and surrogate mothers in a male couple, but such offspring are not genetic duplicates of both parents, although cultural shaping may come from both parents. Transcultural nurses can influence others to act on selected processes involved in family shaping.[39–41]

Transcultural nurses need to continue studying the changing cultural norms and values related to mating as these norms influence biologic aspects as well as cultural care patterns to provide culturally competent and responsible care.[42–44]

Genetics Within a Biocultural Framework

Genetic factors influence biocultural caring and are especially critical in reproducing a family. Transcultural nursing focuses on cultural beliefs and practices of what is observed — *the phenotype* — such as the physical characteristics of the ideal male or ideal female. Yet within this framework are also the cultural beliefs important to birthing a child. Transcultural nursing research tends to focus on culture caring meanings and practices of birth, but more attention needs to be directed toward the inheritable characteristics being carried forward from one generation to another. In fact, within the human gene pool today remains the inheritable characteristics of all our ancestors since the begining of the human species.[45] Transcultural nursing has a great interest in the inheritance and the caring patterns passing from one generation to another. The genetic structure of the culture remains important to study and learn more with current genetic research findings.

Current genetic research findings are topics of daily newspapers, but interest in inheritance has been longstanding. Prior to the establishment of Mendelian Law of Inheritance in the late 1880s there was an interest in ancestry, but understanding of inheritance was unclear and often guided by myths and folktales. Understanding genetics has become more urgent as research about genetics and disease and diversity in human population has increased dramatically following World War II.[46]

Part of the increased interest in diversity relates to the rapid increase in migration of people throughout the world. Humans have always been migratory creatures, but once they found ways to grow their food supplies, humans were largely tied to the land so they could plant, harvest, and practice animal husbandry. This transition from hunting and gathering migrations meant the family had to stay physically in one place. Marriage patterns were shaped to keep the working group — the family — within close physical contact, and everyone had clearly defined roles for all the work to get done.[47] However, following World War II the numbers of people migrating worldwide have been astonishing. One reason was that agricultural work became industrialized, and fewer people were needed on the farm, so they left the land to find work in the city. Another reason for migration was globalization of democracy that meant continents such as Africa and Asia were decolonized, resulting in large populations moving, sometimes as a result of war or tribal conflicts. An example in the United States was the civil rights movement in the 1960s, which promoted large numbers of farm workers in the south moving to industrial cities in the north. Now globally, groups are migrating not just within countries but between continents. Such cultural movements have challenged many of the former rigidly held rules about preferred marriages, raising many issues about ancestry. An intellectual movement concerned with ancestry was called *eugenics*.

Eugenics began in late 19th century England as social thought, linking the study of human biology and evolution for the betterment of humankind. Several scientists of that era such as Galton, Coon, and Davenport had presumably humanitarian goals for improving humans by proposing selective breeding or mating.[48] The first eugenics movement died out around 1910. Today, some are hesitant to study genetics in the

United States and Europe because of the visible abuse of genetics during the eugenics movement in the totalitarian Aryan aims of Nazi Germany in the 1930s and 1940s. Lashley,[49] a nurse and a molecular geneticist, has written a stellar second edition textbook, *Clinical Genetics in Nursing Practice*, in which she notes there are two types of eugenics: the negative and positive. The *negative* type seeks to reduce the number of undesirable persons who possess "unfit" traits, and the *positive* type tries to improve the genetics of a species by encouraging selective mating. In the United States a Eugenics Record Office was established in New York in 1910 with the goal of preserving the "racial welfare" of the United States; those people who were considered "fit" were of Anglo-Saxon or Nordic extraction and of high moral character. The procreation of these "fit" people was encouraged through all types of social programs and support; however, on the other hand, "unfit" persons were discouraged from even coming to the United States. One way to control "unfit" persons from immigrating occurred through an Act in 1924 that restricted immigration to only 2% of the number of each nationality listed in the 1890 census. For instance, if there was a meager number of immigrants coming from Togo, Africa in 1890, that number would continue to be very restricted with only 2% of the original number being allowed as immigrants to enter the United States after 1924. In contrast to this prejudicial restriction, "fit" Anglo-Saxon and Nordic folks were able to continue to immigrate up to 2% of their "generous" 1890 census, while other groups "unfit" were controlled to their minimal number. It may be surprising that this unbalanced immigration pattern existed until the passage of the Celler Act in 1965 — the beginning of the civil rights movement.[50]

Compulsory Sterilization Laws Affecting the Reproduction Pool Compulsory sterilization has been another way of preventing the reproduction of the "unfit" such as paupers, the insane, alcoholics, orphans, epileptics, and even chicken thieves.[51] The first state to pass sterilization laws was Indiana in 1907, and by 1935 thirty states had passed such laws. By then about 20,000 sterilizations had been performed. Abuses to involuntary sterilization are well known, and, unfortunately, nurses have been active participants in some of these sterilization movements. However,

nurses also have been responsible for the cessation of many others.[52] Entering the 21st century, nurses hopefully have become "enlightened" to assess moral and ethical issues through transcultural values.[53] Such issues as discriminatory practices toward some cultures still remain. In some parts of the United States, indigent welfare mothers (and some who are working poor) who are uninsured are given no choice — either have a Norplant birth-control devise implanted or are taken off of any type of state financial support. Is this a type of modern-day eugenics to control the reproduction of poor and indigent people? What are the moral and ethical implications? Transcultural nurses continue to investigate some of these culture care ideals that influence or control procreation. Cultural control of populations to protect the rights of some over others is a crucial transcultural nursing issue.

Mapping the Human Genome: a Cultural Change Influencing Biology A growing and important dimension influencing families is the *genome* factor related to family procreation. It is a relevant domain of inquiry for nurses working in transcultural areas to pursue. Probably no cultural change involving genetics has been so great as the international program to map the human genome. The genome consists of all the genetic material of the genes that make up the 46 chromosomes of human beings (23 from each parent). This mapping has great potential for transcultural nurses to understand and consider in work situations. The genome idea and major project began in 1953 when the double helix structure of the DNA was proposed by Watson and Crick, and in 1965 the genetic code was cracked. The first successful DNA cloning experiments began in 1972, in 1975 the first monoclonal antibodies were produced, and by 1977 the first human gene was cloned. By the mid 1980s there was international talk about mapping the entire human genome, and in 1990, with the financial assistance of Wellcome Trust of England and United Nations Education, Social and Cultural Organization (UNESCO), the 15 billion dollar collaborative international project was begun. The Human Genome Project is housed at the National Center for Human Genetic Research, later renamed the National Human Genome Research Institute of the National Institutes of Health (NIH) with James Watson and Francis S. Collins as the first and second directors.[54] Fogarty International Center of NIH remains a key player for maximizing international collaboration. Twenty-two centers across the United States have been established to help map the genome, and there are collaborative centers throughout the world. The goal to have the entire human genome mapped by 2005 seems to be realistic as early reports have been optimistic. Many commercial organizations are trying to maximize the benefits of being the first to discover some aspect of the genome for their commercial advantage — such as developing new drugs and vaccines.[55] As of December 1999 one chromosome has been entirely mapped.[56] Others are currently being mapped.

Genome research and projects related to it are a vital part of the biocultural basis of transcultural nursing. In a national survey only a few schools of nursing offered complete courses in genetics. The consequences of gene therapy can have great impact on health with the potential elimination of some disorders plaguing humankind.[56] Knowledge about the chemical parts of over 100,000 genes that make up the human genome are known, but far less is known about the actual *process* functioning between these parts.[57] Much is to be learned and many questions need answers such as the following: How do errors in DNA replication that become known as mutations go unnoticed unless a genetically related disease actually occurs? Can we carry mutations from one generation to another without consequence yet with potential harm to our offspring?

Generally, humans do not suffer any harmful effects from such inherited genes as humans carry two copies of almost all of our genes — one set from each parent. Genetic disease, however, actually occurs only if a set of defective recessive genes are received from both parents such as occurs in hemophilia. However, receiving a single dominant defective gene from one parent may also result in disease.[58] Since transcultural nurses focus on cultural diversity and similarities with the theory of Culture Care, they should have a major interest and leadership role in the Human Genome Project.[59]

Gene Therapy Human-Made Environment   Gene therapy is a human-made environment of importance. It is the technological method by which a missing or defective gene is actually replaced with a correct gene. For instance, people with hemophilia can now re-

ceive genetically engineered clotting factors that allow them to avoid the risk of exposure to transfused blood products.[60] Also, the locus for schizophrenia has been located that will be studied more definitively as it possibly explains a different clinical pattern in males than females.[61] Cystic fibrosis, muscular dystrophy, polycystic kidney disease, diabetes mellitus, Alzheimer's disease, and some cancers are other diseases and disorders that are targets for gene therapy. The potential for helping people seems great; however, the strengths and weaknesses need to be continually studied as there are many adverse views about gene therapy. In the Fifth Annual Report of Genetic Diseases it is estimated that 12% of adults and 30% of children admitted to hospitals have a genetic component to their illnesses. Fifty percent of all spontaneous abortions appear to be caused by chromosomal disorders. Thus, genetic factors play a critical role in morbidity and mortality.[62] What role will transcultural nurses have in gene therapy as they work directly with different cultures in providing direct and intimate care? What are the ethical aspects?

Ethics of the Genome Project   Nursing has a leadership role in the Human Genome Project. The Nursing Institute for Nursing Research (NINR) and the Human Genome Institute (HGI) are the two institutes of the National Institutes of Health (NIH) sharing in the overall research plan for the Human Genome Project. The role of NINR is to provide leadership in the area of ethical concerns. When the Genome Project was first established, a counterpart institute, the Ethical, Legal and Social Institute (ELSI) was also established.[63] Leading scientists and scholars developed the agenda for protecting human rights related to the international mapping of the human genome. Nursing's leadership in client and family counseling was recognized early and promoted with the Project.

The National Coalition for Health Professional Education was formed in 1997 under the leadership of the American Nurses Association (ANA) and the American Medical Association (AMA) and the National Genome Research Institute;[64] the Coalition's goals are to ensure that health care professionals are prepared with knowledge and resources to integrate the new genetic findings into their practices. The National Institute for Nursing Research (NINR) has been designated as the institute of NIH in which research studies related to the use of genetics, genetic counseling, and social issues will be reviewed and processed.[65] In 1998 a State of the Science of Genetics for Nursing was a Symposium offered with the School of Nursing, Johns Hopkins Center. There is an international nurses' organization: The International Society of Nurses in Genetics at http//www.147.134.150/isong that has an important function in building the knowledge base for genetic nursing.[66] Transcultural nursing needs to become actively involved for care phenomena with the beliefs, values, and meanings of specific cultures to be included and to ensure that ethical standards are held as primary concerns.

Biotechnology and Transcultural Nursing

Another human-made environment that is currently influencing transcultural nursing is biotechnology. This cultural technology has been greatly changing the face of health care in the United States in prevention, in treatment and care modalities, and in changing the courses of wellness and illness.[67-71] Indeed, the whole field of biopharmaceuticals has expanded in many ways through vaccines that prevent disease transmission. The use of biotechnological products at home, for pregnancy testing, and cholesterol screening; the glucose sensor for monitoring blood sugar; and all other uses are evident. Biotechnical products are increasing daily and influencing the interaction between biology and culture. In addition, health care is moving toward replacement of diseased organs with genetically engineered organs such as a pancreas in the treatment of diabetic patients or genetically engineered neuromuscular devices to aid those paralyzed or immobile with diseases such as Parkinson's or from accident injuries. What is the cultural care meaning and response to these products? In what ways is biotechnology influencing illness, health, and well-being? How has it changed caring practices? And are these meanings different in diverse cultural groups? How do transcultural nurses broker between the wishes of a dying patient and the technology used to extend life? Transcultural nurses are at the central focus dealing with biotechnologies that may be greatly feared, greatly welcomed, or even viewed as cultural taboos. There are many conflicts that transcultural nurses daily encounter, including moral-ethical and religious concerns.

One example of a conflict can be noted as debates are raised about the biotechnology of genetically altered food supplies. In the area of food production there are great differences in the acceptance of such technology. For instance, with the promise of expanding the world's food supply there is also a down side — that of making poor, developing nations more and more dependent on large, international, agricultural corporations that sell farmers in these countries genetically altered grains. Some of these grains are altered to make them sterile so that the farmers must buy new seeds for each planting rather than saving some seeds from the harvest for planting the next crop. Such a practice creates an increased dependency of the farmers on the genetically altered seeds and keeps them unable to gain economically and raise their natural and familiar geographic and cultural products.

Another area of concern is that the use of some altered grains appears to have long-term effects on the ecology. For example, when honeybees were fed on a concentrated solution of protein expressed by a genetically engineered grapeseed, those bees could not distinguish between the smell of flowers, and, alas, these bees died sooner than unexposed bees. As a response to the early death of bees, plants were not pollinated and could no longer reproduce, thus eventually diminishing the food supply in that area. As a result of some of these alterations and fears of disasters to their food supplies, the European Union (EU) has mandated that genetically modified foods must be labeled, whereas the United States government still opposes mandatory labeling. The EU goes farther as it prohibits imports of unapproved varieties of genetically engineered foods.[72] Transcultural nurses remain concerned and need to be continually alert to unethical practices that link the biologic and cultural practices of all people.

■ Transcultural Nursing Biocultural Contributions in the 21st Century

During the 20th century transcultural nursing has contributed greatly toward competent health care of culturally diverse people, bringing knowledge, understanding, and meaningful caring to many cultural groups. It is through understanding the essential tenets of Leininger's Culture Care Theory that transcultural nurses will continue to discover new dimensions of cultural lifeways.[73,74] This chapter has focused on the synthesis of biology and culture within theoretical frameworks supporting the biocultural basis of transcultural nursing. This broad, holistic synthesis can lead to the best possible choices for all of humankind.[75,76] Emerging challenges of biotechnology and gene therapy need transcultural nurses' rigorous research into the negatives and positives of changing norms, values, meanings, and practices. Globalization brings cultural conflicts and change into sharp focus that need theories like Culture Care to discover knowledge to provide culturally congruent care practices.

In summary, by using a broad biocultural framework for assessing needs and implementing care, we acknowledge the importance of understanding this synthesis as part of Leininger's quest for substantive and relevant transcultural nursing knowledge. Biocultural interactions may be beneficial or, on the contrary, detrimental to health. Examples of mating, genetics, and biotechnology were used in this chapter to stress the importance of using a holistic framework in transcultural nursing research and practice. Transcultural nursing remains the intellectual and transformative link in nursing to know, understand, and respond to diverse human behavior, as well as to search for ethical solutions to health problems.

References

1. Leininger, M., *Culture Care Diversity and Universality: A Theory of Nursing*, New York, NY: National League for Nursing Press, 1991.
2. Leininger, M., *Transcultural Nursing: Concepts, Theories, Research & Practice*, 2nd ed., New York, NY: McGraw Hill, Inc., 1995.
3. Leininger, M., "Overview of the Theory of Culture Care with the Ethnonursing Research Method," *Journal of Transcultural Nursing*, 1997, v. 8, no. 3, pp. 32–52.
4. Leininger, op. cit., 1995, p. 68.
5. Moore, L., P. Van Arsdale, J. Glittenberg, and R. Alrich, *The Biocultural Basis of Health*, Prospect Heights, II: Waveland Press, 1987.
6. Leininger, op. cit., 1991.
7. Andrew, M.M. and J.S. Boyle, *Transcultural Concepts in Nursing Care*, 3rd ed., Philadelphia: J.B. Lippincott Company, 1999.
8. Leininger, op. cit., 1991, p. 48.
9. Moore, et al., op. cit., 1987.
10. Glittenberg, J., "NIDDM (Non-insulin Dependent Diabetes Mellitus): A Biocultural Comparative Study of Gila River and Seri Pima Indians," paper presented at the American Anthropology Association Annual Meeting, Washington, DC, November 21, 1993.
11. Hogle, H.F., "Transforming 'Body Parts' into Therapeutic Tools: A Report from Germany," *Medical Anthropology Quarterly*, 1996, v. 10 no. 4, pp. 675–682.
12. Armelagoa, G.J., T.L. Leatherman, M. Ryan, and L. Sibley, "Biocultural Synthesis in Medical Anthropology, *Medical Anthropology Quarterly*, 1992, v. 14, pp. 35–52.
13. Baer, H.A., "Toward a Political Ecology of Health in Medical Anthropology. In Critical and Biocultural Approaches to Medical Anthropology: A Dialogue," *Medical Anthropology Quarterly*, 1996, v. 10, no. 4, pp. 451–454.
14. Kleffel, D., "An Ecofeminist Analysis of Nursing Knowledge," *Nursing Forum*, 1991, v. 26, no. 4, pp. 5–18.
15. Zimmerman, M., "Feminism, Deep Ecology and Environmental Ethics," *Environmental Ethics*, 1987, v. 9, no. 1, pp. 21–44.
16. Moore, et al, op. cit., 1987.
17. Glittenberg, J., *To the Mountain and Back*, Prospect Heights, II: Waveland Press, 1994.
18. Marks, J., *Human Biodiversity: Genes, Race and History*, New York: Aldine de Gruyter, 1995.
19. Overfield, T., *Biologic Variation in Health and Illness: Race, Age and Sex Differences*, Boca Raton: CRC Press, 1995.
20. Marks, op. cit., 1994.
21. D'Adamo, P.J. and C. Whitney, *Eat Right for Your Type*, New York: G.P. Putnam's Sons, 1996.
22. Ibid.
23. Brothwell, D., "Disease, Micro-Evolution and Earlier Populations: An Important Bridge Between Medical History and Human Biology," in *Modern Methods in the History of Medicine*, E. Clarke, ed., London: The Athlone Press, 1971.
24. D'Adamo, op. cit., 1996.
25. Ibid.
26. Ibid.
27. Ibid.
28. Glittenberg, op. cit., 1993.
29. Glittenberg, J., "A Comparative Study of Fertility in Highland Guatemalo: A Ladino and an Indian Town," unpublished dissertation, The University of Colorado, Boulder, CO, 1976.

30. Singer, M., "Farewell to Adaptationism: Unnatural Selection and the Politics of Biology," *Medical Anthropology Quarterly*, 1996, v. 10, no. 4, pp. 496–515.

31. Harris, M., *Theories of Culture in Postmodern Times*, Walnut Creek, CA: Altmira Press, 1999.

32. Leininger, M., op. cit., 1995, Gadsup Chapter, pp. 559–589.

33. Fisher, H., *Anatomy of Love*, New York: W.W. Norton and Company, Inc., 1992.

34. Jankowiak, W.R. and E.F. Fischer, "A Cross Cultural Perspective on Romantic Love," *Ethnology*, 1992, v. 31, no. 2, pp. 149–155.

35. Mead, M., *Male and Female*, New York: William Morrow, 1949.

36. Rosaldo, M.Z. and L. Lamphere, *Women, Culture and Society*, Stanford, CA: Stanford University Press, 1974.

37. Glittenberg, op. cit., 1993.

38. Glittenberg, op. cit., 1993.

39. Corbett, K.S. "Infant Feeding Styles of West Indian Women," *Journal of Transcultural Nursing*, 1999, v. 10, no. 1, pp. 14–21.

40. Kendall, K., "Maternal and Child Care in an Iranian Village," *Journal of Transcultural Nursing*, 1992, v. 4 (1 Summer), pp. 29–36.

41. Morgan, M., "Pregnancy and Childbirth Beliefs and Practices of American Hare Krishna Devotees within Transcultural Nursing," *Journal of Transcultural Nursing*, 1992, v. 4, no. 1, pp. 10–14.

42. Leininger, op. cit., 1987.

43. Leininger, op. cit., 1995.

44. Leininger, op. cit., 1997.

45. Goodheart, A., "Mapping the Past," *Civilization*, Library of Congress, March–April, 1996, pp. 14–20.

46. Lashley (Cohen), F.R., *Clinical Genetics in Nursing Practice*, 2nd ed., New York: Springer Publishing Co., 1998.

47. Glittenberg, op. cit., 1976.

48. Marks, op. cit., 1994.

49. Lashley, op. cit., 1998.

50. Ibid.

51. Ibid.

52. Ibid.

53. Leininger, op. cit., 1988.

54. Lashley, op. cit., 1998.

55. Glittenberg, J., "Mapping the Human Genome Across Millenia: Searching the Roots of Disease," paper presented at the American Anthropology Association Annual Meeting, Washington, D.C., 1999.

56. Hetteberg C.G., C.A. Prows, C. Deets, R.B. Monsen and C.A. Kenner, "National Survey of Genetics Content in Basic Nursing Preparatory Programs in the United States," *Nursing Outlook*, 1999, v. 47, no. 4, pp. 168–174.

57. Glittenberg, op. cit., 1999.

58. Lashley, op. cit., 1998.

59. Leininger, op. cit., 1991.

60. Lashley, op. cit., 1998.

61. Wei, J. and G.P. Hemmings, "Searching for a Locus for Schizophrenia Within Chromosome Xp11," *American Journal of Medical Genetics*, 2000, v. 96, pp. 4–7.

62. Lashley, op. cit., 1998.

63. Ibid.

64. Ibid.

65. Ibid.

66. Ibid.

67. Casper, M.J. and B. Koenig, "Reconfiguring Nature and Culture: Intersections of Medical Anthropology and Technoscience Studies," *Medical Anthropology Quarterly*, 1996, v. 10, no. 4, pp. 523–536.

68. Hess, M., "Technology and Alternative Cancer Therapies: An Analysis of Heterodoxy and Constructivism," *Medical Anthropology Quarterly*, 1996, v. 10, no. 4, pp. 657–674.

69. Kaufert, P.A. and J.M. Kaufert, "Anthropology and Technoscience Studies: Prospects for Synthesis and Ambiguity," *Medical Anthropology Quarterly*, 1996, v. 10, no. 4, pp. 675–689.

70. Leininger, op. cit., 1995.

71. Pfeifer, P.B. and M.R. Kraft, "Biotechnology Overview: From Science Fiction to Reality," in *Biotechnology Nursing Core Curriculum*, Pitman, NJ: National Federation for Specialty Nursing Organizations, 1995.

72. "Seeds of Change," *Consumer Report*, July 1999, pp. 41–45.

73. Leininger, M., *Care: The Essence of Nursing and Health*, Detroit: Wayne State University, 1988.

74. Leininger, op. cit., 1995.

75. Greaves, T. "Declaration on Anthropology and Human Rights," *Anthropology Newsletter*, September 1988.

76. Harris, op. cit., 1999.

7

Western Ethical, Moral, and Legal Dimensions Within the Culture Care Theory

Elizabeth Cameron-Traub

Cultural beliefs, values, and meanings often guide the thought and behavior of people in diverse cultures and underpin their moral, ethical, and legal codes. Nurses and other health professionals need to have culture-specific and universal ethical, moral, and legal cultural knowledge to guide their care decisions and actions in ways that are justifiable and defensible. Leininger's Theory of Culture Care Diversity and Universality challenges nurses to explore the domain of inquiry concerning the ethical, moral, and legal dimensions of culture care in relation to culture-specific or universal codes of moral behavior.[1,2] Cultural diversity underscores the importance of nurses gaining culturally ethical and moral care knowledge to provide culturally congruent care within varied care contexts.[3–6] The origins of the words "moral" (i.e., Roman) and "ethical" (i.e., Greek) indicate that they relate to "habits, customs, and ways of life, especially when these are assessed as good or bad, right or wrong."[7] The word *legal* relates to rules or laws, and sanctions made by a governing body. Moral or ethical values and norms, together with legal systems, provide frameworks to guide and make moral judgments about people's behavior in various situations, including health care. In this chapter the domain of inquiry is explored using a philosophical approach to identify areas of congruence between Western ethical, moral, and legal orientations and features of professional caring within Leininger's[8,9] Theory of Culture Care Diversity and Universality. Selected orientations, themes, and principles in Western moral philosophy, ethics, and bioethics relevant to contemporary health care provide a framework for a thematic analysis of ethical, moral, and legal aspects of culture care within Leininger's theory.

Cultural Aspects of Morality, Ethics, and Caring

All societies, large or small-scale, tend to have ethical systems based on values and principles that can be used to interpret people's behavior that has implications for others and affects their moral judgments about this behavior.[10] When people's duties or obligations in a social or cultural context conflict, general principles can assist them to resolve or arbitrate matters,[11] serving as moral or ethical codes, or reference points to guide moral decisions and actions, and setting standards of behavior.

Cultural systems or codes may provide rules and conditions that guide societal caring and maintain the social fabric, for example, by limiting injustices that are inconsistent with sociability and social well-being. Although moral codes or laws in a given society may change over time, they are generally binding on members and can be of great importance to people in their activities and life experiences, including health care. Leininger[12–14] encourages nurses to identify differences and similarities, or universals, in moral and ethical aspects of care and caring. These phenomena may be found in the cultural worldview — social structures and lifeways of cultures — to provide culture care that is morally, ethically, and legally congruent for people from diverse cultures.

Culture, Ethics, Relativism, and Universality

The cultural relevance of moral, ethical, and legal codes or systems may suggest that morality and ethics are whatever different cultures or societies depict. However, while there may be differences, there are also similarities or universals between cultures. It is an essential task for philosophers and others who have concern for morality and ethical behavior in human interaction to identify standards or rules of morality that would apply across cultures. It is argued that ethical relativism (i.e., that which is good or right depends on the group) is not a defensible philosophical position and that a universal viewpoint is required in ethics.[15] Condemnations of some societal actions with moral implications of universal significance (e.g., persecution, torture, victimisation, war crimes, and ethnic cleansing) in many ways transcend culture-specific views of morality and judgments about right or wrong, good or bad actions and indicate the need for universally accepted moral standards. Issues related to human rights and international codes of practice, for example, in health care[16–19] or biomedical research[20] concern identification and application of universal principles to guide critical moral actions and decisions. Efforts to introduce or enforce universal principles to protect human rights, however, do not suggest that for all ethical views, actions, or decisions to be right or good they have to be universal, regardless of historical or social contexts. On the contrary, the idea of ethics being universal refers to the logical defense of a moral judgment, whereby, if a principle is accepted in one case or situation, then it applies to all similar circumstances.[21]

Principles that guide moral action, or resolve moral problems, tend to have certain characteristics.[22–24] First, the principles or rules consider more than the interests of the individual; that is, they go beyond self-interest and determine a moral decision or action in a given situation. Second, they are expected to be applicable across all such cases or situations (i.e., universal). Third, they provide culturally shared reasons to support or defend the decision or action. Indeed, cultural beliefs and values provide "moral presuppositions," whereas ethics generally refers to a "formal normative framework" for moral decisions and actions.[25]

 ## Ethics and Moral Philosophy: Western Approaches

Moral philosophy and the field of ethics, as known in Western cultures, have been affected by various social, cultural, historical, economic, and political influences on Western thought and reasoning and the outcomes of diverse and intensive philosophical discussion and debate extending over many centuries. As a systematic study of morality and moral behavior, ethics is characterised by moral reasoning and rational argument to provide support for, or to defend, moral choices made between a number of alternatives. There are two fields of study in ethics. First, the area of *prescriptive* (or *normative*) ethics seeks to determine what "ought" or "should" be done, and second, the field of *descriptive* ethics describes what "is" done.[26] It is generally accepted within pluralist societies that ethical viewpoints and arguments are diverse and reflect many different values. In contrast, in a society characterised by culturally shared values, beliefs, and practices, descriptive ethics can reflect moral expectations that are essentially normative for that society.

Approaches to Western Moral Argument and Ethics

Philosophical or normative (Western) ethics tends to address two main questions. One question relates to how people ought (or should) behave and thus the duties they have, whereas the second question asks what is the value and desirability of actions, and what relative good arises from them.[27] These questions correspond to two main approaches or viewpoints in philosophical debate. One approach is called *deontological* and focuses on the importance of *duty* and the inherent rightness (or wrongness) of a moral action. The other approach is identified as *teleological* (i.e., purposive) or *consequentialist* and focuses on the *value* (good or bad) of anticipated consequences of moral action.[28]

Debates in moral philosophy also address whether ethical or moral reasoning can be based on rules, laws, or principles that would apply to all moral acts of a certain kind regardless of context, or alternatively, on the nature of a particular act in a given situation. This distinction between moral argument based on rule or act may seem to be important in health care since health professionals typically make clinical decisions that pertain to clients, generally on a one-to-one basis. However, as noted above, it is generally accepted that reasons supporting a moral decision are based on at least one ethical principle that would apply to all similar cases or situations.[29–31]

Ethics in Professional Health Care

The diversity of moral or ethical codes and viewpoints in Western normative ethics (e.g., bioethics) is consistent with a tolerance of pluralist societal beliefs and values. Multiple philosophical viewpoints in ethics may suggest that the area is rather academic and abstract and of dubious relevance to ethical or moral issues or concerns that are encountered by nurses and other health professionals in their practice. However, the two main approaches do provide focal points for discussion and ethical debate in health care. A *teleological* (or consequences) approach to ethical health care decision making is characterised by primary consideration of the purpose of the action and the anticipated outcomes (or good). In contrast, health care decisions made from a *deontological* (or duty) viewpoint focus on the nature of the action itself, whether it is right or desirable, in addition to, or more so than, the expected effects or outcomes. For example, the nurse who argues against abortion or euthanasia may do so on the grounds that these are acts of killing, and so they are wrong, and that moral action is to preserve not to take life (deontological argument). Alternatively, the nurse may argue that the outcomes or consequences of the abortion or euthanasia will be inevitably bad and outweigh any supposed good, and that therefore the procedure should not be done (teleological and primarily utilitarian argument).

Principles in Bioethics

Beauchamp and Childress[32] identify four principles to guide ethical or moral decision making in contemporary health care. These principles are *respect for autonomy* (to act in respect of another as an autonomous person); *nonmaleficence* (to act so as not to inflict harm); *beneficence* (to act to benefit another); and *justice* (to act fairly). It will be noted again that these principles have been determined within a Western moral philosophical framework. Later in this chapter I will consider how these principles may relate to professional practice and culture care.

Cultural Diversity and Ethical, Moral, and Legal Considerations in Health Care

Practice by health professionals generally takes place within a Western biomedical cultural framework.[33–35] It is argued that nursing should shift from a predominantly unicultural orientation to transcultural practice to meet the special needs of people, for example, in Australia.[36–44] The ways nurses and other health professionals tend to think about ethical issues or dilemmas may correspond to dominant cultural values underpinning professional health care and practice orientations.[45–49]

Western ethical and moral values, meanings, and practices may not be congruent with those in non-Western cultures.[50–53] There may also be marked differences in meanings or interpretations of ethical, moral, or legal phenomena between countries within the Western tradition.[54] Thus, views and arguments in ethics may require careful consideration of cultural differences to avoid or prevent cultural conflict, imperialism, or imposition. First, the decision itself and the underlying ethical reasoning supporting it need to be examined for congruence with reasoning and ethical or moral expectations, values, and meanings within the client's culture. Second, the manner in which the client, or family, is informed of the decision must be addressed within the context of the client's culture for values, meanings, patterns, and practices of professional care to be culturally congruent for the client. Third, ethical, moral, or legal aspects of the client's culture may need to be considered and incorporated into decision making if the decision or act itself, or expected effects or outcomes, are to be morally acceptable to the client or family. Indeed, the application of any ethical or moral principles from a professional viewpoint may require a great deal of cultural knowledge and sensitivity for the decisions and actions to be rendered as culturally congruent in meaning and significance and as acceptable within another culture.[55–57]

The legal frameworks of importance to the client may extend beyond the formal legislation prevailing in a society, or dominant culture, in which the person or family lives. Cultural rules or laws that determine the acceptability of behavior, and punishment or retribution for morally unacceptable behavior, may be very important to the client. For example, tribal law in some societies can be critically binding on members of the group and can be considered more important, or more fearful, than legal matters determined by a dominant culture. Cultural care would address legal matters that are culturally significant for the client.

 ## Ethical and Moral Care Themes in Culture Care Theory

Ethical, moral, or legal aspects of culture care can be explored within Leininger's[58,59] Theory of Culture Care Diversity and Universality. The following discussion identifies some theoretical themes and predictions that illuminate aspects of ethical, moral, and legal culture care to guide and inform professional nursing and health care practice. This analysis involves selected orientations, concepts, and principles in Western moral philosophy and ethics.

Philosophical Orientations in Culture Care

Leininger[60] states that the purpose of the theory is "to discover human care diversities and universalities in relation to worldview, social structure, and other dimensions cited, and then to discover ways to provide culturally congruent care to people of different or similar cultures in order to maintain or regain their well-being, health, or face death in a culturally appropriate way." Furthermore, "the goal of the theory is to improve and to provide culturally congruent care to people that is beneficial, will fit with, and be useful to the client, family, or culture group healthy lifeways."[61] Finally, in terms of outcomes, Leininger[62] states that "the findings from the theory would be used toward providing care that blends with culture values, beliefs, and lifeways of people, and is assessed to be beneficial, satisfying, and meaningful to people of designated cultures."

These definitions of purpose, goal, expected outcomes, and value are consistent with a *teleological* orientation to moral and ethical determinations in regard to culture care. The statement of purpose explicates the intention, focusing on the importance of theoretically guided inquiry and discovery pertaining to culture care. The goal, again a purposive (or teleological) statement, identifies the expected value or good related to culturally congruent care. The purposive approach is further reinforced in the statement of expected outcomes. A teleological ethical orientation in the Theory of Culture Care Diversity and Universality is not surprising, since professional health care is expected to have beneficial outcomes, and the theory explicates how these may be affected and what they should be.

A *deontological* orientation can also be found with- in Leininger's Culture Care Theory, although it is implicit rather than explicitly stated. The theory predicts that culture care combines or synthesizes professional (or *etic*) care with generic (or *emic*) care for a given client. If professional care fails to incorporate cultural care information, then the care would not be morally or ethically defensible; that is, the professional duty would not have been fulfilled. Nurses have a duty of care, and thus a duty or obligation to seek and obtain all relevant information (including cultural) pertaining to their clients and to develop relevant competencies and skills, again guided by the theory, to meet requirements for professional practice. Thus, deontological aspects of ethical, moral, and legal culture care can be identified within Culture Care Theory and highlight its importance as a guide to professional nursing and health care.

 ## Using Leininger's Sunrise Model and Bioethics

Leininger's Sunrise Model[63] provides a framework to explore ethical, moral, and legal dimensions of culture care. Cultural phenomena revealed through the worldview, language, ethnohistory, and various social and cultural factors may indicate moral, ethical, or legal codes, values, meanings, patterns, and practices that should be addressed in determining provision of health care for people from a given culture. For example, a requirement in professional practice is that a client consenting to a biomedical or nursing procedure is fully informed of the purpose, possible risks, actions to be taken, and expected outcomes. The nature and validity of informed consent may be affected by a number of cultural phenomena, including worldview, language, ethnohistory, and the environmental context, as well as educational, technological, religious, social and kinship, political and legal, or economic factors. The cultural adequacy of the client's consent needs to be ensured in the professional care context. Cultural implications of the client's potential choices may relate significantly to specific care values and meanings that would be addressed in the process of the client's decision making if informed consent is to be valid and professional care defensible from moral, ethical, and legal viewpoints.

Principles in Bioethics and Culture Care

Ethical and moral aspects of culture care, using Leininger's Theory of Culture Care, will now be considered against the four principles for bioethics referred to above. If these principles define orientations that assist health professionals to approach care decisions and actions, then one would expect them to be congruent with care themes and dimensions within the Theory of Culture Care, a theory of professional nursing and health care.

Respect for Autonomy

Culture Care Theory reflects a deep respect for people from diverse cultures and the need for care decisions to respect the client's choices, guided by and consistent with their cultural care values, expressions, and meanings. Although autonomy and the related concept of self-determination are Western values and not necessarily universal,[64,65] the significance of this ethical principle is reflected in the prediction that culturally congruent care would be provided when the client's cultural care is incorporated into nursing care decisions. Thus, professional care would involve respect for the client's autonomy, including care values, expressions and meanings, and their choices.

Respect for autonomy of the client means that the health professional would actively include the client's cultural viewpoints and that culture care would be coestablished between the nurse and client, as indicated in the theory. A conflict between professional (*etic*) and client (*emic*) moral codes would be resolved through culture care. Finally, respect for autonomy in health care would include the nurse or other health professional acting to prevent decisions and actions that are culturally incongruent. Acting in accordance with the principle of respect for autonomy in regard to all clients would assist professional decision making in transcultural health care situations.

Beneficence and Nonmaleficence

There are several indications that Culture Care Theory is focused on guiding professional practice that would produce beneficial outcomes and that any nonbeneficial actions or those of maleficent intent would be avoided, minimized, or eliminated. Philosophical discussion about the theory in relation to beneficence and nonmaleficence would go well beyond the scope of this paper. To encapsulate the main ideas, the reader is referred to the Leininger's[66] theoretical statements, especially those relating to the purpose, goal, and expected outcomes of culture care. There are three areas of importance in relation to professional intentions that would be characterized as beneficent and nonmaleficent in transcultural nursing and health care. First, the nurse who does not have cultural care knowledge should obtain it before making care decisions or taking actions in the care of clients. Second, cultural knowledge alone is not enough; the nurse should use this knowledge during processes of caring and should seek information from the client to guide, confirm, or refute actions and care decisions that the nurse considers from a professional viewpoint. Third, the nurse who practices only from a professional (or *etic*) viewpoint would not be fulfilling the ethical principle of beneficence, since Leininger's theory predicts that culture care is required to provide beneficial and satisfying care. Fourth, the nurse, or other, who denies the importance of cultural knowledge in professional caring, or fails to use it, may not satisfy the principle of nonmaleficence, since the theory predicts, and substantial research has shown, that culturally incongruent care is detrimental to the health or well-being of clients. Cultural conflict and imposition may result in cultural pain when professional decisions and actions are inconsistent with client's cultural values, patterns, and practices.[67] Therefore, the principles of beneficence and nonmaleficence as guides to ethical professional practice are highly consistent with themes and professional intentions within Leiningers' Theory of Culture Care Diversity and Universality.[68,69]

Justice

As for most moral, ethical, or legal principles the concept and practice of justice may be socially and culturally constructed and expressed in culture-specific and universal ways. In general, it is a principle pertaining to fairness, and it may be considered in regard to rights, retribution, and the distribution of good, harm, or resources, including in health care.[70–73] The main theories in contemporary philosophy focus on justification by entitlement or need, and each raises concerns in terms of adequacy.[74] Alternatively, justice in relation to good can be explored within the framework of natural law theory.[75] Although there may be no conclusive philosophical approach to justice, nevertheless, it is a concept that often underpins contemporary thinking in terms of what is right, good, proper, or fair. For example, judgments of fairness are made every day in regard to the allocation of resources for people seeking professional health care in hospitals or clinics or community care services.

Themes related to justice such as entitlement and need may be found in Culture Care Theory. Culture care would be entitlements for people from different cultures; it may also be required to meet client's health needs effectively and in satisfying ways. Thus, fairness to people from cultural backgrounds different from the care context may require a culture care approach. In other words, from the client's viewpoint culture care would be a necessary condition for professional care to be morally, ethically, or legally defensible in regard to the principle of justice. If the societal expectation of health professionals is to consider care for each client as an individual human being, then justice in professional practice includes attention to cultural phenomena pertaining to the client. Holistic caring is justice oriented.

Ethical, Moral, and Legal Decisions and Actions Using Culture Care Theory

Leininger's[76] theory postulates three modes for nursing decisions and actions to "assist, support, facilitate, or enhance" culturally congruent care for people from diverse cultures. These three modes are 1) *culture care preservation and/or maintenance*, 2) *culture care accommodation and/or negotiation*, and 3) *culture*
care repatterning and/or restructuring*. Using cultural knowledge, competencies, and skills, the nurse will arrive at appropriate uses of the action modes. Multiple and varied cultural phenomena and factors, as indicated by Leininger's theory and reflected in the Sunrise Model, may influence the use of the action modes.

Where there is evidence of similarity or congruence between ethical, moral, and legal aspects of care from the professional viewpoint, and from the cultural viewpoint of the client, the action mode of *culture care preservation and/or maintenance* would be appropriate. Moreover, decisions or actions that are consistent with universal moral or ethical views, principles, or codes of conduct would be taken in relation to this action mode.

When there are different or conflicting cultural view- points, the nurse may use the action mode of *culture care accommodation and or negotiation* to help the client to "adapt to, or to negotiate with, others for a beneficial or satisfying health outcome with professional care providers."[77] For example, the nurse may use this action mode to obtain a required consent for treatment for a female client from a culture in which the husband's consent would be required within the cultural framework of ethical and legal responsibility. Transcultural approaches to professional practice may need to be taken, for example, when informing a client of "bad news" such as malignancy or terminal illness.[78–81] The nurse or other health professional would need to seek culturally congruent ways to meet the client's care needs.

In situations where cultural differences would have ethical, moral, or legal implications that may impact in nonbeneficial ways on the health or well-being of the client, the nurse would use the action mode of *culture care repatterning and/or restructuring*. The nurses would coestablish with the client how to "reorder, change, or greatly modify their lifeways for new, different, and beneficial health care pattern while respecting the client(s) cultural values and beliefs."[82] For example, the nurse may need to use cultural care knowledge to ensure that a client is informed of possible consequences of accepting or refusing treatment (e.g., blood transfusion, chemotherapy, surgery, diagnostic tests, or immunization) in culturally congruent ways. Through extensive and consistent examination of culture care phenomena for the client, and others affected by decisions and actions, the nurse would seek to provide ethical, moral, and legal culture care. There are many challenges in contemporary health care that raise ethical, moral, or legal concerns, for example, issues related to withdrawal of treatment (not for resuscitation orders), organ donation, organ transplantation, reproductive technology, surrogacy, genetics, reproductive rights, abortion, euthanasia, female circumcision, clinical trials, and any issue pertaining to human life or death, health, or well-being.

Conclusion

Moral codes of thought and behavior are inextricably linked with culture. All health professionals are challenged to be open and responsive to culturally different viewpoints, values, expressions, and meanings that have significance and meanings in different cultural contexts. Moral, ethical, and legal dimensions of culture care can be readily identified as themes in Leininger's Theory of Culture Care Diversity and Universality. Western ethical orientations and principles are highly congruent with moral and ethical themes in the theory, highlighting its relevance as a guide to professional health care practice for nurses and others who are concerned with human care and caring. Culture care that addresses moral, ethical, and legal orientations within varied care contexts is critical for health professionals to practice from defensible moral, ethical, and legal viewpoints and for their care decisions and actions to be consistent with culturally specific or universal moral codes.

References

1. Leininger, M., "Leininger's Theory of Culture Care Diversity and Universality: A Theory of Nursing," *Nursing Science Quarterly*, 1988, v. 1, no. 4, pp. 152–160.
2. Leininger, M., "The Theory of Culture Care Diversity and Universality," in *Culture Care Diversity and Universality: A Theory of Nursing*, M. Leininger, ed., New York: National League for Nursing Press, 1991a.
3. Leininger, M., "Culture: The Conspicuous Missing Link to Understand Ethical and Moral Dimensions of Human Care," in *Ethical and Moral Dimensions of Care*, M. Leininger, ed., Detroit: Wayne State University Press, 1990, pp. 49–66.
4. Leininger, M., "Transcultural Care Principles, Human Rights and Ethical Considerations," *Journal of Transcultural Nursing*, 1991b, v. 3, no. 1, pp. 21–23.
5. Leininger, M., "Ethical, Moral and Legal Aspects of Transcultural Nursing," in *Transcultural Nursing, Concepts, Theories and Practices*, 2nd ed., M. Leininger, ed., New York: McGraw-Hill, 1995, pp. 25–314.
6. Stitzlein, D., "Phenomenon of Moral Care/Caring Conceptualized Within Leininger's Theory," paper presented at the 25th Annual Transcultural Nursing Society Conference, Snowbird, Utah, October 1999.
7. Lacy, A.R., *A Dictionary of Philosophy*, 2nd ed., London: Routledge, 1986, p. 154.
8. Leininger, op. cit., 1988.
9. Leininger, op. cit., 1991a.
10. Silberbauer, G., "Ethics in Small-Scale Societies," in *A Companion to Ethics*, P. Singer, ed., Oxford: Blackwell Reference, 1993, pp. 14–28.
11. Midgley, M., "The Origin of Ethics," in *A Companion to Ethics*, P. Singer, ed., Oxford: Blackwell Reference, 1993, pp. 3–13.
12. Leininger, op. cit., 1990.
13. Leininger, op. cit., 1991b.
14. Leininger, op. cit., 1995.
15. Singer, P., *Practical Ethics*, 2nd ed., Cambridge: Cambridge University Press, 1993a.
16. Leininger, op. cit., 1991b.
17. DeVries, R. and J. Subedi, eds., *Bioethics and Society, Constructing the Ethical Enterprise*, Upper Saddle River, NJ: Prentice Hall, 1998.
18. Moskop, J.C. and L.Kopelman, eds., *Ethics and Critical Care Medicine*, Dordrecht: D. Riedel Publishing Company, 1985.
19. Pellegrino, E., P. Mazzarella, and P. Corsi, eds., *Transcultural Dimensions in Medical Ethics*, Frederick, MD: University Publishing Group, 1992.
20. Vanderpool, H.Y. ed., *The Ethics of Research Involving Human Subjects: Facing the 21st Century*, Frederick, MD: University Publishing Group, 1996.
21. Beauchanp, T.L. and J.F. Childress, *Principles of Biomedical Ethics*, 3rd ed., New York: Oxford University Press, 1989.
22. Shaw, W.H., *Social and Personal Ethics*, Belmont, CA: Wadsworth, 1993.
23. Singer, op. cit., 1993a.
24. Beauchamp and Childress, op. cit., 1989.

25. Pellegrino, E.D., "Prologue: Intersections of Western Biomedical Ethics and World Culture," in *Transcultural Dimensions in Medical Ethics*, E. Pelligrino, P. Mazzarella, and P. Corsi, eds., Frederick, MD: University Publishing Group, 1992, pp. 13–19.
26. Lacy, op. cit., 1986.
27. Ibid.
28. Ibid.
29. Beauchamp and Childress, op. cit., 1989.
30. Singer, op. cit., 1993a.
31. Singer, P., *A Companion to Ethics*, Oxford: Blackwell Reference, 1993b.
32. Beauchamp and Childress, op. cit., 1989.
33. Leininger, M., *Nursing and Anthropology: Two Worlds to Blend*, New York: John Wiley & Sons, 1970.
34. Leininger, M., *Transcultural Nursing: Concepts, Theories and Practices*, New York: John Wiley & Sons, 1978.
35. Leininger, op. cit., 1995.
36. Cameron-Traub, E., "Meeting Health Care Needs in Australia's Diverse Society," in *Contexts of Nursing*, J. Daly, S. Speedy, and D. Jackson, eds., Sydney: MacLennan and Petty, 2000.
37. Cameron-Traub, E., and A. Stewart, "Clients from Eastern Countries: A New Worldview in Australian Nursing," in *Issues in Australian Nursing 4*, G. Gray and R. Pratt, eds., Melbourne: Churchill Livingstone, 1995, pp. 115–128.
38. Harrison, L. and E. Cameron-Traub, "Patient's Perspectives on Nursing in Hospital," in *Just Health, Inequality in Illness, Care and Prevention*, C. Waddell and A.R. Peterson, eds., Melbourne: Churchill Livingstone, 1994, pp. 147–158.
39. Kanitsaki, O., "Acculturation—A New Dimension in Nursing," *The Australian Nurses Journal*, 1983, v. 13, no. 5, pp. 42–53.
40. Kanitsaki, O., "Transcultural Nursing: Challenge to Change," *The Australian Journal of Advanced Nursing*, 1988, v. 5, no. 3, pp. 4–11.
41. Kanitsaki, O., "Transcultural Human Care: Its Challenge to and Critique of Professional Nursing Care," in *A Global Agenda for Caring*, D.A. Gaut, ed., New York: National League for Nursing Press, 1993, pp 19–45.
42. Omeri, A. and E. Cameron-Traub, *Transcultural Nursing in Multicultural Australia*, Deakin, ACT, Australia: Royal College of Nursing, Australia, 1996.
43. Omeri, A. and V. Nahas, "Working with a Multicultural Community: Cultural Care Nursing Assessment," in *Issues in Australian Nursing 5, The Nurse as Clinician*, G. Gray and R. Pratt, eds., Melbourne: Churchill Livingstone, 1995, pp. 149–162.
44. Pittman, L. and T. Rogers, "Nursing: A Culturally Diverse Profession in a Monocultural Health System," *The Australian Journal of Advanced Nursing*, 1990, v. 8, no. 1, pp. 30–38.
45. Johnstone, M.J. and O. Kanitsaki, "Rationalization of Interpreter Services for NESB and Health Care: A Question of Human Rights," *Health Issues*, 1991b, v. 27, pp. 9–11.
46. Rickard, M., H. Kuhse, and P. Singer, "Caring and Justice: A Study of Two Approaches to Health Care Ethics," *Nursing Ethics*, 1996, v. 3, no. 3, pp. 212–223.
47. Eliason, M.J., "Ethics and Transcultural Nursing Care," *Nursing Outlook*, 1993, v. 41, no. 5, pp. 225–228.
48. Gorman, D., "Multiculturalism and Transcultural Nursing in Australia," *Journal of Transcultural Nursing*, 1995, v. 6, no. 2, pp. 27–33.
49. Kikuchi, J.F., "Multicultural Ethics in Nursing Education: A Potential Threat to Responsible Practice," *Journal of Professional Nursing*, 1996, v. 12, no. 3, pp. 159–165.
50. Leininger, op. cit., 1991b.
51. Leininger, op. cit., 1995.
52. Pellegrino, et al., op. cit., 1992.
53. Singer, op. cit., 1993b.
54. Marshall, P., D.C. Thomasma, and J. Bergsma, "Intercultural Reasoning: The Challenge for International Bioethics," *Cambridge Quarterly of Healthcare Ethics*, 1994, v. 3, no. 3, pp. 21–328.
55. Leininger, op. cit., 1990.
56. Leininger, op. cit., 1991b.
57. Leininger, op. cit., 1995.
58. Leininger, op. cit., 1988.
59. Leininger, op. cit., 1991a.
60. Leininger, op. cit., 1991a, p. 39.
61. Ibid.
62. Ibid.
63. Leininger, op. cit., 1991b, p. 43.
64. Glick, S.M., "Unlimited Human Autonomy—A Cultural Bias?" *The New England Journal of Medicine*, 1997, v. 336, pp. 954–956.
65. Klessig, J., "The Effect of Values and Culture on Life-Support Decisions," *The Western Journal of Medicine*, 1992, v. 157, no. 3, pp. 316–322.

66. Leininger, op. cit., 1991a.
67. Leininger, M., "Understanding Cultural Pain for Improved Health Care," *Journal of Transcultural Nursing*, 1997, v. 9, no. 1, pp. 32–35.
68. Leininger, op. cit., 1988.
69. Leininger, op. cit., 1991a.
70. Beauchamp and Childress, op. cit., 1989.
71. Johnstone, M.J., *Nursing and the Injustices of the Law*, Sydney: W.B. Saunders/Bailliere Tindall, 1994a.
72. Johnstone, M.J., *Bioethics, A Nursing Perspective*, 2nd ed., Sydney: W.B. Saunders/Bailliere Tindall. 1994b.
73. Thompson, I.E., K.M. Melia, and K.M. Boyd, *Nursing Ethics*, 3rd ed., Edinburgh: Churchill Livingstone, 1994.
74. MacIntyre, A., *After Virtue, A Study in Moral Theory*, London: Duckworth, 1981.
75. Finnis, J., *Natural Law and Natural Rights*, Oxford: Clarendon Press, 1980.
76. Leininger, op. cit., 1991a, pp. 48–49.
77. Ibid.
78. Beyene, Y., "Medical Disclosure and Refugees, Telling Bad News to Ethiopian Patients," *Western Journal of Medicine*, 1992, v. 157, no. 3, pp. 328–332.
79. Brotzman, G.L. and D.J. Butler, "Cross-Cultural Issues in the Disclosure of a Terminal Diagnosis, a Case Report," *The Journal of Family Practice*, 1991, v. 32, no. 4, pp. 426–427.
80. Jecker, N.S., J.A. Carrese, and R.A. Pearlman, "Caring for Patients in Cross-Cultural Settings," *Hasting Center Report*, 1995, v. 25, no. 1, pp. 6–14.
81. Takahashi, Y., "Informing a Patient of Malignant Illness: Commentary from a Cross-Cultural Viewpoint," *Death Studies*, 1990, v. 14, pp. 83–91.
82. Leininger, op. cit., 1991, p. 49.

Special Topics in Transcultural Nursing

CHAPTER 8

Cultures and Tribes of Nursing, Hospitals, and the Medical Culture

Madeleine Leininger

If health professionals are to function effectively and humanistically with people of diverse cultures, then one must understand one's own culture, the culture of one's profession, the culture of the workplace and community and other cultures. Such insights are imperative to respond appropriately to others. LEININGER, 1975

With the advent of transcultural nursing in the mid 20th century, there were new challenges and insights for nurses and the nursing profession. It was at this time that the author as a nurse anthropologist realized that there were cultural differences among health professional cultures as nursing, medicine, and others, which needed to be studied to understand the major features of each profession. Such insight could help nurses with comparative reviews of their particular values and norms. This challenge seemed long overdue as nurses, physicians, and other health professional groups had functioned together for more than 100 years. Moreover, this knowledge could help in understanding the tendencies and expectations of each profession, as well as the conflicts, tensions, and concerns of diverse professionals. Most importantly, nursing was often caught in the middle of medicine, social work, and other disciplines as the direct care provider. This led me to begin studying nursing's culture and medicine, and I wrote about the culture of nursing and other health cultures, which were the first writings on this subject for nurses.[1]

In this chapter, the culture and tribes of United States nursing will be discussed along with the hospital culture and a few perspectives about the culture of medicine. In addition, some glimpses of other nursing cultures such as Australia, Great Britain, and others will be presented to obtain a comparative nursing perspective. Much could be written about the early and current culture of each, but hopefully these ideas and others will stimulate additional studies in all health professions. In the past decade, the cultures of nursing and medicine have been of considerable interest with the realization of the importance to know much more about these cultures. It is, of course, well to start with one's own culture and know it before moving to others.

Culture of Nursing

To understand the culture of nursing, the nurse is in a central and unique position. Figure 8.1 provides a view of nurses' unique role.

In the diagram, the nurse appears in the center of many cultures. However, it is important to first understand one's own personal and professional cultures and then to become knowledgeable about the nursing culture and other cultures. The professional nursing culture has its patterned beliefs, values, norms, and practices that can have a significant influence on one's self and others. Soon, however, the nurse realizes the influence of the cultures of medicine, hospital (or agency culture), and other professional cultures as the nurse interacts with them in any typical day or night. These cultures can not be overlooked, but need to be reflected on to establish and maintain good interpersonal relationships and for better client care. Each professional culture has

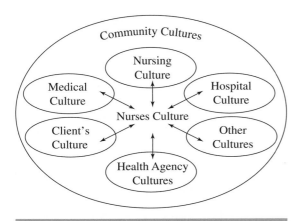

Figure 8.1
The nurse and other cultures.

different values, beliefs, and norms that guide their actions and decisions.

The idea of studying the culture of nursing in the 1950s and 1960s was, however, unknown to most nurses, and some nurses held it was useless and unimportant. They said that it had limited relevance to the practice of nursing and that other areas were more important to study. Yet the culture of nursing became more important as I observed, listened to, and watched many nurses in their interaction with other nurses, physicians, social workers, clients, and hospital representatives. Knowledge of these diverse cultures or subcultures with identifiable norms, values, and behavior was clearly influencing the way others responded and in their work roles and lives. Even of greater importance was the thought that the culture of nursing, medicine, and other health professional cultures needed study for their interactional influences on people. This area was long overdue, as well as how the client's culture was influenced by professional cultures.

Most importantly, the long range goal to establish ultimately a body of *comparative* transcultural nursing knowledge about different nursing cultures worldwide could bring forth some extremely useful transcultural nursing knowledge. It could facilitate better communication, deeper understanding of people, more effective collegial professional work, and understanding of transcultural care practices and outcomes. What are the cultural beliefs, values, norms, and practices of nursing cultures worldwide? What might be some

universal cultural norms, values, and beliefs of nursing cultures? In what ways could such knowledge be used to advance humanistic care knowledge and practices of nursing worldwide? A whole new area of discovery was unknown to nurses in the mid 20th century. Of course, nurses talked occasionally about aspects of their cultural travel experiences earlier, but nurses' culture values, beliefs, and practices needed to be identified, documented, analyzed, and synthesized. It seemed like an urgent need for the future success and advancement of nursing.

I recall that in the early 1960s when I first began to explore with nurses the lifeways and patterns for the United States culture of nursing, I received some interesting comments such as, "This is useless knowledge for every nurse, is highly individualistic, and there are no commonalities"; "How can we use such knowledge as all situations are different in nursing and each nurse is different?"; "There is more important and practical work to do such as giving patients medicines and treatments"; and "You're wasting your time studying nurses as a culture — I don't know what this means." Nonetheless, I continued to observe, interview, and talk with nurses about their values, beliefs, and recurrent patterns in nursing, but was also attentive to listen to nurses from other countries. This first work led to the paper, "Cultural Differences among Staff Members and the Impact on Patient Care" (1968)[2]; then to the next paper, "The Tribes of Nursing in the United States" (Leininger, 1985)[3]; and to two creative major papers entitled, "Grisrun and Enicidem: Two Tribes in the Health Professions." (Leininger, 1976).[4] These studies became of great interest to nurses and especially to see documented differences among the cultures of the clients, nursing, and medicine with intercultural patterns of variations across the United States and some shared commonalities. These studies helped nurses to realize the importance of studying the culture of nurses and nursing worldwide. Based on this work, the author has remained alert to commonalities and differences of nursing cultures and changes that occur over time and in different places in the world of nursing.

Reasons to Learn About the Culture of Nursing

Why should nurses be interested in and learn about the culture of nursing? There are several major reasons.

First, knowledge of the culture of nursing can assist nurses in the profession to understand some of the dominant, recurrent, and patterned features of nursing. Accordingly, it can help nurses to reflect on their nursing behaviors and gain fresh insights or perspectives about the beliefs and practices of the nursing profession. Second, such knowledge serves as a valuable historical guide to reflect on changes in the nursing profession over time and speculate about possible reasons for any changes. Today and in the past, nurses need to realize that nursing as a culture can change over time in varying ways, or it can remain relatively stable.

Third, knowledge of the nature, beliefs, and characteristics of diverse and similar cultural features of nursing is essential to provide sensitive and understanding nursing care practices. Nurses' cultural behavior can influence the clients. Gaining knowledge about the culture of nursing can be enormously helpful to guide nurses in their interactions with clients and health personnel whose personal culture values may be quite different from those of the nurses. In fact, the cultural values, beliefs, and practices of medicine, social work, pharmacy, physical therapy, and other health professions are different from those of the nursing profession and often different from the client's.

A fourth major reason for the nurse to understand the culture of nursing is to appreciate differences and similarities among nursing cultures regionally, nationally, and worldwide. Such knowledge is invaluable to help nurses realize that not all nursing cultures are alike. Such transcultural nursing knowledge has been helpful to nurses traveling and working in many different places in the world such as in Europe, Korea, China, Japan, Australia, the Middle East, and Papua New Guinea. Nurses often experience cultural shock when they discover that their own values, norms, and standards may be very different from those of other nursing groups in the world. From current transcultural nursing findings, there is evidence of more diversity than similarities among nurses and nursing cultures worldwide.[5] Yet, amid these diversities are always some commonalties. Hence, it is imperative for nurses to learn about differences and similarities among nursing cultures in the world to serve clients effectively and to work well with other nurses. Tolerance and flexibility is essential today for nurses to meet such cultural differences. An appreciation of the cultural history and diverse factors that have influenced nursing cultures

helps the nurse to understand specific differences and similarities among professional nurses. Indeed, knowledge of cultures has become essential today for nurses to function with people in any culture and society and to remain effective. For without such knowledge and awareness, nurses can encounter a host of intercultural problems and stresses without understanding why these stresses occur and how to take appropriate actions.

Fifth, knowledge of one's own nursing culture and those of others in the world can stimulate nurses to pursue comparative research on diverse cultures transculturally. Discovering comparative features and speculating about the reasons for differences and similarities can lead to many new insights to guide professional nursing practices and thinking.

Amid the transcultural diversities, the author predicts that there are probably some universally shared, cultural nursing values that characterize the nature, essence, and dominant attributes of nursing as a profession and discipline. The commonalities or universal culture of nursing, however, has yet to be discovered. As transcultural nurses and others pursue this goal, it may be a rich discovery. If established, this could provide valuable knowledge to nurse scholars and students for educational practice and research. The author predicts that this goal will not be reached until well into the 21st century after studying many nursing cultures worldwide and within a past and present perspective.

■ Definition of Culture and Subculture of Nursing

Culture of nursing refers to the learned and transmitted lifeways, values, symbols, patterns, and normative practices of members of the nursing profession of a particular society. In contrast, a *subculture of nursing* refers to *a subgroup of nurses who show distinctive values and lifeways that differ from the dominant or mainstream culture of nursing.*[6,7] Cultures and subcultures are dynamic and abstracted entities that tend to change over time in different ways; however, they also have patterns and general characteristics that provide distinct stable features over time. It is the stability or constancy of cultures over time that help nurses to know and understand people.

Cultures also have ideal and manifest features that are usually recognizable and can be studied and transmitted to others. An *ideal culture* refers to attributes that are the most desired and preferred or the wished for values and norms of a group, whereas *manifest culture* refers to what actually exists and is identifiable in the day-to-day world such as patterns, values, lifestyle patterns, and expressions.[8] For example, nurses may ideally say that they value and respect elderly people in a nursing home and that the elderly get "good nursing care." This ideal philosophy and image of "good nursing care" may not always be manifest or what actually exists as a reality. The manifest cultural reality is that elderly clients may receive rather inadequate or even negligent nursing care and may not always be respected by nurses. Noticeable differences may exist between the ideal and the manifest culture of any group and especially within the culture of nursing. Furthermore, the emic or the insider's expressions and patterns of a culture may be limitedly known by its members, whereas the etic or outsider's views or public knowledge about a culture may be well known and described by others. These definitions are important to guide nurses in their pursuit of identifying and understanding the culture of nursing and medicine and other cultures or subcultures.

Identifying the Culture(s) of Nursing

In the process of studying the culture of nursing in the United States, the author recalls several experiences that helped her to learn about the culture. For example, in the early 1960s the author was attending a national nursing convention in Chicago. As she entered the hotel, she said to the hotel receptionist, "Could you tell me where the nurses are meeting?" The two female receptionists quickly replied, "Yes, there are nurses here." They gave the author directions to the convention room. As the author walked to the convention room with the receptionist, the latter kept talking about nurses and how well she knew them. The author asked, "Could you describe more about how you know nurses and how they differ from other professional groups that come here for conventions?" She replied, "Well, nurses are quite different in that they tend to stay together in a group, talk about hospital, school work, and physicians. They generally wear similarly styled clothes." She continued, "They are friendly and eager to help others, but they are not too assertive or politically astute. Nurses tend to be silent, are generally passive, kind,

and do what is expected of them as nurses. They do not seem to have any power to deal with those doctors in our city hospital." She then told about her hospital experiences with nurses and said, "When I was hospitalized, nurses were very busy persons and hard workers. They always seemed to be doing things for the doctor and sometimes less for some patients and other nurses." She told how in 1964 nurses were attentive to fulfill physicians' requests and that nurses "strictly follow doctors' orders." This American lay citizen's views indicated that she knew about the culture of nursing as an outsider to the profession. The author was amazed how much she knew about nurses and could describe the culture of nursing with her image. These accounts and others reinforced the author's desire to discover the culture of nurses nationally and to study nurses across the United States and in other countries.

In identifying the culture(s) of nursing, the researcher searched for the patterns, rules (norms), and values of nurses within the general culture and society such as the American culture with its dominant features. The culture of nursing within the society with their special features that make them different from those of the rest of society was the challenge. Most assuredly, the norms, values, and action modes of the larger society and of other cultures also could influence the culture of nursing. Identifying any commonly shared values and beliefs among nurses is helpful, but one should remain attentive to areas of diversities.

An important consideration in identifying a culture of nursing is to study the past and present history of nursing in which patterns and values of nursing can be identified and abstracted with specific examples. The cultural history is extremely important because it provides specific facts and patterns that help to establish the credibility of the culture of nursing over time. The study of images of nursing is another way to discover aspects of nursing culture, which will be highlighted next.

Historical Images of Nursing from the Kalischs' Research

During the past several decades two American historians have systematically and extensively studied American nursing using historical documents, audiovisual media, and other data. These outstanding scholarly leaders are Philip and Beatrice Kalisch, who have devoted almost a lifetime to studying images of American nurses. They are well known for their detailed and rigorous work on the past and changing image of nursing from the days of Florence Nightingale until the present.[9] Their mass media image data have included the printed media (200 novels; 143 magazine short stories, poems, and articles; and 20,000 newspaper clippings), as well as newer nonprint media (204 motion pictures, 122 radio programs, and 320 television episodes).[10] Since this research work they have continued to study general changes in the image of nursing. The author has known these scholars over several decades and has seen their creative, detailed, and systematic work on nursing images. Indeed, the Kalischs' many publications have provided some of the most substantive, scholarly, and rigorous documentation of nursing knowledge from the images of American nurses and the nursing profession.[11,12]

In the Kalischs' historical research on the image of nursing, they identified six images of nursing. While these images are *not* the culture of nursing per se, they provide meaningful data to support some features of the American culture of nursing. They are presented to provide knowledge and special insights about the images of nursing as another perspective of the author's focus on the culture of nursing from transcultural nursing and anthropological viewpoints. The research is included here as it is scholarly and valuable for nurses to understand and appreciate the evolutionary images of nursing over time.

The first image identified by the Kalischs is the *Angel of Nursing*, in which the nurse is portrayed as "noble, moral, religious, virginal, ritualistic, and self-sacrificing."[13] This image prevailed from 1914 to 1919 and concluded with World War I when nurses were viewed as heroic and noble. While it was held that Florence Nightingale reflected this image, she also showed other features such as her noteworthy leadership, altruism, and direct efforts to make nursing a respected profession.

The Kalischs' second image, called *Girl Friday*, prevailed as an image from 1920 to 1929. The nurse was portrayed as "subservient, cooperative, methodological, dedicated, modest, and loyal."[14] This image showed the nurse as a handmaiden and revealed some decline in nursing educational standards resulting from the proliferation of hospitals with nursing students being exploited to staff hospitals under poor working conditions and receiving no salary.

The third media image was called *The Heroine*, which covered 1930 to 1945. This image portrayed the nurse as "brave, rational, dedicated, decisive, humanistic, and autonomous."[15] The Kalischs drew heavily on the biographies of Edith Cavell, Florence Nightingale, and Sister Kenney to reveal this image.

The fourth image portrayed the nurse as a maternal, sympathetic, passive, and domestic person, called the *Mother Image*, from 1945 to 1965. In this period it was believed that married women nurses should be in the home and function as dutiful and conscientious lay mothers rather than as professional working people.

The fifth image was the most negative, in which the nurse was viewed as a *Sex Object*, who was "a sensual romantic, hedonistic, frivolous, irresponsible, promiscuous individual."[16] This sexy image was seen recently as in television programs such as *M*A*S*H* and *Trapper John*. This image failed to portray nurses as professionals or intellectually self-directed persons.

The Kalischs' sixth image was *The Careerist* (after 1965 to mid 1980s), which they described as "an intelligent, logical, progressive, sophisticated, empathic, and assertive woman who is committed to attaining higher and higher standards of health care."[17] These six images discovered by the Kalischs' provide some valuable image characteristics of nurses obtained largely through the mass media in specific historical periods from 1920 to the mid 1980s.

 ## The American Culture of Nursing: Early (1940–1974) and Recent (1975–2000) Eras

Realizing that the nursing profession had not been studied as a culture, it was necessary to study this area of the nursing profession. From a transcultural nursing and anthropological perspective, the author conducted research by examining major past and recent periods in nursing using ethnonursing and ethnographic methods. The author focused on two major contemporary periods of nursing, namely, the Early (1940–1974) and the Recent (1975–2000) Eras of the nursing culture (Table 8.1). Data for these findings drew on the author's continuous and active, lived-through personal experiences of nearly 50 years using the research methods cited. With the ethnonursing method, extensive observations and participant experiences along with interviews of many key and general informants provided a

Table 8.1 Dominant Comparative Patterns of the United States Culture of Nursing

Early Era (1940–1974)	Recent Era (1975–2000)
1. Caring for patients with interpersonal skills and commitment.	1. Serving clients by relying mainly on high-tech skills and efficiency modes.
2. *Other-care* practices based on altruism, self-sacrifice and vocation calling with professional responsibilities.	2. *Self-care* practices of clients to alleviate mainly psychophysical stresses with "symptom management."
3. Professional dedication to work (overworked, underpaid, worked long hours) and "was responsible."	3. Self-gains and interests with better pay, shorter hours and financial gains for professional and personal gains.
4. Limited material supplies and equipment (improvisation to give care).	4. Modern, high-tech equipment, a lot of materials and supplies (very limited improvisation) for client care.
5. Interdependence among nurses for comprehensive or total care.	5. Independence and some autonomy of nurses for primary care, but less with managed care.
6. Deferent and compliant to authority except for strong nursing leaders.	6. Competition with authority and limited deference and compliance.
7. Politically passive, but strong leaders used diverse management strategies.	7. Politically active with open and direct confrontations and "female empowerment."
8. Male dominance and patriarchal systems (nurses as handmaidens to physicians).	8. Pursuit of equal sex rights with rise in feminism and women's issues and rights.
9. Limited competition among nurses (get along and work together), males and females.	9. Increased nurse competition with female status seekers, assertiveness and jealousy. Male nurses asserting their rights.
10. Relationship ties tested over time.	10. Sociopolitical ties and alliances.
11. Innovative leadership ideas with practice breakthroughs and limited grant funds.	11. "Bandwagon" leadership patterns in competing for grants and awards.
12. Recognition of a few highly respected and true scholars.	12. Recognition of mainly sociopolitical leaders, self-promoting goals, and pseudo-scholars evident.

lot of rich data to identify and substantiate the dominant features of the culture of American nursing.[18–20] The data analysis went beyond nursing images to broad perspectives and abstractions about the culture of American nurses over the past 50 years. The ethnonursing method, drawing on emic (insider's) and an etic (outsider's) data, was especially rich to abstract and substantiate comparative data of differences in nurses' values, beliefs, and practices over the two periods.

 Dominant Comparative Core Features of the American Culture of Nursing

The past and present cultural eras were identified to show mainly dominant themes and contrasts in values, beliefs, and practices from an earlier to the recent day

culture. In fact, all nurse informants used the terms "early" and "recent" to describe the periods in nursing. For example, one nurse said, "In the earlier days we would never do that, but today we do." Table 8.1 provides a comparison of dominant themes based on patterns to capture the culture of American nursing over the two eras. By studying these dominant patterns, the nurse learns about general features that characterize the culture of nursing that can be helpful as the nurse works with nurses from the different nursing eras. Such comparative data gives changing patterns of the professional nurse over several decades. There is no intent to offer evaluative judgments about what is "good" or "bad" within each era, but rather it is a means to share knowledge of past and present eras of the American culture of nursing. Most importantly, there is no intent to stereotype but rather to identify common themes or patterns in each cultural era. Of course, not all nurses as individual themes rigidly characterize the era, but there remain general patterns abstracted from the data over time.

In the Early Era, the culture of nursing showed a commitment in common and recurrent sayings, that is, "I gave good care, total care, and comprehensive care whether in the home or in the hospital." Nurses had a deep sense of pride and commitment to provide comprehensive and total care to patients. In the early 1940s to the 1960s private duty nursing was widespread, and nurses were frequently employed to give private duty care to patients in a home context, and a few nurses were on private duty while caring for patients in the hospital. The author remembers that in 1948 she was often called to do private duty nursing in home and hospital settings. She developed close relationships with the families and was often referred to by the family as "our positive feedback from the client's family about their nursing care practices." Nurse informants offered many stories and narratives about their direct nursing care experiences with patients and how satisfying it was "to give total care." Nurses knew all "their patients" and often spent time with them in their home or room.

Nurses in the Early Era showed many signs of being self-sacrificing for others. They would often sacrifice personal gains or interest for the "good of the patient" or for "the good of nursing." Such behavior fit with nursing as a vocational and religious calling and for the professional commitment to serve others. Some nurses held it was part of their religious beliefs to serve God by serving others who needed help. Giving the best care possible was being a competent, dedicated, and responsible professional nurse. Unquestionably, nurses in this era were underpaid and overworked.

In the Early Era, some very outstanding nurse leaders showed autonomy and strong leadership in their decision making and in being responsible for professional actions and goals. A number of these leaders were clear about what should or ought to be done to become a professional nurse. These leaders were excellent exemplars to help nurses see a strong and active leader in action. Many of these nurse leaders held top positions in schools of nursing. Leaders of this era valued personalized care of patients, but also sound education for nurses to become professional nurses. Young nurses were greatly inspired by these strong nursing leaders who could handle difficult situations. Moreover, many of these leaders were quite effective in handling male physicians with their oppressive dominance and authoritative ways. Indeed, there were many physicians who were unreasonable, pompous, and authoritative over patients and staff, and even tried to run schools of nursing. However, many strong and effective nursing leaders maintained their roles and seldom let physicians rule over them. They demonstrated how nurses could maintain their rights with male administrators and outsmart them in female-male situations. A few male nursing administrators were among these nurse leaders, but the majority were females. The male leaders were more readily accepted than females and even today. Being assertive and autonomous were not universal features of all nurse leaders in this Early Era of the culture of nursing.

In contrasting the Early Era with the Recent Era, one finds that nurses since 1975 have been known as active doers to and with clients. Since 1975 nurses have been known as "high tech" and "low touch" nurses. Most nurses are technologically competent and confident of their technical skills, especially in acute care settings. Nurses keep busy administering many medications and giving high-tech treatment, fulfilling physicians' orders, and meeting normal hospital expectations. The hospital is where nearly 80% of all American nurses work today.[21] Amid nursing practitioners are clinical specialists who have been prepared through graduate master-degree nursing programs. These nurses are generally known for their clinical competencies and leadership to manage client care symptoms. Most are generally knowledgeable about the use of modern electronic or computerized equipment that pervades most modern hospitals and emergency clinics in the United States. Most clinical nurse specialists are grounded in physiological nursing and are intrigued with high technologies and their efficacious uses in different treatment modalities. Nurses who work in critical care nursing units have many opportunities to learn high-tech skills and managed care. The ability of nurses to function in high-tech emergency and critical care units with a focus on physiological and medical treatment regimes is clearly evident today.

Since the early 1990s nurses are functioning in "managed" care hospitals and some in community settings. Physiological assessment skills and competencies in handling high-tech equipment are evident with managed care and are used to get clients out of the hospitals as soon as possible. While these nurses are competent in medical-technological areas, few are prepared in cultural nursing and still fewer have had preparation in transcultural nursing. Family nurse and primary care practitioners are evident. The current trend in primary nursing is difficult until nurses become knowledgeable about culturalogical care needs of the diverse cultures.

These primary and clinical specialists with high-tech skills are known for their efficiency and ability to manage symptoms and hospital situations, but they are few in number. The "cult of efficiency" and high-tech competencies characterize the acute care settings in which hospital specialists work and monitor machines. The era of high technology prevails in the present culture of nursing, and nurses can manage diverse technologies and new equipment in very modern technological hospitals in the United States and the world. Life-and-death situations are often contingent on the competencies of critical care, high-tech nurses. Many of these high-tech nurses experience "burn out" in hospitals because of such intense monitoring of acutely ill clients with high-tech, complex equipment, and this leads to an acute shortage of nurses. Providing culturally competent care is not an area of competence for most of these nurse specialists or symptom-management nurses.

During the 1960s an emphasis on discovering human caring knowledge and action modes was initiated by the author and slowly captured the interest of a cadre of care scholars. I held that care was the essence and central and dominant domain of nursing.[22,23] To be a discipline nursing needed a substantive knowledge domain to explain nursing and as a basis for actions and decisions. The absence of care scholars in academia and clinical areas made it difficult to redirect nursing into caring from their heavy focus on medical ideologies, symptoms, and diseases. The author and a small cadre of nurse scholars took a definitive stand to study human caring and study care phenomenon.[24–26] The Transcultural Nursing Society, the National Care Conference Group, and the International Association of Human Caring were the major organizations to support the study of humanistic and scientific care in nursing since the mid 1970s. Still today, too few nurses value and use caring research theory and knowledge in clinical practices. While the words of care and car-

ing are used today with practitioners of nursing care, constructs such as comfort, compassion, presence, nurturance, and others are not explicitly used.

Another trend characterizing the culture of nursing in the Recent Era has been an emphasis on self-care ideology, theory, and practices. This trend began in the mid 1970s with Dorothea Orem's self-care theory.[27] Self-care is largely an Anglo-American middle- and upper-class philosophy and practice mode. It has been used by Anglo-American nurses who value self-reliance and independence. Orem's theory emphasized nurses providing self-care where "self-care deficits" could be identified. This deficit need was largely of a psychophysical nature, and high-tech nurses rely on patients to be self-care managers. The knowledge of many self-care nurse advocates in using transcultural nursing perspectives of cultural differences is very limited. The absence of such culture care knowledge has raised problems using self-care practices with cultural groups where it does not fit.[28] The author's research and that of others in transcultural nursing has revealed problems with the use of the self-care theory and practices when other-care expectations and beliefs are dominant in several cultures.[29] Resistance from non–Anglo-American clients has been identified by transcultural nurses because self-care ideology leads to conflict with the cultural norms and values of people who rely upon *other-care* practices and not self-care beliefs and practices.

Still another area of contrast between the Early and Recent Eras in the culture of nursing is that nurses of the latter era tend to be centered more on their self-interests and economic gains than on professional values of being fully dedicated and committed to nursing. The nurses' self-interests and gains have often been an important means to improve the economic professional image and status of nursing. Better salaries and more favorable working conditions are firmly upheld by many nurses today. Self-interests, status, and gains have led some female nurses to pursue top executive positions to advance their personal and professional interests. Most importantly, female nurses are seeking comparable pay for comparable worth positions that have been traditionally held by males in many societies. It is encouraging to see female and male nurses advancing themselves with advanced master's and doctoral nursing education and certification. They are seeking new positions in nursing, as well as honors and recognition.

Thus a focus on autonomy, self-gains, assertive behavior, empowerment of women, and achieving top professional and corporate positions are helping to make American nurses visible and publicly recognized. This trend has been a major pattern in the new era of American nursing, especially during the past two decades. Struggles remain, however, for female nurses to get and retain top positions because of budget cuts, recessions, and competition with males for such positions. The current catchwords or metaphors of "cut backs," "economic crunches," "the bottom line is cost reduction," and an emphasis on "managed care" all have symbolic meaning of continued struggles and of changing economic and sociocultural conditions for nurses at the present time. A critical issue is the current shortage of nurses as the older generation retires or leaves nursing. Managed care has lead some nurses to leave nursing. Interprofessional competition was evident in the mid 1990s with nurse leaders and consultants being released from some of the high-salaried positions for other male executives. Master's or doctorate prepared nurses were also released because of budget cut backs and other reasons. This recent trend of dismissing or laying-off female nurses remains of concern, as their expertise is much needed in all health systems but especially in corporate organizational cultures. A few American female nurses have broken the glass ceiling with some valiant efforts. Thus, the self-gain, self-interest, and seeking of top positions are important and contrast with nurses of the past era whose interests were different. In fact, self-interests and gains in the past era were largely a cultural taboo or viewed almost as counter to being a professional nurse. Let us look at more comparative, specific culture of nursing values, beliefs, and practices in the two eras (Table 8.1).

 ## Authority Relationships and Female Rights

In the Early Era of nursing most nurses were socialized to be deferent to and respectful of those in authority. Nurses were generally taught to yield to male physicians, hospital administrators, presidents, religious leaders, and others in authority roles.[30,31] Males were in authority roles. Male physicians were viewed as knowing what was best for women, especially nurses. Physicians held almost complete power to enforce their authoritarian roles in hospitals, clinics, and university medical systems. They controlled the clinical and hospital settings and wanted to control nurses and nursing education. However, the strong female nurse leaders discussed earlier knew how to handle most of these hegemonic male leaders. In fact, some nurse leaders were quite clever in getting what they needed, often indirectly so as to not unduly threaten or make male physicians and hospital administrators too defensive. Some nurses listened to males, but remained firm and authoritative at the appropriate times. Nursing leadership successes included holding male leaders "in their places" in hospitals and preventing physicians from taking over schools of nursing, which was quite a feat in the Early Era. The author and many other nurses witnessed these attempted power and control takeovers by male physicians in many situations, but succeeded to hold their stance during the Early Era of nursing culture.[32,33]

Political nursing was not a topic for discussion in the Early Era, nor were ideas published until the author introduced one of the first articles in nursing written on political nursing in the mid 1960s and published in the 1970s.[34] Since then, political aspects of nursing are now a dominant and frequent topic in hospitals and schools of nursing in the current era. Unquestionably, female political strategies were clearly needed for survival and for the full development of nursing as a profession and discipline amid male medical and societal dominance. Interestingly, most of the strong and successful political administrative nurse leaders who made pathways for future nursing leaders never relinquished their goals to achieve what was believed best for the profession. These female leaders of the Early Era could be viewed as exemplary role models, as many were quite skilled politically at handling male issues, retaining their administrative positions, and keeping schools of nursing going despite major hurdles. Unpublished creative management strategies and uncanny leadership skills were important to establish a number of significant directions in nursing education and service. Some of our strongest nurse leaders of the past and current eras should be studied with oral and written histories to discover more fully how female leaders have succeeded in highly patriarchal and political systems since the 1940s in the United States and also in other places in the world.

The feminist movement in nursing was an outgrowth of biases, discriminatory acts, and oppression by male leaders in health care systems and other organizations. Female leaders made their concerns known and took steps to alleviate problems that had greatly limited nursing achievements and progress. Most assuredly, cultural values, norms, and organizational practices had to be changed in most situations to help nurse leaders to be heard, recognized, valued, and respected in health care systems. The author, then dean of the School of Nursing at the University of Washington in the late 1960s and early 1970s, recalls how very difficult it was to raise the salaries of nursing faculty and female deans and to establish the first departmental structures in nursing schools in the United States because of male physicians and administrative leaders trying to control nursing. It was clear across the United States (prior to 1970) that female professions and schools had lower salaries, and yet some nurses had more education, expertise, and experiences than their male counterparts. Slowly, salary and power inequities began to change, but often only after legal suits and persistent nursing actions. It was not until the early 1980s that nursing salaries began to increase in the United States.[35]

Today, equal rights and respect for women nurses are gradually being acknowledged by other health disciplines and in the public sector. Valuing nurses' experiences, skills, and creative contributions remains important and is a frequent topic for discussion by nurses in the United States and in many places in the world where nurses' rights and work merit equal attention with males'. There are female nurses today who struggle to obtain favorable salaries, working conditions, employment benefits, and basic institutional recognition. There are also some cultures in the world where women are well respected, have equal rights, and can make decisions in domestic and public arenas. Transcultural nursing research has helped nurses to expand their database of these realities and to pursue comparative cultural knowledge and experiences, especially related to gender roles in Western and non-Western cultures. This remains critical as transcultural nursing becomes in great demand in this 21st century.

In the Early Era in the United States there was no question that nurses were overworked and underpaid. The author remembers that her beginning staff-nurse salary in 1948 was $5000 per year. Through the active political and economic leadership of the American Nurses Association, the National League for Nursing, American College of Nursing, and other organizations, better salaries and other benefits have been forthcoming to staff nurses, administrators, faculty, and others in nursing. This active stance has also contributed to a better working environment for nurses. In 1999 the beginning staff-nurse salary in large science centers or hospitals was reported to be near $60,000, and clinical specialists and primary nurse practitioners with master's and doctoral degrees in nursing earned close to $65,000 to $85,000 in the United States, but in the rural areas salaries are much lower.[36] These are noteworthy changes affecting the image, worth, respect, and status of professional nurses in the United States. These cultural changes sharply contrast with the Early Era in which nurses seldom complained about their salaries, took limited political action to change their economic status, and often accepted what they were given. Today, nurses are taught to become politically active and use empowerment strategies to negotiate and bargain for ways to improve their salaries, employment rights, and work environment. Some noteworthy strides are evident.

One would be remiss not to identify that in the Early Era many American hospitals and schools of nursing had working conditions for nurses that were often undesirable. Nurses usually had very limited or undesirable space to do their work in clinical and academic facilities. They not only had limited space to prepare medications but also limited space for staff conferences and in-service meetings within the hospital. Schools of nursing often had to use buildings undesired by medicine or other disciplines, until federal monies were obtained by the courageous nurse leaders of the era. By the mid 1970s, United States hospitals and several schools of nursing had comfortable modern conference rooms, well-lighted nurses stations, teaching facilities, and other conveniences with federal funds. Working conditions and salaries have gradually improved largely as a result of action by the American Nurses Association and the American Colleges of Nursing while improving morale and the self-esteem of nurses.

In the Early Era, hospital staff nurses were often exploited by working many additional hours with low salaries. Nursing students were also exploited as they were expected to provide major nursing services to hospitals with no or very limited pay and sometimes with limited faculty guidance. Many hospitals were largely maintained by nursing students (3 year, non-degree) in which students provided direct patient care without pay. This exploitation of hospital nursing students continued in the United States until nursing education programs moved into institutions of higher education, that is, colleges and universities. When this occurred, nursing students became learners with educational opportunities comparable with other university students on campus. Today, the apprenticeship role of nursing students in hospitals has nearly disappeared in the United States and nursing. Students are valuing university preparation with livable salaries on graduation.

Political Power and Politics

As indicated earlier, one of the major contrasts between the Early Era and today is that many nurses today have become politically active and informed about political power and politics. Some professional nurses have become politicians and know how to confront political leaders, legislators, and other politicians about their health and nursing platforms and issues. Many nursing students are politically active in nursing affairs through nursing organizations such as the National Student Nurses Association, the Transcultural Nursing Society, and the American Nurses Association. A few registered nurses are holding legislative and key government positions in the United States. These are noteworthy cultural changes from the Early Era and in sharp contrast with the Early Era when most nurses were politically inactive.

In the Early Era, *politics*, *religion*, and *sex* were generally three cultural taboo areas in nursing seldom discussed in the pre-1960 era. As the first full-time President of the American Association of Deans of Colleges of Nursing from 1970 to 1978 I led a group of deans to the Office of Budget Management in Washington, D.C., to let government officials know of nursing's critical need for capitation funds for schools of nursing. This event became known as the "First March of Deans on Capital Hill." It was successful and led to nursing schools receiving capitation funds to support nursing education. At that landmark meeting with government leaders, the deans learned about the politicians' views and images of nurses as "pillow fluffers"

in their direct care giving and managing of client care. Such shocking gaps of knowledge by top governmental officials about nurses in service and education awakened deans and faculty of schools of nursing to the importance of becoming politically active. Today, faculty teach about politics and benefits of political action in nursing service, in education, and in communities.

There are also a number of nurse lawyers functioning in top leadership positions in nursing associations and educational systems, which has helped change the culture of nursing to advance political, professional, economic, and legal skills of nurses. Transcultural comparative political and legal knowledge in Western and non-Western cultures continues to be discovered, but much work lies ahead in this new era.

Still today, there are far too few males in nursing (about 9%), even though one of the first schools of nursing in the United States was for men on the East Coast. Male nurses also have their struggles in nursing with the dominance of female nurses. Some females feared earlier that males would dominate the nursing profession, but this did not occur. Recently, male nurses have become organized with a national association that encourages discussion of "male concerns including male abuses" and other political and professional issues that are influencing their roles and rights, especially with strong nurse feminists or others. It is reasonable to predict that cultural backlash with legal suits by male nurses in the future will occur as male nurses seek ways to protect their rights within the largely female profession. Thus gender issues in nursing are evident with role changes in the American culture of nursing.

Competition and the Culture of Nursing

Another comparative feature noted in Table 8.1 has been the cultural value of *competition*. While competition for human and physical resources has always existed among nurses in service and education arenas, today there is more open and active competition among American nurses and colleagues for scarce resources in relation to perceived needs. Competitive behavior among nurse administrators and educators is expressed through direct confrontation, managing resources, and group alignments. Negative gossip and putting nurses out of favor to get control of something or a position generally requires competitive moves and social alliances. Presently, there is a strong desire for nurses to be socially recognized among female peers and others to gain prestigious awards or to gain access to top positions within and outside of nursing. While some degree of competition is usually healthy and expected among human beings, sometimes female nursing competition becomes destructive, demeaning, unnecessary, and unethical. This concern has been more covert and limitedly discussed among female nurses. Statements are made such as, "Nurses are their own worst enemies"; "You can never trust your best nurse friend when it comes to what some nurses will do to get what they want"; "You scratch my back and I'll scratch yours"; and "You got to fight for your rights to survive among female nurses." Female jealousy and the need for public and peer recognition are major professional issues that merit attention. It is of deep concern that some of our most outstanding and true nurse scholars, leaders, educators, clinicians, and administrators often do not get recognized, promoted, or rewarded. A strange norm exists in nursing to give recognition to unqualified or less capable nurses, including minorities, when social ties keep them out. This trend appears related to female competitions, female jealousies, and close sociopolitical ties among female nurses whom they wish to mainly recognize and support. In the United States culture of nursing more attention needs to be given to truly outstanding scholars and leaders in nursing who are making substantial breakthrough contributions to nursing and worldwide, but who are limitedly recognized.

It is interesting that competition among United States nurses in the present era appears related to nurses establishing strong sociopolitical ties with other women whom they view as influential friends and powerful advocates to gain status, recognition, or positions in highly desired professional roles. Nurses in key positions often bring their next closest friend into a related position within the same agency, hospital, or academic institution so that social and political alliances can be found, especially in the perceived prestigious American Academy of Nursing. From several nurse observers, nurses are often sponsored by and voted in through their social friends who have done favors or promoted them in the past. This further increases social and political alliances and decreases opportunities

to get outstanding nurses in the organization. Hence, some of the most scholarly and outstanding nurse leaders may not be in the Academy or in the sociopolitical Institute of Medicine. Likewise, scholarly nurses may not be in Sigma Theta Tau awards because they have no social or political nurses to sponsor them. As a consequence, some nondistinguished scholars and sociopolitical competitive leaders become evident in these nursing organizations. Minorities are sought to increase the numbers of minorities in nursing associations; some of these nurses may or may not be outstanding, but rather "token members" to increase the representation of minorities in the organization. Such issues prevail with challenges to recognize such dynamic factors in the culture of nursing in establishing desired norms and images.

In the Early Era of nursing, there were a number of outstanding and distinctive nurse leaders who had achieved their status as unique leaders with patterned and established contributions over time. These leaders were recognized and respected for having advanced nursing in unique ways such as Lillian Wald, Lavinia Dock, Isabel Hampton Robb, and Mary Brewster. These leaders were well known because of their unique leadership ability to make substantive and noteworthy contributions to nursing. In the culture of nursing and from an anthropological perspective, these were the *achieved leaders*, whereas today there are some leaders who are *proclaimed or ascribed leaders* by virtue of the sociopolitical position of friendship ties. Thus our most outstanding breakthrough scholars and leaders in nursing are essential to advance the discipline and profession of nursing.

Finally, there is also a tendency of American nurses and those in other places not to recognize outstanding leaders or scholars until they are dead. This may be related to female jealousy or to avoiding problems with outstanding or controversial leaders. Some of these late-recognized deceased leaders are among the most outstanding, successful, and provocative leaders in nursing who were great risk-takers and willing to fight for nursing goals.

Unquestionably, USA nurses have long valued higher education as a means to help nurses gain knowledge and skills to become competent in their profession. There have been some highly invocative, talented, and creative USA nurses who have been innovators in nursing education and services for many decades and have influenced nursing worldwide. Many of these outstanding leaders need to be fully recognized in their homelands and worldwide. Sometimes, these nurses may not be recognized as a "prophet in one's homeland" or in USA culture, but are well known and respected in other countries for their outstanding leadership in education and research and for promoting worldwide advances in nursing.

 ## Glimpses from Other Cultures of Nursing

It has been of great interest for the author to be a participant-observer with nurses in other countries as they share their views and knowledge about their nursing cultures. Some overseas nurses were quick to compare "American" nursing with their own cultural values and action modes. In the author's extensive studies and travels, there is the view that American nurses are friendly and the innovative leaders in the world of nursing. However, some nurses contend that American nurses are a bit too ethnocentric and fail to value nurses' contributions in other countries. Generally, nurses from other countries are highly laudatory of USA nurses because of their willingness to educate and share information and because of their generosity and willingness to help nurses in other countries. Nurses from other countries expect USA nurses to be prepared in transcultural nursing in their homeland, *before* trying to establish educational contracts, visits, or exchanges. They also hope USA nurses will learn to speak different languages, especially that of the culture in which they will be visiting or working, so that they can better understand the new cultures. Most overseas nurses have been quick to see the importance of transcultural nursing and culture care and are eager to have shared experiences. They question why many USA nurse leaders fail to get prepared in transcultural nursing, but students eagerly study the field.

Australian Culture of Nursing

Probably the greatest challenge for Australian nurses and other nurses worldwide is to realize that there are cultural differences and some similarities among nurses in the world that must be studied and fully rec-

ognized. It is the cultural diversities that can stimulate nurses' thinking; and it is the commonalities that help to link nurses together in areas of mutual interest. At the present time, the diversities appear more evident worldwide. The author has discovered in her several visits to Australia that Australian nurses tend to act independently and speak frankly about outsiders. They seem to feel confident about "what is best, or right" about certain issues. Australian nurses are comfortable speaking out, confronting, and challenging other nurse leaders and generally in a frank and direct manner. It is of special interest that Australian nurses tend to cut down figuratively what they call a "tall poppy" or a nurse leader who moves too fast in leadership or becomes too pompous in attempting to move into certain prestigious positions or roles.[37] Australian nurses know how to "cut off the stem of the tall and wild poppy" to symbolically curtail the growth of a leader or a "wild nurse." There is a covert cultural practice in Australia to reduce a nurse's pompous leadership when it appears to be getting out of hand. In so doing, it puts the nurse back into an egalitarian status with other Australian nurses, controls nurses who might exert too much leadership, and controls nurses before other nurses are ready to move in the new direction. Such a phenomenon was fascinating for the author to discover in talking with Australian nurses and in observing aspects of this cultural norm. Street's work offers further insight about the culture.[37] The Royal College of Nursing Australia (RCNA) has been an excellent means to strengthen nursing across all of Australia with strong leadership. Transcultural nursing has had a slow development in Australia, but with differences in each province, transcultural nursing courses have been established.

British Nursing Culture

One would be remiss not to give a brief glimpse of the British nursing culture, which the author has had the opportunity to observe, experience, and read about with British nursing associates over time. The British culture of nursing reflects great pride and respect for their strong, early leaders in nursing who helped to shape the profession. Florence Nightingale remains extolled in British nursing. As a consequence of their pride, they have great difficulty and reluctance to recognize other significant and outstanding leaders such as Jeanne Mance of Canada, whose significant work preceded Nightingale's by more than 200 years.[38] Florence Nightingale's image reigns strongly and protectively in Britain. British nursing ethnocentrism is evident, which has made some nurses reluctant to learn about other nurses in the world who have made contributions to nursing equal or sometimes greater than Nightingale, but unrecognized. British nurses are also proud of their own nurse leaders and praise their work.

Since British nurses highly value their historical legacy, there are signs to maintain the status quo in nursing and not change except for urgent or imperative changes mandated by a few top leaders or the government. Several British nurses told the author, "If changes are being promoted, one finds traditional nurse leaders remaining as the powerful conservative in-group to control what exists and not to make any major changes." They continue, "Older British nurses are quite conservative and very guarded about making any new, drastic, or sudden changes in nursing or in the existing health care system." As key British nurse informants said, "We do not want to upset the British apple cart or to lose our treasured, traditional ways." There are, however, young British nurses and nurses from other countries who are eager for changes in British nursing. These nurses say it is difficult to change outdated British nursing practices or to implement modern values because of strong historical and traditional values of older nurses. They contend that some outdated and dysfunctional practices have been used for years, but need to be changed to fit the modern world. Younger nurses with counterculture ideas are trying to modernize British nursing and to be more like modern American nursing, but they feel they have limited authority and power to do so. Maintaining order, normative standards, and preserving the past are valued and important in the British nursing culture. British nurses value controversy and intellectual arguments. They are willing to discuss matters that are worthy of debate and discussion. British nursing with a *colonization* ethos has had a great influence on nursing practices in many places where people were under their rule. European unification plans are a recent issue. Non-British nurses are concerned about unification of Europe fearing that British nurses will dominate nursing as the country did in the earlier colonial times. The diversity of nursing across greater Europe challenges the idea of unification within nursing. British nurses are proud of their Royal College of Nursing with its counterpoint in Australia. English and Australian nursing rival in their differences. Transcultural nursing programs have not yet been established in Britain.

Canadian Nursing Culture

In considering the culture of Canadian nurses, there are some similarities to the USA nursing culture, yet there are more differences. Since the author's first consultation visit and keynote addresses in Canada in the early 1960s, she has found that Canadian nurses are realists and also visionaries who forge ahead and take action when necessary. Jeanne Mance's mid 17th century pioneering hospital work in Montreal along with the Grey Nuns of the mid 18th century have served well as role models for many Canadian nurses.[39] These great leaders held to the spirit of preserving human life, practicing caring, and nourishing the spiritual needs of people served. Throughout the history of Canadian nursing, nurses have been resourceful and adventuresome in establishing important nursing goals. Canadian nurses have had strong nursing leaders who have served well their profession and country. While Canadian nurses have been influenced by British and American nursing, still they have developed their unique ways to help people in their homelands and overseas. In recent decades, Canadians have become more intensely interested in helping with nursing care practices in West Africa, South America, China, and other places in the world. Professionalism permeates the Canadian nursing culture in lifeways, standards, values, and actions. Their organized nursing groups such as the Canadian Nurses Association, the provincial nursing associations, and nursing unions adhere rather firmly to professional roles and responsibilities as they continue to shape Canada's nursing destiny and future.[40] There are many signs of assertive thinking and acting in their culture amid severe economic constraints.

Canadian nurse leaders have been struggling with provincial legislation in their efforts to move master's and doctoral nursing programs forward. For example, it has taken several years to get master of nursing degrees (M.S.N.) and doctoral nursing programs (Ph.D.) established in Canada.[41] Canadian nurses have also struggled with provincial governments to get funds and to maintain their self-regulatory professional goals. They have had to function within large professional bureaucracies and work in public institutions rather than private ones. As Canadian nurses function within their national health program, they have struggled to make transcultural nursing a reality for reasons discussed in another chapter in this book. Canadian nurses need to provide health care to many transcultural population groups and need leadership and financial resources to support such work. In general, the Canadian culture of nursing reflects nurses who are strong foragers and persistent leaders who struggle with serving many native cultures and immigrants in their vast land. While other cultures of nursing could be identified, the above examples illustrate how important it is for nurses to have some holding knowledge of nursing cultures in the world and the ways they may be similar or different.

United States Tribes of Nursing

Since the author first wrote about the tribes of nursing in the United States in the late 1960s and 1970s, nursing students and others have frequently requested this information. The idea of "tribes of nursing" came to the author with her anthropological interests during her frequent consultations, visits, and interactions with nurses in different regions of the United States.[42] The anthropological concept of tribe seemed appropriate to identify cultural variations among nursing groups within the United States culture of nursing. A *tribe* refers to a large number of people who claim common group identity and are generally loosely organized, but who remain an identifiable large group with shared values and lifeways. Accordingly, during the 1970s, the author identified four major nursing tribes in different regions in the United States with anthropological views and reality nursing experiences.[43–46] What follows shows cultural variations *within* a country such as the United States, and yet commonalities of dominant cultural themes.

The *first tribe* identified by the author in the 1970s was found in the Southern region of the United States. The author appropriately called these nurses the "*Friendly Tribe*" because they were friendly to outsiders and maintained an open and hospitable attitude toward strangers. Nurses of this tribe had a positive view about people, life, and what they were doing in nursing. They showed an easy-going and conservative

pace of living and working. They welcomed and wanted other nurses to join them in their nursing culture with its Southern lifeways. Most of these tribal members were Southern women who had been born and lived most of their lives in the Southern region of the United States. Besides being exceptionally polite to strangers, they tried not to offend, confront, or make trouble with anyone. They would use Southern jokes, stories, and expressions of humor to ease any tensions or controversies and to maintain positive relationships with others.

While serving as a visiting professor at one of the major Southern universities, the author also learned that deans of schools of nursing knew the best ways to get what they needed from their male university colleagues. Their approach was interesting as they used a warm and friendly greeting with common Southern courtesies and chitchat. They would remain polite and interested in male viewpoints. They avoided any open confrontation with male leaders, as they held such behaviors to be inappropriate to their cultural practices. These nurse leaders knew that aggressive female behavior often turns Southern males off, resulting in negative outcomes. Interestingly, these female nursing deans were quite successful in getting what they most desired from their male academic and most hospital leaders in early 1970s.

Nurses from the Southern tribe were closely attached to their families and to home life values, which they firmly upheld. The tribal members seemed relaxed about domestic, political, and economic nursing issues in their conversation, even though there were a number of serious political and economic matters to address. The Southern tribe was quick to state and reinforce their cultural values and lifeways when working with nurses from other places in the United States. They would speak of "how they did things in the South and how they differed from the Yankee nurses in the North." A nurse from New York spoke about such cultural differences. She said, "I sure see a lot of differences between Northern and Southern nursing practitioners, especially the way we practice nursing in New York City. I have lived in this Southern area for 2 years and I find the nurses are very different. They are too passive, kind, relaxed, and conservative for me. They are also too deferent to males." Another nurse from Minnesota said, "These nurses are friendly and good nurses, but we live and act differently in the North. We live a faster and more competitive and assertive pace of life than these Southern nurses." She continued, "We Northerners are far more work-oriented and get more done in one nursing shift than most of these easy-going Southern nurses do in 3 days." These non-Southern nurses were also concerned about losing their clinical skills and returned to their Northern homelands within a short span of time. Such comments and other similar ones commonly heard by non-Southern nurses provided some important comparative variations about differences in cultural lifeways, values, and practices of the Southern nursing tribe with other outside nurses.

The *second* nursing tribe identified in the United States by the author was called the *"Novel Tribe."* This tribe has many members dispersed along the West Coast of the United States, with the largest numbers found in California. This tribe is distinct in that they tend to view themselves as establishing and promoting new ideas and novel approaches to old issues or problems in nursing. Although there was variability among these tribal members, still a dominant feature of the nurses was to do something quite different from what most nurses were doing in other places in the United States. Their tribal leaders wanted to make their ideas known publicly as novel ones and to market and sell them to nurses across the United States and overseas. In fact, some nurses from the Midwest Tribe often said to the author, "Whatever these Western nurses develop, it tends to get lots of written and oral publicity as something entirely new or novel, but some ideas are not really that new." The concern was that their ideas diffused rapidly across the country and tended to be adopted in a short span of time. The Novel Tribe members are competitive in making their ideas known to many nurse leaders so that their ideas would be used widely by many nurses. These tribal members believe their ideas are some of the most exciting and advanced in nursing and deal with national problems. Other nurses held that this Novel Tribe needed to give in-depth thought to their ideas and refine them before "selling them" as the ideas were often viewed by outsiders as premature and needing further research or documentation. Nonetheless, the Novel Tribe usually got national recognition for their innovations or special contributions. These nurses often proclaimed, "We were the first in the United States with that idea, theory, or practice mode and want other nurses to use our ideas to move nursing forward." Some

Western tribal members are not only highly competitive and maintain elitism, but often isolate themselves as being too different with questionable soundness. It should be noted that amid these innovative Novel Tribe members, there were some very conservative nurses who disliked such progressive, liberal, or novel advocates. These nurses were found in small rural communities in Oregon, Washington, and California. Their conservative views are known to the Novel members, but they seldom "win" on their ideas. Interestingly, many of these conservative nurses are immigrant nurses living in small rural communities and working in nearby general hospitals. Another distinctive feature of the Novel Tribe was the tendency to dress in the latest fashions, wear bright colors, and present some of the latest fashions such as "exotic" earrings, belts, head pieces, and dresses. Many of these San Francisco and Los Angeles nurses were identified when they attended national conferences, and they differed in dress from their conservative sisters.

The author called the *third tribe* the *"Historic Tribe."* This tribe was firmly committed to preserving their nursing heritage, as well as their regional artifacts, at all costs. Most of the members mainly lived on the East Coast, particularly in the northeastern and eastern coastal areas of the United States such as in Maine, Connecticut, New York, New Hampshire, and Massachusetts. These tribal members make firm claims about, "Holding the history of American nursing." They greatly treasure ways to preserve the traditional features of the nursing profession. Most of these nurses were born and had lived in the area most of their lives. These nurses are eager to tell or show strangers about their rich cultural history, influencing nursing leaders with their practices and material artifacts. The native members were proud to say, "We are true Bostonians, Connecticut, or New York nurses who have preserved the American nursing culture for years." They also said, "This is the best place to live and practice nursing, as we have the rich American history of nursing here." While these tribal nurses may leave the area for various reasons, they prefer not to be gone very long and are always eager to return to their tribal area. The Historic Tribe not only cherish and preserve what they held as true American nursing values and practices, but they make future related contributions. They are eager and sensitive to transmit their cultural heritage to succeeding generations of nursing students and to outsiders. Their historical respect for their nursing leaders is clearly evident, as well as archival materials, places, and symbols of past nurses and nursing practices in their historic settings.

Nurses who have been born and reared in the Historic Tribe often have some difficulty with the idea of transculturalism and adopting other cultural lifeways, beliefs, and norms because of proud heritage and ethnocentrism. For example, several nurses from Connecticut, West Virginia, Massachusetts, and New Jersey told the author, "We have always had lots of strangers and immigrants come to this area, but they are very different from us in many ways." Another key informant said, "Why would anyone want to live here if they did not value and appreciate our great American historical roots and places." They know that many European immigrants and nurses came to their region early in American history, and they have tried to help them become acculturated to the region. They feel a deep obligation to teach them about the rich cultural heritage here and *how much* of the history of the United States began in this part of the country.

Interestingly, the Historical Tribal members have many old nursing documents and artifacts to reaffirm their cultural identity. When nurses from other tribal areas come to visit or to work with members of this tribe, they are quick to show these cultural artifacts and to share stories and special events about them. For example, a nurse from the Novel Tribe was employed in one of the historical hospitals for 3 years. She told the author, "I am ready to go back to California as these nurses are far too conservative, ethnocentric, and too protective of their traditional lifeways and historical nursing roots." She found that nothing pleased these tribal nurses more than to talk about their cultural heritage, historic artifacts, and the places to visit in the area. In general, the Historic Tribe emphasized that nurses need to be active to preserve historic places and to value nursing's early, pioneering work in America and many noteworthy contributions. Within this Tribe there were, however, some younger-generation nurses with different values who were eager for major changes from the past preoccupation with historical views and traditional perspectives. The young generation feels it is almost impossible to change nursing and native-born nurses in the area. Instead, the youth say, "We do what

was historically proper, acceptable, and valued as characterized by this Historic Tribe." These Tribal nurses remain powerful political leaders and advocates to preserve nursing's legacy.

The *fourth* major nursing group the author called the "*Blue Collar Tribe.*" These nurses reside in the Midwest or the midlands of the United States, largely in rural agricultural areas and in cities such as Chicago, Detroit, Minneapolis, Pierre, Omaha, Iowa City, and Kansas City. The term "Blue Collar Tribe" reflects that these nurses are hard workers with commonsense ways to do things. They are usually employed in industrial, urban, or rural health care places in the region. Besides being oriented to agricultural and industrial lifeways, they are known for their ability "to pitch in and get things done soon," rather than delaying to get tasks started. These nurses are capable of handling a great variety of different nursing roles, tasks, and jobs. They are known for their ability to improvise, adapt to new tasks, and achieve specific practical goals. These Tribal nurses are frequently referred to by outsiders as the "down-to-earth nursing folks who know how to get work done and can make a difference in nursing practices."

The Blue Collar Tribe is economically and politically astute because of their long history of dealing with strong labor unions, the poor rural folks, and politically motivated urban nurses. Most of the urban nurses are knowledgeable about collective bargaining and negotiating modes with labor groups and organizations and are united by a strong work ethic. They have learned how to deal with unions and complex bureaucratic organizations and with competitive groups. They also know how to adapt to terrible agricultural and industrial losses caused by many factors such as droughts, floods, industrial layoffs, and many other conditions. Generally, the Blue Collar nurses know "their people" in the rural communities and in suburban communities outside urban areas. They deal with low- and high-context cultures. Rural nurses are usually challenged by urban nurses on professional issues and trends, but the rural give urban nurses some reality shock in health care.

Having been born in Nebraska and lived for 16 years in Michigan and Ohio, the author found Blue Collar tribal members tend to give far more medications under physicians' standing orders and rely more on high-tech modes to care for clients than nurses in other areas in the United States. The administration of many medications and the use of many different kinds of high-tech equipment were often explained as "our nursing care practices" in an industrial and union area. Nurses' strikes and boycotts were also viewed as essential to prevent economic losses to nurses and to improve employment practices. Most nurses prefer to fight rather than acquiesce to standards of practice that were unfair, unfavorable, or not desirable to nursing. Such practices and values were explained as being part of their long-term physician-nurse relationships in industrial urban settings, by union philosophy, and by many high technologies in their hospital or industry.

The Blue Collar Tribe had many female nurse executive administrators and supervisors until the mid 1970s, and until 1985 they distinguished themselves by wearing two-piece business suits while working in hospitals, academic settings, and top administrative positions. The business suits are often similar to male executive styles and symbolize the nurses' desire for power, for businesslike endeavors, and to be like patriarchal leaders. Staff nurses wore white or blue two-piece pant suits while working in hospitals and community agencies. Several tribal nurses told the author, "If a nurse wears bright colored dresses, suits, or uniforms (except in children's units), one knows these nurses are probably 'outsiders' or from the West Coast as this is not their usual dress."

The Blue Collar tribal members generally have local group or union nurses as their friends and coworkers who can be relied on in times of need. This is also evident among rural nurses because interdependence and group work is valued in professional role expectations. Rural nurses are generally viewed as "very practical" and less aggressive than urban nurses. Rural nurses are the exceptionally hard workers who know how to improve and deal with rural situations. Most Blue Collar tribal members who have lived and worked in the areas for some time are awarded for being practical and getting things done quickly and effectively. Although cultural variation exists among the rural and urban tribal members, still there are common bonds that make them feel connected to and supportive of one another—many through their strong Christian beliefs and practices.

In sum, the Blue Collar Tribe has not been a "showy tribe" and does not push for publicity or to make their achievements known quickly and in dra-

matic ways. They are moderately conservative in their viewpoints and actions. They are also known for their persistent attitude, diligent work ethic, and their ethical and moral viewpoints. Blue Collar nurses have only recently begun to market their unique skills and contributions in a way comparable to the Novel Tribe of the West Coast. The sharing of ideas among the Blue Collar Tribe occurs when friendship and professional ties are well established, trusted, and respected. These tribal members have been recently advocating for and encouraging nurses to seek power, to "empower female" nurses, and to remain active in political-legislative affairs. They too are becoming interested in transcultural nursing and entrepreneurial practices and critical of managed care practices.

The above four American Tribes of Nursing, namely, the *Friendly*, *Novel*, *Historic*, and *Blue Collar Tribes*, have been presented in this chapter as another way of learning about variability patterns within the United States culture of nursing. All of these tribes share with each other some common values and practices, particularly with respect to valuing independence, autonomy, self-reliance, dependence on high technologies, rights of women, and power to advance professional nursing—all part of the USA cultural values.

Such information among the four tribes within the American culture of nursing can assist nurses who frequently travel or take positions across the United States. Nurses need to understand factors that can facilitate or hinder their entry into new nursing communities, institutions, and diverse employment arenas. Different cultural values, beliefs, and nursing practices impacted nurses' personal and professional work rate and life. Cultural shock, cultural conflicts, and cultural clashes along with a host of other problems can occur as nurses work with other nurses, clients, and health personnel from different regions. Through advanced study in transcultural nursing, nurses can be aware of such differences and their influence on professional success. In the future, nurses will continue to relocate at a more rapid pace than in the past 50 years, and they will need holding knowledge about diverse cultures within American nursing and in other places in the world. Knowledge of transcultural differences and similarities can lead to better nurse images, better role performance, and more satisfying and congruent professional experiences. Of course, some changes may occur in regions, but patterns of stability occur because of desired values and practices. As the number of nurses from foreign countries increases in the United States, United States nurses need to realize that cultural variability continues and that they should practice cultural accommodation and maintenance modes.

United States Hospital Culture

In this section some general features of hospital culture in the United States will be highlighted. Hospitals are cultures, and the *hospital culture influences the way nurses, clients, staff, and others function and make decisions and influences the public views*. Urban and rural hospitals are cultures that become known to the public for what they value and believe and how they contribute to society. Urban hospitals and health science centers have become large cultural organizations that tend to function like businesses and corporate industrial bureaucracies. These organizational structures and cultures influence the work of nurses and associates, but especially the clients' health and well-being. Sociologists have studied hospital structures and anthropologists have studied a few health cultures with their norms and practices in mental hospitals and nursing homes.

Currently, American health care practices in hospitals and other health services are undergoing changes to make health care more accessible, acceptable, and less costly to Americans.[48] Universal health care has been promoted by some health professionals and politicians for years, but is not a reality yet. While American hospitals are some of the most modern in the world, they are not always the most accessible and affordable to many people, especially immigrants, the poor, and many minorities who may have no health insurance or money for hospitalizations or short treatments. The use of modern technologies and many medical and nursing specialists have markedly increased in hospital care in the United States during the past decade (1990–2000), as have the cost of medical and surgical services. As a consequence, hospital costs and services are being regulated by managed care and many insurance companies. Health care reform and patients' rights are the cry today and will increase in the 21st century.[48–50]

Nurses remain the largest health professional group who are employed in United States hospitals,

about 83%. There are, however, a great variety of workers who are called "nurses," such as practical nurses, registered nurses, clinical nurse specialists, nursing case managers, primary and tertiary nurses, nurse researchers, and many more with nurse labels, but only a few are professional registered nurses in many hospital and clinic settings today because of the shortage of nurses. The wide diversity of educational preparation of nurses makes it difficult for the average health consumer to know who is the professionally registered nurse and who can be relied on for competent care practices. Clients from foreign cultures who have never been in the hospital are often confused and feel uncertain about nurses and their roles because there are so many different kinds of nurses and nonprofessional aides. They are also confused on entering and leaving hospitals because of all the paperwork.

Debates are occurring about the actual and anticipated health care costs of current and future hospitals. There are many uninsured clients such as the poor, homeless, elderly, teenagers, and many immigrants and minorities who need health care services but have no money. As a consequence, structural reorganization, staff cutbacks, and different management schemes plus other practices are under study. Some professional nurses have lost their positions, and some are being replaced by aides and practical nurses to obtain "cheaper" services—all of which is endangering client health care needs because of the lack of professional nursing care services. Some nurses are seeking positions in other fields for higher salaries and stable positions. Some are retiring early and others are frustrated with managed care and not being able to practice nursing in holistic or therapeutic ways. A critical shortage in nursing has occurred in the United States today, and even more critical shortages are expected in the near future. Thus these are unsettling times for hospitals, clinics, and professional nurses and some nursing administrators in hospitals. It is also unsettling as the shift of health care providers to work in homes, community health centers, and in new kinds of alternative health care services is much needed. This would serve diverse cultural and population needs in their natural and familiar home environments and avoid costly and unfamiliar hospital services for many cultures.

The United States urban hospitals have become very complex organizational structures with a wide variety of health services and specialties that are costly. Surgical centers, outreach health centers (or satellites of health centers), walk-in emergency centers, and other innovations exist across the United States. The high costs of hospital services, health care specialists, technologists, therapists, and many nonprofessional staff have markedly increased the complexity and problems with hospital services. Clients and especially cultural strangers who enter big urban hospitals find many new technologies and all the paperwork overwhelming. They often feel helpless and uncertain, and some are frightened by seeing so many different employees and high-tech equipment. As predicted in 1978, as high-tech increases, impersonal care and mechanized practices will occur in hospitals and other agencies.[51] Hospitals are busy places that can make new clients and their family feel less important and less involved unless the professional nurse is present to help them feel safe, respected, and wanted. After admission, clients are often sent to many different departments, clinics, or different places for tests and treatments. Some can get lost going from one service to another despite instruction, signs, and directional color line markers in the hallways. Clients are also aware of many different technologies used on them and different personnel coming "to do something to or for them" such as taking blood samples, obtaining lots of strange information, taking vital signs, or giving medications. Sometimes, people enter the hospital reluctant to ask questions, as staff are too busy with many matters and monitoring machines. An ethos and a caring attitude may not prevail, and so for many clients they may fear the hospital as it is strange, impersonal, and frightening, despite some modern homelike furnishings and modern equipment.

As one reflects back to the Early Era (1950s and 1960s), patients (as they were called then) were sometimes met by the nurses or a hospital attendant at the entrance of the hospital or in the parking lot. Nurses visited with clients and their family or friends and then oriented them to the unit and spent time visiting with them. The physician also visited with the patient in a fairly friendly and informative manner. Nurses gave complete care related to feeding, bathing, and often walking with patients and knew the patient quite well and professionally. The nurse of the Early Era used her caring skills of presence and concern such that clients valued the nurse as "their nurse." There was also less movement of patients to diagnostic and special treatment places than today. If patients went off the unit for special therapies, the nurse often accompanied the patient and stayed with them or returned them back to the unit.

Today, clients are admitted with many documents to sign. They may be gone for several hours for extensive diagnostic and laboratory work and different kinds of treatment for cancer and other illness. The client has contact with many different kinds of therapists and specialists, including nurses, physicians, pharmacists, radiologists, occupational and physical therapists, and many others, some with nonprofessional skills. The client's care and treatment may be the responsibility of many team members and/or managed care regime. With managed care and control of costs, clients stay only 2 to 3 days in the hospital and are sent home for recovery. The goal is to diagnose and treat clients quickly, and they receive limited care. As a consequence, clients' early dismissals have not always had positive outcomes. Most concerning is that cultural immigrants, refugees, and the poor may not get help because they have no health care or insurance to cover even a short stay.

While there are claims that the United States has the best and most modern health care system in the world, these views may not be supported with other developments worldwide. The United States has some excellent health services, especially for those who have money or insurance and can afford expert physicians, as well as treatments, medications, and other needs, but there is a big gap between the poor and the wealthy. With no national health program, so many clients are not covered for health care. Major changes are being proposed, but the outcome remains uncertain because of strong bipartisan political party interests and goals and a lack of well-conceived plans for diverse cultures.

Nurses are acutely aware of the health crisis situation as they work directly with clients and families. They are concerned about early dismissals and trying to arrange referral services. Nurses have very heavy client care loads because of the shortage of nurses. Nurses have to monitor vital signs, machines, and respond to physicians', specialists', technicians' and clients' requests. They often have limited time to spend with clients or to provide direct caring modes such as presence, sustained surveillance, and comfort, and other caring measures essential for health and well-being.[52]

This inhibits the nurse from giving good nursing care practices that are culturally congruent, meaningful, and beneficial. Moreover, some nurses have contact with clients from as many as thirty different cultures in one day.

Currently, metaphors predominate in hospitals as symbolic and meaningful expressions such as "Time is money"; "The bottom line is cost savings"; "Staff management is our goal"; and "That's all I can do now for anyone."[53] Such metaphors have become common linguistic expressions that convey a visual image of the practice modes in hospitals. Nurses and hospital staff need to reflect on these metaphors as part of the hospital culture and to be alert that such metaphors get communicated to clients with different meanings and concerns, especially to clients from other cultures.

Cultural client care differences are also a source of problems that can lead to client dissatisfactions and slow recovery. Nurses' "common sense" or "being kind" are not adequate to care for the culturally different as some clients need culture-specific care practices. With many hospital staff having limited or no preparation in transcultural health care, communication, treatment, and caring problems can be noted in rural and urban hospitals. Until staff are prepared in transculturism, the quality of care is threatened or unsafe, and even destructive services can occur as a result of cultural ignorance.[54]

The concept of "managed care," "case management," and "symptom management" are the latest popular language in hospitals and clinic settings. These terms imply managed control of clients and largely of money resources. Managed care is questionable and is incongruent with humanistic transcultural nursing care practices. Minorities, the poor, and others are deprived of care because of lack of health funds. The author predicts managed care will be extinct and in a short time. Instead, transcultural nursing care and coparticipation care with a focus on wellness and prevention must be considered for the welfare of clients.[55] Transcultural nurses have been active in supporting this trend, but it is difficult when other staff do not understand these important goals from a transcultural caring perspective.

Today and in the future, hospitals, clinics, and new health services must change to provide culturally congruent, safe, and meaningful care to the culturally different. This need is already in demand in the 21st cen-tury as more and more immigrants, refugees, homeless, poor, and elderly from diverse countries come to live in the United States. Health care can no longer be focused on traditional Anglo-American services, but will need to accommodate multicultural groups and individuals. This will pose great problems for health personnel who are not prepared in culturally diverse caring modes. Culture shock, cultural problems, and legal suits can be anticipated unless hospitals, community, and other health services are transformed to a multicultural one working closely with people of diverse cultures. For example, some Greek Americans are afraid to come to the hospital unless absolutely necessary and believe that it is difficult to get well and stay well in a hospital context. African Americans and Mexican Americans have expressed similar concerns with the former, often fearing surgery or taking powerful medications they believe could kill them, make them weak, or unable to function. High-tech equipment is often greatly feared by cultures such as the Old Order Amish, and Japanese women fear the use of ultrasound and CAT scans. Arab Muslim women fear being in hospitals if they are cared for by male nurses and physicians, and they fear being left alone in the room with males. Other clients fear they will not get the right foods to eat and so their cultural food taboos will be neglected, which could lead to sickness and death while in the hospital. Korean clients often fear that their "good family blood" will be taken from them and given to nonkin people. These glimpses from transcultural nursing research knowledge need to be given full consideration to attain and maintain culturally congruent care.[56] Such available transcultural nursing research has not been used in many health services in the United States.

The United States Culture of Medicine

Much could be written about the United States culture of medicine in relation to the culture(s) of nursing (the Early and Recent Eras) covered in this chapter. It is a fascinating and important area but limitedly studied in a systematic and in-depth comparative perspective. Because of space limitations only a general overview is offered to stimulate nurses to consider further study and research on the subject. Some dominant cultural differences between the culture of nursing and medicine will be identified to understand potential and actual areas of cultural clashes, conflicts, imposition practices, and other nurse-physician recurrent patterns of professional relationships.

Since the beginning of modern health services, nurses and physicians have worked together or been in close contact with each other. Both professions have had direct contact with clients and have been committed to help people. In fact, the Cultures of Nursing and Medicine have been influencing one another in direct and indirect ways, and in favorable or less favorable ways, for many years, and written about since the early 1970s.[57] Amid these interactions, gender power plays (or games) and status differences have been major areas for conflict and tension. In addition, perceived and public identity differences between the two cultures in roles and practices have been another source of concern, especially for nurses.

The Culture of Medicine is well known to value and practice strong autonomy and independence and to show hegemonic power in decisions and actions. The Medical Culture is known for its actual or perceived power over other health disciplines, clients, and often health organizations. Indeed, medical participants in the United States profession have many outstanding experts in many specialty fields frequently receiving public awards for their achievements. Most assuredly, they are the experts in the diagnoses, treatment, and prognoses of diseases and *caring* practices. Accordingly, most consumers expect physicians to be experts in medical diseases and in diagnosing and treating largely pathological and psychopathological conditions or diseases. This is an important societal contribution of physicians in the United States and with other world cultures. In a complementary position, nurses are expected to provide expert nursing caring to clients in relation to their caring and health needs. Nurses are expected to help clients attain, preserve, and maintain healthy outcomes or to provide compassionate caring for the dying through caring processes. Interpersonal conflicts tend to occur when nurses (largely female) exert their power and independence in decision making related to the therapeutic caring modes with physicians. Physicians may be threatened and try to control or interfere with nursing's independent area of contributions to clients. Physicians' use of power and control over nurses along with their egocentrism often is annoy-

ing. Physicians tend to communicate that they "always know what is best" for the client, even though they see the client very little in hospitals and other care settings except for a few minutes. Respecting and facilitating female nurse experts' professional decisions and actions for the care of clients is extremely important but often difficult for some physician and the medical associates to accept or recognize.

More problems occur when nurses fail to be committed to the nursing care and health (healing) model and imitate physicians as "mini docs" and follow the medical disease-treatment and symptom management model. More than ever, some physicians want to control nurses and limit or regulate their actions and often creative ways to practice using appropriate emic client data and professional etic data for culturally congruent care. Medicine as largely a male profession and nursing as largely a female profession enter into both overt and covert views related to gender, power, and professional dominance conflicts.

The Culture of Medicine has a strong public image with discoveries and technological advancement immediately brought into public awareness in prestigious magazines and public media. In contrast, while nursing has made many unique and outstanding innovations and breakthroughs in caring, helping, and developing unique ways to serve the public, these advancements rarely become known in the public arena. Medical discoveries dominate the public media. Nursing's unique and valuable discoveries such as in generic care, breast-feeding, positioning of clients, home care, sleep-rest strategies, and many other valuable contributions toward people healing and well-being, are seldom made known or publicly recognized. Hence, such discrimination or differential recognition leads to cultural pain and distrust and the perpetuating of medicine's hegemonic practices, and decreases interprofessional relationships and trust. It is a point of interest that in the last decade the public image of medicine is waning, and practices are being ethically challenged in the United States. So, while the public is holding this questionable view of medicine, a positive image of nursing is emerging. Perhaps the public is discovering nurses' tremendous contributions to society and the world, and perhaps someday a Nobel Prize will go to a nursing leader.

The Culture of Medicine also dominates and controls the hierarchical structure of most hospitals, agencies, and any new health centers. There are very few female nurses in CEO positions in health organizations. An egalitarian and lateral partnership model with consumers has been sought and written about by nurses since the early 1970s. Hopefully, health care reform and health institutional changes in access, costs, and policies will bring forth favorable opportunities for nurses in this 21st century. It is also encouraging that, with nurses continuing to be prepared in institutions of higher education and holding baccalaureate with master's, doctoral, and post-doctoral degrees or certificates, these nurse leaders, educators, researchers, and practitioners will bring about favorable control and participatory change practices between medicine and nursing. Nurse entrepreneurship such as transcultural nursing, wellness clinics, and other innovations are opening new and attractive ways for nurses to shape and establish client-centered care and in turn to increase nurses' salaries, images, and practices.

While many other cultural features could be identified as differences and as similarities between the Cultures of Nursing and Medicine, this overview will suffice. The reader is, however, strongly encouraged to read the author's 1970 and 1995 articles on the two changing cultures entitled, *"Grisrun and Encidem: Two Strange Health Tribes in Acrimena,"* to get a full picture of the two cultures over time.

Summary

In this chapter, the cultures and tribes of United States nursing have been discussed with reference to the Early and Recent Eras in nursing and from a transcultural and anthropological perspective. The tribes of nursing in different regions in the United States provided knowledge of geographic and cultural variation among nurses. In contrast, a few non-United States cultures of nursing were presented to show global variabilities among nursing cultures. In addition, the hospital culture was featured with ways it can influence the client, nurse, and other professional cultures working within the hospital environment. Finally, a brief on the United States Culture of Medicine was tapped to highlight some major areas of differences and sources of tension between the Nursing Culture and the Culture of Medicine. With such differences between the Cultures of Nursing and Medicine, it leads to cultural clashes, tension, and hegemonic power problems for both professionals. However, understanding such cultural differences between key professionals are important for working toward satisfying, nonstressful, understandable relationships in the future. Transcultural nursing has the unique obligation to continue to study and guide nurses in discovery of diverse health cultures and in arriving at explanatory factors. Undoubtedly, the study of different health cultures will steadily increase in the 21st century as there is a growing transcultural global world in need of quality-based health care services.

References

1. Leininger, M., "The Traditional Culture of Nursing and the Emerging New One," in *Nursing and Anthropology: Two Worlds to Blend*, M. Leininger, ed., New York: John Wiley & Sons, 1970, pp. 63–82.
2. Ibid.
3. Leininger, M., "Culture of Nursing and the Four Tribes," *Health Care News*, Detroit: Detroit Receiving Hospital, 1985.
4. Leininger, M., "Two Strange Health Tribes: Gnisrun and Enicidem in the United States," *Human Organization*, v. 35, no. 3, Fall 1976, pp. 253–261.
5. Leininger, M., "USA Tribes of Nursing," *Journal of Transcultural Nursing*, v. 6, no. 1, 1994, pp. 2–5.
6. Leininger, M., *Transcultural Nursing: Concepts, Theories, and Practices*, New York: John Wiley & Sons, 1978.
7. Leininger, M., *Transcultural Nursing: Concepts, Theories, Research and Practice and Health*, New York: McGraw-Hill, 1995, p. 208.
8. Ibid., p. 208.
9. Kalisch, B. and P. Kalisch, "Anatomy of the Image of the Nurse: Dissonant and Ideal Models," in *Image-Making in Nursing*, C. Williams, ed., Kansas City: American Academy of Nursing, 1982, pp. 3–23.
10. Ibid., p. 5.
11. Kalisch, B. and P. Kalisch, "Improving the Image of Nursing," *American Journal of Nursing*, v. 83, no. 1, 1983, pp. 48–52.
12. Kalisch, B. and P. Kalisch, *The Changing Image of the Nurse*, Don Mills, Ontario: Addison Wesley Publishing Company, 1987.
13. Ibid., p. 7.
14. Ibid., p. 11.

15. Ibid.
16. Ibid., p. 17.
17. Ibid., p. 21.
18. Leininger, op. cit., 1970.
19. Leininger, M., "The Culture of American (USA) Nurses," unpublished paper, Seattle, 1992.
20. Leininger, M., "Cultural Differences Among Staff Members and the Impact on Patient Care," *Minnesota League of Nursing Bulletin*, v. 16, no. 5, November 1968, pp. 5–9.
21. *The American Nurse*, Washington, D.C.: American Nurses Association, 1994.
22. Leininger, M., *Care: The Essential Human Need*, Thorofare, NJ: C. Slack, Inc., 1981 (republished, Detroit: Wayne State University Press, 1988).
23. Leininger, M., *Care: The Essence of Nursing and Health*, Thorofare, NJ: C. Slack, Inc., 1984a (republished, Detroit: Wayne State University Press, 1988).
24. Ibid.
25. Gaut, D., "Conceptual Analysis of Caring," in *Care: An Essential Human Need*, M. Leininger, ed., Thorofare, NJ: C. Slack, Inc., 1981, pp. 17–24.
26. Watson, J., *Nursing: Human Science and Human Care: A Theory of Nursing*, New York: National League for Nursing, 1988.
27. Orem, D.E., *Nursing: Concepts of Practices*, 2nd ed., New York: McGraw-Hill Book Co., 1980, p. 35.
28. Leininger, M., "Editorial: Self-Care Ideology and Cultural Incongruities: Some Critical Issues," *Journal of Transcultural Nursing*, v. 4, no. 1, Summer 1992, pp. 2–4.
29. Leininger, M., "Selected Culture Care Findings of Diverse Cultures Using Culture Care Theory and Ethnomethods," in *Culture Care Diversity and Universality: A Theory of Nursing*, M. Leininger, ed., New York: National League for Nursing Press, 1991, pp. 345–368.
30. Leininger, op. cit., 1970, pp. 70–82.
31. Ashley, J., *The Hospital's Paternalism and the Role of the Nurse*, New York: Teachers College Press, 1976.
32. Leininger, M., "Leadership in Nursing: Challenges, Concerns, and Effects," in *The Challenge: National Administration in Nursing and Health Care Services*, Tempe, AZ: University of Arizona, 1974, pp. 35–53.
33. Ashley, op. cit.
34. Leininger, M., "Political Nursing: Essential for Health and Educational Systems of Tomorrow," *Nursing Administration Quarterly*, v. 2, no. 3, Summer 1978, pp. 1–15.
35. American Nurses Association, "Salary Report," Kansas City, MO: ANA, 1994, pp. 3–4.
36. Leininger, op. cit., 1991.
37. Omeri, Akram, personal communication, Omaha, 2001.
38. Kerr, J. and J. MacPhail, *Canadian Nursing: Issues and Perspectives*, Toronto: McGraw-Hill Ltd., 1988, pp. 1–65.
39. Ibid.
40. Baumgart, A. and J. Larsen, *Canadian Nursing Faces the Future: Development and Change*, St. Louis: The C.V. Mosby Co., 1988, pp. 1–18.
41. Kerr and MacPhail, op. cit., 1988.
42. Leininger, op. cit., 1985.
43. Ibid.
44. Leininger, op. cit., 1970.
45. Leininger, M., "Two Strange Health Tribes: The Gnisrun and Enicidem in the United States," in *Transcultural Nursing: Concepts, Theories, and Practices*, M. Leininger, ed., New York: John Wiley & Sons, 1978, pp. 267–283.
46. Leininger, op. cit., 1978a, pp. 1–35.
47. Ketter, J., "Restructuring Spurs Debate on Staffing Rations, Skill Mix," *American Nurse*, July/August 1994, pp. 26.
48. Leininger, M., op. cit., 1995, pp. 236–246.
49. Leininger, M., "Future Directions in Transcultural Nursing in the 21st Century." *International Nursing Review*, 2001, v. 14, no. 1, pp. 19–23.
50. Grady, T., "Profound Change: 21st Century Nursing." *Nursing Outlook*, 2001, v. 49, no. 4, pp. 182–186.
51. Leininger, M., op. cit., 1978.
52. Leininger, M., op. cit., 1991.
53. Stein, H.F., *Medical Metaphors and Their Roles in Clinical Decision Making and Practice*, Boulder: Westview Press, 1990, pp. 61–93.
54. Leininger, M., op. cit., 1995.
55. Ibid.
56. Leininger, M., *Care: Diversity and Uses in Clinical Community Nursing*, Thorofare, NJ: C. Slack, Inc., 1984b, (republished, Detroit: Wayne State University Press, 1988).
57. Leininger, M., *Nursing and Anthropology: Two Worlds to Blend*, New York: John Wiley & Sons, 1970.

9

Transcultural Food Functions, Beliefs, and Practices*

Madeleine Leininger

Unquestionably, food beliefs and practices have intrigued human beings universally and persistently over time and in different geographic places. It is a subject that our early ancestors must have talked about in their daily search for food to survive each day in different environments. Today, the topic of food is popular and pervades our lives at home, in social gatherings, and in virtually every place where people live and work. From an anthropological perspective food is more than a biological source of nutrition as it has social, economic, political, religious, and cultural meanings and uses. From a transcultural nursing view, food remains essential for human growth, health, and cultural survival. Food has long been used as a powerful means to establish and maintain relationships with individuals and groups. It can make people feel physically better and psychologically good, but food also has many cultural and social functions. In general, food has always had multiple functions and uses with its special symbols and meanings in different cultures. Such knowledge is extremely important for nurses to learn so they can provide culturally acceptable, congruent, and beneficial nursing care.

In this chapter the importance of nurses to understand food beliefs, functions, symbols, and practices is discussed from a transcultural nursing perspective. Differences and similarities related to food functions and uses among selected Western and non-Western cultures are discussed. The relevance of food meanings, uses, and functions is emphasized to help nurses understand the role of food in keeping people well and in aiding recovery from illness or disabilities. Since culture strongly influences food beliefs and uses in health and wellness, nurses will come to realize the significant part cultural factors can play in the care of clients from specific cultures. Gaining an understanding of specific transcultural food beliefs, functions, and practices can help the nurse to provide for culture-specific and congruent care practices.

At the outset, several universal and diverse food questions need to be considered not only by nurses, but also by nutritionists, physical anthropologists, ecologists, social scientists, health personnel, and others interested in helping people of diverse cultures. They are as follows:

1. What are the basic nutritional needs of people transculturally?
2. How do religion, worldview, emotions, education, and social and ecological factors influence food uses and consumption transculturally?
3. Are there common foods that tend to be eaten or avoided in different cultures when well or sick?
4. What foods tend to support wellness patterns over time in different cultures?
5. What factors often lead to changes in food patterns of production, consumption, and usage?
6. What foods tend to be most beneficial throughout the lifecycle for infants, children, and adults transculturally?

*This chapter has been revised and updated from an earlier article published in the second edition of *Transcultural Nursing: Concepts, Theories, Research and Practices*, 1995, pp. 187–204.

7. What is the role of nurses and other health personnel in helping clients to remain well or through appropriate food uses to prevent illnesses?
8. Do food beliefs and practices change over time in different cultures? If so, why?

The Nurse's Role in Nutrition Uses

One of the most important functions of the nurse is to take an active role in helping clients maintain a favorable nutritional status within their culture. The client's daily well-being and nutritional needs in illness depend considerably on the nurse's knowledge, decisions, and actions to provide appropriate nutrients to clients. Helping the client recover from illnesses, diseases, and disabilities through appropriate food uses that are acceptable in the culture is an important part of nursing. The nurse as a primary care provider is in a unique position to help clients establish and maintain good health through food uses daily and throughout the lifecycle.

To be effective in maintaining the health of clients and preventing illnesses, the nurse needs to be knowledgeable about different cultural foods, the client's food likes and dislikes, and the cultural context in which food is prepared, served, and eaten. It is essential and important to know about food nutrients and what foods are generally acceptable by clients in their cultural lifeways. The nurse should also understand the uses of foods for ceremonial purposes at birth, marriage, religious events, and death as it makes a difference in communicating with and helping individuals and groups of specific cultures. Transcultural nursing requires that nurses learn about cultural explanations such as the "hot-cold" theory to provide effective ways to use these foods with professional health care practices. In general, the nurse needs to know that cultural foods are a powerful means to facilitate family relationships, communication, well-being, and illness conditions. Becoming alert to different foods in diverse cultures, the eating patterns of cultures, and the ways foods are used to help individuals either stay well or when they are ill is essential. Let us turn next to some transcultural universal (or common) and diverse food functions and their uses in selected cultures worldwide.

Universal Functions and Uses of Foods

Food for Biophysical Needs

First, food has been used universally since the beginning of *homo sapiens* to *provide essential nutritional needs to help people maintain body functions and energy and survive.*[1] Food provides energy for humans to keep well, grow, work, communicate with others, and socialize. Transculturally, there still exists considerable variability among different cultures regarding what constitutes "the essential" or basic nutritional needs of human beings in different ecological settings. Bogan has identified some essential nutrients for human evolution, but intercultural and intracultural variability still exists.[2] How nutrients are used depends on the taste and how foods are produced, processed, and prepared for consumption. How food nutrients are metabolized in the body and used varies transculturally. The way foods are prepared and served also influences food uses. These factors are important to consider while working with clients of different cultures in their home, the hospital, or other places.

Nutritionists and physical and cultural anthropologists have discovered that cultures tend to require different amounts of food depending on their biological, genetic, social, cultural, and ecological factors. If infants and adults do not get sufficient basic food nutrients, signs of nutritional deficiencies, illnesses, inability to function, and even death occur. For example, *kwashiorkor* is a nutritional disorder seen in children, especially in poor countries, caused by a protein-scarce diet.[3] This condition was first described in West Africa, but it is frequently found in other non-Western tropic countries where the diet consists largely of starchy foods such as cassava, yams, and taro. A few conditions have been seen in the United States and other Western countries. With *kwashiorkor*, the child's legs and body are edematous as fluid is retained and the child becomes withdrawn and whiny largely because of low protein intake. Children with *marasmus* have slightly different symptoms than children with *kwashiorkor*, but they also show signs of low protein and calorie intake and reflect a failure to grow.[4] Every culture over time has developed what they believe are essential and preferred foods in their diet and also have patterned ways to prepare foods for children and adults.

Sometimes, cultures may not have balanced or highly nutritional diets as known in the Western world, but these foods are desired and eaten. For further study on the physical nutrient needs of cultures, the reader is encouraged to read McElroy and Townsend[5] and Bogan's[6] comprehensive and insightful publications on this subject, including the evolution of food nutrients with preferred foods in different cultures.

Food for Human Relationships

A *second* universal function of *food is in establishing and maintaining social and cultural relationships with friends, kinfolk, strangers, and others.* Many social friendships and professional ties have been initiated and maintained with the sharing of food. Food is a universal means to link and maintain relationships for communicating ideas among individuals, family members, groups, and human organizations. Food is a symbol to indicate special social and cultural patterns and to test or maintain relationships. Food rituals are important to unite people and/or to initiate and maintain cultural beliefs and values. Relationships with strangers that are tense and questionable are often tendered through food offerings and social uses. For example, in the United States coffee or beverage breaks have become a significant social ritual to relax people or to discuss problems or gossip about others. Morning, afternoon, or evening beverage breaks have become well institutionalized in the United States, Canada, Europe, and Scandinavia with a variety of ritual practices at work and for pleasure. Beverage breaks are imperative to give employees a brief recess from their intense or routine work worldwide. However, beverage breaks have different cultural functions besides a rest break, as some are for hospitality, for friendships, and to communicate work happenings or to plan work strategies each day. Thus "ritual beverage breaks" often serve as more than a nourishment or rest break, but are important social and cultural functions in cultures worldwide.

Procuring and distributing foods are often closely linked with cultural status and prestige functions related to work, marriage, achievements, and with birth and death ceremonies. In our industrialized Western world, if an individual gets an award, a new job, or is promoted, dinner celebrations or cocktail parties often occur. At these dinners special, prestigious foods are often served in fancy ways with special people present.

Tables are often decorated with a special tablecloth and flowers. Expensive foods are usually served such as steak for Anglo-Americans, lamb for Britains, veal for Greeks, and special bean and rice foods for Mexicans and other Hispanics. For North American Indians, a potluck feast with native food exchanges would occur. At these social and ritualized gatherings, the honored guest is often toasted with preferred cultural beverages or foods to acknowledge achievements or change in status. These food feasts reinforce social and group cohesion, recognize the new status of those honored, and strengthen cultural identities using preferred cultural foods and beverages.

Cultural foods are especially evident at wedding feasts, religious holidays, and at particular lifecycle events or "rites of passage." The Jewish bar mitzvah for young boys and bat mitzvah for girls are important lifecycle religious events. These celebrations have great symbolic religious significance of entry into adulthood and are more important rituals than the nutritional aspects of the food. Christians' Christmas, Easter, and other religious times reflect the preparation and use of special food dishes to celebrate each occasion. The food preparation and the arranging of the time, place, guests, and context for the celebrations are very important to foster a special cultural experience in Christian countries.[7]

Food has, therefore, universal functions in all ceremonies and cultures for prestige, to exchange wealth, and to renew bonds of friendship, solidarity, and religious functions. These functions in food ceremonies are evident in Western cultures, but are often more impressive in non-Western cultures. For example, in many non-Western cultures people gather large amounts of food that they have produced and saved to honor supernatural spirits, ancestors, and gods and to express thanksgiving for their good harvest. Harvest food festivals are often annual occasions in non-Western cultures. The festivals are very colorful, happy, and often spiritual occasions with people wearing bright colored outfits. At these food festivals people dance, perform certain rituals, show their talents, and express appreciation for the food, family, and cultural ties.

Birth ceremonies are often special occasions in many non-Western cultures that love children. Special foods are prepared and used to symbolize a child's entry into the family, community, and culture. Family and friends gather to celebrate the infant's arrival and to see the child as a future active participant in their culture. In many cultures there are big birth celebrations with males because of their ascribed statuses. This is especially true in Middle Eastern and Pacific Islands cultures. For the Gadsup of Papua, New Guinea, all infants are warmly welcomed into the world with a special birth ceremony after two months but especially males. During the Gadsup birth ceremony the infant's father's brother holds the male infant and places small, soft particles of garden food in his mouth.[8] In the female birth ceremony, food is given to her for her future work role in the garden. As the father's brother places the food on the female infant's tongue, he says, "We give you these Gadsup foods from our female gardens so that you will want to grow them like other women in the village as they have done in the past." This beautiful but simple birth ceremony uses food to signify that the female infant is special and has a special future role when she becomes an adult. Likewise, male Gadsup children are given meat foods to taste that are related to their gender role, namely, to hunt and gather foods as an adult.

Universally, foods are used for ceremonial feasts, but vary in expressions and rituals. Usually, rare, exotic, expensive, and highly preferred foods are used to make the ceremony a special day to long remember. Most food ceremonies require considerable time to collect, prepare, and ritualize for ceremonial purposes. In most cultures, ceremonial food must be prepared, served, or distributed properly with attention to cultural food taboos and preferences, especially those associated with the invited guests and the special occasion. For example, the Gadsup would spend several weeks collecting food that they had grown, store it, and then display it in piles at the large group ceremonies. Displaying these foods increased the village's status and prestige and brought great honor to the villagers, tribe, and community. Food ceremonial competition existed between villages, especially for harvest and lifecycle events. One can think of many similar preparations of special foods and saving money to collect and prepare food for wedding and birth ceremonies in North and South American, European, and Southeastern cultures of the world—some very elaborate and lasting for days.

It is extremely important to recognize food taboos associated with ceremonies. Many cultures may abstain from eating foods that are generally choice, highly desired foods. Some foods cannot be eaten by males or females at ceremonies in non-Western cultures because they are believed to bring harm, illness, or reduce one's importance. Religious groups often have strong food taboos and strict ritual observances in which the "sacred" (of religious significance) and the profane (worldly and often viewed as unclean or dangerous) are observed. For example, at Yom Kippur, Jews observe a 24-hour fast. In keeping with their religious beliefs, all pig products are taboo as are fish without fins and scales, and only hooved animals that chew a cud and have been ritually slaughtered may be eaten. Milk and meat dishes must never be mixed at the same meal. Some similar food taboos are practiced by Muslims in that pork or pig products are taboo, and they can only eat food from animals that chew a cud and that are virtually slaughtered (*halal*). The Muslim fast of Ramadan is observed during the ninth month of the lunar year. During this time, food and drink are taboo between sunset and dawn for Muslims who are of the "age of responsibility" (12 years for girls and about 15 years for boys). These strict food taboos are associated with religious beliefs and yearly ritualized ceremonies.[9,10]

Lifecycle initiation rites remain fairly universal in using food for symbolic purposes. There are, however, cultural variations with lifecycle rites, and some cultures have reduced their importance for a variety of reasons. Where they prevail, the ceremonies are used to recognize that an individual has moved from one lifecycle period to another with changes in social status. For example, in many Papua New Guinea villages in the past and some today, lifecycle rituals are important for the transition from a young boy to becoming a man.[11] Before the initiation ceremony, the boy initiates were expected to observe strict food taboos by not eating eel and cassowary meat. At the end of the intense, long male ritual ceremony, the boys had become men and were now strong enough to eat these "powerful male foods." Today, these initiation ceremonies have been simplified, but special foods and activities are still used to help male children as they change role, status, and gain privileges to be a man. Becoming a man means that a Gadsup boy may marry and have children and assume other adult male roles.

Although most Western cultures do not have such definitive lifecycle initiation rites as the Gadsup, still one can find different forms, expressions, and interpretations. For example, in Western cultures when a boy or girl reaches adolescence, or is 21 years of age, parents help celebrate this occasion by preparing a special dinner with favorite cultural foods, that is, meats, cakes, and vegetables. They may also honor them with gifts and sometimes a social gathering with their peers or friends. The lifecycle event is also acknowledged by the adolescent usually obtaining a driver's license, car, or other material cultural symbols. Most Western lifecycles are not as elaborate, prolonged, and ritualized as those of non-Western cultures, but special foods and material goods are used.

Food to Assess Interpersonal Distance

A *third* function of *food is to assess social relationships or interpersonal closeness or distance between people*. Universally, foods are often used to determine the extent of friendship or distrust between individuals, families, or groups. An example of this function comes to mind from my ethnonursing field study with the Gadsup of New Guinea.[12] I began my field research as a complete stranger to the Gadsup and entered their world as a white, single woman. Initially, the people perceived me as a potential sorceress—or a stranger who could harm them. They distrusted me and watched me carefully until I became a friend. During the first 6 weeks, a few village men and women brought me small amounts of withered, dry, and scrubby-looking sweet potatoes, fruits, and greens. They would cautiously give me the food and quickly leave. The food was of poor quality and reflected that they distrusted me and, therefore, did not want to give their best foods to an unknown stranger or sorceress. Later, as the villagers got to know me (about the second month), they began to bring me better quality fruits and vegetables and, occasionally, fresh foods from distant places. By the end of the first year the Gadsup brought me lots of fresh pineapple, vegetables, and even rare foods that they had obtained by walking nearly 20 miles. So, as I became their friend, the quality of food markedly improved and the quantity increased. This example shows how food was used to reflect cultural stranger-to-friend interpersonal relationships.

Transculturally and universally, food use often reflects the social stratification of society and indicates which persons are to be respected or held in positions of higher authority or status. Often, stratified cultures with castes, classes, gender, and hierarchies determine who gets what foods and how the foods can be used by people of particular statuses. In some stratified societies such as India certain foods are highly restricted for certain castes, and food is regulated by the rules of the caste system. People in higher castes such as the Brahmins often are given high-quality food. Food also becomes a powerful means for regulating social and political controls and maintaining cultural norms and rules of behavior. In stratified societies, cultural diversity prevails because of economics, politics, and the way a society is organized and controlled by cultural norms and statuses.

Food to Cope with Stress and Conflict

A *fourth universal function and symbolic use of food is to cope with emotional stresses, conflicts, and traumatic life events*. In many cultures in the world, foods and diet patterns are used to relieve anxiety, tensions, and interpersonal conflicts or frustrations related to work at home, at the office, or in daily living. The way cultures deal with emotional stresses and conflicts varies considerably in Western and non-Western cultures. Western cultures such as Anglo-Americans, Europeans, Canadians, and Australians often rely on eating to relieve their stresses and in ways they may not be fully aware of until weight gain occurs. Some people tend to almost constantly eat or nibble on food or drink to relieve their anger, frustrations, or anxieties. Some individuals hoard food to have it readily available when they get upset. Compulsive eating and hoarding of food to relieve tensions or anxieties are largely learned and patterned from cultural practices. Compulsive eating to relieve tension tends to occur more frequently in Western cultures where food is more readily available and conspicuous than in non-Western cultures. In non-Western cultures where food is often scarce, seasonal, and cannot be stored in refrigerators, people relieve their anxieties by activities such as running, hunting, fighting, or being aggressive at political and cultural gatherings. In these cultures one seldom finds obesity problems and depression because they have other ways to deal with stresses and are often thin and some malnourished.

In some Western American and European cultures, individuals may handle their anxieties and tensions by avoiding eating. These individuals under stress who will not eat food are often depressed, have low self-esteem, and are not interested in eating anything, or they do not feel worthy to eat or receive foods. They may, instead, take drugs, drink alcohol, or become very active or withdraw. In Western cultures, the mental health conditions of anorexia nervosa and bulimia exist, especially in teenagers. Individuals with anorexia nervosa usually refuse to eat anything or gorge food and vomit it. As a consequence, these persons become very thin and underweight. The individual with bulimia who gorges large amounts of food will soon after vomit and not retain the nutrient values of the food. These conditions are well-known in Western cultures, but are limitedly found in non-Western cultures, thus reflecting global differences.

Nurses with preparation in transcultural mental health are alert to such cultural variations related to cultural patterns of overeating or undereating and can observe, listen to, and counsel the client. The nurse can help the individual, group, or family work toward resolving their problems within their cultural lifeways and values. Most cultures have prescribed ways to relieve feelings of boredom, disappointments, dissatisfactions, and depression, which the nurse uses in therapy with clients. Foods such as sweets and drinks are commonly used in the United States by adults and children to handle anger, emotional frustrations, and disappointments, whereas vegetables and daily outside activities are generally used in non-Western cultures. Smoking is also used in many cultures to relieve stress, but is decreasing because of health threats in past decades.

Food for Rewards and Punishments

A *fifth universal function of food transculturally, but with some cultural variations, is the use of food to reward, punish, and influence the behavior of others.* In most cultures in the world there are norms and practices of the ways children and adults are rewarded, punished, or receive positive or negative sanctions with food. Foods have long been used by humans to regulate cultural and social behaviors that they want rewarded, maintained, or curtailed. Moreover, cultures know which foods have highly favorable rewards and which ones communicate dislikes or negative rewards. For example, Anglo-American children are often rewarded for good behavior with all kinds of sweets, that is, candy, sugared cereals, drinks, and cookies. In contrast, the Gadsup children were rewarded for desired cultural behavior with nonrefined foods such as vegetables, nuts, taro, fruits, fish, or forest meats if available. Lots of sweet foods consumed in America have led to dental caries, diabetes, and other health problems over time. Infants and children are quick to learn how parents and other adults use foods for rewards and punishment, and so food-giving becomes a symbol of children's "likes and dislikes" in cultures. Children may also try to control and test parents by the uses of foods in their culture. If food is eaten in a culturally and socially unacceptable way, parents often become embarrassed with their child and may view themselves as inadequate parents. Parents or surrogates are often expected in most cultures to reprimand children with foods to get them to act in culturally appropriate ways. For example, an 8-year-old boy was eating food with his fingers at a formal dinner. The parents reprimanded him gently at the table, but later the child was harshly reprimanded at home because the parents were extremely embarrassed by the child's "terrible" behavior. It reflected "poor upbringing" by the parents. The child enjoyed the food with his fingers.

Food to Influence Status

A *sixth universal function of food is to influence the political and economic status of an individual or a group.* Transculturally, food has great economic importance and political uses, and these two aspects are closely interrelated. Food has been used to build political alliances with people and for economic gains. Politically and economically, food can reaffirm and sustain traditional power ties and establish new power alliances. Sometimes, food has been used to test political relationships and to test the strength of alliances. Serving food before, during, and after political meetings often leads to friendly and congenial outcomes. Food tends to "soften" political group behavior and ease questionable relationships. In some cultures political leaders are offered rare and very choice foods or drinks before political meetings to ease a strong leader's potential aggressive or polemic disposition. Food has been a means to build and maintain smooth relationships, to gain votes, and to foster desired political alliances and support. Some examples to support this general function will be offered.

The non-Western Gadsup, for example, carefully selected foods given to one's political friends and to enemies at political gatherings. The Gadsup spend a lot of time getting some of their choicest foods for their "true and trusted" political friends to maintain good ties. They will, however, also get choice foods for enemies to prevent further hostilities, accusations of sorcery, or to reestablish favorable political relationships. If the Gadsup did not give the best quality food to their friends or enemies, they could be accused of sorcery, which might lead to illnesses and deaths in a village. Traditional enemies are usually strong in political power, and so foods offered and eaten at the public gatherings impress the politically oriented "big men" of different villages. Foods that are not fresh or look of questionable quality are always suspected by enemies as potentially harmful and will be avoided. Such political uses of foods exist in other cultures such as Africa and South America with different food meanings, uses, purposes, and ritual giving practices.

In many European countries and in the United States, gift-giving occurs regularly and in different ways among political and social interest groups to promote positive relationships and to win over new political and social friends. Presidents and prime ministers of countries often receive lavish or expensive gifts, which reaffirm their political, economic, and social status and their relationships with the public and other countries. Such gifts to special people are usually displayed in visible places but always under protected security.

Economically, food is important in exchanges to maintain basic food supplies and to provide diversity in the people's diets. The distribution of food is of great concern worldwide and so the economic production, accumulation, and distribution of goods and services are given much consideration. Farmers and peasants of different cultures often know the best ways to maintain their economic lifeways; however, they often have limited political and economic power with bureaucrats and dominant cultures. Cultures learn what food other groups need or desire. They try to increase the demand in trade exchange patterns for economic benefits. For hundreds of years people have made food exchanges to support political ties, provide essential foods, and to strengthen one's economic position. Essential food im-

ports and exports, whether of small or large amounts, are central to the development, maintenance, and survival of cultures worldwide. An imbalance in the production and distribution of foods can cause serious problems in any society and can ultimately influence the health status of people. As frequently seen in Africa, thousands of people have died of hunger as a result of war, political feuds, economic greed, and poor distribution of foods. Food taken to international food distribution points may never reach its goal because of political groups taking the food, such as was the case in Somalia, Africa, in 1993, 1994, and 1999. Hungry and dying people may never receive the food. Hence, charitable organizations that try to help starving people may never see their food received by those who so desperately need it. The cultures of poverty and affluence exist worldwide.

Periods of drought, floods, earthquakes, tornadoes, and other environmental conditions continue to have a devastating impact on the production and distribution of foods in many countries. Farmers in the United States, Canada, and other countries often fail to get their surplus foods exported to "have not" countries because of government politics and poor marketing policies and practices. Moreover, farmers struggle to get fair or adequate prices for their food products to meet their farm production costs. There is a very close relationship between politics and economics in most cultures that transculturally oriented nurses need to realize when working in foreign countries or in local, rural, or urban communities, and such factors influence food and health care worldwide.

Food to Treat and Prevent Illness

A *seventh and major universal function of food is to access, treat, and prevent illnesses or disabilities of people transculturally.* Anthropologists have long observed and studied how food is used as a means to diagnose, treat, and deal with illnesses and stresses in different cultures.[13] Practically all cultures today still rely on both folk (generic) and professional caring and curing of illnesses. Some cultures have skilled folk diagnosticians (or diviners) who assess the health and illness states of their people before considering professional services. Folk practitioners often use symbolic figures and foods to assess the health or illness status of their people. Cultures know what foods people should eat and why some foods should be rejected because of certain physical illnesses and sociocultural conditions. In most non-Western cultures, folk diagnosticians look for cultural reasons for illnesses; whereas in Western cultures professional diagnosticians often seek physical or emotional causes rather than cultural ones. Such practices are important to know as nurses work with different cultures worldwide.

Transculturally, food is also used to explain why certain illnesses occur or conditions exist. Food is used to predict possible illnesses, reasons, and consequences for both professional Western diagnosticians and non-Western folk diviners and healers. For example, if a client drinks milk and complains of intestinal discomfort (e.g., abdominal pain, cramping, diarrhea, and vomiting), Western health personnel may or may not identify this as a sign of lactose intolerance.[14] This condition has been found in nearly two-thirds of the world's population after early childhood and is caused by problems with the production of the enzyme lactase.[15,16] In contrast, folk healers will often diagnose this condition in relation to disturbances in social ties and breaking cultural rules.[17] Food is the medium to diagnose cultural factors that can initiate or aggravate biophysical and other illnesses. Lactose intolerance is important for the nurse to know as it is found in many cultures and can aggravate a client's health status markedly.

Food products are often used by folk diagnosticians to warn people of potentially unfavorable sociocultural relations with friends or strangers in a culture. It is believed that favorable or malevolent behaviors can lead to illnesses, which most health personnel fail to see or understand because of the lack of knowledge and the disbelief that cultural factors can lead to illnesses. Western scientific medical and health practitioners are quite determined to view all illnesses as resulting from genetic, biophysical, or emotional causes related to cell, organ, and body dysfunctions. Until physicians, pharmacists, nurses, and other health personnel become knowledgeable about comparative generic health and illness, they will continue to use their explanations and not cultural ones.

In many cultures food remains important to prevent and cure certain illnesses such as hypertension, diabetes mellitus, peptic ulcers, coronary diseases, aging, and other conditions or disorders. In the United States, Canada, Europe, Japan, Australia, and other Western cultures, large sums of money are spent on radio, television, and internet advertisements to promote optimal health by eating "the right kinds of foods" and avoiding others. Food tends to dominate the Western mass media so that people are almost obsessed with food interests and ways to live by what is being advertised, promoted, marketed, and studied. Some of these food values change over time, leaving non-Western cultures baffled about Western "food facts." Today, most Western cultures believe that eating the right foods, exercising, and regulating one's own food intake leads to health. In contrast, non-Western cultures tend to be more concerned about procuring and distributing food among their kin, social, political groups, and getting enough food for daily survival. Malnutrition prevails in many non-Western cultures today.

■ Generic Food Theories and Uses

Non-Western cultures such as Southeast Asians, Mexicans, Caribbean, and related Latin Americans are attentive to assessing and using "hot and cold" foods, beverages, and medicines. The *hot and cold theory* is a very old belief that originated in non-Western countries and in ancient Greece with the desire to balance body fluids or humors between perceived hot and cold substances.[18] If an imbalance of hot and cold body fluids occurs, this is believed to cause illnesses and even death. Foods, beverages, and medicines remain classified as hot and cold by many people in these cultures to prevent and treat illnesses. In general, hot or warm foods are believed to be easier to digest than cold or cool foods. To treat human conditions, it is important to assess the substance taken or to be used to provide usually the opposite effect, that is, one counters too much exposure to cold substances with hot foods and beverages or medicines, but cultural variations remain on uses. For example, an upset stomach condition may be caused by eating too many cold foods, and so warm foods are needed to correct the imbalanced state. In general, foods and medicines are classified and used by cultures in different ways. Nurses need to study such cultural beliefs and classifications with their meanings and how they vary transculturally.[19–21] These beliefs and practices exist today.

Interestingly, the Chinese according to the ancient philosophy of Taoism have, for nearly 3000 years, been attentive to the *yin* and *yang* elements to maintain harmony and balance in the universe.[22] *Yin* signifies the cold, female, and darkness element, whereas *yang* signifies the hot, male, and light element. Accordingly, when foods are digested, they can lead to either *yin* or *yang* conditions. The important principle is to balance *yin* and *yang* components of foods to maintain good health. Excesses or imbalances of either *yin* or *yang* can lead to illnesses, diseases, or unfavorable conditions. To provide culturally congruent and competent care, nurses need to be knowledgeable about hot and cold (*yin/yang*) theories and others related to food, drinks, and medicines in healing, caring, and curing.

It is also especially important to realize that many professional medications, surgical operations, or medical treatments such as chemotherapy are usually considered to be "hot" and powerful. Clients of different cultures are sometimes baffled as how best to counteract such "hot" professional treatments or avoid them. Clients may be noncompliant or refuse medicines and treatments because they are too hot or cold. Noncompliance and uncooperative behavior of clients, with their refusal of nursing care, medicines, and treatments, can be related to cultural fears, clashes, or uncertainties, which some health personnel need to understand. Nurses and other health professionals may demean and offend clients who hold beliefs about foods and their favorable or less favorable uses.

Cultural Preferences

Most importantly, the nurse who has studied transcultural differences in the uses of foods will be attentive to the food preferences of cultures to promote health and prevent unfavorable responses of individuals and families to foods. Since cultures have specific food preferences and dislikes, which can make a difference in caring for clients of different cultures wherever they reside, the nurse assesses these foods and their nutritional values within the client's health needs to provide culturally congruent care. It is extremely important to ask the client or family to tell about these foods rather than guessing or using an inaccurate source. To facilitate recovery from illness, maintain health status, and prevent illness, cultural knowledge within a holistic perspective is imperative. For example, the nurse should understand that Vietnamese people like fish, rice, fresh vegetables,

and herbal teas. Unless fully acculturated, they may consistently refuse hamburgers, potatoes, carbonated beverages and other Western foods. When Vietnamese are served their cultural foods, it is wonderful to see them smile and eat "their foods." Eating culturally desired foods can lead to a quicker recovery from illness and greater client satisfaction than when these clients are expected to eat strange or taboo foods. Most nurses realize that when one is ill or under stress, there is a longing for foods that one knows about and likes. Indeed, American hospitals waste far too much good food because clients from other cultures dislike certain foods as strange or cannot be eaten for cultural reasons. Such hospital food wastes are difficult to accept; however, they occur because the food was culturally taboo or inappropriate. Transcultural nurses need to know what cultural foods should be served and what clients will eat and need. They need to help other nurses and staff to make use of culture-specific foods for their health and to be acceptable. Today, hospital staff need to be educated about cultural food likes and dislikes through in-service education and academic courses on transcultural nutrition and health care.

Although considerable variability exists with African Americans as a result of economic and acculturation factors and where they have lived (North or South), many African Americans enjoy their traditional foods as vegetables, greens, pork, legumes, chicken, cornbread, and soul foods. Hot breads and fried or boiled foods are popular. The author has found these preferences remain strong from her 40 years of study and living near African Americans in urban and rural areas of the United States.[23] With some of the current and serious African American health problems related to stroke, hypertension, and general cardiovascular conditions, nurses and other health professionals need to be aware of food uses by African Americans and especially by those who have limited income and are living in poor areas. Bailey's study of African Americans in a large urban context, in which he used both anthropological and transcultural nursing principles and theories, provides invaluable insight about these problems and ways to alleviate them.[24]

Although Mexican Americans' and Puerto Ricans' preferred foods vary, they tend to like foods such as beans, chicken, chili peppers, tomatoes, onions, squash, and herbal teas, especially chamomile tea when ill or experiencing cultural pain or stresses. Mexicans in California, the South, and Southwestern areas of the United States enjoy enchiladas, tostados, tamales, chili con carne, chicken, and chili dishes. These common cultural foods will be acceptable and generally beneficial to clients of health care services.

Native Americans in Canada and the United States were the first to introduce foods such as maize, beans, and squash into Anglo-American diets. The many Native Americans of different tribes have different food choices, which are related to their ethnohistory, environmental context, and traditional food and spiritual rituals. Generally, though, Native Americans like fresh fish, fruits, berries, corn, beans, squash, wild greens, root foods, and game meats. Since more are moving to urban areas, they often miss their traditional and highly valued foods because they are closely related to their religious or spiritual beliefs and to their natural environment. As the nurse becomes knowledgeable about the close interrelationship of the Native Americans in Canada and the United States, they will discover that foods are extremely important for diverse reasons. Food uses and consumption must be harmonious with them and their environment. Food practices bear on these realities with their close relationship to their sacred beliefs and lifecycle rituals and survival.

Environmental Influences

As nurses become more sensitive and competent about transculturalism, their ability to provide culturally congruent care will increase. Knowledge about the people's environment with an understanding of what foods are raised or available is important as one counsels clients about food resources and uses. How foods are produced and used largely depends on the agricultural resources and their distribution, as well as the cost at markets. Geographic environments and climates generally determine which foods will be raised, sold, and used and which can be relied on for daily health maintenance or restorative processes. The climate, soil, amount of rainfall, seasonal plants and animals, available technologies, and human resources in any ecosystem greatly influence food values and uses over time in cultures. Some cultures live on day-to-day gardening and hunting foods or have limited daily subsistence

food supplies. Other cultures may live on Western foods obtained from supermarkets and other outlets. Western cultures today rely heavily on frozen foods, including meats, fish, fruits, and vegetables, or those that are seasonally fresh and available to them. Nurses working with clients need to assess holistic transcultural care food factors, along with social structure and environmental factors such as natural disasters (floods, hurricanes, or fires) that influence food uses, functions, and health outcomes.

Genetic Factors: Newest Emphasis

Another fascinating factor that needs to be mentioned is that the genetic, constitutional, and metabolic processes of human beings may differ considerably with different cultures and have different consequences. Nutritional anthropologists, biologists, geneticists, and biochemists continue to study these factors. Cultures have found that some imported "new" foods brought into their areas can aggravate and/or threaten the health of the people. Sometimes, missionaries, health personnel, and lay people who have good intentions may not realize the foods were not so good for the people. The reasons may be related to metabolic, genetic, and cultural intolerance. For example, Brunce reported about a metabolic disturbance found in northeast Brazil in which the population was predisposed to any aggravation of vitamin A deficiency.[25] Dried milk was introduced into the community, which caused the people to experience sudden growth. However, this led to a rapid depletion of the existing meager supply of vitamin A. As a consequence, an outbreak of night blindness, xerophthalmia, keratomalacia, and irreversible blindness occurred. Brunce offered a warning to people who have the good intention of improving dietary inputs in undernourished countries because the foods may be highly disruptive to the normal metabolic functions of the people. Other studies have been done, but more of the consequences of introducing new foods into a new or different cultural area and environment are needed.

Summary Reflections

Considering the above facts, principles, and research studies related to food universals and nonuniversals, the nurse prepared in transcultural knowledge can be a care facilitator to help clients with their food needs and appropriate uses. Nurses of tommorow, however, must increase their knowledge of cultural uses and abuses of foods in diverse cultures. Transcultural nursing insights about general aspects of the client's food culture is essential to making appropriate culture-specific and culturally congruent care in most cultures in the world.

In the process of doing a culturalogical care assessment (see Chapter 4), the nurse identifies food preferences, beliefs, and practices within the different areas of the Sunrise Model, that is, kinship, cultural values, etcetera, as they relate to care and well-being. As mentioned above, the transcultural nurse may need to help other nurses and health personnel to use this model with clients, families, or groups to get an accurate food and health picture.

In the future, one can anticipate more demands for culture-specific foods to increase healing, reduce illnesses, improve health care, and avoid food wastes. Far more attention is needed in hospitals to the way clients want their foods served (i.e., hot or cold) and to give serious attention to client and family ideas of what helps them to keep well or become ill. The nurse should be sensitive not to force clients to eat certain foods just because of professional beliefs that they are "good for the client" because of professional reasons. There is much professionals have to learn about cultural food uses and their nutritional benefits. The color, form, shape, and nutritional value of the food often determine if a client will eat and retain the food. For example, the color red may be a taboo color in a culture, and so red foods are not acceptable. How foods are prepared and served influences acceptance or rejection of the food. Cultural enthnocentrism with imposition practices by the nurse can lead to psychophysical illnesses and cultural pain such as vomiting, gastrointestinal upsets, high anxiety, and passive-resistive behaviors. An important transcultural nursing principle is always to talk with the client and family about their food likes and dislikes and how they prefer to eat the foods, that is, raw, cooked, fried, etcetera. It is also wise to talk about foods that keep them well or tend to make them ill (or uncomfortable), especially when they return home from a hospital experience or have had outpatient treatments. To provide appropriate advice or direct services in an acceptable way, the transculturally oriented nurse tries to enter the food world of the client and understand how they view and use foods.[26] Remaining sensitive to client's food interests and needs is an extremely important means to effective and therapeutic nursing care practices and to promote the well-being of those whom nurses serve. The nurse with transcultural caring knowledge about food uses and functions and flexible caring skills is invaluable to promote client or family well-being and recovery from illnesses and to maintain daily functioning in our changing multicultural world. The use of the three modes of care with the *Culture Care Theory* and with the ethnonursing method can be very helpful in assessing and making decisions with clients on foods, as well as to assess outcomes. In sum, the nurse should keep this message in mind: *Culture defines food uses, functions, and benefits over time and in different places in the world. The nurse's challenge is to discover this reality and to use foods congruently with cultures and therapeutic modes.*

References

1. Kottak, C., *Anthropology: The Exploration of Human Diversity*, New York: McGraw-Hill Co., 1991, p. 176.
2. Bogan, B., "The Evolution of Human Nutrition," in *The Anthropology of Medicine*, 2nd ed., L. Romanucci-Ross, D.E. Moerman, and L.R. Tancrei, eds., New York: Bergin and Garvey, 1991, pp. 158–195.
3. McElroy, A., and P.K. Townsend, "Nutrition Throughout the Lifecycle," in *Medical Anthropology in Ecological Perspective*, 2nd ed., Boulder: Westview Press, 1989, pp. 207–216.
4. Ibid.
5. McElroy, A., and P.K. Townsend, "The Ecology and Economics of Nutrition," in *Medical Anthropology in Ecological Perspective*, 2nd ed., Boulder: Westview Press, 1989, pp. 166–202.
6. Bogan, op. cit.
7. Helman, C., "Diet and Nutrition," in *Culture, Health, and Illness*, Bristol: John Wright PSG, 1990, pp. 31–54.
8. Leininger, M., "Culture Care of the Gadsup Akuna of the Eastern Highlands of New Guinea," in *Culture Care Diversity and Universality: A Theory of Nursing*, M. Leininger, ed., New York: National League for Nursing, 1991, p. 231–280.

9. Leininger, M., "Transcultural Eating Patterns and Nutrition: Transcultural Nursing and Anthropological Perspectives," *Holistic Nursing Practice*, v. 3, no. 1, 1988, pp. 12–26.

10. Helman, op. cit., pp. 32–36.

11. Leininger, op. cit., 1988, pp. 18–24.

12. Leininger, op. cit., 1991, pp. 231–280.

13. McElroy and Townsend, op. cit., 1989, pp. 243–289.

14. Brunce, G.E., "Milk and Blindness in Brazil," *Natural History*, v. 78, no. 2, February 1969, p. 44.

15. McElroy and Townsend, op. cit., 1989, pp. 180–181.

16. Davis, A.E., and T.D. Bolin, "Milk Intolerance in Southeast Asia," *Natural History*, v. 78, no. 2, February 1969, pp. 53–55.

17. Leininger, op. cit., 1991.

18. Manderson, L., "Hot-Cold Food and Medical Theories: Cross Cultural Perspectives," *Introduction to Social Science and Medicine*, v. 25, no. 4, 1987, pp. 329–420.

19. Boyle, J., and M. Andrews, *Transcultural Concepts in Nursing Care*, Boston: Scott, Foresman, and Co., 1999, pp. 335–337.

20. Leininger, op. cit., 1988a.

21. Leininger, M., *Culture Care Diversity and Universality: A Theory of Nursing*, New York: National League for Nursing Press, 1991.

22. Manderson, op. cit., 1987.

23. Leininger, M., "Southern Rural Black and White American Lifeways with Focus on Care and Health Phenomena," in *Care: The Essence of Nursing and Health*, Detroit: Wayne State University Press, 1988, pp. 195–217.

24. Bailey, E., *Urban African American Health Care*, Lanham, MD: University Press of America, Inc., 1991.

25. Brunce, op. cit., 1969.

26. Leininger, M., op. cit., 1988, pp. 16–25.

CHAPTER **10**

Life-Cycle Culturally Based Care and Health Patterns of the Gadsup of New Guinea: A Non-Western Culture*

Madeleine Leininger

A n important part of becoming a transcultural nurse or health care provider is to learn about Western and non-Western comparative practices of how human beings are enculturated to become members of a culture and society. The enculturation process varies in Western and non-Western cultures in birth to death life-cycle practices, in how humans are raised, and in how they develop. All too frequently Western nurses, physicians, and others are taught specific theories and facts about how children and adults become human and survive based on dominant Western theories or stages of development such as Erickson's, Maslow's, and Bronfenbrenner's theories or the Kubler-Ross theory of phases of death and dying. However, as one becomes immersed in studying non-Western cultures from emic lived-through experiences, one often discovers major differences and new information about life-cycle patterns and processes. Very serious ethical and moral issues can be identified if health personnel make assumptions and decisions based on Western child and adult rearing practices when they do not fit non-Western cultures. Nor can one assume that these non-Western or "underdeveloped people" and even some minority cultures will develop and become Westernized sooner or later to fit our theories or standards of enculturation practices.

 ## Researcher's Interests in Non-Western Culture

This chapter provides in-depth emic life-cycle enculturalation patterns of a non-Western culture discovered anew by the author, a social and cultural nurse anthropologist. By living immersed in the daily lifeways of the Gadsup people of the Eastern Highlands of New Guinea (a non-Western culture) for nearly 2 years in the early 1960s, I discovered many new insights that were strikingly different from Western cultures. These discoveries were confirmed by the people in their linguistic meanings and actions and made me realize the extreme importance of nurses and other health personnel knowing non-Western lifeways, human caring, and the enculturation process of human beings. Such discovered knowledge is essential for assessing and making care and cure (or treatment) plans with clients. Granted, all cultures change over time, but some retain certain values, beliefs, and life-cycle practices for justified reasons. In fact, many non-Western minorities, subcultures, and other groups tend to reinforce traditional practices that lead to health and survival as shown in the author's writings over time.[1,2]

Andrews & Boyles' book, *Transcultural Concepts in Nursing*, offers some examples and general guides to help nurses work with clients of some Western and non-Western cultures, particularly related to life-cycle differences in religious, ethical, and general cultural concerns.[3] However, this chapter presents in-depth life-cycle content of one specific culture with a theoretical

---

*This is an edited, expanded, and updated version from earlier chapters in the 1978 and 1995 books on *Transcultural Nursing*. It was written in first person to capture the lived-through, direct observations and experiences of the author over four decades.

217

and experiential transcultural nursing focus over extended time. It should help the reader to understand how the Gadsup develop and live in their Gadsup world.

During the early 1960s I lived with and studied the Gadsup of the Eastern Highlands of New Guinea, who lived thousands of miles from the West Coast of the United States.[4] I wanted to study a non-Western culture to gain new insights, knowledge, and practices essential for nurses to function in perhaps a very different culture from Western cultures. I was interested in how a Gadsup became one from birth into adulthood—especially the life-cycle caring focus. Since I was also developing my theory of Culture Care and the ethnonursing method, I wanted to examine the theory systematically in a non-Western culture to see if the tenets of the theory could be upheld or refuted.

After completing nearly 4 years of rigorous doctoral study at the University of Washington in Seattle, I was ready to do both ethnographic and ethnonursing field research and to identify differences and similarities. I was especially interested in ethnonursing to explicate knowledge about the culture care and health of the Gadsup. The concepts of emic (insider's viewpoints) and etic (outsider's viewpoints) were of much interest to me. I wondered how these concepts could be used to discover covert generic and professional care knowledge. Most of all, I was curious about specific care, illnesses, and wellness ideas of the Gadsup. The concepts of ethnocare and ethnohealth were new ideas in nursing that I had coined to study transcultural nursing phenomena.[5] I also knew that nursing and medicine needed to change from their unicultural viewpoints to a multicultural stance. It was imperative for the future to have such knowledge of a non-Western culture. Moreover, comparative life-cycle practices between cultures was essentially a new idea in nursing in 1960, but well known in anthropology. Anthropology literature and a caring faculty had greatly stimulated my thinking about caring life cycles of cultures. My goal, however, was to develop ultimately a body of knowledge worldwide for the discipline of transcultural nursing for the 21st century with Gadsup non-Western findings.

Before leaving the United States in the early 1960s, several questions came to me: Would it be safe for me to live alone as a single female with the proclaimed "headhunters" (Gadsup) of New Guinea? Could I work in a very different culture over an extended period and make sense out of the people's lifeways? What would I

eat and where would I live in this nontechnical village? Since there had been no outside women who had lived alone in the village without a spouse, would the people kill me or permit me to live under those conditions? Whom could I contact with no Western neighbors, no phone, no car, or no mail service? How would I allay my parents' and family's concerns? When Margaret Mead was at the University of Cincinnati in 1959, she told me she always had some Americans who lived with and helped her while she was doing fieldwork in a northern village in New Guinea. The Papua New Guinea officials told me I needed a gun to protect myself from "headhunters as the Gadsup had been headhunters and could kill you." Such messages were of concern, but I refused having a gun. I believed my Nebraska rural life experiences, anthropological and psychiatric nursing skills, along with my faith in God and prayers would help me.

Entering and Living with Gadsup

I took two small suitcases and a sleeping bag and departed for the Gadsup. My entry into the Gadsup land was initially a cultural shock as everything I saw and experienced was very different from my lifetime experiences in the United States.[6] My Irish and German American cultural heritage along with many diverse life experiences gave me a tenacious work ethic (German) and the ability to know how to "make the best out of life and enjoy it" (Irish). The Gadsup and their environment were very different. The language had not been recorded and was difficult to understand and learn.

The Gadsup were small, dark brown skinned people with very dark brown eyes. The average height of the women was five feet four inches; the men were about five feet and seven inches tall. The women and young children stayed close together in the village, while the young men strayed away from the village each day. The Gadsup lived in bamboo huts with no electricity or modern appliances such as refrigerators and stoves. There were no clocks or watches in the village, so no one lived by a mechanical clock, nor did they keep rigid time schedules. This was strange for me having come from a highly time-centered, United States work-schedule culture. The Gadsup water supply was carried in bamboo tubes from a mountain stream about 2 miles from the village. It was drunk and used without boiling. There were no modern indoor hut toilets but only external "toilet holes" on the edge of the village.

There were no coins or money. Instead, garden and forest products were valued and exchanged under certain rules and conditions until the mid 1970s.

This culture had limited outside contacts in the early 1960s. There were no village health personnel such as nurses, dentists, physicians, pharmacists, or social workers. There were no village schools with professional teachers. There were, however, native or Gadsup folk caregivers and folk curers who provided for the health care needs of the people in the two villages. There were no Western people or Australians living in or near the villages. The Gadsup were quite isolated from the outside world in the 1960s and only knew their village neighbors as traditional friends or enemies.[7] These factors and others made me realize that the Gadsup had a different way of living and valuing from mine.

I began my research by observing and listening about the Gadsup's daily lifeways and lifeworld, using my theory of Culture Care and the enthnonursing and ethnographic methods.[8] The men went into the forest area for hunting birds and small animals; the women worked in the gardens each day. I identified particular beliefs, taboos, values, and practices of the Gadsup, but initially could not understand the meanings. Their lifeways were like a puzzle that had to be put together to make sense to me. Initially, I tried to interpret their strange actions and practices in Western ways, but soon stopped this as nothing fit. It took time, patience, language learning (verbal and nonverbal), and trust in the people to know the Gadsup. Living in the two Gadsup villages I studied (about 10 months in each) was essential to discover the totality of the Gadsup lifeways.

At first, I was an object of curiosity to the Gadsups, as the majority of the people in the two villages had never seen a white woman. The people followed me wherever I went, and they observed everything I did or tried to do! This was strange to me, as I had never had twenty to fifty people watching or trailing me each day and evening. My life was not private but open to all the Gadsup, and I understood this. There was no way of being completely private in my bamboo hut, for even at night the people peered through the lattices of the bamboo hut to watch me. I discovered that my feelings about the lack of privacy and my American values of independence, privacy, and autonomy were clearly different from the Gadsup who valued openness and a totally shared community life. The people were curious about me as a "different" woman and wondered about my white skin and light brown hair. They would touch my skin and stare at my nonkinky hair. Some were cautious about coming to me during my first few months in each village. They stared at my tennis shoes and pant skirts and blouses I wore each day, which contrasted with the Gadsup who wore no shoes. The women wore grass skirts, and the men wore shorts or laplaps. The Gadsup often asked me "what tribe I came from." Later some Gadsup told me that they first saw me as a ghost because my skin was so white, and because I came from an unknown place. I learned to be sensitive to their actions and voice inflections, viewing me as a potential sorceress. My own initial survival was at stake.

Since there was no recorded Gadsup language, I had to learn and record their non-verbal language expressions. The language was tonal and very difficult. At first, I used Melanesian pidgin (a lingua franca, or limited conversational language), but found only two or three men in the village who could speak this language. I observed firsthand the people by their daily and nightly interactions and participated gradually in what they did. They watched me almost constantly during my months in the two Gadsup villages, because I was slightly different. Both villages had traditional enemies and friends, and in the past they had been friends with each other. I learned about how the Gadsup got along with their clans, subclans, and lineages and about their social ways of living together or apart at times.

After 3 months, the villagers became more comfortable and trusted me. They began to share ideas and gradually became protective of me by telling me what I needed to do or avoid. Protective caring and surveillance caring became evident as dominant modes of caring for "true friends." In time, I became their "trusted true friend," and they did not watch me closely. I used the *Observation-Participation-Reflection Enabler* and *the Stranger-Friend Enabler*, which were extremely useful to examine my own behavior and the villagers in both places.[9] In addition, my *Culture Caring Semistructured Gadsup Enabler* guide was essential to study life-cycle events with their meanings and expressions. My domain of inquiry was to discover what could be culturally congruent care decisions and practices as the goal of my study. The use of my Sunrise Model (explained earlier) was most important to guide my study of the different influences on the life cycle and general lifeways of the two Gadsup villages. The Sunrise

Model became a constant mental image to cover the total lifeways of the people with social structure and other holistic features. In both villages I learned much about my own Western cultural behaviors and expressions and what seemed to be troublesome to the Gadsup about me and vice versa. Learning about self through others remained the first important principle in transcultural nursing, which helped me grow and helped the people to share their world with me. Being open to the villagers was essential. Having no privacy was difficult, but I gradually learned to be comfortable with it.

 ## The Gadsup Environment and Social Structure Factors

The Gadsup live in the Eastern Highlands of New Guinea and about six degrees south of the equator. It is a tropical environment with day temperatures of 80 to 85 and 72 at night in the dry season. The Island of New Guinea is shaped like a large bird with its tail and feet toward Australia and the bird's head looking to the Pacific Ocean on the east. The island is about 1500 miles long and 500 miles wide. It is marked with high mountain ranges of nearly 12,000 feet above sea level and many valleys and rivers. There are also large, open grassland areas between the mountainous ranges.[10] The Gadsup frequently walked for miles across these grasslands and mountainous areas to visit their kinsmen in other villages, to hunt birds and animals, or to explore new areas for tribal or political reasons. Young boys and men often walked 10 miles or more to hunt, to gather fruits, and to meet other friendly "tribal brothers." The Gadsup had no cars; however, a few Europeans or Australians who lived and worked for the government would drive by the village, giving them an awareness of automobiles and their uses.

The Gadsup build their huts on the top of flat mountain ridges to protect themselves from their enemies and to prevent their huts from being washed away by torrential rains during the wet season. The country is picturesque with the high mountains in the distance, beautiful lush green trees, tall grasses, and many large wildflowers such as bright red poinsettias growing in their fields and villages. The round huts on the ridges of the mountains are built from bamboo, local trees, and grass. They are remade about every 10 years with all villagers participating, especially those of one's lineage.

There are two main seasons each year, namely, a wet season from December to April, and a dry season from May to November. The average rainfall for the area is about 85 inches per year. During the wet season, hard rains frequently washed away the crudely built Gadsup roads, walking paths, and man-made bridges. Small streams rise and drain into the nearby valleys to produce a tall grass called *kunai*. In the dry season the people enjoy warm and sunny days with temperatures of 80 to 90 degrees Fahrenheit in the daytime, but can drop to 68 to 75 degrees Fahrenheit at night. In the rainy season, there was a 15 to 20 degree temperature difference from the dry season. The temperature in the rainy season sometimes dropped to 57 degrees at night. Such marked changes in temperature often led to infant respiratory conditions and occasionally to death for infants and older Gadsups.[11]

Each Gadsup village plaza was comprised of 20 to 40 small dwelling huts that were made of native bamboo. The roofs of the huts were covered with a tall grass called kunai. Gadsup huts had two or three partitioned rooms, and a raised or ground-floor fireplace to cook native foods, and to keep occupants warm during the wet season. Smoke often filled the hut when the door was closed, as there were no windows. During the dry season, the foods were cooked outside the hut, and the indoor fireplace was seldom used.

The Gadsup in the early 1960s were hunters and gatherers, and so their daily life was spent producing, gathering, and distributing foods to maintain daily sustenance. What they raised, they used each day with limited accumulation or storage of extra foods. They had no way to refrigerate or store large amounts of foods. Food producing and gathering was central to their lifeway. Food was used not only for their physical needs, but for social, political, and ceremonial purposes. Gardening was the important daily activity for the women and young girls. Men participated by clearing and building new gardens. Wild birds and animals were sought in the forest by young Gadsup boys and men. The men were also involved in a great variety of political meetings, doing "walk-abouts" to their neighboring villages, and conducting ceremonial life-cycle activities and village rituals. Garden and forest products were the main exchanges between kin groups within and outside the village. Coffee and tea raising was for some economic gain as these products were sold to

Australians. The people used this small, irregular income to buy small amounts of rice, canned goods, and other material items that were available at a small hut store about 5 to 10 miles from each village.[12] The little stores were new developments in the Eastern Highlands of New Guinea in the mid 1960s and have decreased as small towns became established later.

Kinship and Family Ties

The kinship ties of the Gadsup were complex with many kinship terms to guide social and cultural relationships. The important kinship themes and family behaviors were the following:

1. Gadsup adults carefully regulate their behavior according to whether the individual or group was close or distant to them and to the lineage and clan they belonged to over the years. It was a patrilineal kinship with extended lineages.
2. Male and female behaviors had different expectations and were closely related to kinship expectations, family roles, and cultural values and beliefs.
3. Care and health practices were embedded in their kinship behaviors, responsibilities, and expectations and were critical for caregiving.
4. Kinship and lineage ties strongly organized the Gadsup lifeways and directly influenced care and health practices through their extended family.

It was interesting to discover that if a child or adult became ill or exposed to sorcerers, there were natural built-in care providers from the lineage family (often 20 to 40 people) and even from clans and subclans (hundreds of people). Finally, the tribal group (which was the largest Gadsup cultural group) could be called on if the illness was caused by outside enemies or sorcerers.[13]

This was very different from Western health-illness practices. It was a unique culturally based social and caring system with different role expectations that sharply contrasted with United States nuclear-family structures with approximately two children. The Gadsup culture care structure was a unique, powerful, and effective generic care system in that they received care from their extended kinsmen and lineage groups. There were also choices for the children to get help

from both men and women of their familial lineage. The Gadsup often told me, "We are all one big family," "We come from one source," and "We belong to each other." Their daily behavior supported these statements and showed the differences among the involved groups. Aggressive or violent acts were largely regulated by kinship, clan, and tribal rules. The assurance of culture care continuity was a regulatory cultural norm and contributed to their state of well-being and to their ability to function without a lot of physical stresses or even mental illnesses.

The roles of the kinspersons were guided by the particular environmental-historical context and by well-known gender roles. For example, there were appropriate times and places to give foods, conduct life-cycle ceremonies, provide direct care to others, help the sick or dying, protect villagers from strangers, and give advice to their people. Gadsup children learned at an early age to know these cultural modes of conduct and rules of behavior. The Gadsup kinship structure with its caring expressions had a powerful influence on the health and well-being of the people throughout the life cycle and on their expectations to be good people.

The Political and Religious Lifeways

The political system was complex because kinship and politics were closely linked together. Male and female gender roles were regulated by village politics and political norms. Political groups varied in size and function according to the clans, lineage, subclans, and tribes. The men maintained the most active public roles in all political affairs such as conducting village affairs (largely food gift exchanges), ritual male life-cycle ceremonies, pig festivals, daily political debates in the village, religious activities, and all affairs with strangers or traditional enemies. These political roles constituted much of the men's daily activities in the village, but they always had time to hunt, which was usually a political and social activity among males. The Gadsup women had some influence on political thinking and actions of men in covert and subtle ways but not by public decrees. When upset, they made loud pronouncements in the village plaza, and the men listened to the women and generally heeded their concerns.

With *respect to religion*, the Gadsup believed in their deceased *ancestors*. It meant that they worshipped their deceased kinsperson as their life spirit or an essence that lived in them. This life spirit became an ethical and moral guide to govern the daily actions and judgments of children and adults. They talked about their ancestors and their moral values and how they should live according to them. Moral values were usually a positive guide for young children and adults in many of their daily actions and life-cycle affairs. The adults taught the children about their ancestors and how they lived according to "the good Gadsup values of brotherly caring and protective caring." The children were rewarded or negatively sanctioned according to whether their acts were like those of their ancestors. Thus their ancestral religion was most meaningful and a powerful moral and ethical guide for all villagers. It was interesting that in the early 1960s a Western Lutheran group came to the Gadsup villages. The Gadsup struggled to understand the Christian beliefs such as faith, God, heaven, and hell. These concepts and the associated beliefs were very strange and impersonal to the Gadsup because they did not fit with their ancestral beliefs, and some were frightening to them and difficult to accept.[14] By the mid 1980s, some adapted Christian beliefs.

 ## Life-Cycle Phases: Values, Beliefs, and Practices

There are few cultures today that have as sharp a dichotomy between the gender roles and activities of men and women as the Gadsup. Male and female Gadsup secrets pervaded their beliefs throughout the entire life span in the early 1960s and into the 1990s. Sex role activities clearly organized men and women's social, economic, political, and religious activities. The villagers enculturated their children with appropriate male and female role behaviors early in life, which were respected and maintained throughout the life cycle.

The Gadsup had many male and female beliefs and secrets about the life cycle related to conception, birth, growth, marriage, and death. These beliefs were kept within each gender group as it was taboo (or forbidden) to discuss sex secrets with members of the opposite sex. For example, the men had traditional beliefs and secrets about their sacred bamboo flutes that had religious, health and illness, and sociocultural significance.[15] Men were not permitted to talk about

their bamboo flutes to the women, and if they did, it could lead to unfavorable consequences such as sickness, death, or village feuds. Likewise, women had their secrets about birth, child and adult care, and ways to deal with men's behavior and their use of male sacred flutes. The women believed that the men had originally taken these sacred flutes from the women. The flutes symbolized fertility, sexual power, social relatedness, and procreation. The men wanted the flutes to get some female sexual power. It was interesting to discover these beliefs, as there had been a traditional emphasis in the anthropological literature that only males had sexual power over women. However, I found the Gadsup women had more sexual power that the men traditionally wanted. Males developed female symbols such as *found with the male* sacred flutes and other female objects they used to express their sexual power. Female menstruation, childbirth, and child rearing knowledge were sources of sexual power and secrets that the women kept away from the men in the village. The importance of gender secrets and keeping them secret created sexual identity differences and pride. Male-female ceremonies were separate but fit the daily patterns of Gadsup living, eating, playing, and sociopolitical activities. In a later visit in the 1990s I found that some of the old Gadsup gender secrets were not as strictly guarded as in the past.[16] However, these secrets and other values, beliefs, and practices were still a major influence on the Gadsup gender interactions and on life-cycle ceremonies, which will be discussed next.

 ## Pregnancy Through Childbirth Phase

While living in the two Gadsup villages, I carefully observed and documented the prenatal, natal, and postnatal activities of birthing women. Perhaps most striking were the tremendous physical strength and the role expectations of young, middle-aged, and older women. The Gadsup women were short with strong muscular development. They were physically strong as they had rigorous daily physical activities such as daily gardening, cleaning the village plaza, walking great distances to their gardens, carrying infants and garden tools or firewood on their backs, and doing daily family or clan chores. While pregnant, the women maintained a physically very active daily work schedule. There were no pregnancy complaints or signs of morning sickness with the women in either village. There was no pampering of women during pregnancy as pregnancy was a normal and a highly desired life experience for women. Young girls were expected to get married, become pregnant, and raise healthy children. These were the hallmarks of becoming a respected Gadsup woman. There were no unmarried girls in the village beyond the age of 19 years. Indeed, a girl becomes a woman *only* when she is married and gives birth to her first child. Marriage and childbearing lead to a highly desired social status and recognition for women. Likewise, boys become men *only* if they are married and have at least one child. Marriage and having the first child make Gadsup "complete human beings" and socially recognized by all Gadsup in the lineage, clan, and tribe.[17]

Gadsup married women viewed pregnancy not only as highly desired, but also as a symbolic expression of maintaining the continuity of Gadsup. It reaffirmed a woman's fertility, her femininity, her social role and respect in the village, and power. Gadsup women desired four living children per husband and most women had four or five children. The women held that through their long history they were the "real culture carriers" as they had the power to bear children, while men did not have this sexual power. Female and male secret sexual legends and beliefs confirmed these beliefs and action patterns. Gadsup men, however, held that they determined the viability and healthy status of the child by their semen and strong male physical condition. Thus a comparative and complementary gender status prevailed between males and females with their sexual abilities and offspring. It was of interest that the number of children per couple remained fairly constant by the genealogies over three generations.

Gadsup males and females were married between the ages of 17 and 21 years. There were very few Gadsup divorces as divorces were unacceptable. A boy who was unmarried by 18 years was an extremely restless male who often asked adult villagers to help him find a good wife. The first child was born usually within the first 2 years after marriage. The birth was a happy occasion. The succeeding children were born 2 or 3 years apart, which the women said they regulated by using indigenous plants as contraceptives. The Gadsup confirmed their manhood and womanhood statuses by marriage and children. They loved children, and the

first child was especially warmly welcomed as this established their adult married status.

A married girl who did not bear a child early in marriage faced the possibility of divorce or separation, which was viewed as most unfortunate. When a Gadsup female knew she was pregnant, she happily told her mother and close kinswomen. A small informal female gathering occurred to rejoice that the girl would soon be a woman and that she would be a desired Gadsup in the village with a child. During the course of my research a few young girls were anxious and afraid of becoming pregnant. These girls were counseled by the older and experienced Gadsup women about their concerns. Some counseling occurred before pregnancy, but only a few weeks before, by the use of personal accounts or stories by older women who functioned like lay midwives. When the woman knew she was pregnant, she told her female kinswomen but not her husband or any males. This was to be kept as a surprise to males and to protect the unborn infant from male magical harm.

While Gadsup males believed they influenced whether the child would be strong and healthy, the women believed they had the strongest procreation abilities and powers to ensure a live infant in utero and thereafter. It was the woman's belief that she determined the sex of the child and whether the child would survive during pregnancy and the critical first year of life. The males believed that their semen takes hold after the first year of life and makes the child a strong Gadsup person so that in utero and early infancy the female sexual powers then take hold.[18]

During pregnancy women often crave rare foods, and so the Gadsup spouse and his kinsmen are expected to get special foods for the pregnant wife by complying and walking great distances for their wants. Foods craved by pregnant women were usually fresh fruits, nuts, bird meat, taro, and greens—all foods they seldom have in their daily diets. There were no accounts of the Gadsup men experiencing pregnancy symptoms or food cravings while their spouse was pregnant. Foods that normally are associated with males were taboo during the wife's pregnancy. These foods are special male foods used for ceremonial and political gatherings such as eel and forest meats, and pregnant women cannot eat these foods. It was believed that if the woman ate these foods she would become deathly sick and the child would probably die because these are male power foods and far "too strong" for women and the infant. Instead, nurturing female foods such as sweet potatoes, taro, greens, fresh fruits, and nuts are eaten for a healthy child. Women who had eaten male taboo foods were reported as becoming very sick, and their children were often deformed or physically handicapped. The pregnancy period strongly emphasized the woman's procreative and envied fertility abilities. Foods were eaten to have a healthy and active baby in utero and shortly after the birth.

Of the twenty Gadsup women (key informants) studied in-depth, none complained of morning sickness during their pregnancy.[19] A pregnant woman went to her garden to work each day until a few hours before she delivered her child. The daily work schedule of the pregnant woman included routine garden labor, cooking, and childcare. The pregnant woman occasionally paused to relax and feed a child while in the garden, but she worked hard each day in the garden and at home for about 10 hours. Of the twenty pregnant women in both villages (one-half were primiparous and one-half multiparous), none had swollen extremities, signs of toxemia, or unusual prenatal problems during their pregnancy. These women were in good physical health and seemed relaxed about pregnancy, and this seemed to contribute to a healthy and normal pregnancy. Moreover, I would hold that their lifelong strenuous physical activities (since approximately the age of 4 years) put them in good physical and mental condition for pregnancy and delivery. In addition, their positive attitude about pregnancy and wanting children supported their pregnancy and influenced favorably the birth of a healthy infant. Abortion was generally seldom desired and rarely occurred.

The Delivery Event

As the day of delivery approached, the expectant mother continued to work hard in her garden—planting seeds, pulling weeds by hand, digging, and cleaning vegetables. She stooped over and dug plants or sat on the ground to do her garden work. She only paused for short rest periods to care for or feed children. During pregnancy the wife is also expected to provide daily foods for the family and to help around the village from early in the morning until late at night. Interestingly,

she does these activities to maintain her female role and village status. Gadsup males do not assume any female roles or helping female activities before, during, or after the birth of the child. The pregnant woman may talk to lay midwives about her expectations and pregnancy signs while they work in the gardens or while they prepare food in the woman's hut or village place. Delivery guidance is largely based on traditional intergenerational beliefs and stories of women in the village and how they have a healthy child.[20] There was much pride in sharing these secrets with young girls during the last phase of their pregnancy.

The following incident was fairly typical of Gadsup childbirth practices. Anu was a 20-year-old mother ready to give birth to her second child. Her first female child, Annurunu, was 3 years old, and her husband was 22 years of age. It was about 10 p.m. when Anu's mother knocked on my door and told me, "We go now to the forest." Anu was having regular uterine contractions about 15 minutes apart. On this night, there were earthquake tremors of about 4.5 in intensity, and it was the dry season with the night temperature at 68 degrees Fahrenheit. Anu's mother, her grandmothers, father's sister, and myself left the village for the forest delivery hut on a bright moonlit night. We walked up and down mountainous terrain for about 3 miles until we reached the delivery hut located in a densely forested area. It took about 1 hour to walk the 3 miles with Anu and her maternal kinswomen. I had expected that Anu would probably deliver along the way as her labor pains became closer together, stronger, and more regular. We stopped only twice along the way to rest briefly and to look at the moon. There was limited talk among the women as we walked fairly vigorously to the delivery hut.

After arriving at the hut, the three Gadsup kinswomen (like lay midwives) quickly moved to prepare the area for Anu's delivery. Anu sat outside the delivery hut as the women swept the dirt floor inside and started a fire to heat some water, which they had carried in bamboo tubes to the hut. Then Anu came inside (about 10 minutes later) and knelt on a pandanus mat on the floor. She was told to grasp a wooden post that was fixed in the center of the hut. She used the pole to help her bear down with each labor contraction. The midwives showed Anu how to use her arms in a crossed position over her abdomen to bear down on the abdomen and facilitate the labor contractions. Soon the child's head appeared (within 10 to 15 minutes), and the midwives guided the infant gently from the vaginal orifice. A large, 7-pound male infant was born and was shown immediately to the mother. The placenta was soon delivered by the skilled lay midwives. The infant and the placenta were smoothly delivered without complications such as excessive bleeding or great pains. (There were no delivery complications with any of the seven deliveries I witnessed.) The actual delivery took about 20 minutes. Great joy was expressed by the women in their quiet ways with the infant. Anu seemed very happy to have a second child, especially her first male child. Since the Gadsup love and are overjoyed to have children, the delivery was a big event.

Immediately after birth, Anu was laid on a big pandanus mat with the infant in her arms and across her abdomen. The mother and midwives held the infant closely to their bare skins. Women in the hut cleaned the floor, while one woman stayed close to Anu. The women gave Anu an herbal (nonalcoholic) drink about 20 minutes after the delivery. Anu did not show signs of being exhausted or ill. Instead, she appeared relieved and pleased with her well child. Anu's husband and his kinsmen were not allowed to be present during the delivery—a cultural taboo. If males were present, this could bring unfortunate ill effects to the child and mother and could reveal the secrets of the women. This point has significant nursing implications and contrasts with American and European nursing practices in which fathers are taught "to bond with the infant" immediately after birth. For the Gadsup such bonding or attachment practices would be a cultural taboo as they are not congruent with their cultural values.[21] American nurses would need to be aware of and respect such cultural differences and use culture care maintenance or preservation mode rather than forcing parents to bond with their infant. Transcultural nurses would support culturally congruent care for the health and well-being of the family.

Postnatal Ethnocare Expressions and Practices

The postnatal period begins after the infant is born and the placenta delivered. The Gadsup midwife used a bamboo knife to cut the cord. The knife had been sterilized by the women by moving it over an open hot fire. The women told me this technique had been used for many years by the Gadsup midwives. The mother's sister then buried the placenta under a tree near the delivery hut to symbolize the perpetuation of women's fertility or procreative abilities and continuity of the lineage. The placenta must not be buried in a garden as the woman's blood is so powerful, it would contaminate the food and make males and children ill. Their cultural taboo and belief is that female fertility blood can produce illness and death in males because it is so powerful and harmful to men's bodies. At no time can female blood get into the garden. The danger of female blood was a major reason the delivery huts are always built a far distance from the village. After the placenta was buried, the kinswomen carried the new infant in the mother's new net bag. The adults all walked back to the village, which was approximately a 1-hour walk. I walked with Anu and the baby up and down a rugged mountainous terrain. We rested only occasionally to check the infant on my request. I was most impressed with the strength of the mother to walk such a great distance so soon after delivery of the infant. This practice was not unique to Anu, as I found it was common with several village mothers studied.

When the mother and infant returned to the village, the husband, father, and other males did not come near the woman even though they were extremely eager to see the newborn child. It was a cultural taboo to have males close to a woman who had just delivered as she is "full of blood that could be harmful to men and kill them." Several Gadsup men explained this interpretation to me, as well as the women. The father of the child and male kinsmen live with their father and away from the hut (usually in a nearby hamlet) during the postdelivery period. This is the time that the mother and infant establish a close "bare-skin relationship" with no cloth between infant and mother while she feeds and cares for the infant. The mother holds the infant close to her breast and body as she sits and does daily household tasks. Sometimes the infant may also lay in the mother's lap as she works at preparing taro, sweet potatoes, and other foods for a family meal.

Gadsup infants are breast-fed for 2 or 3 years. There are no cow's milk or infant-feeding bottles. The mothers said they would not like to use "such things" as bottles as they enjoy breast-feeding and holding their infants. Some wet kin-mothers feed other infants in the village because of the absence, illness, or death of a mother. In caring for the infant, the mother does a lot of touching and holding the infant, but she seldom coos or gives a lot of facial communication to the infant as found with American or Western mothers. The mother, her close kinswomen, and young girls in the village provided the primary care to the newborn infant for months. The bare skin contact of the infant with the mother is valued to feel and to assess the child's wellness. *Caring is nurturance* and includes *touching* and *being close* to the infant as the major caring modes to help the infant grow and survive. The midwives or maternal kinswomen remain close to the mother to provide protection, surveillance, direct help, and other nurturant care expectations.[22] While the mother is able to provide for her own care and that of the infant, she also expects her kinswomen and young daughters to provide "other care" acts for her and the infant.

As the child grows, the mothers hold their infants on their crossed legs while sitting on a pandanus mat outside their hut and continue to work. The mother never leaves the infant alone or out of her sight until after the third or fourth week. She frequently breast-feeds the baby as she believes the infant needs mother's milk to grow and to soothe when the infant cries or is restless. The breast is viewed by the mother as consoling care to the infant but also the key source of nutrients. While the mother is nursing her newborn infant, a 2- or 3-year old child may also want the mother's breast, and so the mother gives the breast to the child for a few minutes. The child suckles and soon runs away. This action tends to allay and meet the sibling's need and prevent sibling tensions. After 3 months, breast-feeding is decreased and new supplemental soft masticated foods are gradually given the infant. At all times the newborn female infant is wrapped in a grass skirt to cover genitals, whereas the male child's genitals are not covered and he receives no clothing until about the age of 5. The early childhood phases of development were known by the way girls and boys are dressed and cared for by the villagers.

The Gadsup people believe it is extremely important for the infant and small child to relate to his immediate physical and local village environment. When the mother and her infant sit outside the hut, other women in the village come to see and hold the child and talk to the mother. These women hold the small child close to their bare-skinned bodies and use hand-touching to stimulate the child, which is important in care-taking. Small male children are held and touched by mother and kinswomen. However, males over 7 years are not encouraged to touch infants for fear of sickness to themselves and to the infant. This is because older boys (over 7 years) are held to have some powerful female blood in them that could cause illnesses until they undergo male initiation rites around the age of 7 to 10 years.

In the village small pigs or dogs are permitted to come close to the infant and are seldom chased away. The Gadsup believe these animals are part of their child's natural and familiar environment, so it is important for the child to see and hear these animals early in life as part of their environment. The mothers usually have an environmental "test" for the small infant (under 3 months) that consists of placing the infant on a pandanus mat on the ground to see if the child becomes ill. This test tells the mother if the child will be healthy and if it will respond to Gadsup land on which he or she is to live and survive. The mother assesses the child's response and predicts the potential wellness or illness of the child. If the child is active (strong movements), he or she will survive and be healthy. If there is a weak or no body response to the cool ground, the child will be ill and may not survive the rigors of the Gadsup environment.[23]

Small Child Phase   When the child is about 6 months old, the wife's kinsmen present the child to the biological father, to his male kinsmen, and to her kinspeople. This presentation symbolizes the child's entry and acceptance into the Gadsup village and especially to all the parents' kinsfolk. This is a greatly anticipated event that brings the new child fully into the community. There is very little physical touching of the child, but instead the villagers make statements of praise, joy, and pleasure such as "He is like us Gadsup," "He is good and strong," "He is our brother," "He is one of us," and so on. The female relatives touch and hold the child to protect the child's health and well-being as *protective* and *nurturant caring* of the vulnerable infants. Males have limited nurturant abilities according to women villagers.

After the infant is presented to the villagers in a formalized and ritualized ceremony, cooked food is shared among the villagers. This is the mother's first presentation of the child to all kinsmen and villagers, and so her kinswomen and children bring foods from their gardens.[24] The husband is expected to get food from the forest areas and give to his close female kinsmen. Bundles of food such as bananas, sugar cane, taro, pit-pit, sweet potatoes, and, occasionally, some fruits from the Markham Valley are offered. At this special occasion it is the father's oldest brother (social father) who makes a speech indicating that the child comes from their Gadsup lineage and so the food is a gift to their lineage. Small piles of food are formally presented to the husband's kinsmen and to the wife's kinsmen. This ceremony signifies an appreciation for and recognition of the status of the kinspeople and of their contribution to the Gadsup culture and their lineages. During this ceremony the wife and newborn child sit near the piles of food (often in the center of the village). The mother shows the child to the kinspeople as they casually come to view the child (mostly women admirers come close and touch the infant, whereas the men are afraid to get close to the mother and child for fear of causing illnesses). This ceremony signifies that the child is now an integral part of the village and has a legitimate relationship and status with all Gadsup villagers, but especially kinsfolk. The child is, therefore, an accepted human being belonging to a large extended family-lineage social network and the Gadsup community. This child ceremony contrasts with United States Anglo-Americans in many areas but especially that American children belong to their parents. The Gadsup child is presented into the larger community or social group at a very early age for acceptance and identity.

During the infant village presentation, it is the father's brother who holds the child and offers a small taste of garden or forest foods. A male child is given a taste of male foods such as sugar cane and forest meat as "his foods," whereas a female is given food such as sweet potatoes and female foods. When the father's brother presents the food to the child, he says, "I give you these foods so that you will taste them and always want them. You will work hard to get these foods as you grow in our place." This symbolic ritual ceremony has economic and sociocultural significance as it imprints on the Gadsup villagers their sex roles, symbolic foods, and a division of labor for males and females with their anticipated sociocultural roles.

Infant Baby Phase   During the first year of life the infant's most intensive relationship is with the mother and her extended kinsmen. The infant sleeps with the mother who also stays close to the child as she works in her garden or near the hut. The villagers show interest in the infant by stimulating him or her to respond to them as they hold and nurture the small child. The child learns to respond to diverse kinspersons, animals, and the total environment. The child relates to other children in the village and is often cared for by girls of approximately 7 to 12 years. On the basis of Western theories one might expect that there would be a lot of sibling jealousy and rivalry with the young child, but this is not the case. This seems related to the belief that the child *always belongs to the villagers*, and *all villagers share in caring for or about the new member* in their cultural world. The child, too, learns that all the Gadsup are interested in helping him or her become a responsible, morally good person in the village.

During the early child-rearing period, the mother breast-feeds the infant whenever the child expresses the need for food or cries. There is no rigid time to feed the child, whether on the breast or soft foods. At night, the child sleeps with the mother cuddled under her arms or on one side of her bare-skinned body. The husband sleeps in another hut away from the mother and child for about 6 to 8 months after the child is born. The infant becomes attached to women's voices, touches, and other stimulating care modes. There is no "bonding of the child to his or her biological parents" per se or to the sociolegal father because of the cultural taboos that the child must relate to and be part of many villagers' lifeways.[25]

When the child begins to walk (about 10 months to 1 year), the mother lets the child explore the village area. Infants are not expected to crawl but rather standup and walk for many cultural reasons. The female kinspersons provide surveillance as good and expected child care. Surveillance as caring means to *watch over* and to *protect* the child from external harm in the environment, including people, animals, and natural forces. Young female siblings provide most of the surveillance and protective caring to the child along with the mother and her kinswomen in the village. *Surveillance as caring* was important as women watch the infant explore his or her social, cultural, human, and physical environment at short and longer distance ranges.[26] When the mother works in the garden (usually 3 months after delivery), the infant is hung in a handmade pandanus net bag on a nearby garden fence. The child sleeps in the pandanus bag until he awakens or needs to be fed. When the mother is in her hut, she places the infant on a pandanus mat or hangs him or her in the net bag on an internal house post. Small children are free to run about in the garden, home, or village and learn what areas are safe to explore and to touch and hold with the mother present.

Gadsup infants and children seldom cry, but when they do, female siblings come to them. Mothers tend to let children cry until they have finished whatever they are doing. Mothers believe it is important to let children cry and not be overly responsive to them or to feed them every time they cry. Since Gadsup mothers are extremely busy, hard-working, and responsible for their village roles, the child must fit his rhythm of life to the daily role activities of the mother. Nonetheless, the child is never unduly neglected, ignored, or abused. Disciplining of the child fits with Gadsup cultural values, norms, and taboos and is seldom too harsh or inappropriate.

As already noted, the Gadsup early stages of development are different from what many Americans or Westerners learn in child development courses, and they do not fit well with Piaget's or Erikson's stages of development. From my nearly 2 years of daily and direct observations in both villages, from interviews, and from first-hand participant experiences, the following are the *Gadsup phases of development in their linguistic terms.* The first stage of child development is called the *tiny baby stage.* During the tiny baby stage, the infant is weak and vulnerable and must be cared for through *surveillance* and *protective care* acts by the mother and other village females. The dominant care behaviors to ensure a healthy baby were *surveillance, nurturance, protection, stimulation, and avoiding breaking of cultural taboos* to prevent illness and death. These care modes are essential for the infant's survival, growth, and remaining well. The tiny baby needs protection from sorcery, damp or cold weather, and especially strangers who can cause illness by their careless acts or words. Older mothers gave young mothers advice on ways they must be surveillant to protect the vulnerable child. Many nurturant acts such as holding, encouraging activity, and breast-feeding were ways to help the

infant grow. Interestingly, the small child is exposed early to many different noises and the sounds of people and animals in the village environment (See Color Insert 10).

Comparative analysis of the two Gadsup villages revealed only slight differences in the "tiny baby" and early child care phases largely because Gadsup women married into other Gadsup villages. Gadsup intervillage child-rearing care practices and values by females were similar, but some techniques and expressions of caring showed slight variations. For example, in one Gadsup village, the infant was fed solid foods 2 months after birth, whereas in another village the infant was 4 to 5 months old before given solid foods. In both villages the mothers premasticated bananas or sweet potatoes to feed the infant along with offering their breast milk. I documented that infants who received solid foods 2 to 3 months after birth grew more rapidly, cried less, and were more content than infants who were given solid foods after 5 or 6 months. There were also no signs of allergy or difficulty with the infant taking premasticated foods. In both Gadsup villages infants were breast-fed frequently for 6 months, but some continued for the 2 years. The techniques of feeding the infant solid food showed slight variation as some mothers would use their fingers to feed the infant, whereas others would let the child pick up the food and eat by themselves, (no spoons were in the villages). Very small infants during the first 3 months received premasticated food from the mother as she placed it in the child's mouth.[27]

The Gadsup mothers highly valued breast milk as the best and most essential infant food. Cow's milk was never used or brought into the villages. A religious group brought goats into the village, but the people would not milk the goats, eat the meat, or give goat's milk to infants. The Gadsup found the goats were a nuisance, and they called them the "Seventh Day Pigs" to reflect the fact that the Seventh Day Adventists brought the goats into the village. With the Gadsup women breast-feeding their infants, there was no contamination of milk, and breast milk was readily available to the child for food and as comfort care practices.

Although pinworms existed in the village, only a few children were ill because of these pinworms. The mothers were more concerned about cultural factors that might cause illnesses to small children such as sorcery and harm from outsiders rather than biological factors. Decreases in infant mortality and morbidity rates were largely the result of the *excellent female care-giving*, using the *care values* of *protection, nurturance, surveillance, and other cultural ways to keep children well*. Young girls (ages 8 to 14 years) and older kinswomen were also active care providers for infants and young children. Older females and males who could no longer work in their gardens or go to the forest took care of young children and enjoyed caretaking role responsibilities. The mothers, young girls, and maternal kinswomen were the primary caregivers of small infants and children in the two villages, and they valued caring for infants.

Gadsup children generally remained well unless a respiratory or sorcery condition occurred. If the child became ill, the mother and her kinsmen used folk generic remedies and folk-care methods to care for the child. There were no professional health services in the two villages. If the infant became acutely ill and died, the mothers and maternal kinsmen were often viewed as inadequate caregivers and protectors. During my years in the two villages, I saw only one infant die in each village, which was caused by a very chilly rainy season that led to pneumonia. If a child died, the Gadsup were deeply saddened and greatly mourned this loss. The genealogical history of 15 and 30 key informants revealed that fewer than three infants died in each village per year, and there were 20 to 25 births per year in each village in the early 1960s.

During my stay in each Gadsup village in the early 1960s there was one Australian public heath nurse who came to a distant patrol post to weigh infants and checked on the mothers, but most Gadsup women did not use or value this service. This nurse did not understand the Gadsup and their care practices. The one-day clinics were poorly attended by Gadsup mothers as they viewed the nurse as a potential sorceress and the clinic as a harmful place to go. It was a high risk to take an infant or sick child outside the village to a potential sorcery place, as this would be a source for illnesses or death for any vulnerable child. The government officers encouraged the Gadsup to use the infant and child road clinics, but few would go. The informants said it was "too dangerous" to go because of sorcery potentials. When the nurse came, most mothers stood away from the nurse and were very reluctant to give their children to her to be held, examined, and weighed. The

nurse could not speak the Gadsup language and was unaware of the Gadsup child-rearing cultural beliefs and practices. Hence, professional nursing service was of limited help to the Gadsup mothers and infants in both villages.[28]

Small Child and Young Girl and Boy Phases   The *second stage* of Gadsup development was the "*small child.*" In this stage the Gadsup child usually learned how to walk by 10 months *without crawling* first. Gadsup mothers and other caretakers encourage children to walk as early as possible. Learning to walk was a major task but expected in this phase. Children were warned not to leave their village by themselves until after the age of 5 or 6 years. If the child left the village, he or she was always accompanied by an adult kinsperson as the child was very vulnerable to sorcery and possible dangers by potential Gadsup enemies. Prevention of illnesses was achieved by limiting the child's territorial areas to avoid sorcery and outside harm. There was less emphasis in both villages on teaching the child to talk. Informants told me that their children will learn Gadsup naturally. Children begin to focus on talking the Gadsup language by 10 months and mastered it around 2 years.

After the tiny infant phase (from birth to 1 year) and the small child phase (from about 1 to 3 years), the other phases of development with their names are the following: the *little girl and boy phase* (about 3 to 6 years); the *companion phase* (about 10 to 14 years); and the *exploring and courting phase* (about 14 to 20 years). The *becoming a man or woman phase* was after marriage and having one child when they became fully recognized as a Gadsup man or woman. Since the Gadsup have no Western calendars, the ages of the villagers had to be estimated from special events, observations, genealogies, and views of key informants. Because of space constraints these remaining phases will be briefly highlighted with their major characteristics but realizing that tiny infant and small child phases were viewed as extremely important for the next little boy and girl phases.

The little girl and boy phase covered the ages of about 3 to 6 years and was characterized by the girl beginning to work closely with her mother and maternal kinsperson in the gardens and in all female village activities. Likewise, the little boy phase began when he followed his father and male kinspersons into the nearby forest or grassland areas and learned directly from them. During this time the small boy was never completely separated from his mother and maternal kinswomen as the Gadsup believe that small children of both sexes need their mother for nurturance and protection along with other maternal caring acts. The father and male villagers were always excited and very eager to have the little boy with them in the forest while hunting. They would show him how to hunt birds and mammals with handmade bows and arrows and how to know the secrets of the male world, including the natural forest and other male friends. Some sacred male objects were introduced to the boy. The little girl was socialized early and continuously into a female work role and was taught by the village women how to share female role responsibilities. In the garden and in the villages, the little girl would collect food, firewood, and watch infants. The little boy activities were directed toward exploring the village and had the limited emphasis on male work roles.[29]

During the next *phase* known as *young girl and boy phase* (roughly 6 to 10 years), the girls assumed a heavier work role than in the previous phase, but little boys remained free to roam about the village with or without male kinsmen. During the little boy phase, the boys spent most of their day playing with other young and older boys, interacting with villagers, and going to the forest with adult men. I discovered that young boys in this phase learn how to be highly innovative as they are free to explore and express themselves in the Gadsup village environment. Young boys made creative toys such as seed popguns, clay animals, and hunting bows. In contrast, the young girls did not have free time to explore and create. Instead, they worked almost a full day closely with female kinswomen and had virtually no time for free play. Their task was to focus on child care-taking and adult women's work roles as they were expected to be responsible, good women who knew how to work and care for children.

Companion Phase   During the companion phase (about 10 to 14 years), the girls had "pals" and kept together, whereas the boys had companionship groups (often four to six in a group). The companion boy's group activities included going far into the deep forest area to hunt birds and cassowaries. Gadsup boys

would sit and visit together, wash themselves in the small stream, and have "walkabouts" to nearby villages. This phase was highly exploratory and an exciting time for the boys to develop social friendship ties. The girls had small pal groups (two or three) who would walk together to the gardens and work close to each other and small children in the village. Girls of this age would talk, laugh, and enjoy each other while working together. It was common to observe boys and girls putting their arms around the neck or waist of companions of the same sex as they walked around the village, garden, or forest. While some might be tempted to call them "homosexuals" in Western terms, they were not. There was no sexual play, intercourse, or intense unisexual affection expressed. These companion groups were viewed as important to learn "good village friendship but not sexual activities." Boys and girls developed strong social relationships, learned about appropriate sex roles, and had fun "walking about" together. They learned about cultural activities of adults within and outside the village area, but stayed close to the Gadsup village.

Courting Phase   The courting phase (10 to 18 years) was characterized by young boys making themselves attractive to girls as potential spouses. It was fascinating to observe young boys (still not called men) during this phase go to the stream to wash themselves (without soap, as none existed in the village), wash laplaps, or go to a trade store for new laplaps or trouser-like apparel. They would also look within and outside the village for young girls whom they thought might be good wives and mothers and would have brief talks with the girls. The boys sang courting songs to the girls they would like to court. He would toss a pebble at her and the girl would respond by looking to see who tossed the pebble, and then she would decide if she wanted to see him. This was an emotionally exciting experience for boys who took active steps to find and court girls they hoped would be their wives. Interestingly, the girls were not active pursuers of young boys, but waited for boys to seek them out. The girl, however, had to decide if she wanted to know and be courted by the boy with the intent that he should be a future husband. The young girls were the decision makers and were in control of whom they courted and with whom they wanted to be or to make Gadsup love. If the girl agreed to see the boy, the boy would sing love songs outside her hut, and if acceptable, a love tryst would probably occur in which they would hug each other or occasionally sleep with one another. Premarital sexual intercourse was a cultural taboo and not sanctioned. Active courting was, however, acceptable. The girls and boys enjoyed this phase and were often found together in their groups talking about good wives (or husbands) they would value as spouses. Giggling, making themselves look attractive, and making brief "tough and go" encounters characterized this phase. It was a phase that helped the young girls and boys develop gender identity, responsibilities, and confidence in themselves. There was limited interference from married spouses or biological parents unless they broke cultural norms by "stealing married women or men." The later was a serious cultural taboo and violation. This phase led to spouse selection and to the next phase of getting married, which all young boys and girls desired and adult villagers expected.[30]

Becoming a Man or Woman Phase The phase of becoming a man or woman referred to the person who was married and had a child. Gadsup could not be called a man or woman unless they were married and had an offspring. Great pride and excitement were evident in both villages as young boys and girls decided on their marriage partners. For the boys, it meant achieving new status in the village as a man. Becoming a man meant having certain rights, responsibilities, privileges, and cultural acceptance as an adult. For the young girl, it meant she achieved new rights and responsibilities as a wife and mother. For both boys and girls, it legitimized their full adult status as Gadsup. Girls knew it meant that when they got married, they would be leaving their village to live in their husband's village (called neolocal residence). Married women lost much of the earlier protection, surveillance, and nurturant support of their mothers and maternal kinsfolk. It was, therefore, common to see young girls and later brides cry before and during the wedding ceremony as they would lose their close kin ties in the village. As the boy became a spouse, he was very happy and especially at the marriage ceremony because he no longer needed to search for a wife. Courting periods were often long to find a "good" wife, and especially because of a shortage of girls in both villages. The marriage ceremony

symbolized uniting people from different villages as the bride usually came from another village than the groom's. There was also an exchange of foods and bride price goods. Divorce was rare in both villages but by 1993 divorce was becoming more common with women wanting to divorce their spouse more often than the men. Wife abuse incidents were reported to me in 1993. Most men had only one wife, but some had two or more.[31] In the second village, I found one man who had eight wives, and he said "he kept all rather happy." However, I heard many stories of violent fights among the wives for the one husband.

Becoming Recognized as a Gadsup Adult The last phase of becoming recognized as a Gadsup man or woman meant that the married couple were now married and would soon have offspring to legitimize their status. The couple knew they were to serve as "true and good Gadsup" embodying Gadsup ideals and values. They were to reflect the right ways of living and respect adults and their ancestors who served as their moral and ethical guides to proper living. The married couple regulated their behaviors to get and retain cultural approval, recognition, and sanctions by the villagers and extended lineages. Gadsup who behaved properly were often chosen for special village roles. Some males were chosen as village orators, leaders, and "big men." Women were recognized and respected as "good women" because they had healthy children, pigs, and good gardens. This life cycle of becoming a man or woman was only fully recognized and sanctioned by the villagers when the couple had a child. If they did not have a child, they were not called "man" or "woman" and did not have full rights and privileges. The first child was, therefore, a joyous occasion and legitimized full adult social and cultural status as Gadsup. It was a life-cycle phase greatly desired by young adults, especially prior to 1990.

Old Age Phase The elders were viewed as people with knowledge of the past and today. They are respected and honored for their past roles. The older women stop working when they no longer have "strong muscles." They did not go to the gardens but stayed in the village plaza and took care of children and pigs. The older men no longer hunted in the forest as they were no longer "strong muscle men." They remained in the village and protected the villagers from strangers while guarding grandchildren from cassowaries that might come into the village to harm children. The men live to about 75 to 78 years and women to 83 to 86 years. Most of the aged died "naturally" in their sleep, but some from pneumonia (called "hard to breathe") and a few from malaria (due to "hot fever"). I saw or heard of no heart attacks. A few elderly had emphysema. All aged over 70 years became very thin and had a malnourished appearance. Death was feared only if they offended their ancestors and villagers. The Gadsup do not resent caring for their aged.[32] In 1999 a few AIDS and HIV conditions were reported in the Highlands. The people viewed these conditions as caused by sorcery and were very afraid of them. Outsiders were viewed as introducing and causing the AIDS condition.[33]

 ## Culture Care Findings and Uses

The above life-cycle data generated and analyzed by the use of the theory and the ethnonursing research methods has many culture care implications. From the author's theory of Culture Care, it was predicted that cultural patterns, expressions, structural froms, and meanings would be discovered by studying these data from the Sunrise Model, looking for differences and similarities.

Dominant Care Constructs and Meanings

Many new insights and specific findings were forthcoming from the author's study of the two villages. The following *dominant care meanings and daily action patterns* were documented and remain valued by the Gadsup over several decades:[34]

1. *Care meant nurturance*, which referred to the ability to help people grow, live, and survive throughout the life cycle.
2. *Care meant surveillance*, which referred to watching others attentively, but especially those who were vulnerable to preserve their well-being and health and to prevent accidents, disabilities, or untimely death.
3. *Care meant protection*, which referred to different ways to guard against outside harmful people or acts or thoughts by others, and especially to maintain cultural taboos and avoid sorcery.
4. *Care meant prevention of illness or harm to others*, which referred to being attentive to culturally prescribed norms, taboos, and values and by living the right way to remain healthy or well as known by ancestors and elders in the village.
5. *Care meant touching*, which referred to the importance of using one's hands or body on another Gadsup to heal and console or to help others become well, healed, or secure.

These major care constructs were recurrent and dominant findings in both Gadsup villages. They were recurrently observed and confirmed by the people in their emic language and general lifeways. Besides the above definition of Gadsup care, there were many additional findings that came from key and general informants about each care construct and about their lifeways, which will be briefly highlighted next.

Care as Nurturance   *Care as nurturance* was known to the Gadsup as the way the people helped others to grow and to be strong and well. By being attentive to the total needs of children, adolescents, and the elderly, care as nurturance was valued, especially to help infants and children grow and survive. Gadsup women had the major responsibility to provide nurturance by periodically providing for the child's growth and eating patterns, and helping the young to become healthy Gadsup adults through the life cycle. Nurturant expressions and patterns were observed as the Gadsup gave fresh garden food to the child each day, told children not to break cultural taboos, encouraged children to handle new roles or difficult tasks, and followed moral codes of what the ancestors had lived by to be healthy and "good" Gadsup. Gadsup women took active steps to monitor the nurtuant status of infants and children as they ate, played, and slept and in other daily activities. The women often talked about what was needed to keep children and adults healthy throughout the life cycle and of ways to have strong and healthy Gadsup. Women displayed more nurturant acts than men. These nurturant acts and patterns of living would need to be *preserved* and *maintained* as critical to care for the Gadsup so they could grow and remain well and healthy.

Care as Surveillance and Protection   The *second and third* dominant Gadsup care *constructs of surveillance and protection* were closely related concepts.

Surveillance as care meant actively watching over those who might be vulnerable to external harm, that is, harm from outsiders such as sorcerers, strangers, bad food, environmental conditions, and bad influences. Surveillance was closely linked with protective care. The Gadsup believe that if you gave good surveillance to Gadsup "brothers or sisters," you would be protecting them and ensuring their well-being, safety, and health. The Gadsup adult men and women stressed surveillance and protection of young children and the necessity of protecting them from harm such as poisonous snakes, sorcerers, and many potential physical accidents or natural disasters. External sociocultural factors were of more concern to Gadsups than internal mental, physical, or emotional factors because cultural forces were powerful and active forces that if neglected could lead to serious illnesses and even death. The Gadsup watched where their children went and warned them of dangers if they strayed too far from the village. Such surveillance was important as children are believed to be highly vulnerable to external malevolent forces that can lead to illness and death, especially from sorcery or by witchcraft practices. Surveillance as caring also meant being a good parent and protecting children, the lineage, or clan. Older women who did not go to the garden each day were often providers of surveillant care for the young and others needing protective care. Protecting children from cassowaries that came into the village was important as these animals could claw a child to death. Children needed to be protected from deadly snakes that could kill children (and adults) in a few minutes. Unquestionably, the care value of surveillance was very important, and thus nurses would need to preserve and maintain these protective and surveillant activities to care for Gadsup.[35] A non-caring nurse in these areas could lead Gadsup to sickness and death. Care as nurturance and protection were very closely related to surveillance, but separate constructs. Protective care measures were needed to be maintained and preserved as an action mode of the nurse. The construct of protective care as a major ideal became evident with this culture and had not been identified in nursing.

Preventive Care   The *fourth dominant care construct was prevention of illnesses with counseling.* Preventive behaviors as a caring modality were observed in many daily-life activities and from the cultural history of the people over time. Gadsup depended on ways to prevent sociocultural illnesses and harm from within or outside the village. They practiced *preventive care* by giving specific advice to adults and children to prevent sorcery, which causes illness. Adults warned children not to break Gadsup cultural taboos. They taught them to prevent illnesses by properly handling fecal materials, nail and hair clippings, and other human products to prevent sorcerers or sorceresses from doing harm to individuals or the whole village. Gadsup women in both villages talked about ancestral spirits and the need not to displease their ancestors by breaking cultural rules or showing disrespect to them. If a child or adolescent was too aggressive, ancestral admonitions were recited to prevent deviant behaviors. Counseling at different times helped to modify any deviant person's behavior and ultimately to contribute to his or her well-being. Hence, prevention, like surveillance and protection as caring modalities and values, prevented illness and promoted well-being and health. Preventive measures would need to be *maintained* and *preserved* with Gadsup. In addition, the nurse needs to consider ways to do *culture care repatterning or restructuring* with deviant behaviors or sorcery accusations for the health and well-being of the villagers by altering distructive patterns.

Care as Touching to Heal   The *fifth care value of touching* was important but only in different contexts and occasions throughout the life cycle. Touching was very important during infancy and young adulthood. Mothers touched children's genitalia and kissed infants and children. Bare skin maternal touching was used with infants and children when they got real upset or angry. Both maternal and paternal kinspersons would firmly hold or shake a child by the arm if the child acted badly. Male Gadsup were not to show affection or touch women in public, but only in private. Touching with body hugs among Gadsup kin was frequently observed, but touching strangers was avoided or done cautiously. If one touched a stranger, it was done to discover if one liked them or could trust them. A few adult Gadsup's sorcery fights were violent and led to fractured limbs, cuts, and bruises for both sexes. Domestic quarrels were usually related to major conflicts about women's infidelity, stealing garden foods and pigs, and harming children unduly. Bodily touching and hitting of an aggressive nature was observed and reported with domestic night fights. Nonviolent body "brother hugs" among men (and seldom among women) were observed in political greetings.

■ Major Cultural Gadsup Values

Nurses working with the Gadsup would need to consider the above Gadsup care concepts to provide culturally congruent care. In addition, the following general cultural values would need to be understood to provide culturally congruent care practices. The major Gadsup cultural values identified by the researcher and confirmed by the villagers were as follows:[36]

1. *Respecting sex role differences*
2. *Acknowledging strong kinship ties among extended family and lineage members*
3. *Valuing the concept of "brotherhood" and egalitarianism*
4. *Valuing land, women, children, and pigs*
5. *Giving birth to healthy children and keeping children well.*

To implement these values, the nurse would first need to be cognizant of *marked differences in sex roles and functions* of men and women. All Gadsup activities were sex-linked and reinforced by the people's political, religious, kinship, and cultural values. For example, if the nurse were a strong feminist and wanted to promote equal sex rights, she or he would encounter serious cultural conflicts and stresses with the Gadsup. Such ideas and practices would be culturally incongruent and lead to serious village problems. If a Western nurse attempted to change women's roles in infant and child care practices, this could seriously jeopardize Gadsup women's lifeways. Maintaining sex role differences as women and men is expected for respective functional roles. A Western nurse might also be tempted to make Gadsup women more politically active in the village and in ceremonial activities. This would be questioned and resisted as several are already politically active in their home in domestic areas. There are beneficial complementary outcomes with both sexes in performance of their male and female political and power roles. *Women have domestic political power*, whereas *men* have more *direct and overt*

public power to influence decisions and actions. The researcher documented several times how the women's domestic power was frequently respected and expected by men in public decisions and was effective.

If a Western female nurse were functioning with the Gadsup, she would need to realize that she might be viewed as a sorceress. Knowing how to respond to such beliefs or comments would be important. One might not convince the people that she was not a sorceress, but it is more important to observe cultural taboos in the village and larger community for nurse's protective care.

Another dominant cultural value is to *acknowledge strong clans, subclans, and tribes*. Kinship ties designate the expected relationship among and between groups inside and outside the village and determine who are the "real" Gadsup and the fictive kinspeople. They influence who cares for whom throughout the life cycle. For example, Gadsup females provide much of the *nurturant* and *surveillance care* to infants and adults. In contrast, the male kin provide outside *protective care* to the villagers, children, and vulnerable elderly. Gadsup men are also the external curing specialists, whereas females are domestic family carers. Gadsup women such as the mother's and father's sisters and their female kin are important lay midwives to provide prenatal, natal, and postnatal care to mothers and newborn infants. These lay midwives were competent in birth deliveries using care as surveillance and nurturance. Outsiders who are not viewed as "Gadsup brothers" with its linkage to clans, subclans, and lineages need to be understood to provide beneficial and acceptable generic and professional care.

The cultural value of *respecting Gadsup land, women, children, and pigs* is very important. Caring for land, women, children and pigs has been valued throughout their life cycle and long history. Land and women have been fought for in past feuds and wars. Gadsup want and love their children and lands as they perpetuate their culture. One woman said, "Without healthy children and our land, no people would exist in the future." Women took great pride in having healthy children, and they admonished women who had ill or weak children. Children represented the future life and preservation of the Gadsup. Some domestic fights occurred over pigs, land, and women while the researcher lived in the villages, but were usually resolved by political discussions in the local village.

Another dominant cultural value was that the Gadsup *treat each other as "brothers" who are equal in social and cultural relationships*. The Gadsup frequently state they are "brothers," which reaffirms their bonds of unity and solidarity. The concept of "brother" generates feelings of warmth, respect, belonging, nurturance, and caring among Gadsup.[37] It is a highly desired and a favorable idea to treat others as a "brother" and to include even "safe" strangers in supportive and helpful relationships. While in the Gadsup culture, I discovered patterns of care and cure with outside carers and curers. Male curers often came from *non-Gadsup* villages to cure acutely ill villagers. These outside curers had an ethical responsibility to assist other Gadsup tribal brothers. In return, the curers usually received gifts of food, material goods, or reciprocal services. The village *female carers* were responsible for assisting others by listening, counseling, or providing direct caring services to those who were well or sick. Adult female carers were highly effective in ways to help men, women, and children avoid illnesses, recover from their cultural sicknesses, and maintain patterns of wellness. The Gadsup female carers were expected to perform these roles to please their ancestral spirits and to perpetuate "good Gadsups" over time. Maintaining cultural taboos and values were a powerful means to keep Gadsup well and to perform their expected daily role activities. The ethical norm to prevent killing Gadsup villagers was viewed as another means to prevent ancestor revenge. The caring sensitivity of female carers was noteworthy, as well as the skills of outside Gadsup curers.

▇ Using the Three Care Modes

To provide *culturally congruent care, cultural care maintenance and preservation* is highly essential to preserve their generic care patterns of surveillance, nurturance, prevention of illnesses, and other positive and beneficial caring modalities for Gadsup health and well-being. Caring practices that maintained cultural taboos would be essential for Gadsup well-being. The nurse might cautiously use *culture care accommodation* to change care practices that would improve their well-being such as new medications and selected professional treatments for illnesses or to clean wounds and prevent infections. The author found that some of

their folk practices for treating open wounds were not effective and could be improved by culture care *accommodation or negotiation strategies*. Culture care *repatterning and restructuring* would be limitedly considered unless the people wanted to change some practices that were dysfunctional or causing village deaths as AIDs, HIV infections, or specific childhood and elder illnesses. Prevention of AIDs would require that the nurse understand sorcery practices, social structure factors, and specific cultural values before repatterning or restructuring anything. Social structure factors were very closely linked to health, illness, and beliefs. With recent contacts since the 1990s with Western health personnel, the Gadsup traditional folk system was being threatened, and the quality of care was less positive than in 1960s, 1970s, and 1980s. AIDs and other new illnesses were thought to be linked to Western sorcerers who killed people with their illnesses.

Still another consideration in caring for the Gadsup people *would be to blend generic (emic) folk care rituals with professional (etic) practices where acceptable to the people*. Gadsup ritual behaviors such as the festival for the birth of a new baby were especially beneficial and satisfying to the Gadsup with many positive health benefits. The symbolic food rituals for helping the infant grow were essential to protect and nurture the infant through kinship support. The cultural ritual of putting small amounts of white ashes on the head of newborn infants to protect them from evil spirits could be maintained with professional counseling and body hygiene. Pregnant mothers had cultural taboo rituals such as not leaving the home village unless accompanied by other women. The men had many protective care rituals that protected the villagers. *Community caring cultural rituals were important to the people* to ensure and provide a healthy environment for children, young adults, and the aged.

Finally, to provide culturally congruent care to the Gadsup, professional nurses and other health providers would need to know how to *use the local native foods* and understand their value in health maintenance practices. The majority of the Gadsup in both villages were quite healthy except for intestinal parasites and occasionally malaria. Gadsup native foods were different in taste from many Western foods such as their greens, sweet potatoes, bananas, passion fruit, taro, and seasonal nuts. The Gadsup have lived for hundreds of years on these native nutritious foods with many grown in their local gardens and forests. There were no canned foods, no butter, and no table salt. There was also very little meat except for occasional wild game and park. With no nearby lakes or large rivers, fish was not available. One may wonder how these people survive without meat and fish in their diet, but they have and were quite healthy on vegetables, fruits, and nuts. There were no signs of hypertension, obesity, diabetes, cardiovascular disease, or psychoses in the early 1960s, but today evidence of AIDs and HIV cases is threatening the Gadsups and many other areas in the Eastern Highlands.[38]

Another interesting discovery was the absence of animal milk or any milk products except for infants taking breast milk for 12 to 20 months. Gadsup never expressed a desire for milk. I later discovered the Gadsup had lactose intolerance, which was a rather new discovery in the early 1960s. All food practices were closely linked with many cultural ceremonies and rituals, which would require *culture care accommodation and maintenance* practices by the nurse. Eating cultural foods with the people helped to reinforce a trusting relationship with strangers and to gain new insights about their foods and their lifeways. Professional nursing and medical services have limitedly reached the two villages, and so generic care and treatment are major health services. The ethnoscience method was also valuable so identify carers and healers to maintain health and was the first used and modified for nursing.[39]

◼ Summary Comments

In this chapter ethnonursing and ethnographic data were presented from my research study as an in-depth, lived experience with the Gadsup of the Eastern Highlands of New Guinea beginning in the 1960s with follow-up visits and observations in 1978, 1987, and 1992. The focus of this chapter was primarily on the life cycle of the Gadsup in two villages. It was the first transcultural nursing study using the evolving Culture Care Theory as an anthropologist and ethnonurse researcher. Unquestionably, it was one of my richest learning and discovering life experiences, especially of a non-Western culture.

I learned much from the Gadsup as they became my teachers and friends over the past four decades. I discovered how different the non-Western world was from the Western world and the importance to become fully immersed with the people in their culture and natural environment. Observing, listening, and learning directly from the people about their cultural daily and nightly lifeways for nearly 2 years was invaluable to substantiate my findings. I observed many details in their lifeways and lifestyle, and especially their "cultural secrets" after I became their trusted friend. They helped to confirm or refute my observations, interpretations, or findings in ongoing ways. Although I was warned initially by outsiders that these Gadsup were "dangerous headhunters," I discovered that this was not true. Instead, they took actions to protect me at time and to defend their culture from persons who failed to know their concerns. I became increasingly sensitive to what could be shared and what were cultural taboos within each village. It was, indeed, a special privilege and opportunity to live with them and to become ultimately their "true and trusted friend."

My theory of Culture Care Diversity and Universality was a well substantiated and valuable guide to obtain a wealth of in-depth, descriptive, covert, and often embedded knowledge of the people. It was also evident that the theory and the Ethnonursing Enablers were essential and would need to be used in future studies of cultures. The ethnonursing research method of focusing on data within the nursing perspective contrasted sharply with the ethnography method in many areas with different outcomes. This study confirmed for me that the ethnographic method is *not* needed for nursing students as ethnonursing is targeted research. Both the theory and the ethnonursing method were major breakthroughs in nursing and in transcultural nursing with contributions also to anthropology. Since this was the first transcultural ethnonursing qualitative and life-cycle research study in nursing, as well as a longitudinal study, it was valuable to bring entirely new findings to nursing. Culture variability existed in the two villages, but there were Gadsup commonalities (universals) that were shared in both villages. This comparative study was informative and revealing to contrast lifeways within and between cultures in life-cycle practices. For it is the cultural lifeways with the focus on birth to death that is extremely important for nurses to study in the prevention, healing, and helping processes.

References

1. Leininger, M., *Transcultural Nursing: Concepts, Theories, Research, and Practices*, Columbus, OH: McGraw-Hill College Custom Series, 1978 (reprinted Columbus, OH: Greyden Press).
2. Leininger, M., *Transcultural Nursing: Concepts, Theories, Research, and Practice*, 2nd. ed., Columbus, OH: McGraw-Hill College Custom Series, 1995.
3. Andrews, M. and J. Boyle, *Transcultural Concepts in Nursing Care*, 3rd ed., Philadelphia, PA: J. B. Lippincott, 1999.
4. Leininger, M., *Nursing and Anthropology: Two Worlds to Blend*, New York, NY: John Wiley & Sons, 1970.
5. Leininger, M., "Gadsup of New Guinea: Child Rearing, Ethnocare, Ethnohealth, and Ethnonursing," in *Transcultural Nursing: Concepts, Theories, Research*, and *Practice*, 2nd ed., M. Leininger, ed., Columbus, OH: McGraw-Hill College Custom Series, 1995, pp. 559–589.
6. Leininger, op. cit., 1978, pp. 375–399.
7. Leininger, M., "Ecological Behavior Variability: Cognitive Images and Sociocultural Expressions in Two Gadsup Villages," unpublished doctoral dissertation, Seattle, University of Washington, 1996.
8. Leininger, M., *Cultural Care Diversity and Universality: A Theory of Nursing*, New York, NY: NLN Press. Distributed by Jones and Bartlett Publishers, 1991, pp. 5–73.
9. Ibid., pp. 82–83.
10. Leininger, op. cit., 1995, pp. 559–589.
11. Leininger, M., "Gadsup of New Guinea: Early Child-Caring Behaviors with Nursing Care Implications," in *Transcultural Nursing: Concepts, Theories, Research, and Practices*, M. Leininger, ed., Columbus, OH: McGraw-Hill College Custom Series, 1978, pp. 375–399 (reprinted Columbus, OH: Greyden Press).
12. Leininger, op. cit., 1995, pp. 559–589.
13. Leininger, op. cit., 1978.
14. Ibid.
15. Leininger, op. cit., 1994, pp. 559–589.
16. Leininger, M., "Gadsup of New Guinea Revisited: A Three Decade View," *Journal of Transcultural Nursing*, v. 5, no. 1, 1993, pp. 21–29.
17. Leininger, op. cit., 1978.
18. Ibid.
19. Leininger, op. cit., 1995.
20. Leininger, op. cit., 1978, pp. 375–399.
21. Ibid.
22. Leininger, M., "Culture Care of the Gadsup Akuna of the Eastern Highlands of New Guinea," in *Cultural Care Diversity and Universality: A Theory of Nursing*, M. Leininger, ed., New York, NY: NLN Press. Distributed by Jones and Bartlett Publishers, 1991, pp. 231–280, 358.
23. Ibid.
24. Leininger, M., "Some Cross-Cultural Universal and Non-Universal Function, Beliefs, and Practices of Food Dimensions of Nutrition," *Proceedings of the Colorado Dietetic Association Conference*, J. Dupont, ed., Fort Collins, CO: Colorado Associate Universities Press, 1970, pp. 153–179.
25. Leininger, op. cit., 1991, pp. 231–280.
26. Ibid.
27. Ibid.
28. Leininger, op. cit., 1978, pp. 559–589.
29. Ibid.
30. Leininger, op. cit., 1991, pp. 231–280.
31. Leininger, op. cit., 1993, pp. 21–29.
32. Leininger, op. cit., 1995, pp. 559–581.
33. Personal letter of communication, John Orami, Gadsup native, Port Moresby, New Guinea, 2001.
34. Leininger, op. cit., 1991, p. 358.
35. Ibid., pp. 231–280.
36. Ibid., pp. 231–280, 358.
37. Ibid.
38. Orami, op. cit., 2000.
39. Leininger, M., "Ethnoscience: A New and Promising Research Approach for Health Sciences," *Image: Sigma Theta Tau Magazine*, v. 9, no. 1, 1969, pp. 2–8.

11

Transcultural Mental Health Nursing

Madeleine Leininger

Without the inclusion of explicit cultural and care-health research-based knowledge, mental health nursing will have limited meanings and beneficial therapy outcomes. LEININGER, 1995

As an early pioneer in psychiatric nursing and the author of one of the first comprehensive psychiatric nursing textbooks, *Basic Psychiatric Concepts in Nursing*, in 1960, it has been encouraging to see some changes in psychiatric mental health nursing.[1] However, some major changes are needed to incorporate cultural care dimensions of mental health to meet client's cultural expectations. The cultural needs became clearly apparent to me while trying to use Western Euro-American psychoanalytical and other general psychiatric concepts to care for disturbed children and adults of different cultures in the mid 1950s. It was these children with their cultural expressions and uninhibited comments or actions that told me there were differences among African, Jewish, German, Appalachian, and Anglo-American children that needed to be recognized. Transcultural differences among the children in daily caring experiences were extremely difficult to overlook or deny. As an experienced psychiatric nurse specialist interested to help people, this reality left me in culture shock and feeling helpless and concerned. My basic and advanced psychiatric nursing education had been inadequate and incomplete with the absence of cultural factors in therapy. Transcultural nursing theory, research, and practice were clearly missing until the advent of transcultural nursing. Still today, this need remains critical and must be addressed worldwide.

■ Discovery of the Need for Changes

The above culture-shock experience led me in the 1950s to study cultural and social anthropology. Anthropological concepts and research from diverse cultures were needed to help nurses understand and change psychiatric nursing knowledge, research, and practices. Following 5 years of doctoral study in anthropology and as the first nurse with graduate preparation in nursing to complete a Ph.D. program in cultural anthropology, I began in the 1960s to research and teach about different cultures with diverse beliefs and mental health and illness conditions. I became deeply concerned that clients in psychiatric hospitals or in private psychotherapy were often misdiagnosed, misunderstood, or not cared for appropriately as a result of Western ethnocentric psychiatric viewpoints and practices and the absence of cultural knowledge. Major differences in cultural care needs, expressions, and beliefs related to mental health and illness were of concern to me since most psychiatric nurses largely focused on diagnosis and symptoms of Freudian and neo-Freudian psychiatric conditions to be a competent clinical specialist or therapist in psychiatric nursing. It also became apparent that psychiatric nurses should no longer rely only on mind-body, genetics, or psychophysical aspects without inclusion of cultural factors. Psychiatric nurses and others needed to incorporate comparative culture care into psychiatric nursing in the mid 20th century and still today.[2,3]

Ethnocentric and narrow Western psychiatric perspectives of the APA nomenclature with prescribed treatment regimens were also inadequate for multicultural clients in the mid 20th century with the increased global migrations and immigrations of clients. Major cultural value conflicts and stresses with psychiatric clients along with problems related to misdiagnosis and mistreatment of cultural strangers were clearly evident in the mid-century. Indeed, the Western APA nomenclature with rigid diagnostic categories and treatment regimens was far too narrow and failed to accommodate many non-Western immigrants. These clients' "strange behaviors" noted in the mid 20th century are still largely misunderstood today. However, in the 1994 APA Diagnostic and Statistical Manual of Mental Disorders, a supplement has been added attempting to deal with some cultural factors.[4] There remains, however, an urgent need for mental health diagnosticians and therapists to study in a systematic, qualitative, and quantitative way the diverse expressions and caring modalities of people from diverse Western and non-Western cultures for accurate assessments and therapies. Most assuredly, mental health and other clinicians need to become aware of the importance of culture in defining, influencing, and shaping mental health and illness conditions. As our world becomes intensely multicultural, one can predict more signs of cultural clashes, misunderstanding, violence, and stresses between client and therapist and where cultural, developmental, and current lifeways play a significant role in these "mental" conditions.[5]

From my ethnostudies of fifteen cultures over 40 years in Western and non-Western societies, many mental health concerns and issues have become evident such as the following:[6-9]

1. Mental pathologies in the Western world do not universally exist in non-Western cultures.
2. Western diagnostic categories, symptoms, and treatment outcomes are difficult to use or fit in a number of cultures, but Western therapists or assessors often try to impose these categories as Western phenomena.
3. Some cultures do not explain, define, and know mental illnesses as identified by Western psychiatric staff as their culture cognitions, explanations, and epistemic knowing.

4. What is "normal or abnormal" is usually very difficult to define in dualistic terms because of cultural influences and variabilities.
5. Many cultures do not use psychological language terms to explain cultural phenomena.
6. Culture-bound conditions exist with cultures, and their functions may have nonpsychological and nonbiological terms to describe and explain them.
7. The Western dualistic mind-body focus is often most difficult to use in non-Western cultures and subcultures that rely on holistic data.
8. Most cultures have generic (folk or indigenous) ways to help their people with emotional concerns or conditions when they become evident.
9. Indigenous cultural care modalities for therapeutic healing outcomes are generally the least known and understood by mental health practitioners and especially by nurses and physicians.
10. In-depth study of cultures from a holistic social structure, worldview, gender, class, language use and in environmental cultural context are essential to grasp accurate expressions of mental illness, health or another human conditions and to develop effective therapies.

Nurses prepared through graduate study in transcultural nursing with courses in anthropology need to study further the issues identified above and develop appropriate knowledge and competencies in the new area of *transcultural mental health*. Traditionally oriented psychiatric nurses should join transcultural nurse specialists to study holistic culture care within the broad and yet particularistic areas of culturally based therapies. Mental health can best be understood as the learned *totality of the human cultural lifeways* and not as a separate mental phenomenon. Transcultural mental health care needs to also be understood within naturalistic and familiar cultural contexts of living and dying. Indeed, most cultures dislike compartmentalization of their mind from their holistic ways of knowing and living. These ideas and others challenge traditionally oriented psychiatric nurses to shift to a transcultural nursing perspective along with other psychiatric professionals.

Today, the most critical issue is to help psychiatric nurses shift from a Western and largely unicultural perspective to a transcultural broad and comparative viewpoint to serve many people of diverse and similar cultures. A broad and yet specific cultural care approach related to the human condition in different cultural contexts based on in-depth transcultural knowledge of Western and non-Western cultures must be instituted in the immediate future to deal with societal and worldwide problems related to lifespan, violence, homicide, suicide, hostilities, abuses, and to many other major concerns found in diverse societies. Nurses prepared in transcultural nursing and anthropology are in a unique position to deal with these global concerns.

Questions for Reflection to Develop and Advance Transcultural Mental Health Nursing

In shifting to a transcultural mental health nursing perspective, the following questions are important to consider:

1. What are the universal (or common) and diverse mental stresses, conflicts, and behaviors that reoccur in different cultural contexts?
2. What are the expressions and meanings of clients' interpretations of these stresses or conflicts and the ways clients believe these concerns could be reduced or altered?
3. What are the emic (insider's) knowledge and the etic (outsider's) interpretations of specific cultural conditions, clashes, or conflicts that lead to mental illness?
4. What factors lead to mental illness or to well-being in specific cultures such as the Turks, Arabs, Mexicans, Italians, Russians, Czechs, and in many non-Western cultures?
5. What beliefs, explanations, and interpretations are offered in diverse cultures about mental health, illness, treatment, and culture care?
6. What similarities and differences exist between Western and non-Western cultures related to mental health that could provide guidelines and principles for transcultural mental health nursing?
7. What generic folk care practices need to be incorporated into transcultural mental health nursing practices, and how do these practices differ from traditional or current professional psychiatric practices or therapies?
8. Can and should generic and professional mental health nursing practices be used effectively with clients?
9. What problems exist with the present-day use of nursing diagnoses (NANDA or others) to identify, understand, and accurately care for clients from diverse cultures?
10. Why do some cultures or subcultures resist or never use psychiatric care?
11. What culture-specific mental illnesses exist in specific cultures?
12. What are the potential benefits of culture-specific mental health nursing?
13. What factors limit mental health care to clients of diverse cultures and why?

These questions can lead the nurse to a wealth of new discoveries related to transcultural care practices. The theory of Culture Care Diversity and Universality with the Sunrise Model can serve as a valuable guide to discover holistic and comparative transcultural mental health knowledge and ways to provide care practices that are culturally congruent and beneficial.[10] Research studies focused on the meaning of mental health and illness in different cultures are very important to provide mental health therapy goals. Psychiatric nurses with traditional professional education will need to reexamine their own personal and professional cultural myths, biases, and practices in light of extant transcultural nursing concepts, principles, and research findings about diverse cultures. The use of emic and etic interpretations and experiences offers many stimulating challenges and rewards for nurses who use the theory of Culture Care Diversity and Universality. Let us look next at some fundamental principles in transcultural mental health nursing for further reflection and consideration.

Fundamental Principles for Transcultural Mental Health Nursing

Currently, transcultural mental health nurses can draw on the body of transcultural nursing knowledge to guide them in their teaching, research, and practice.[11,12] A comparative focus on mental health differences and similarities among cultures helps the nurse to think anew about ideas and practices of transcultural nursing concepts such as cultural imposition, cultural blindness, cultural conflicts, cultural values, cultural beliefs, and cultural lifeways to provide information to understand clients and develop meaningful transcultural mental health nursing practices. There is a growing body of transcultural research knowledge from diverse cultures that can be used or considered in developing and transforming traditional mental health practices.[13] Such knowledge can also be found in many chapters in this book and in other reference sources.

The first transcultural nursing principle is to understand and respect cultural differences and care for clients from any culture as human beings. To understand the "why" of beliefs and actions helps the nurse to know why many differences exist transculturally. The nurse needs to recognize that differences have meanings that can generally be discovered from clients and from transcultural nursing and anthropological knowledge. Understanding cultural differences means the nurse is aware of using ideas appropriate to ideas with specific cultures. Recognizing cultural variabilities and similarities of "mental" expressions is difficult and complex without some cultural holding knowledge to reflect on in an assessment or therapy session. Interactional data may be helpful, but may be of limited assistance to understand specific cultural values, beliefs, and practices.

The second important principle is that the nurse should endeavor to understand her (his) own culture values, beliefs, and lifeways to make accurate client assessments and interpretations. Without awareness of the nurse's own culture, misinterpretations and inaccurate decisions and actions can readily occur, which often leads to unfavorable consequences. Cultural informants are generally sensitive to how their beliefs and actions are interpreted and of professional biases, prejudices, and disbeliefs of the clients' views. It is often difficult for clients to convince health personnel to regard their beliefs as "normal" and accurate from their perspective, as well as to understand what is "abnormal" or distorted in their culture. Nonetheless, the transcultural mental health nurse needs to make sense out of diverse behaviors and reflect on cultural norms and rules of the client's culture, as well as the therapist's cultural interpretations. Misinterpretation of cultural background factors can lead to cultural destructiveness and to many unfavorable outcomes. Most importantly, the nurse must understand her (his) cultural values and behaviors to make accurate assessments and to work effectively with clients.

The third principle is to identify and work with a transcultural nurse mentor to help the nurse practitioner or specialist to become effective in therapy. Transcultural nurse mentors can be of great assistance to help novice nurses reflect on their own cultural attitudes and practices to consider the context of behavior and what may be relevant to help the client or family. Learning about nonverbal and verbal cues from clients is essential to understand and accurately interpret what clients say or do *within their cultural frame of reference and context.* Making mental health nursing practices meaningful within the client's cultural context from the initial contact until the end of the relationship is essential and depends on the nurse's knowledge of the culture and the use of mentor's insights. Rigid professional attitudes, policies, or the lack of accommodation to meet the client's cultural needs can lead to disturbing, violent, and uncooperative behavior. The three modes from the Culture Care theory are excellent guides in transcultural nursing therapies, namely, 1) culture care preservation or maintenance, 2) culture care accommodation or negotiation, and 3) culture care repatterning or restructuring. They are also meaningful therapeutic guides for nursing action and interaction in the care of the mentally ill client and his (her) family.[14]

The fourth transcultural nursing principle is to learn about the client's cultural lifeways, multiple social structure factors, worldview, and environmental context as influencers of mental health behaviors. Understanding the cultural context of the mentally ill means grasping the totality of the client's environment and situation. What makes the client upset or ill is usually context specific and often a violation of cultural taboos. The nurse considers *high cultural context* in which the clients give a lot of verbal explanations and use many words and symbols to convey their ideas. In contrast, a client from a *low cultural context* will have very limited verbal comments, but will expect the nurse to quickly understand them without using a lot of verbal explanations. Usually, clients of low cultural context reflect more traditional values, beliefs, and explanations that are readily known to people in the community but less to high-context therapists. Knowledge and assessment of high and low cultural contexts have enabled nurses to discover other ways of communicating and assessing client's cultural behaviors.

The fifth principle is to allow time and to be patient as one works with clients whose language and behavior are different in beliefs, values, and lifeways. Adjusting to a client's language may be stressful and difficult for the nurse as it requires alertness, sensitivity, a conscious centering on the client's culture, and responding appropriately to verbal and nonverbal communication modes. Periodic assessment of the client alerts the nurse to changes in the client's behavior and often needs. To use the client's cultural data in thoughtful and appropriate ways necessitates active listening, patience, reflective thinking, and being aware of the cultural situation while being responsive to the client's modes of communicating and acting.

Sixth, the nurse learns about the different cultural-bound illness and wellness states of cultures and subcultures and responds to these conditions in a sensitive, knowing, and appropriate way. Since the Western *APA Diagnostic and Statistical Manual* may not include and explain culture-bound illnesses, syndromes, or conditions such as running amok, susto, evil eye, intentional death, spiritualism, stoicism, and other cultural specifics,[15,16] the nurse needs to study these non-Western and other culture-bound conditions. Cultures also tend to have different thresholds and times for expressing particular deviant behaviors, which they may not consider to be pathological, psychotic, or even neurotic. Hallucinations and delusions are often not expressed in the same transcultural manner as other cultures. Most importantly, it is often the cultural context, situation, or event that influences or determines whether cultural behaviors are viewed as "normal" or "deviant." Some cultures tend to accept specific and unusual behaviors more readily than others and without fear or concern. Transcultural mental health nurses need to be open and recognize such diverse cultural expressions as normal or abnormal in a culture.

Cultural variability exists, which may make the nurse uncomfortable when clients change their behaviors in varying ways in different contexts and with different people because of cultural status expectations. Some Western psychopathological conditions may not exist in some cultures or may be expressed differently in non-Western cultures.[17] Assertive, aggressive, and some forms of violent behavior are often viewed quite differently in cultures as "normal," adaptive, and desired behaviors for survival or to fulfill social and cultural obligations. For example, counter-revenge feuds and "game-like" aggressive actions may be an integral part of a New Guinea (Melansian) cultural lifeways and not viewed as illness. Major discrepancies and variations with diagnosis and symptoms of clients of non-Western cultures can be baffling to mental health nurses unless knowledgeable in transcultural nursing. Thus, discrepancies in the treatment, prognosis, and care of clients may greatly vary in diverse cultures. Making symptoms and signs of Western categories fit non-Western cultures or nomenclatures often leads to inaccurate and nontherapeutic therapy and care practices.

It is also important for the mental health nurse to know that psychological and medical anthropology are branches of anthropology. Researchers in these fields have been studying mental illnesses and diseases in different cultures for many decades and often focus on what constitutes "normality" and "abnormality" of different cultures, such as Marsella's research on depression.[18,19] Anthropologists focus in-depth on social structure factors such as politics, religion, and cultural beliefs to assess the impact of these factors on the client. They study the functions of the healers and curers in different cultures in treating cultural conditions.[20] Psychological anthropologists remain interested in the effect of forced and general migrations of refugees, of urbanization, and of cultural environmental and ecological changes on clients. The impact of medicalization and high technologies on people of different cultures has been of interest to transcultural mental health nurses for several decades, which needs to be considered with other ideas related to biochemical, physiological, and genetic (DNA) factors. Specific life-cycle illnesses and cultural coping strategies with cultural adaptations to life experiences and the prevention of mental stresses need far more emphasis.

Currently, several psychiatrists tend to be holding to the stance that mental diseases are genetic or caused by biochemical factors. The search for chemical, DNA factors, and brain dysfunctions have been found with ADHD (attention deficient hyperactive disorder) and the use of Ritalin medication for hyperactivity for nearly 20 years. Unfortunately, cultural factors and the cultural contexts of ADHD have been limitedly investigated. Transcultural nurses usually seek culture-specific factors first, or factors often external to the mind-body focus, but must remain interested in physical and chemical discoveries. It is most important to remember that there is a close relationship of culture to mental illness that tends to define what is "normal" and "abnormal" and the way mental illnesses are recognized, explained, and treated by members of specific cultures. Transcultural nurses are expected to focus on this important premise with direct observation in different cultural contexts. At the same time, they also remain focused on human caring, environmental community living factors, and how people remain well or become ill from a holistic perspective.[21]

 ## Psychocultural Specific Mental Health Conditions

During the past several decades much has been written by transcultural nurses, anthropologists, psychologists and some psychiatrists about culture-specific expressions of mental illness and the relationship of culture to personality. The works of Helman,[22] Marsella et al., Ciborowski,[23] Peterson,[24] Peterson et al.,[25] Leininger,[26-28] Mead,[29] Glittenberg,[30] Barnauw,[31] Moore et al.,[32] Tripp-Reimers,[33] Kennedy,[34] Kavanagh,[35] and Zoucha[36] have all been important contributions to establish culturally based knowledge and research practices.

Psychiatric nurses have been generally slow to recognize and systemically study mental health and illness from a transcultural nursing perspective. The author contends this is largely because of the lack of preparation in anthropology and transcultural nursing and the close identification of psychiatric nurses with Western psychiatrists' work and therapies. Many psychiatric nurses remain absorbed in studying psychiatric medical diseases and psychoanalytical modes of therapy to institute independent or collaborative treatment practices with psychiatrists and other disciplines. Still today psychiatric nurse therapists tend to rely on psychoanalytical interpretations of data and established psychotherapy practices rather than transcultural nursing care theories and modes. Psychoanalytical, neo-Freudian, and other psychiatric schools of thought have greatly influenced psychiatric nursing education and services in the 20th century. The cultural dimensions, cultural therapies, and theories have been neglected except for work of a few transcultural nurses with anthropological and graduate transcultural nursing preparation.

The author's early study of the Gadsup of the Eastern Highlands of new Guinea in the 1960s documented the absence of schizophrenic and Western psychotic behavior in the two villages where she lived and studied for nearly 2 years.[37,38] The Gadsup had short-term, transient, depressive behavior that was usually related to the deeply felt loss of a loved kinsman, child, spouse, elder, or significant village leader. The absence of many Western illnesses was apparent and could be explained from ethnographic and ethnonursing research findings related to the cultural context and to culturally constituted values, beliefs, and therapies. A caring ethos and nurturant childcare by women with strong protective care by men among their kinsmen and lineages were other important prevention factors.[39] In addition, the rhythm of Gadsup daily life was quite regularized and predictable. This gave them security and confidence in knowing what to do and the rules of living to follow with clear expectation for action toward self and others in the community. Intertribal feuds and sorcery acquisitions existed, which were related to normative protective beliefs and explicit village rules of action for all Gadsups. They were not labeled as deviant and abnormal behaviors.

In recent years, the Gadsup have had increased contact with outsiders or strangers from other countries and cultures who are held as "invading and taking their land." The author found in her visit in 1992 signs of retaliation, unrest, violence, paranoid-like behaviors, and extended family anxieties, as well as signs of being confused. Group stresses were identified as the villagers related to these foreigners in their villages or nearby. One could identify growing paranoid-like and/or suspicious behavior, which the Gadsup rascals felt was justifiable because of outsiders encroaching on their lands, lifeways, and use of their natural resources. These outsiders "took" without giving anything in return to the Gadsup villagers. In fact, a young male group known as the "rascals" had launched an aggressive movement toward foreigners with violent acts to regain their indigenous rights, land, and money.[40] Rascal behavior could be viewed as understandable and necessary for protective care action and to retain the village's healthy lifeways (see Chapter 10 in this book for more on the Gadsup lifeways).

In the next section some culture-specific psychocultural expression and research related to mental health will be highlighted to help the reader understand the influence of culture on mental health or illness in different cultures. Many of these culture-specific findings come from the author's research and those of doctoral transcultural nursing students or faculty.

Culture-Specific Mental Conditions

Appalachians

Appalachians come from the rural mountains and hills of the eastern United States. Many are moving to urban areas to seek employment for survival. The complex and fast-moving large-city culture often makes Appalachians feel alone and depressed. They experience what they call the "blues," but usually do not become psychotic. They have a deep sense of being separated from their kinsmen and friends in the rural "hollows" of their homeland when in the city.[41] Appalachians often talk about the fear of urban crime and not leaving their homes at night unless absolutely necessary. Elderly Appalachians are especially afraid to go out at night in the urban environment. The Appalachians often talk about a "case of nerves" or of trying to understand how to cope with urban violence, stresses, and a different environment. The author's research revealed that many of the urban Appalachians were seen as "neglected and unknown white people" by health personnel. These Appalachians were experiencing great poverty and isolation in the large urban communities. They had limited financial resources, and many lived below the poverty level of $5000 per year in 1988. Appalachians said they were generally uncomfortable with Anglo-Americans and multicultural urban values, beliefs, and lifeways because they were so strange to them "and made them nervous." Their need for transcultural caring values consisted of the following: 1) keeping close ties with kin from their home hollows, 2) relying on their personal fiends and kin, 3) using folk remedies, and 4) protecting themselves from harmful strangers. These care needs were desired and important for Appalachians to maintain their mental health and survival in an urban context. Appalachians wanted transcultural nurses to understand their cultural values and lifeways and to remain active listeners to them. Hence, moving to large cities can make this culture "nervous," anxious, and "very uncomfortable" but not necessarily mentally ill.

African Americans

Psychological, psychiatric, and some anthropological literature on African Americans or "Blacks" show considerable mental health variability in research findings and interpretations. Nursing students and others are encouraged to read extensively on this subject because this short account is in no way complete enough to show variabilities among a large and growing African American culture. Moreover, controversial issues exist related to mental health and illness with African Americans. Hence, only a brief summary of a few dominant themes is given here.

In general, there is a great lack of in-depth understanding about African Americans (and those who are called "Black") because of cultural, biological, racial (phenotypes and genotypes), and diverse life experiences. The transcultural mental health nurse must study acculturation and ethnohistorical factors in-depth to grasp the general picture and the change in African Americans and their culture over time. One must go beyond hair, body size, and skin color differences and study the past and present cultural life experiences influencing African Americans living in different places over time. The Culture Care theory, with the Sunrise Model with the worldview and diverse social structure factors, is valuable to assess the mental health of African Americans. There are also differences between rural and urban African Americans who experience different kinds of mental stresses as they move from rural to urban environments often under stressful conditions and limited money.

Ronan and Bailey's studies show that the major mental health problems for urban African Americans are related to alcohol and drug abuse, which have led to street deaths, homicide, and major diseases such as hepatitis, liver cirrhosis, heart disease, cancer, and a host of other pathological conditions.[42,43] Some studies hold that the urban African American extended family no longer exists and family instability is evident. The lack of strong African American male and female sex role identification and survival skills is often related to crime in urban society. Today, many African American fathers and mothers are absent from their homes because of outside work for economic survival. This has undoubtedly had a major influence on maintaining their cultural values and helping children survive and cope with life in a persistent changing and different world. In the past, African American families provided food, shelter, clothing, counseling, and environmental support through extended family ties. With the absence of family stability and ties in urban homes, Bailey's study showed how this influenced the mental health and well-being of African Americans.[44]

The growing increase of human immunodeficiency virus (HIV) infection in many large African American urban communities is a serious threat to the people's mental and holistic health. Hypertension, stroke, and other pathological conditions have frequently been traced to cultural, social, economic, and political factors, which have had a deleterious impact on the general mental health and survival of African Americans in large urban contexts. As the transcultural mental health nurse remains knowledgeable about current sociocultural, political, economic, and other factors influencing African American lifeways, one focuses on specific cultural care values, beliefs, and lifestyle practices, as well as folk beliefs that may be related to witchcraft and voodoo practices and less to restore their health. One must understand hexes and voodoo practices in relation to mental illness and health. Voodoo teaches that illness or death can come to an individual or group through supernatural forces.[45] It may be referred to as root work, black magic, being hexed, fix, a spell, or witchcraft. The affected person may talk about being nauseated, vomiting, having diarrhea, or having muscle weakness or convulsions. "Falling out" may also be identified by African Americans as a sudden collapse, inability to talk, and sometimes paralysis. These culture-specific expressions often lead to misdiagnosis and inappropriate treatment and nursing care actions when behavior is not understood. Nurses can identify these kinds of cultural conditions influencing African American holistic health and well-being. Drawing on African folk (emic and etic) knowledge and experiences is extremely important to understand the client and the family and their use of cultural healing to relieve mental stresses. Voodoo, hexing, and other cultural forms may mimic some mental diseases, but are different and require emic folk healing modes.[46]

Vietnamese

Traditionally oriented Vietnamese generally find that Western psychiatric treatment and mental health care are strange and questionable. If Vietnamese are seen in a psychiatric setting, their concerns are often misinterpreted or misdiagnosed by nurses and physicians who

fail to understand Vietnamese culture values, beliefs, and lifeways. Vietnamese hold that the mind, body, and soul are integrated and cannot be viewed as separate entities. The idea of psychiatric nurses or physicians separating the mind, body, and soul is disturbing to Vietnamese immigrants and refugees if they seek Western psychiatric help. The idea closest to Western mental illness would be a "case of nerves" or having "something wrong with their nervous system." Some Vietnamese view mental conditions as mainly a "weakness of the nerves." Most important, the head is sacred with many different spirits and must be considered sacred with any treatment regime.[47]

Many traditional Vietnamese clients that the author and other transcultural nurses have studied have encountered great difficulty with hospital personnel because of value differences, language, and staff cultural ignorance.[48] Traditional Vietnamese tend to suppress or deny their feelings about problems because nurses and physicians are viewed as strangers. They will often talk about somatic concerns rather than spiritual and private cultural life situations, feelings, and family losses. Experiencing "cultural pain" as defined by the author has been typically found with Vietnamese refugees who have endured severe cultural tensions and hardships. For refugees, spending time with the Vietnamese client and family to help them get comfortable with the nurse is important. With trust, they will talk about their losses and concerns and how to use their folk remedies, foods, herbs, and teas. When they trust health personnel, they share their cultural lifeways, both past and present. Posttraumatic stress disorder (PTSD) is commonly used by psychiatric staff to fit Vietnamese refugees into a Western diagnosis. Nurses using the Culture Care theory will want to focus on the assets or strengths of Vietnamese clients and especially their families when dealing with life stresses or conflicts. Cultural pain is often caused by loss of kinship or family members, inability to get work, and lack of respect. Nurses will also need to deal with feelings of loneliness and separation that refugees experience, as well as leaving their homeland and adjusting to a very different culture.

Feelings of hopelessness, distress, grief, fatigue, mood swings, and somatic complaints can be found as dominant mental concerns with many Vietnamese refugees and immigrants. Vietnamese culture care values related to kinship factors, religious beliefs, and their present or past ethnohistory and environmental contexts are important care areas for the nurse to focus on with Vietnamese. This broad holistic approach reflected in the Culture Care theory and the use of the Sunrise Model can be extremely helpful guides to the nurse in discovering and understanding their concerns, stresses, and present life situations and needs. The Vietnamese traditional beliefs, values, lifeways, and folk healing can prevent illness, as well as respect cultural taboos. Helping Vietnamese to maintain or regain their integrated mind-body-soul holistic equilibrium (or balance) should be a major goal in nursing care. Western psychiatric disease labels and nursing diagnostic categories (NANDA) are usually inappropriate for Vietnamese clients unless fully acculturated to Western ways. Providing silence and a quiet area for reflection and talking is useful, and avoiding negative criticism (saving face) is important. Clients should be encouraged to share ideas about their family or work situations. These suggestions and others contribute to providing culturally competent and beneficial care.

Mexican Americans

Mexican Americans tend to have fewer incidences of mental illnesses, which is largely the result of their close extended family ties, direct support for their cultural values and beliefs, and importance of religion and kinship to allay anxieties, stresses, and unnecessary conflicts.[49] Mexican Americans' stresses are often related to poverty, unemployment, and urban conflict problems, which can bring about periods of depression, overweight conditions, and potential suicide. Research among Mexican Americans reveals that alcohol is frequently used by males to relieve male stress and to express *machismo*. With machismo, men take too much alcohol to express their masculinity, bravery, or power and to repress their frustrations. Mexican American women tend to relieve mental stresses or conflicts by relying on direct family support, using folk healing modes—herbal drinks, and eating fatty Mexican foods. Some Mexican American women talk about panic expressions, which they blame on external societal forces that lead to family problems and societal difficulties. Mexican Americans also pray and petition to God, their Lady of Guadalupe, and specific saints to help them

cope with daily stresses, needs, and cultural problems, especially those related to death, losses, and family poverty. The cultural phenomenon of *susto* (magical fright) can be precipitated by sudden or unexpected accidents or critical social and family life situations. Casting the *mal olo* (evil eye), *nerios, zar, susto*, and *ataque de nervios* are other cultural conditions that can lead to minor or serious mental illnesses unless treated culturally. The evil eye occurs when strangers as nurses and physicians overpraise or envy a newborn or another person.[50] This cultural condition is often caused unintentionally by health personnel who do not understand the Mexican cultural beliefs and lifeways and leads to harm by their actions and words. This, as well as other conditions, can be prevented by generic *emic* care and ritual Mexican practices. (See other chapters in this book.)

Guest Researchers Zoucha and George

In this last section, Drs. Zoucha's and George's (both transcultural mental health nurses) research is shared. Zoucha's research is first discussed, which is on a cultural condition with Mexican Americans. This is followed by George's transcultural nursing research study with the chronically ill living in an urban community.

Mexican American Care (by Dr. Zoucha)*

Mexican Americans are of a culture that transcultural nurses need to understand in the promotion of mental health and well-being. Mexican Americans have had a long history of being under-served regarding mental health services and misunderstandings of their cultural expressions by health care professionals. Understanding their folk beliefs, religious faith, and mental illness is difficult without considerable holding knowledge of the culture. For many Mexican Americans, mental illness is a family matter and must be understood and treated within the family context. Sometimes, the

---

*Dr. Rick Zoucha is a transcultural mental health nurse who has done research with Mexican and African Americans since 1989. He is an Associate Professor at Duquesne University in the School of Nursing at Pittsburgh, Pennsylvania.

family members are unable to care for a sick family member, and so nurses and other health care professionals are expected to help them. Nurses prepared in transcultural nursing are in a unique position to serve as a cultural bridge to help the Mexican Americans experiencing mental illness within the extended family context. During times of extreme stress and anxiety, nurses need to provide *protective care* so the client will not harm himself or others. The transcultural nurse is also expected to work with the staff to provide culturally based congruent care for the client and the family.

The transcultural nurse must be knowledgeable about cultural-bound mental conditions such as *sustos*, *nervios*, and others. *Sustos* is the belief that the soul was frightened out of the body, which has led to unhappiness, depression, and sometimes to death.[51] *Nervios* refers to stress brought on by difficult life situations that lead to somatic expressions, the inability to function, sleeplessness nights, and loss of appetite. There are also other expressions and conditions of mental illness such as being hexed or marked by a social-cultural taboo.

An example of *sustos* is offered with a transcultural nursing assessment and actions for therapeutic outcomes. Juana Luz is a 30-year-old Mexican American female who was seen in the outpatient mental health center for symptoms of depression, anxiety, sleep disturbances, and loss of appetite. Juana is of the first generation of Mexican Americans living in the United States. She works as a Spanish language interpreter at an insurance company and is fluent in Spanish and English. Juana has been married to Ricardo for the last 8 years and the couple has two children, namely, a 7-year-old daughter and a 3-year-old son. Juana reports during the second interview that she is experiencing *sustos*. She states that her symptoms started when she came out of the house to look for her daughter and witnessed a near miss between a city bus and her daughter who was playing in the yard and went after a ball. She believes that "her soul was frightened out of her" and since then has been experiencing depression, anxiety, loss of appetite, and great difficulty sleeping. Juana believes that because she witnessed such a potentially horrible event that her soul has left her body. She feels she will not feel better until her soul is reunited with her body.

In this situation, it is important that the transcultural nurse understands the cultural context in which

sustos occurs. Nurses should assess the family concerns and encourage family involvement in helping with care and treatment. Religious factors need to be considered as they are often linked to mental disturbances related to violating cultural taboos. At the individual's or family's request, mental health treatment usually includes both professional (etic) and generic (emic) folk care with nurses acting as the cultural bridge between professional and folk healers. With Juana it is important to know if she is currently being treated by a *curandera* or a folk indigenous healer. Today, Mexican Americans will seek treatment from both the Western professionals and their familiar folk carers and healers. In the folk system of care, the *curandera* is viewed as the healer and will often try to treat culture-bound mental illness drawing on the family caregivers. Treatment and nursing actions for Juana include an integrated approach of using *generic and professional* care services. If Juana requests the treatment of a *curandera*, it would be culturally appropriate to work in consultation with the faith healer and with the family's endorsement. A combination of family/individual therapy with folk and professional treatment often occurs. Treatment for *sustos* may include healing rituals that reunite the soul and body. The ritual includes the use of religious prayers as the holy cross and holy water with other indigenous practices. Reuniting the body with the soul may be adequate to reduce the symptoms of depression and anxiety; however, antidepressant medications and/or antianxiety medication are often indicated today in conjunction with generic care. The main transcultural concern for the nurse is the ability to negotiate cultural care that is appropriate and congruent with the culture of the individual and family. Filial direct care, prayers, and holy water along with generic care are often used to alleviate *sustos*. The transcultural nurse would be wise to use Leininger's theory with her three modes of care actions, especially culture care accommodation for the health and well-being of Juana and her family.

Other transcultural nursing concerns are understanding the client's language and medication needs. Many Mexican Americans speak Spanish as a first language and English as a second. During times of stress, some clients resort to the language that is most comfortable to them. Transcultural nurses should know and speak some Spanish today with the marked increase in Hispanics in the United States and elsewhere.

Language use greatly facilitates care to the Mexican American client and is important to effectively give medications or treatments. Culture care accommodation is made to provide safe and culturally appropriate care and to give medications effectively.

The relationship between the individual, family, and nurse is critical to promote and maintain the mental health and well-being of Mexican Americans. The researcher found that confidence in the relationship between nurses and clients leads to healthy outcomes. If the individual and family have confidence in the nurse, this will support actions to promote mental health and well-being.[52] Transcultural nurses need to understand the emic views of mental illness and the use of both professional (etic) and folk (emic) health care with Mexican Americans. Transcultural nurses also need to maintain their role as a cultural bridge with the client and the family to *successfully use both professional and folk care practices for culturally congruent care outcomes.*

Dr. George's Research with the Chronically Mentally Ill*

This ethnonursing study was focused on the chronically mentally ill in the community as a subculture. It was the first study to use the theory of Culture Care Diversity and Universality and the Sunrise Model to explicate care meanings, expressions, and experiences of the chronically mentally ill in a midwestern United States community over a 1-year period.[53] The study focuses on using Leininger's Culture Care theory with the ethnonursing qualitative research method.[54] Data were collected with a total of 54 interviews with 15 key informants and 24 general informants. Eleven months of observation and participation were done with members of a public community mental health day/partial treatment center. This center served approximately 90 chronically mentally ill persons who lived in the community in a midwestern city with a population of approximately 90,000. Data analysis was directed on the

domain of inquiry and using the Leininger Phases of Ethnonursing Analysis. The ethnonursing domain of focus was on care meanings and expressions of these chronically mentally ill in the community.

As predicted by the Culture Care theory, the worldview, cultural and social structure factors, ethnohistory, and environmental context greatly influenced the informants' behavior and lifeways. For example, the ethnohistory of mental illness influenced the subculture of the chronically mentally ill in the community in many ways as informants repeatedly told of their long hospitalizations. One key informant said that her mother had spent her entire adult life in a mental institution. Several informants described how long hospitalizations fostered a passive institutionalized mindset. They found that deinstitutionalization profoundly affected their lives. However, one general informant said that care and treatment settings today are very different than they were in the distant past. He stated, "In the past, if they had (client) someone in the family who was mentally ill, they hid that person. Now you see these people on the street."

Each key informant told at length the history of their life experiences with mental illness. Some commonalities were noted among informants of care experiences such as the onset of symptoms during their teens or twenties; multiple hospitalizations; severed ties over time with family relationships; the lack of a long-term partner in life; the difficulties in socializing with others; and the relinquishing of career and family aspirations. The informants said these were replaced with a focus on attempting to meet basic needs and acceptance of their ongoing need for psychotropic medications.

From this long-term in-depth study, six major themes were identified and formulated from the multiple descriptors and abstracted patterns of the data.[55] The dominant care themes with meanings were as follows:

1. Care as listening and giving presence is meaningful to the chronically mentally ill.
2. The chronically mentally ill have a strong desire to give care to others.
3. The chronically mentally ill in the community are a subculture with shared social structure factors, cultural norms, values, and lifeways that differ from those of the dominant culture.

---

*Dr. Tamara George is a transcultural mental health nurse and an Associate Professor of Nursing at Calvin College in Michigan. (Dr. Leininger was her research mentor for this doctoral dissertation study at Wayne State University.)

4. Mental illness carries a public stigma in the dominant culture.
5. The chronically mentally ill desire culturally congruent care modalities that help them meet their needs and support their potential with care practices that are flexible and growth promoting.
6. The chronically mentally ill value normalcy and strive to develop "normal" lifeways, but they fear rejection and failure in the large culture.

All of these themes have multiple implications for transcultural mental health nurses and other mental health providers. This study has been published with full discussion of these themes and the reader is encouraged to study it.[56] Most encouragingly, the chronically mentally ill in the community were able to articulate their ideas and stories clearly about care and its meanings. The findings from this study led to the discovery and formulation of three care constructs that can be used by nurses in conjunction with the three modalities of action as theorized by Leininger, which can provide meaningful and helpful care to members of this subculture. The three dominant and newly discovered constructs were *survival care, constructive care,* and *inclusive care,* which are defined and discussed in the study.[57] The researcher concluded that culture-specific care for the chronically mentally ill could potentially increase their feelings of well-being, reduce the frequency and length of hospital stays, and lead to more positive interactions with others in the larger community.

 Summary

In this chapter a number of critical issues, trends, and practices have been discussed of traditional and current aspects related to the discovery and the need for care that fits with or is congruent with cultures and their mental health conditions. As an early and contemporary nurse in mental health, the author has set forth several challenges for traditionally oriented psychiatric nurses in the mental health field to become prepared through graduate courses and programs in transcultural nursing to provide culturally competent and meaningful care to clients of diverse cultures. While many nurses in other clinical areas have prepared themselves in transcultural nursing, psychiatric nurses have

been slow to do so; they need to realize how powerful culture care factors are in mental wellness and illness. An in-depth study of cultural factors influencing human caring and mental health is essential to alleviate current problems related to violence, depression, suicide, homicide, and other mental health conditions in homes, schools, and community settings. Indeed, it is difficult to assess biophysical, psychosomatic, and other conditions and to help clients in appropriate ways without cultural knowledge and research. To be called a "mental health nurse therapist" is questionable without knowledge of specific cultures and their human care knowledge. Ethnohistory, religious or spiritual beliefs, kinship and social ties, cultural values, worldview, language, gender roles, and other emic and etic knowledge dimensions need to be integrated into the new and future focus of transcultural mental health practices to be a competent mental health therapist.

Most importantly, it is time to conduct research and further develop transcultural mental health knowledge, assessments, and therapies that fit Western and non-Western cultures. The dominance of Western diagnostic categories with predetermined symptoms and treatment modes often fail to fit non-Western cultures for beneficial client outcomes. Nurses prepared in transcultural mental health nursing need to give leadership and to use their knowledge and skills to guide other interdisciplinary mental health practitioners toward culturally congruent mental health services. Theoretical perspectives are essential to study and explain outcomes of mental health care research. The theory of Culture Care Diversity and Universality has already generated rich and new holistic care insights to help clients of diverse and similar cultures and those with mental health stresses. This theory with the ethnonursing method and enablers continues to be most appropriate for many transcultural mental health nurses today in arriving at culturally relevant, meaningful, and beneficial practices as demonstrated in this chapter and others in this book related to holistic human health and well-being.

Finally, mental health nurses, psychiatrists, and others need to realize that with most cultures in the world it is generally unacceptable and inappropriate to separate the mind from either the body or the diverse spiritual (soul) aspects as such separatist practices greatly limit understanding and meaningful services to clients from diverse cultures. It is my contention that, as traditional *emic* cultural knowledge is interwoven with selected and appropriate psychiatric professional etic research-based knowledge, there will be major changes in the assessment, care, and treatment of clients with diverse life experiences and mental conditions. Indeed, *all* psychiatric diagnostic, care, and treatment modes need to become culturally grounded with Western and non-Western transcultural perspectives to provide therapeutic and culturally congruent client practices in our growing and intense multicultural global world.

References

1. Hofling, C. and M. Leininger, *Basic Psychiatric Concepts in Nursing*, New York: John Wiley & Sons, Inc., 1960.

2. Leininger, M., *Transcultural Nursing: Concepts, Theories, and Practices*, New York: John Wiley & Sons, Inc., 1978.

3. Leininger, M., "Caring for the Culturally Different Necessitates Transcultural Nursing Knowledge and Competencies," *Cultura De Los Cuidados*, Portugal, Alicante: University of Alicante Press, v. 3, no. 6, 1999, Semestre 1999, p. 5–9.

4. American Psychiatric Association, *Diagnostic and Statistical Manual*, 4th ed., New York, 1994.

5. Leininger, M., *Transcultural Nursing: Concepts, Theories, Research and Practice*, 2nd ed., Blacklick, Ohio: McGraw-Hill Custom College Series, 1995, pp. 279–292.

6. Leininger, M., *Nursing and Anthropology: Two Worlds to Blend*, New York: John Wiley & Sons, 1970.

7. Leininger, M., *Culture Care Diversity and Universality: A Theory of Nursing*, New York: National League for Nursing Press, 1991.

8. Leininger, M., op. cit., 1978.

9. Leininger, M., op. cit., 1995.

10. Leininger, M., op. cit., 1991.

11. Leininger, M., op. cit., 1995.

12. Leininger, M., op. cit., 1991.

13. Leininger, M., 1997, "Transcultural Nursing Research to Transform Nursing Education and Practice: 40 Years," *Image: Journal of Nursing Scholarships*, v. 29, no. 4, Fourth Quarter, 1997, pp. 341–347.

14. Leininger, M., op. cit., 1991.

15. Kottak, C., *Anthropology: The Exploration of Human Diversity*, 5th ed., New York: McGraw-Hill, Inc., 1991, pp. 354–367.

16. Helman, C. G., *Culture, Health, and Illness*, London: Wright, 1990.

17. Marsella, A., R. Tharp, and T. Ciborowski, eds., *Perspectives on Cross-Cultural Psychology*, New York: Academic Press, 1979.

18. Marsella, A., et. al., "Cross-Cultural Studies of Depressive Disorders: An Overview," in *Culture and Depression*, Kleinman & B. Good, eds., Berkeley, CA: University of California Press, 1995, pp. 299–324.

19. Kottak, C., op. cit., 1991.

20. Kottak, C., op. cit., 1991.

21. Leininger, M., *Discovery and Uses in Clinical and Community Nurses*, Detroit, MI: Wayne State University Press, 1984 (reprinted by Charles Slack, 1988).

22. Helman, op. cit., 1990.

23. Marsella et al., op. cit., 1979.

24. Peterson, P., *Handbook of Cross-Cultural Counseling and Therapy*, Westport, CT: Greenwood Press, 1985.

25. Peterson, P., N. Sartorius, and A. Marsella, *Mental Health Services: The Cross-Cultural Context*, Beverly Hills: Sage Publications, 1984.

26. Leininger, M., "Witchcraft Practices and Psychocultural Therapy with Urban United States Families," *Human Organization*, v. 32, no. 1, 1978, pp. 73–80.

27. Leininger, M., "Transcultural Interviewing and Health Assessment," in *Mental Health Services: The Cross Cultural Context*, P. Peterson, N. Sartorius and A. Marsella, eds., Beverly Hills: Sage Publications, 1984, pp. 109–135.

28. Leininger, M., "Transcultural United Health Nursing Assessment of Children and Adolescents," in *Psychiatric and Mental Health Nursing with Children and Adolescents*, C. Evans, ed., Gaithersburg, MD: Aspen Publishers, Inc., 1990.

29. Mead, M., *Coming of Age in Samoa*, New York: New American Library, 1961, (originally published 1928).

30. Glittenberg, J., "Cultural Heroes Aid in Coping," unpublished paper, *Psychiatric Nurse Clinical Symposium*, Denver: April 18, 1979.

31. Barnauw, W. V., *Culture and Personality*, 4th ed., Homewood, IL: Dorsey Press, 1985.

32. Moore, L., P. VanArsdale, J. Glittenberg, and R. Aldrich, *The Biocultural Basis of Health: Expanding Views of Medical Anthropology*, Prospect Heights, IL: Waveland Press, 1989.

33. Tripp-Reimer, T., "Cultural Diversity in Therapy," in *Mental Health Psychiatric Nursing*, C. Beck, R. Rawlins and S. Williams, eds., St. Louis, MO: C. V. Mosby, 1984, pp. 381–398.

34. Kennedy, M., "Cultural Competence and Psychiatric-Mental Health Nursing," *Journal of Transcultural Nursing*, v. 10, no. 1, January 1999, p. 11.

35. Kavanagh, K., "Transcultural Perspectives in Mental Health," in *Transcultural Nursing*, 3rd ed., M. Andrews and J. Boyle, eds., Philadelphia: J. B. Lippincott, 1995, pp. 223–261.

36. Zoucha, R., "The Experiences of Mexican Americans Receiving Professional Nursing Care: An Ethnonursing Study," *Journal of Transcultural Nursing*, v. 9, no. 2, 1995, pp. 34–44.

37. Leininger, M., op. cit., 1978, pp. 375–397.

38. Leininger, M., op. cit., 1995, pp. 559–589.

39. Ibid.

40. Leininger, M., "Gadsup of Papua New Guinea Revisited: A Three Decade View," *Journal of Transcultural Nursing*, v. 5, no. 1, Summer, 1993, pp. 21–30.

41. Leininger, M., "Field Research over Two Decades (1980–2000)." Excerpt from unpublished report, Omaha, 2000.

42. Ronan, L., "Alcohol-Related Health Risks among Black Americans," *Alcohol Health and Research World*, 1987, pp. 36–89.

43. Bailey, E., *African Americans Health in Urban Community*, 1991.

44. Ibid.

45. Campinha-Bacote, J., "Voodoo Illness: A Review," *Perspectives in Psychiatric Nursing*, v. 28, no. 1, 1992, pp. 11–17.

46. Leininger, op. cit., 1995.

47. Tran, T. M., *Indochinese Patients*, Falls Church, VA: Action for Southeast Asians, 1980.

48. Leininger, M., "Vietnamese Culture Care," *Proceedings Community Health*, Baltimore: Maryland Health Department, 1987, pp. 1–7.

49. Leininger, M., op. cit., 1995.

50. Ibid.

51. Zoucha, R. D., "The Experiences of Mexican Americans Receiving Professional Nursing Care: An Ethnonursing Study," *The Journal of Transcultural Nursing*, v. 9, no. 1, 1998, pp. 33–34.

52. Ibid.

53. George, T. B., "Defining Care in the Culture of the Chronically Mentally Ill Living in the Community," *The Journal of Transcultural Nursing*, v. 11, no. 2, 2000, pp. 102–110.

54. Leininger, op. cit. 1991.

55. George, op. cit, 2000.

56. Ibid.

57. Ibid.

12 Transcultural Nursing Care and Health Perspectives of HIV/AIDS

Joan MacNeil

HIV/AIDS is a global illness that requires transcultural caring knowledge, understanding, and practices. The extent of the pandemic demonstrates the need for global human care with a transcultural caring perspective. HIV/AIDS has now been reported in virtually every industrialized and developing country in the world. It has been estimated that at the end of 1998 over 33 million people were living with HIV, about 10% of whom where children. The virus continues to spread, causing nearly 16,000 new infections a day. Although one in every 100 adults in the sexually active age bracket (15–49) today is living with HIV, only a tiny fraction are aware they are infected. Unless a cure is found or life-prolonging therapy can be made more widely available, the majority of those now living with HIV will die within a decade.[1]

While the global picture continues to be worrisome, in the United States HIV infection rates are falling slightly, particularly among homosexual men. However, in some disadvantaged sections of society, AIDS continues to rise. Among African Americans, new AIDS cases rose by 19% among heterosexual men and 12% among heterosexual women in 1996. In the Hispanic community, there were 13% more cases among men and 5% more among women than a year earlier.[2]

The global HIV pandemic continues to be fueled by cultural and economic factors such as increases in migration, political upheavals, economic crises, rising rates of sexually transmitted diseases (STDs), injecting drug use, and violence. As human behavior both prevents and spreads HIV infection, this illness continues to be culturally defined. In addition, as the numbers of infections rise, there is a clear moral and humanitarian obligation to provide whatever care, support, and assistance are appropriate for each person infected and affected by HIV/AIDS.

Nursing, as a transcultural humanistic and scientific care discipline and profession, plays a central role in meeting the care needs of the increasing number of clients from diverse cultures.[3] Regardless of the effectiveness of prevention efforts conducted today and new advances in treatments, the numbers of people becoming ill as a result of HIV infection will dramatically increase over the next few years. As the numbers of infections increase, demands for care will mount globally.[4] Professional nurses who are knowledgeable and sensitive to the transcultural perspectives of the pandemic and who are able to provide culturally congruent care are greatly needed worldwide.

Major Cultural and Social Structure Dimensions

Leininger[5–8] predicted decades ago that cultural beliefs, values, norms, and patterns of caring had a powerful influence on human survival, growth, illness states, health, and well-being. She postulated that care was culturally defined and influenced by specific cultural values, worldview, social structure factors, language, ethnohistory, environmental context, and health care systems. She theorized that all cultures in the world had some kind of generic care system and most had a professional health care system. These two major health care systems were predicted to provide human care that was healthy, satisfying, beneficial, and congruent with the client's culture care values and needs. She believed that carefully combining generic and professional care could lead people to seek health services to attain culturally congruent and beneficial care. She predicted that culturally based care existed, but was minimally recognized by nurses and other health professionals as a pattern of functioning. To fully understand and predict culture caring, discovery of the diverse and similar influencers was needed.

Leininger's Sunrise Model, which presents a visualization of the different dimensions of the theory of Culture Care Diversity and Universality, provides a cognitive map to depict the complex influencing dimensions and to explain and interpret HIV/AIDS health and well-being outcomes.[9] Worldview, social structure factors, and cultural factors with attention to language, ethnohistory, and environmental context are predicted to influence care expressions, patterns, and practices that in turn influence the health, well-being, and care to dying clients. The theory and model can be used to inform nurses and others regarding these different dimensions and to increase our understanding of what constitutes a supportive environmental context for culturally congruent HIV/AIDS care. In this chapter several of the influencing dimensions of the model are discussed in relation to HIV/AIDS care.

While all components of the cultural and social structure dimensions are held to influence care expressions, patterns, and practices, the political and economic factors throughout the span of the pandemic have played and continue to play a pivotal role. Experience has shown that the social and political environments of a country, community, or workplace have a profound influence on efforts not only to reduce the spread of HIV but also to provide care for HIV-infected and affected individuals and their families. Laws, rules, policies, and practices of governments and institutions can either support or constrain the provision of care. For example, restrictions on sex education in schools, condom advertising, needle exchange, and availability of money for drugs and treatments continue to hamper HIV/AIDS protective preventive care programs.

Although many governments, businesses, and institutions have begun to adopt more appropriate HIV/AIDS preventive care policies, progress has not kept pace with the spread of the epidemic. Few countries have responded to HIV/AIDS with comprehensive care programs or have committed resources needed to slow the epidemic. Engaging the interest, concern, and

support of policymakers at early stages of the epidemic continues to be challenging, particularly when prevalence is low and the potential for a future problem may not be apparent. It is also difficult when HIV infections are concentrated among groups in society who may be marginalized or discriminated against such as prostitutes or intravenous drug users.

Once HIV has reached high levels among those likely to contract and spread the virus, containing the epidemic is difficult and requires drastic action. While difficult to contain, drastic political care action and decisions at this phase are not impossible as has been demonstrated in Thailand. Thailand undertook a massive government public health campaign when intravenous drug users and prostitutes were discovered to have high infection rates.[10] This campaign could be considered a form of protective-preventive care, that is protecting people from HIV infection through prevention. A policy of heavily subsidized condom promotion and STD treatment for those with high-risk behavior, supplemented by dissemination of information to the general population, brought down the prevalence of HIV among military conscripts in Thailand within a few years.[11] However, not all countries will have the same political and economic dimensions as Thailand. Each country will develop their own programs to provide preventive care (and within their ethical and moral perspectives). However, this example illustrates the enabling role political dimensions can play in facilitating preventive HIV care.

As people infected early in the epidemic become ill and die from AIDS, governments face growing pressure to spend public resources on care. Responding to these needs compassionately, while keeping them in perspective with the many other pressing human care needs and demands on public resources, is one of the most difficult policy challenges posed by the epidemic. In this instance, both the political and economic dimensions influence how and when HIV/AIDS care and treatment are available.

Increasing Demand and Choices

Increasing demand makes access to care more difficult and expensive for everyone, including people not infected with HIV. As the number of people with HIV/AIDS mounts, rising costs for care leading to increased total health expenditures present societies with difficult choices. Because a large share of increased expenditure is typically financed through public tax revenues, governments and their constituents often confront trade-offs along at least three dimensions: 1) caring for people with AIDS versus protective care to prevent HIV infection, 2) clinical care treatment of people with AIDS versus clinical care treatment of people with other illnesses, and 3) spending for health care versus spending for other objectives.

Choices about the appropriate overall level of public subsidies for health care vary across cultures and are influenced not only by the political and economic dimensions but also by cultural values and ethical beliefs. The fair response, advocated by many, is to offer the same level of subsidy for the care of people with AIDS as the care and treatment of people with other diseases that are expensive and difficult to treat. Denying care to individuals simply because they have HIV/AIDS is unjust to those who are infected and to their families. By the same token, providing a higher level of subsidy for care for people with AIDS than for those with other illnesses is also unfair to the majority of people who are not infected with HIV. As in many countries, the United States government at the national and state level continues to struggle with these choices. These choices in turn influence care practices, including nursing practices, within health care systems.

Cultural, religious, and political dimensions also influence care practices in relation to HIV prevention. Protective care policies that decrease the vulnerability of special groups to HIV should be a priority. In most parts of the world, the majority of new infections occur in young people between 15 and 24 years of age, or sometimes younger.[12] Not only do these infections cluster among youth who are just becoming sexually active, but up to 60% of all infections in females occur by the age of 20. Young people under 20 are frequently not viewed as being vulnerable to HIV or because of cultural beliefs are not thought to be sexually active. All women and men, irrespective of their HIV status, have the right to determine the course of their reproductive life and health. Practical measures should include ensuring access to information about HIV/AIDS and its prevention; promotion of safer sex, including the use of condoms, with moral and religious considerations; and access to reproductive health services. These ser-vices should include family planning and treatment for sexually transmitted infections (STI), which can significantly decrease the risk of transmission.[13–15] Often nurses must overcome resistance to ensure needed services, but they should also recognize controversial issues.

Gender Risk Factors

A woman's risk of HIV infection from unprotected sex is at least twice that of men. Women are more exposed to HIV and STIs through the extensive surface of the vaginal wall. Young women are at even greater risk because of the immaturity of the vaginal cells. In some cultures girls as young as 12 may be married to men three times their age. In addition, girls aged 17 years or younger who have unprotective sex are at increased risk of developing cervical cancer.[16] All these factors make young women especially vulnerable at a time when, culturally, some have limited negotiating and economic power, making them easier targets for sexual exploitation. The situation is worse when more men, especially in high-HIV-prevalence areas, seek out ever younger female partners in the belief that they are least likely to be infected with HIV.

It is often socially unacceptable for a woman in some cultures to seek treatment for an STI because of the stigma attached to seeking services in an STI clinic. In addition, the lack of STI services in traditional family planning or maternal child health clinics, as well as the pressures from other responsibilities, discourage many women from seeking health care. These factors are a care-seeking deterrent for teenage girls in many cultures where it is not considered socially acceptable for girls to be sexually active outside of marriage.

In general, unmarried adolescents may feel unwelcome or embarrassed and make little use of either family planning or STI services. Culturally knowledgeable nurses must be prepared to develop outreach activities, involve communities, and develop care services that are more accessible and culturally acceptable to young people and to women in particular. Confidentiality and privacy need to be assured for young people to be encouraged and to use these services. Transculturally prepared nurses can develop skills and help other staff to deal sensitively with patients of diverse cultures about private matters. One of the commonly cited criticisms by clients of both family planning and STI services is the rude or humiliating attitude of staff.[17] Transcultural nurses can play an important role to repattern care services to meet the special needs of young people and to change negative and biased perspectives through caring modalities.[18,19]

Evolving Transcultural Care Needs as HIV Infection Progresses

No matter where one lives, a diagnosis of HIV is one filled with uncertainties, that is, uncertainty about acceptance by family and friends; uncertainty about ability to continue to be a productive member of society; uncertainty about physical aspects of the infection; and, finally, uncertainty about life itself. Added to this is the uncertainty of HIV disease progression — within an individual HIV disease can be a rapidly progressive illness over 2 years, or it can have limited progression over 10 to 15 years. Unfortunately, such differences occur not only between individuals, but in different contexts with variable resources. Individuals from economically poorer settings often face more rapid disease progression because of limited access to and funds for care. With children, HIV infections usually progress more rapidly. For example, in the United States about 25% of HIV-positive children have a rapidly progressive illness and die within 1 year. However, the majority will survive beyond their first year, and, as in HIV-infected adults, long-term survivors are recognized.[20]

Despite these uncertainties, HIV disease progresses through different stages as immunosuppresion worsens. Experience working with the HIV-infected and their families has revealed that supportive and clinical care needs change during these different phases of the infection. Compassionate care with understanding and continuity must be provided through all stages of HIV infection and in both hospital-based and home-based contexts.[21] Nurses need to be aware of these changing needs and their transcultural implications. In the early phases of HIV infection nurses can assist in identifying culturally appropriate sources of psychological support, facilitating clients' disclosure of their HIV serostatus to families, and providing clients with HIV preventive care. As immunity decreases, nurses can assist clients in maintaining health and seeking early and appropriate clinical care to prevent oppor-

tunistic infections. When AIDS occurs, nurses may assist clients and their families in negotiating a culturally appropriate guardian for their children and facilitate access to ongoing culturally appropriate emotional and spiritual care. In the terminal phase, nurses can support clients in the provision of palliative care.

There must also be coordination and continuity between the professional and generic or folk health care systems. In countries such as South Africa, up to 80% of people may have visited a traditional healer before seeking professional services.[22] In Uganda, AIDS patients often simultaneously seek both generic and professional care.[23] These traditional care services are attractive because they are accessible, culturally appropriate, acceptable, and usually affordable. Generic healers may be able to help their people and help nurses and other health care workers understand their clients' beliefs about illness and caring practices. Generic healers can be valuable partners in HIV prevention and care, and, generally, their knowledge can be combined with professional care practices.

Early HIV Infection

Care during this phase is largely related to identification of the underlying HIV infection and specific disease-management issues. A proactive approach to HIV diagnosis can speed up knowledge, acceptance, and openness about HIV/AIDS. Access to confidential HIV counseling care practices and testing services constitutes a critical first step in dealing with the infection. Clients who are HIV negative are much more likely to accept advice on how to remain HIV negative and to act on that advice. For those who are positive, ongoing psychological and cultural support with counseling are some of the care needs identified at this phase as most HIV-infected people are in, or return to, reasonable health and can resume normal activities.[24]

In a number of different industrialized and developing countries, many people who are counseled and subsequently tested do not return for their results.[25] However, instituting rapid on-site testing allows results to be given within a short time after the pretest counseling care sessions and provides the opportunity for immediate post-test counseling.[26] While not yet common in the United States, this strategy is increasingly used in a number of countries and enables risk-reduction counseling and psychosocial and cultural support to be provided to large numbers of clients. At the same time, nurses who encounter clients from diverse cultures need to be aware that in a number of countries rapid HIV tests are available to people for testing without adequate counseling care and supervision. Migrant workers in southeast Asia are believed to be using such rapid tests before returning home to their regular partners or wives; however, without any counseling and information, they do not understanding that they may be recently infected but, for the present, test negative.[27]

People who are identified early as being infected can benefit from this diagnosis by obtaining early access to care services. Infections can be recognized and treated in a timely fashion before they become complicated. Individuals can be encouraged to engage in protective self-care and other-care by living positively, joining support groups, and taking advantage of any specific antiretroviral intervention or opportunistic disease prophylaxis that is available. In the early stages of infection, nurses can work with families and communities to change pessimistic perceptions and worldviews about the prognosis of HIV/AIDS as a quickly fatal disease.

Another form of protective care, eradicating all vestiges of discrimination against HIV-infected persons, remains an ongoing global need. Unfortunately, in many places, employers, insurance companies, or governments have adopted ad hoc, discriminatory, HIV-testing policies that discourage people from acknowledging their HIV status, seeking care, and acting to protect others from infection. A bias against those with HIV/AIDS can take many forms, ranging from singling out AIDS-specific drug therapies for exclusion from public funding to outright refusal of care services. The case of an asymptomatic, HIV-positive woman who was refused treatment by her dentist in the northeastern United States made its way to the Supreme Court. This led to a judgment that affirmed the respondent's HIV infection was a disability under the American with Disabilities Act.[28] Treating her in the dentist's office was not held as posing a direct threat to the health and safety of others. In making the ruling, the court relied on the national dental association policy on HIV for guidance to ensure both access to care and nondiscrimination.[29] This is a clear example of how policies can facilitate care. Yet at the same time, this case also highlights that

clear policies alone are not enough. Training of health professionals to increase their understanding of HIV protective care and to eradicate all vestiges of discrimination against those infected is also needed. National nursing associations in different countries often play a leadership role through the development of care policies in relation to HIV/AIDS and advocationg for education of their members. The nursing profession, by its caring nature and expectation has the privilege and responsibility to ensure compassionate, safe, and beneficial care of those infected worldwide.[30,31]

Late HIV Illness

Care at this stage involves clinical actions and decisions to treat recurring infections and to provide ongoing psychosocial and cultural support. Economic considerations also play a large role, as recurrent illnesses may limit an infected person's ability to work. New disease problems, which emerge with more advanced immunosuppression, vary transculturally depending on the common pathogens in a region; the shortfalls of existing provisions for care; and the diverse cultural care values, beliefs, and practices. Medication to relieve symptoms and treat opportunistic infections can ease suffering and prolong the productive lives of people with HIV and sometimes at low costs. Treatment for infections such as thrush, toxoplasmosis, and pneumonia/septicemia can extend life expectancy from 1 to 4 years with a drug cost of $30 to $150.[32] These are prices that all but the very poor would probably be willing and able to afford. In addition, palliative care can inexpensively relieve some of the pain and discomfort that otherwise rob people of the ability to enjoy life and contribute to their family and their community. Without symptomatic treatment, dehydration that results from diarrhea and nausea can kill in a few days. The sad reality is that in many places, drugs and treatment modes are often not available.

In many cultures the care and support needs of people chronically ill with AIDS can be better met in the community or the home. Consequently, many initiatives to provide care in the home or community rather than the hospital have been implemented. Homecare provides an important opportunity for nurses to work directly with professional caregivers and families to facilitate the development of skills that caregivers may need to learn to help those living with HIV/AIDS in the home. It also provides opportunities for transcultural nurses to work with communities to promote a more open and honest approach to AIDS with a cultural perspective that takes into focused consideration the beliefs and values of the people of diverse or similar lifeways. Often, the demands of caring for sick family members leads caregivers to neglect their own health care needs or those of others in the household. Most importantly, caregivers can benefit from the support of members of their extended families or communites and from culturally based counseling to address the stigma, isolation, and uncertainty they often feel about the future.

The provision of palliative and terminal care is another care need that has been highlighted by HIV infection. In the final stages of AIDS, analgesics such as morphine to assuage extreme pain can provide relief to the dying patient. However, this essential drug is rarely legally available in poor countries (at any price), and therefore alternative analgesics are needed. Transcultural nurses can work with the families to provide pain relief, management of distressing symptoms, and spiritual and emotional support in ways that respect the patient's and family's cultural care beliefs and values.

Drug Use Issues

While some treatments may ease suffering and prolong life, they ultimately fail to save the patient's life. This is because more treatments do not reach the underlying cause of the illness, and the spread of HIV continues within the body with the consequent decline of the immune system. Recently, a few drugs have dramatically reduced the levels of HIV in the patient's blood below the ability of laboratory tests to detect viral RNA levels. The use of these drugs varies among countries and cultures. The first of these drugs, Zidovudine (AZT), was introduced in the late 1980s and added perhaps 6 months of healthy life for the average patient.[33] New effective therapy involving the use of three antiretrovirals was announced in June 1996. A year later, the U.S. government issued draft guidelines recommending early, aggressive treatment of HIV-infected individuals with triple-drug therapy. Largely as a result of triple thereapy (HAART), the number of people suffering from AIDS in North America and Europe has been dropping at last. However, even if the therapy continues to be generally effective, several substantial problems remain: the cost of the drugs themselves, the costs and difficulty of the monitoring needed for the therapy to be effective, and problems with patient compliance. All of these problems are related to the clients not only receiving and taking the drugs, but also to their following through with the monitoring necessary for successful drug therapy.

The example of AZT for HIV-infected pregnant women provides a dramatic case in point. Five years ago, a randomized control trial on the use of AZT among HIV-infected women in the United States and Europe demonstrated a two-thirds reduction in the risk of maternal-child transmission of HIV.[34] Since that time, AZT therapy has been available to pregnant HIV-infected women in these countries. However, in developing countries where more than 90% of mother-to-child transmission of HIV occurs, AZT therapy has not been available to women because of the cost and the complexity of the regimen. In the United States, identification of HIV-infected pregnant women before or as early as possible during the course of pregnancy and use of this full regimen has been recommended for prevention of perinatal transmission.[35] Despite these recommendations, many pregnant women have been reluctant to be tested for HIV. Transculturally prepared nurses can explore their clients' values and beliefs surrounding pregnancy and childbirth and the cultural meaning of a diagnosis of HIV for an individual client and her partner. This cultural knowledge is essential as a sound basis to provide culturally congruent care.

Because women in poorer countries often have limited or no access to antenatal care, this particular regimen of AZT has not been widely available. Simple and inexpensive caring modes are needed. A recent study in Thailand revealed that a short course of AZT documented a 51% reduction in the risk for mother-to-child transmission.[36] These findings have generated global discussion. Unfortunately, the subsidized cost of US$50 per woman ensures that this treatment is still unattainable for many women in the developing world. However, new research breakthroughs should be forthcoming such as the recent announcement that a single dose of Nivirapine administered during labor and delivery also decreased mother-to-child transmission dramatically.[37] The cost of this medicine is only $7 per dose, and it is less complicated than AZT in administration, which suggest that this can be helpful and more accessible to pregnant HIV-positive women. The likelihood that the use of such drugs will become more common in preventing mother-to-child transmission in diverse cultural settings challenges nurses to use cultural knowledge of childbirth practices to find safe and culturally appropriate ways to administer these medications, especially in home-birth settings.

These drugs represent an important breakthrough in reducing maternal-child transmission, but the dilemma of safe alternatives to breast-feeding continues. Although this is not an issue for most women in the industrialized countries who have access to safe alternatives, providing short-course AZT therapy to breast-feeding mothers without these alternatives may not be beneficial as the infants who escaped HIV infection during pregnancy and in delivery may become infected through breast-feeding. HIV-positive women from cultures where breast-feeding is a cultural norm face a difficult dilemma. With the vital importance of breast milk and breast-feeding for child health and the increasing prevalence of HIV infection around the world, it remains difficult to develop appropriate and feasible nutritional protective care guidelines on breast-feeding for mothers. First, most mothers do not know their HIV status. In developing countries more than nine out of ten HIV-positive women do not know their status.[38] In addition, it is still not possible to determine the relative risks of HIV acquisition from breast-feeding versus the risk of infant and child mortality from unsafe artificial feeding in various settings. In the absence of clear policies, mothers who know or suspect they are HIV-infected are left with the dilemma of trying to weigh the odds of infecting their babies with HIV with its certain mortality versus risking infection and/or death to their babies by inappropriate feeding practices.

Antiretroviral therapy, which has achieved dramatic improvements in the health of some individuals in high-income countries, is currently unaffordable and too demanding of clinical care services to offer realistic hope for millions of poor people infected in developing countries. Nurses who are aware of the disparity of treatments among different cultures and countries can help inform clients of their options and can provide ongoing counseling and cultural support for their choices. In addition, nurses can work through their transnational organizations to raise awareness regarding the issues and advocate for increased treatment options.

Occupational Transmission Dangers

There have been several incidents of occupational transmission of HIV to healthcare workers in the United States.[39] Many of these individuals have advocated nationally against discrimination and for safer workplace practices. These colleagues, often nurses, have risked stigma and loss of confidentiality to educate others. Because of their work health professionals are much more aware that the use of universal precautions and postexposure prophylaxis play a critical role in the care of those who may be infected or who are at risk of exposure to HIV through their occupation. Fear of occupational transmission influences caregiving in a number of ways. In high-HIV-prevalence countries, transmission of HIV through needle-stick injuries within the hospital continues to be a significant worry for many nurses, particularly when protective materials such as gloves and other equipment are in short supply. Consequently, staff recruitment can be adversely affected, and self-deployment can occur away from perceived risky activities such as labor and delivery and the operating room.

There are also the concerns that increasing levels of illness, absenteeism, and death among health workers threatens caregiving in high-HIV-prevalence areas. In Zambia, mortality among nurses increased more than fivefold from 1980 to 1991, which was largely attributed to HIV.[40] Absenteeism resulting from illness among staff and their friends and relatives for whom they have responsibility also contributes to the impact of HIV on caregiving by reducing the number of professional health staff available on any given day.

Children Orphaned by AIDS

By the year 2010 it is predicted that there will be nearly 42 million orphaned children in the 23 countries most heavily infected with HIV/AIDS.[41] These orphans are not evenly distributed across continents, across cultures, within communities, or among families, which makes care needs difficult to address. As nurses work with infected clients and their families, they are in a unique position to assist families in planning for their children's future care in culturally appropriate ways. Transcultural nurses can also play a special role in helping agencies to learn more about these children from different cultures by identifying where they live, who cares for them, and what can be done to help them now and in the future.

Culturally based care is essential to promote the health, well-being, and survival of children.[42-44] Children face problems caused by the fact that HIV/AIDS begins long before their parents die and because they live with sick relatives in households stressed by the drain on their resources.[45] Children in these households face loss of their family and their cultural identity; psychosocial distress; increased malnutrition with loss of health care, including immunizations; reduced opportunities for education; homelessness; and exposure to HIV infection. A study of the Baganda in Uganda[46] found that AIDS orphans without parents or grandparents had some chance of survival providing they had either land or education. Dying parents sought to provide land titles or education for their children as a form of protective care. Another study in Uganda traced 460 children, ages 5- to 15-years-old, who were children of 150 people who had died of AIDS.[47] Results revealed that lacking this type of protective care, one in three children had been abandoned, more than two in three were virtually naked and malnourished, one in 30 had been sexually abused, and two in five showed signs of psychological disorder. Without child protective care that provides counseling and psychological and material support, they face a grim future. Globally, for every ten orphans who survive to age 15, there are three to four children infected with HIV who die much sooner. These children are often quite ill and require special care and attention from their mothers, their families, and the health care system. Nurses can play a pivotal role in helping mothers understand that not all of their children are necessarily HIV-positive and in helping them seek appropriate health care and immunizations. Transculturally prepared nurses can offer special insights for making their care fit with the cultural lifeways

of the children and their families. They can also assess and discover community resources to assist families in caring for their children.

 Conclusion

The continuing global spread of HIV/AIDS requires increasing transcultural human caring knowledge, understanding, and practices to promote equitable resources for both HIV prevention and care, to decrease the vulnerability to HIV of certain groups in our cultures, to erase vestiges of discrimination, and to ensure appropriate care and assistance for each person infected and affected by HIV/AIDS. This chapter has presented a brief overview of some of the major transcultural and health care perspectives of HIV/AIDS. Nurses with transcultural knowledge, who work with clients and communities in diverse cultural settings, have a unique role to play. This role is to ensure that no matter what the cultural setting, for those infected and affected by HIV/AIDS, care is paramount and should be directed toward creative ways to provide culturally congruent care that has been predicted by Leininger to lead to health and well-being or to face death and dying in meaningful ways.

 References

1. UNAIDS, "Report on the Global HIV/AIDS Pandemic," Geneva: World Health Organization, 1999.
2. UNAIDS, "Report on the Global HIV/AIDS Epidemic: June, 1998," Geneva: World Health Organization, 1998a.
3. Leininger, M., ed., "The Theory of Culture Care Diversity and Universality," in *Culture Care Diversity and Universality: A Theory of Nursing*, New York: National League for Nursing Press, 1991, pp. 5–68.
4. MacNeil, J., and S. Anderson, "Beyond the Dichotomy: Linking Prevention with Care," *AIDS*, v. 12, no. 2, 1998, S19–S26.
5. Leininger, M., *Nursing and Anthropology: Two Worlds to Blend*, New York: John Wiley & Sons, 1970.
6. Leininger, M., *Transcultural Nursing: Concepts, Theories, and Practices*, New York: John Wiley & Sons, 1978.

7. Leininger, M., *Care: The Essence of Nursing and Health*, Thorofare, NJ: Charles B. Slack, Inc., 1988. (Reprinted in 1990 by Wayne State University Press, Detroit, MI).

8. Leininger, M., "Culture Care Theory: The Comparative Global Theory to Advance Human Care Nursing Knowledge and Practice," in *A Global Agenda for Caring*, D. Gaut, ed., New York: National League for Nursing Press, 1993, pp. 3–18.

9. Leininger, op. cit., 1991.

10. World Bank, *Confronting AIDS*: *Public Priorities in a Global Epidemic*, New York: Oxford University Press, 1997.

11. Nelson, K., D. Celentano, S. Eiumtrakol, et al., "Changes in Sexual Behavior and a Decline in HIV Infection Among Young Men in Thailand," *New England Journal of Medicine*, 1996, pp. 297–303, 335.

12. UNAIDS, *Facing the Challenges of HIV/AIDS/STDs: A Gender-Based Response*, 1998b. Published by the Royal Tropical Institute: Amsterdam, The Netherlands and the Southern Africa AIDS Information Dissemination Service: Harare, Zimbabwe.

13. Cohen, M., I. Hoffman, R. Royce, et al., "Reduction of Concentration of HIV-1 in Semen After Treatment of Urethritis: Implications for Prevention of Sexual Transmission of HIV-1," *Lancet*, 1997 pp. 349, 1868–1873.

14. Grosskuth, H., F. Mosha, J. Tood, et al., "Impact of Improved Treatment of Sexually Transmitted Diseases on HIV Infection in Rural Tanzani: Randomized Control Trial," *Lancet*, 1995, pp. 346, 530–536.

15. Laga, M., A. Manoka, M. Kivivu, et al., "Non-ulcerative Sexually Transmitted Diseases on HIV as Risk Factors for HIV-1 Transmission in Women: Results from a Cohort Study, " *AIDS*, 1993, pp. 7, 95–102.

16. UNAIDS, op. cit., 1998b.

17. Field, M., "Listening to Patients: Targeted Intervention Research to Improve STD Programs," *AIDSCaptions*, 1996, v. III, no. 1, pp. 16–20. Family Health International.

18. Leininger, op. cit., 1988.

19. Leininger, op. cit., 1991.

20. UNAIDS, op. cit., 1999.

21. Osborn, C., E. van Praag, and H. Jackson, "Models of Care for People with HIV/AIDS," *AIDS*, 1997, v. 11, suppl. B, pp. S135–S141.

22. Gilks, C. K. Floyd, D. Haran, et al., *Sexual Health and Health Care: Care and Support for People with HIV/AIDS in Resource Poor Settings*, London: Department for International Development, 1998.

23. MacNeil, J., "Use of Culture Care Theory with Baganda Women as AIDS Caregivers," *Journal of Transcultural Nursing*, 1996, v. 7, no. 2, pp. 14–20.

24. MacNeil, J., F. Mberesero, and G. Kilonzo, "Is Care and Support Associated with Preventive Behavior Among People with HIV?" *AIDSCare*, 1995, v. 11, no. 5, pp. 537–546.

25. Valdiserri, R., M. Moor, A. Gerber, and C. Campbell, "A Study of Clients Returning for Counseling After HIV Testing: Implication for Improving Rates of Tests Return," *Public Health Reports*, 1993, v. 108, no. 1 pp. 12–18.

26. Centers for Disease Control and Prevention, "Update: HIV Counseling and Testing — United States," *MMWR*, 1995, v. 47, no. 11, pp. 211–215.

27. Wilkinson, D., N. Wilkinson, C. Lombard, et al., "On-Site HIV Testing in Resource-Poor Settings: Is One Rapid Test Enough?" *AIDS*, 1997, v. 11, pp. 577–581.

28. United States Supreme Court, "U.S. Supreme Court June 25, 1998," in *U.S. Supreme Court Syllabus*, 1998, pp. 97–156.

29. American Dental Association, *National Policy on HIV/AIDS*. Washington, DC: American Dental Association, 1991.

30. Leininger, op. cit., 1988.

31. Roach, Sr. S., "The Call to Consciousness: Compassion in Today's Health World," in *Caring: The Compassionate Healer*, D. Gaut and M. Leininger, eds., New York: National League for Nursing Press, 1991, pp. 7–10.

32. World Bank, op. cit., 1997.

33. Agency for Health Care Policy and Research, *Evaluation and Management of Early HIV Infection: Clinical Practice Guideline*, Rockville, MD: U.S. Department of Health and Human Services, 1994, p. 7.

34. Connor, E., R. Sperling, R. Gelber, et al., "Reduction of Maternal-Infant Transmission of Human Immunodeficiency Virus Type 1 with Zidovudine Treatment. Pediatric Clinical Trials Group Protocol 076 Study Group," *New England Journal of Medicine*, 1994, v. 331, pp. 1173–1180.

35. Department of Health and Human Services, *Guidelines for the Use of Antiretrovirals Agents in*

HIV-Infected Adults and Adolescents, Bethesda, MD: National Institutes of Health, June 17, 1998.

36. Centers for Disease Control and Prevention, "Administration of Zidovudine During Pregnancy and Delivery to Prevent Perinatal HIV Transmission-Thailand," 1996–1998. *MMWR*, (March 6, 1998), v. 47, no. 8, pp. 151–154.

37. Jackson, B. and T. Flening, "A Phase IIB Randomized, Controlled Trial to Evaluate the Safety, Tolerance, and HIV Vertical Transmission Rates Associated with Short-Course Nevirapene (NVP) vs. Short-Course Zidovudine (ZDV) in HIV-Infected Pregnant Women and Their Families in Uganda: Executive Summary," *HIVNET 012 Protocol Team*: Makerere University, John Hopkins University, and NIAID, July 12, 1999.

38. UNAIDS, WHO, and UNICEF, "Consensus Statement on Infant Feeding and HIV." *Geneva: World Health Organization*, 1998.

39. Centers for Disease Control and Prevention, "Case-Control Study of HIV Seroconversion in Healthcare Workers After Percutaneous Exposure to HIV-Infected Blood — France, United Kingdom, and United States, January 1988–August 1994," *MMWR*, 1995, v. 44, pp. 929–933.

40. Buve, A., "Mortality Among Female Nurses in the Face of the AIDS Epidemic: A Pilot Study in Zambia," *AIDS*, 1994, v. 8, p. 396.

41. Hunter, S. and G. Williamson, *Children on the Brink*, Washington, DC: United States Agency for International Development, 1997.

42. Leininger, op. cit., 1988.

43. Leininger, op. cit., 1991.

44. Leininger, M., *Transcultural Nursing: Concept, Theories, Research, and Practice*, Columbus, OH: McGraw Hill College Custom Series, 1995.

45. MacNeil, op. cit., 1996.

46. Ibid.

47. Lwanga, J., "Children Whose Parents Die of AIDS (abstract WTR308)," paper presented at the VI International Conference on AIDS in Africa, Dakar, Senegal, January, 1991.

13

Urban USA Transcultural Care Challenges with Multiple Cultures and Culturally Diverse Providers

Beverly Horn

This chapter is focused on issues and challenges related to the fact that urban transcultural care exists largely within a multicultural context with multiple health care providers in the large United States cities. This theme will be presented with the use of discovered culture care constructs within Leininger's theory of Culture Care.[1] The Sunrise Model will be used with the cultural and social dimensions discussed within the urban context with diverse health care providers. All of these factors become part of the decision-making model of the health care team in partnership with clients to achieve culturally congruent care. Culture care preservation and maintenance, cultural care accommodation and negotiation, and cultural care repatterning and restructuring are practice strategies used to arrive at culturally competent care.

Transcultural nursing literature frequently focuses on the interactions of nurses from one culture who are caring for client(s) from a different culture. Frequently, the literature features caregivers that are Euro-Americans caring for persons from a single cultural group that is not Euro-American. Cultural beliefs and values are explored sensitively and in-depth. Most research in transcultural caring in nursing reflects careful use of the ethnonursing method so that transcultural care data about a specific culture are thoroughly documented. Knowledge about cultural care universalities and diversities has contributed to the development of the current body of transcultural knowledge. Transcultural norms, values, and beliefs that affect cultural caring are described.

The reality of urban society in the United States today (as well as in many other countries of the world) is that health care practice requires knowledge of multiple cultures that are constantly undergoing change. The multicultural nature of urban society offers rich and abundant care experiences and challenges for all health care providers. Cultural care competence in these situations involves the ability to function effectively in the context of cultural differences. To practice cultural care competence requires that one first understands his or her own cultural heritage and the roots of his or her care values, beliefs, attitudes, and practices.

A major principle underlying cultural diversity is that there is as much or more intracultural diversity as there is intercultural diversity.[2] This means that within-group differences are as great or greater than differences across groups. Many subcultures exist within a culture, and subcultures exert a great influence on all of us. For example, within the United States subcultures of race, ethnicity, gender, age, and sexual orientation are present.[3] Persons may see themselves as part of many subcultures or predominantly from one subculture. Assumptions cannot be made about anyone until one finds out how he or she views major cultural influences in his or her life. A cultural assessment of caring beliefs and values is essential.

The Context: Multiculturalism in the United States

From the beginning the historical heritage of the United States has reflected a multicultural context. Indigenous people lived on the land that later became the United States. Although today we refer to indigenous cultures as Indian or Native-American Indian, the reality is that indigenous peoples have many different cultures. Although forced to reside in places designated by the federal government in the 19th and 20th centuries, the diversities of these cultures have survived. Today, Native Americans refer to themselves by tribal names that reflect their unique cultural heritages such as the Ojibwa, the Lummi, and the Choctaw Nations, and they are making important contributions to American society and culture.

The history of the United States includes early settling by persons from Northern, Eastern, Southern, and Western Europe in the late 18th and early 19th centuries. Each group brought its own culture, and although English became the official language, early settlers retained many of their own beliefs, values, and practices. Adaptation and enculturation, described in other places in this book, took place. The melting pot ideology that there would be a single American culture with a single language for everyone has never become a reality.

A major cultural influence throughout the history of the American colonies and the independent United States was the introduction of African slaves for economic purposes. Contributions to the fabric of American life by the original slaves and their heirs continue to have a major influence that is much more than economic. Slaves and freed men from African countries brought rich and wonderful cultures, which did not disappear, even under the extreme pressures exerted by slavery. Today, the influence of African cultures is evident in all of American culture in science, the arts, religion, and every other aspect of American life. Also, in the past decade new refugees have come to the United States from East Africa, primarily Somalia, Ethiopia, and Eritrea, and are making their own unique contributions to the American cultural context.

After World War II, during the remainder of the 20th century, and now into the 21st century, the United States has had a constant flow of both refugees and immigrants who often have faced social and political upheaval. Adair et al.[4] point out that today refugees are arriving in the United States at the highest rate since World War II. Recent arrivals have come from Africa, Bosnia, and the former Soviet Union rather than from Southeast Asia or Latin America as in the past. In some parts of the United States, large immigrant pools who are not refugees come from the Pacific Islands such as Guam, the Philippines, Tonga, and others. Again, cultural influences are often profound as these relative newcomers participate in American life. DeSantis noted that ". . . immigration is an ongoing phenomenon that is increasing in magnitude and complexity."[5] Further. As Leininger noted, ". . . there is a growing trend in the Western world to care for clients in diverse community-based health care contexts, and health care will be driven by consumers of diverse and similar cultures."[6]

In summary, health and health care are very much affected by the multicultural nature of American society today. This phenomenon is reflected in both the health care team and in clients. For nursing as a discipline, this influence is clearly evident in cultural care and caring and poses many challenges for the practicing nurse of today and for the future, whether the nurse is a seasoned practitioner or only a beginner in the 21st century.

■ Challenges in Health Care and Caring

Multicultural Health Care Teams

A major challenge for all health care providers today is the multicultural nature of the health care team itself. Not only are health care providers caring for a multitude of persons from cultures other than their own, but also they are in constant interaction with other health care providers from diverse cultures. Such multiculturalism of today's urban centers in the United States influences relationships between and among health care providers and clients.

Some contend that managed care provides unique opportunities for transcultural nurses to influence decision making in a participatory manner in a multicultural health care team.[7] With managed care, many health care decisions are based on population statistics rather than on a client-by-client basis.[8] The cultural context of the client is not taken into consideration in these decisions, unless the transcultural nurse as a partner in the team can provide information about the meaning, for instance, of "cancer prevention" within the client's culture. An example is cancer-prevention education that focuses on breast self-examination, which for some cultures may be a sensitive topic. The challenge for the nurse is to work in partnership in a culturally congruent manner and to have a significant impact on the health care decisions affecting one or many multicultural clients. Uhl Pierce states the following:

> Actually, the multidisciplinary approach required in many managed care organizations has provided the professional nurse a wonderful opportunity to more actively participate in planning, decision making, communicating, and managing cultural care for those they serve.[9]

Urban United States settings are most often multicultural in nature simply because they are large population centers and attract new immigrants for a variety of reasons. Wars, famine, and a desire for a better way of living are just some of the forces influencing the influx of these persons. However, a major force is economic because jobs are more readily available and provide more opportunities for a better life for immigrants and refugee families in the United States than in many other countries. Some immigrants are highly educated and qualified in professional fields such as the health care field. Those who are not qualified often try to become professionally licensed in the United States and then are employed in professional positions. The high value placed on education by many immigrants and refugees has also challenged them to move into the American educational system rapidly, and some have entered the professional health care fields. As a consequence, multicultural dilemmas face health care providers who are also caring for or treating multicultural populations. How can these dilemmas be addressed in a culturally competent manner? Is there a systematic way that one might approach this kind of care in urban settings? Using a model, a theory, or components of a variety of theories may enable nurses and other health care providers to function in a culturally competent manner and provide culturally congruent care. Leininger's Culture Care theory offers one meaningful and helpful approach to this challenge.[10]

Transcultural Nursing Research Findings Applied to Multicultural Situations

Over the past four decades, Leininger's theory of Culture Care Diversity and Universality has helped transcultural nurses to study diverse cultures with a focus on dominant culture care constructs.[11] Twelve dominant culture care constructs have been discovered with extensive research. These care constructs can be applied as common care modalities in urban multicultural health care settings along with particular diversities of findings from the social structure factors. The following are the twelve dominant health care constructs, presented in priority ranking, which have been discovered with Leininger's Culture Care theory as universal or dominant care constructs:[12]

1. Respect for/about (most universal care construct)
2. Concern for/about
3. Attention to (details)/with anticipation of
4. Helping, assisting, and facilitative acts
5. Active listening
6. Giving presence (being there physically)
7. Understanding their cultural beliefs, values, lifeways
8. Being connected to/or relatedness
9. Protection of/for (some gender and kin differences)
10. Touching (how, where, and when varied)
11. Providing comfort measures
12. Showing filial love (family, and love to others)

Using these care constructs can be powerful guides to help with many cultures with common care expectations and needs. This chapter will not discuss how all of them are important in health care encounters, but will focus only on the first universal care construct, which is *respect*. The transcultural nursing research discovery of respect as the most universal care construct is an important discovery. Even if one had very little knowledge about a specific culture, a sense of respect for the other culture needs to be upheld and understood. If the care provider(s) have respect, concern for and about others will undoubtedly occur. An example is a child undergoing a bone marrow transplant for acute leukemia. This child's family was from Greece and the health care team did not understand some of the behaviors of the family. For example, the family asked that the child not be told of her condition. The transcultural nurse as a member of the health care team described in conference how important it was to gain the family's respect and trust. She brought transcultural reading material to the team that helped them to understand and show respect for the wishes of the family. The mother stated to the nurse that she felt everyone on the team respected their manner of doing things. The family then was open to hear what the health care team members suggested as well. The other constructs in practice may be used as appropriate in a specific situation and can be used to evaluate transcultural care and caring. All the care constructs are important, and all build on the universal and major care construct of respect that the health care team members have for one another, for the client, and for the client's family. Thus, in turn, respect is demonstrated by the client for all involved.

 ## Use of the Sunrise Model in Understanding Multicultural Situations

In addition to using the caring constructs, situations that arise in multicultural situations can be systematically addressed by identifying them as components of the Sunrise Model. Leininger's Sunrise Model[13] enables a caregiver to study several cultures simultaneously using the enthnonursing research method. This method, described elsewhere,[14] has proved to be a powerful generator of cultural knowledge and did result in the establishment of the twelve dominant culture care constructs leading to culturally congruent care and health as the goal of the theory. Further knowledge generated in this manner enables caregivers to work in a culturally competent way as they identify situations that fit with one or several dimensions of the Sunrise Model of the Theory of Culture Care. The following discussion will not use the Sunrise Model to explicate the cultural and social structural dimensions of a single culture, but rather to identify some factors that need to be addressed with multiple transcultural care practices. Specific examples will be given. The caveat to the reader is that these are simply culture-specific examples and that generalizations to all cultures cannot be made; otherwise, stereotyping may occur, which is counter to transcultural nursing practices.

Educational Factors

For both caregivers and clients alike, one cannot assume that the Western biomedical model or allopathic medicine is the dominant educational model. Assumptions that caregivers and clients from different cultures

accept the biomedical model can be as deleterious to healthy outcomes as to assume that they ascribe to folk and generic care only. Even though persons are prepared as professionals and meet the requirements for licensure, their model of health care may be quite different from the biomedical model. For example, for many cultures folk and generic care practices are seen as integral to health care and healthy outcomes and not simply alternative modalities. Leininger[15] has discussed that the term alternative was often not acceptable to non-Western caregivers. An example that demonstrated the model, including biomedicine and other practices, was a health care team in a clinic that included a physician from India, a Vietnamese social worker, an Eritrean public health provider, and a Euro-American nurse; the latter was also a transcultural nurse. These health care providers expressed concern that some of the clinic clients might be taking nonprescription herbal remedies and medicines that conflict with prescription medications. To ask clients directly most often leads to client fears and limited or little information. The health care team decided to have focus groups with different cultural groups to find out what kinds of folk and generic care practices were in common use. The focus group leaders were members of the cultural group and became collaborators with the health care team. Based on data obtained, the health care team was able to develop a short guide that had culturally appropriate questions to obtain accurate information about generic and professional care. An educational program for clients regarding drug interactions was the result and was used as an informative and educational guide for persons of diverse cultures.

Economic Factors

Economic factors affect care in powerful ways with multicultural providers and clients. Although the cost of care is important, the economic factors of the cultural systems are addressed here. Social status in many cultures includes financial and other resource holdings such as property, land, and animals. In most cultures a kind of class system exists, and although the class system itself does not necessarily carry over into the United States, the emotional and attitudinal factors are found in most cultures. Further, the transcultural nurse and other health care providers on the team may not know of culture-specific referent factors used in a particular culture. For example, a Somali woman from a wealthy, high-class family in Somalia was alone in a northwestern United States city and about to deliver her first child. She was on Medicaid and thus experienced many of the hassles that Medicaid and government-assisted clients endure. The dietitian and the social worker on the team were also Somali but from a lower class. They had been in the United States longer than the client, were educated in the Western model, and were equally competent in their own cultural model as well. The client needed information on diet, how to get food stamps, and how to obtain food from a food bank. She did not trust the Somalis on the health care team because they were of a different class. The transcultural nurse who was not Somali was able to obtain this information and discuss it with the health care team. The nurse used Leininger's cultural care accommodation/negotiation mode. The nurse arranged to accompany the client to the food bank so that the client could be assisted in finding the place and obtaining the food. Respect and trust existed between the nurse and client as a result of this encounter. However, it was necessary for the client to apply for food stamps through the Somali social worker. The transcultural nurse negotiated with the client to accompany her to the health and human service office to meet with the Somali social worker. The outcomes were most favorable for the client and rewarding for the transcultural nurse to witness. The accommodation/negotiation action/decision mode of the Culture Care theory was clearly and successfully used.[16]

Political and Legal Factors

A complex interplay of political and legal factors exists in almost every urban multicultural health care context or multicultural health care team and with multicultural clients. Lack of awareness of these factors could lead to culturally incongruent care. Health care providers, including transcultural nurses, cannot be expected to know all of these factors for every cultural group. However, "holding knowledge" of a culture and ethnohistorical factors provide valuable insights.[17] For instance, a transcultural nurse should ask, "Who have been political oppressors of whom over the many centuries?" or "What countries have taken over others and occupied

them for years?" Feelings and attitudes generally carry over for centuries. Examples include those countries that have experienced tribal warfare up to the present such as Ethiopia, Bosnia, and Albania. The long wars between Ethiopia and Eritrea have influenced health care interactions in the United States and other places where people from these places have come as refugees. In addition, major differences exist in the cultural care values, beliefs, and practices between Vietnamese and ethnic Chinese Vietnamese persons. Often Korean persons have a residual resentment for Japanese because of Japan's long occupation of Korea.

A common example of cultural diversity within a country in cities with a large Ethiopian population is the use of several different languages. An Ethiopian mother brought her 6-year-old son to a clinic with a high fever. She could not speak English and her native language was Oromo. Although there was a male interpreter present who could speak Oromo, she appeared very uncomfortable and said she preferred her 6-year-old son to be the interpreter for her. The transcultural nurse in this setting was able to elicit from the mother that this interpreter was from another group whose dominant language was Tigrigna, a language spoken by tribes different from this woman. There was another interpreter that was from the mother's tribal group, and the nurse was able to have this interpreter come to interpret for this woman. In this situation the transcultural nurse used cultural care assessment and realized that cultural care accommodation was essential to handle this critical language and caring dilemma.

Cultural Values and Lifeways

Cultural values and lifeways are very important dimensions of the Sunrise Model and the Culture Care theory as cultural values shape one's worldview and behavior patterns. An example of a cultural value that differs markedly among cultures is time. In community-based urban clinics appointments are held as important to care for many clients, and so clients are expected to adhere to a specific time to be at the clinic. Health care providers are also expected to care for clients within a fairly regular time frame. A major conflict regarding time occurred in a clinic where many of the clients were Latino and the providers were Latino, African American, and Euro-American. The African American and Euro-American providers were concerned that the Latino nurse did not adhere to the schedule as well as the other providers did. The Latino nurse was also a transcultural nurse and collected some research papers on the views of time for different cultures and distributed and discussed them with the other providers at a team conference. It was clear that some cultural care repatterning, as well as cultural care accommodation and negotiation, would be needed to provide culturally congruent care. Together the team members decided to change the schedule so there would be 5 to 10 minutes added to each appointment, providing culture care accommodation to meet the cultural needs of the clients and care providers. The clinic stayed open an extra half hour each day to prevent compromising income and also to make the response to cultural differences in views of time an important factor in planning and providing client care. Although not a perfect solution, this approach was respectful of clients' time and values and was most satisfying to Latino clients.

Kinship and Social Factors

Kinship and social factors are critical in successful transcultural nursing and interdisciplinary health care services. Understanding roles and relationships of various family members is essential in providing culturally competent care. A multicultural team whose members have understanding of their own kinship and the significance of social relationships needs to know those factors about the cultures they attempt to serve. An example of a transcultural situation occurred with an outbreak of meningitis among some Mexican migrant workers' children. The health care team obtained the necessary antibiotic preventative medications and delivered them personally to homes in a rather large area and explained to the mothers why their children should take the medicine. On a return visit 1 week later it was found that many children had not taken the medicine. The team consulted a respected older woman in the Mexican community. She explained that the men, who were the decision makers in the family, were in the fields when the health care team made their first visit. The team found out that the men were only home during the evening, and so evening home visits were made stressing the importance to the men of taking the med-

ication. After this was done, all of the children who needed the medication took it. This is an example of using cultural care accommodation that led to a healthy and satisfactory outcome for the children and their families.

Religious and Philosophical Factors

Religious and philosophical factors also play a major role in providing culturally congruent care. In large United States urban areas many religions are found. Often, the care providers may be Christian, Coptic, Orthodox Christian, Jewish, Muslim, or Buddhist and provide care for persons from the same or different religions. With many religions, dietary factors must be taken into consideration when providing health care. Food proscriptions, how food is prepared, who has blessed the food, and times of fasting are very important factors. The meaning of hot and cold foods may or may not be a part of the religious belief system. Life events such as birth, illness, and death have specific religious meanings and involve rituals for each culture. An example of how religious beliefs and practices must be taken into consideration in planning care was a series of parenting classes taught to recently immigrated Muslim women who lived in a housing project. Lunch for mothers and children was an integral part of the educational program for mothers and children and to help mothers understand the kinds of foods necessary to provide nourishment. However, the social worker, who was Muslim, reminded the two nurses that it was the month of Ramadan, and Muslim women could not eat until after sundown. Cultural care accommodation was again the guide for transcultural nursing practices. The nurses planned that Muslim women could take home food and eat it after sundown.

Technological Factors

Technology has a variety of meanings to diverse cultures from the elementary ideas such as dependence on a bicycle for all transportation to airline travel. In urban United States clinics, hospitals, and home visiting agencies multicultural health team members are generally more sophisticated about the language and practice of high technologies than clients. Many of the therapeutic measures require computers and other machinery to be effective. Injections are frequently given for a variety of reasons and are examples of readily understood technology. In one instance, flu shots were being given in a church basement after services on Sunday. Clients lined up, bared their arms and received the injections in their upper arms. A non–English-speaking couple seemed agitated, especially the husband. However, he did know a few words of English, and it became clear that he wanted his wife to have the shot, but did not want her arm bared in public. The nurse in this situation was able to accommodate the couple by having the woman step behind a coat rack where she was not directly visible to others in the large open room. Although this is not an example of complex technology, the interplay of technology and culture are evident in what was a very brief but important health care situation where cultural care accommodation/negotiation was practiced to provide a healthy outcome that was satisfactory to both the woman and her husband.

Summary

In this chapter a few major issues and challenges in urban health care in the United States (with multicultural providers and clients) have been presented. Culturally congruent care involves cultural competence in many contexts and focused on a central goal of transcultural nursing, but is also useful to other providers. In the urban society of the United States today, nurses care for clients from many diverse cultures simultaneously, and the complex interplay of multicultural situations as presented in this chapter can be found in most urban health care settings in the United States. Findings from transcultural nursing research have documented the importance of dominant health care constructs, as well as the use of Leininger's[18] three modes of nursing care decisions and actions to attain and maintain culturally congruent care practices, which are valuable to guide nurses in these complex situations. Leininger also noted that the purpose of the theory of Culture Care ". . . was to discover, document, interpret, explain, and predict multiple factors influencing and explaining care from a cultural holistic perspective."[19] More research is urgently needed in the area of multicultural, multidisciplinary health care in both urban and rural health care settings. The topic of how cultural care preservation/maintenance, cultural care accommodation/negotiation and cultural care repatterning (as the three modes of nursing actions and decisions) assist nurses in providing culturally congruent care requires further study with documented outcomes in clinical contexts and in homes and other settings. In summary, available research already discovered in transcultural caring provides an abundant source of data for nursing decisions and actions, but more research is needed to determine effectiveness and outcomes of transcultural caring in multicultural contexts.

References

1. Leininger, M., *Culture Care Diversity and Universality: A Theory of Nursing*, New York: National League for Nursing Press, 1991.
2. Kluckhohn, F. and P. Brink, "Dominant and Variant Value Orientations," in *Transcultural Nursing*, Prospect Heights, IL: Waveland Press, 1976, pp. 63–81.
3. Erlen, J. A., "Culture, Ethics and Respect: The Bottom Line to Understanding," *Orthopaedic Nursing*, 1998, v. 17, no. 16, p. 79.
4. Adair, R., O. Nwarneri, and N. Barnes, "Health Care Access for Somali Refugees: Views of Patients, Doctors, Nurses," *American Journal of Health Behavior*, 1999, v. 23, no. 4, pp. 286–292.
5. DeSantis, L., "Building Healthy Communities with Immigrants and Refugees," *Journal of Transcultural Nursing*, 1997, v. 9, no. 1, pp. 20–31.
6. Leininger, M., *Transcultural Nursing: Concepts, Themes, Records & Practice*, Blacklick, OH: College McGraw-Hill Series, 1995, p. 20.
7. McKay, T. A., "Managed Care: A Turning Point for Nursing," *Journal of Transcultural Nursing*, 1999, v. 10, no. 4, p. 292.
8. Uhl Pierce, J., "Managing Managed Care: The Next Level for Transcultural Nurses," *Journal of Transcultural Nursing*, 1999, v. 10, no. 3, pp. 181–182.
9. Ibid. p. 181.
10. Leininger, op. cit., 1991.
11. Ibid.
12. Leininger, M., "Special Research Report: Dominant Culture Care (Emic) Meanings and

Practice Findings from Leininger's Theory,"
Journal of Transcultural Nursing, 1998, v. 9, no. 2,
pp. 45–48.

13. Leininger, op. cit., 1991.

14. Leininger, M., "Overview of the Theory of Culture
    Care with the Ethnonursing Research Method,"
    Journal of Transcultural Nursing, 1997b, v. 8, no. 2,
    pp. 32–52.

15. Leininger, M., "Alternative to What? Generic vs.
    Professional Caring, Treatments, and Healing
    Modes," *Journal of Transcultural Nursing*, 1997a,
    v. 9, no. 1, p. 37.

16. Leininger, op. cit., 1997.

17. Leininger, op. cit., 1995.

18. Leininger, op. cit., 1991, p. 39.

19. Leininger, op. cit., 1995.

14

Ethical, Moral, and Legal Aspects of Transcultural Nursing*

Madeleine Leininger

When nurses understand and incorporate ethics of care from a transcultural perspective into all aspects of nursing, we will have achieved one of the greatest and most meaningful services to humankind. LEININGER, 1988

This chapter focuses on selected aspects of transcultural differences and similarities with respect to values, beliefs, and practices of Western and non-Western cultures with nursing implications. Understanding and acting on ethical, moral, and legal values, norms, and practices among human cultures is one of the greatest challenges for nurses today. Some examples of cultural differences are presented to help nurses understand *why* clients may hold firmly to their ethical and moral values in life-and-death situations and why nurses need to respond appropriately. In this chapter "ethics" refers to how *individuals or groups* should or ought to behave, *whereas* "morals" *refers to how individuals or groups need to conduct themselves with respect to what is held to be good, bad, right, or wrong.*[1] "Legal" *describes those claimed rights and acts of individuals or groups that are enforced, maintained, or regulated by law.*[2] Ethical and moral expressions, values, and beliefs tend to be buttressed by multiple social-structure factors, but especially by religious beliefs, philosophical views, and specific cultural values that vary transculturally in meaning and expression.

* This paper has been revised with updated material from *Ethical and Moral Dimensions of Care*, M. Leininger, ed., Detroit, Wayne State University Press, 1988, pp. 49–66 and the 1995 edition of *Transcultural Nursing: Concepts, Theories, Research and Practice*, Blacklick, OH, McGraw-Hill College Series, pp. 295–311.

 ## Worldwide General and Professional Concerns

The topics of ethics, morals, and legal actions or decisions are of interest to all health professionals because they influence the welfare and survival of those served in professional relationships. However, health professionals are not alone, as government officials, politicians, and most scientists and humanists are expected to be knowledgeable about ethical and moral dimensions of their work. Moreover, in recent years, world leaders and citizens have become increasingly vocal about violations of human rights and injustices reflecting unethical behaviors. Many cultures have demanded that unethical or immoral behavior be seriously addressed at local, national, and worldwide levels. Ethical, moral, and legal issues are a growing concern in all areas of health relationships and as worldwide health care issues.

With rapid modes of communication and transportation, people from many different cultures are coming in close contact with one another with intercultural ethical conflicts. Among world strangers are differences in beliefs, values, and actions that often lead to tensions, conflicts, and misunderstandings. As a consequence, ethical, moral, and legal behaviors can often be identified among cultural strangers in business and a variety of work and home-life situations. While one might assume or hope that all humans have similar ethical and moral behaviors to guide their actions, this is not the case. In fact, there seem to be more diversities than anticipated among non-Western and Western cultures worldwide because of different values and lifeways and because of enculturation and acculturation differences. However, it is always important to search for universal or common values amid cultural diversities for human connectedness and relationships. It is imperative for health personnel to learn about transcultural differences and similarities with respect to ethical and moral behaviors among human beings worldwide for appropriate actions and decisions. One must also be aware of the dangers of cultural relativity and stereotyping and should not judge all cultures or situations as totally unique unless adequately documented.

There has been an increased focus on moral, ethical, and legal issues related to nursing care services during the past decade. Many ethical issues have come to the foreground as a result of the marked increase in using a vast array of new technologies, medicines, treatments, and care practices. Many ethical problems arise as the nurse attempts to help clients with their particular concerns and needs from different cultures or subcultures. Today, many clients are also quick to state if their ethical rights have been threatened or violated in health care services. They may seek clarification, pose ethical questions, or seek legal restitution for any ethical violations. Since nurses work so closely with clients in life, death, and in a variety of daily and nightly contexts, they are exposed to many ethical and legal issues. Some nurses are sensitive to violating the client's ethical rights, while other nurses may try to avoid the issue or not be concerned.

Ethics courses are increasing in schools of nursing to inform nurses of ethical and moral issues in education and service settings. It is of interest that in the 1940s to 1960s many nurses had ethics courses in their programs, but in the high technology era of the late 1960s, there was limited time for such instruction. Today, there is a renewed emphasis on nursing ethics because of many consumer professional issues. A number of nurse ethicists such as Aroskar,[3] Carper,[4] Curtin and Flaherty,[5] Davis,[6] Fowler,[7] Fry,[8,9] Gadow,[10] Leininger,[11–13] Ray,[14,15] Veach and Fry,[16] Watson,[17] and Watson and Ray[18] are teaching philosophical and spiritual views, theories, research findings, and principles to help nurses deal with ethical

issues in clinical, research, education, and consultation practices. There are other nurse ethicists who address a variety of nurse/client and other issues. In addition, the scholarly thinking of other ethical and moral theorists or philosophers such as Beauchamp and Childress,[19] Callahan,[20] Gilligan,[21] MacIntyre,[22] Noddings,[23] Pellegrino et al.,[24] and Toulmin et al.[25] continues to influence the thinking and writings of nurses. Western and some non-Western ethical and morality issues are being studied today by health personnel along with many new experimental areas, such as human gene engineering, drugs, and the use of fetal tissue for research. Many additional areas related to birth, living, and dying such as abortion, euthanasia, and assisted suicide include important ethical and moral issues to be studied by nurses.

A most critical and neglected area in teaching and research today concerns transcultural nursing ethical and moral issues. Since the advent of transcultural nursing, only a few research studies have been done, and many schools of nursing have limitedly examined the importance of cultural ethics. How different cultures define, interpret, and practice ethical and moral behavior is only slowly entering nursing and the health professions. The author initiated this focus as an important and essential dimension for nurses' consideration when transcultural nursing was launched and with writings since the 1960s.[26,27] Transcultural nursing is providing nurses with many different ethical insights about illnesses, treatments, and death issues in different cultures.[28] Transcultural leaders are encouraging nurses and physicians to study ethical and moral cultural health care issues and how to resolve or prevent serious ethical dilemmas in clinical practices and research.[29] Interdisciplinary ethical issues have increased as health professionals work closely together.

The Importance of Transcultural Ethical, Moral, and Legal Care Knowledge

The author takes the position that the transcultural ethical, moral, and legal aspects of nursing care are very important issues for professional nurses today. Nurses are challenged to learn how diverse cultures know and practice ethical, moral, and legal aspects of birth, life and death issues. Nurses are challenged to learn ethical decisions and values that are not easy to learn because they are largely embedded into the clients' cultural values, practices, and social structure. Specific examples are often necessary to identify ethical values, beliefs and disparities along with commonalities among cultures.

One of the prevailing myths and beliefs among nurses is that Western and Eastern ethical and moral philosophies are similar worldwide or "should" be alike even though great differences often exist among cultures. Some nurses believe that similar ethical values can be used to care for clients from any culture whether from Africa, the Middle East, Southeast Asia, or South America. This myth can lead to serious ethical and legal problems because there is far more ethical diversity than similarity among cultures. Nonetheless, nurses need to learn about ethical diversities and any universal ethical and moral features among cultures with respect to human values, morals, and legal rights. Otherwise, problems related to cultural impositions and clashes can occur with unfavorable consequences. Ethical client rights can be readily violated by nurses. *Most cultures have their own ethical beliefs, moral rules, and legal standards to guide, interpret, and support their actions and decisions. However, as commonalities or universals among cultures are known and respected, they can be shared. Indeed, transcultural nursing does not support cultural relativity totally but searches for human universals among variabilities.*

Gradually, ethical and moral knowledge of different cultures is being discovered by nurses, which expands their knowledge base and quality of care. Understanding ethical or moral decisions of "right" and "wrong" behaviors for Africans, Asians, Greeks, Jews, and other cultures in the world can facilitate care practices. The theory of Culture Care with the Sunrise Model is extremely helpful for discovering the multiple social structure factors in religious, kinship, legal-political, and other areas to identify the sources of ethical values and actions.[30]

With increased multiculturalism worldwide, transcultural ethical-moral knowledge has become extremely important to provide culturally congruent and ethically responsible care. Ethics needs to be taught early in nursing so that students will be alert to emic and etic client differences in ethical values and practices and with professional nursing cultural values. Clients and their families become upset when nurses are insensitive to or unaware of their ethical beliefs and perform actions that are offensive or inappropriate.[31] Understanding the client's ethical beliefs about birth and death situations are especially important when planning and providing care to clients. Inappropriate ethical decisions and care practices can lead to major legal suits and even destructive actions. Family members often identify when ethical or moral values are violated or not respected, especially in life-death situations.

As nurses learn about cultures and their humanistic ethical care needs, they soon realize that cultures live by different codes, beliefs, principles, standards, rules, and values according to their emic worldview. As ethical values are learned and passed on *intergenerationally*, they give people a stable *anchor or blueprint for living and dying.* Cultural values support ethical and moral decisions by which humans have almost automatic guides to deal with threats of illness, disability, treatment, death, and other life events.

Cultures have *ethical guides that enable them to respond to many situations as a "given" or natural way with strangers and nonstrangers.* Most ethical values are generally derived from one's worldview, religious beliefs, kinship norms, and reinforced cultural values in daily living. Cultural disparities and *variabilities* exist and need to be assessed and understood from cultural and transcultural viewpoints. The term "disparities" has recently come into vogue, but adds little to common and universal differences in almost everything.

As the nurse discovers different transcultural ethical, moral, and legal care knowledge, several questions need to be considered:

1. What are some of the similar and diverse beliefs, meanings, forms, expressions, symbols, metaphors, and values of ethical and moral care?
2. What specific ethical and moral values are universal or common among several cultures?
3. What are the meanings of dominant ethical values to the client, family, and community?
4. What are highly sensitive ethical behaviors or rules that the nurse needs to be alert to for quality care?
5. Are there gender and class differences regarding who carries out ethical or moral duties or procedures?
6. In what ways does the nurse's moral or ethical behavior hinder clients to receive appropriate care?

Such questions and others help the nurse to become sensitive to ethical behaviors that are important to cultures. At all times, the nurse remains an active listener and observer of what clients do, say, and philosophize about life and death situations and their interpretations of them. Current and past stories and religious accounts are valuable ways to learn about ethical and moral values and their importance.

 ## Cultural Differences, Examples, and Concerns

Ethical and moral comparative knowledge can be generated from several different sources, but rich discipline sources come from the following: transcultural nursing research, bioethics, anthropology, moral philosophy and theology, the humanities, and comparative international law and actions. Anthropologists have been studying cultures and ethical moral behavior for nearly a century, and so their work is important for gaining a comparative cultural perspective. The early work of Boas,[32] Herskovits,[33] and Kluckhohn[34] and the more recent work of Downing and Kushner,[35] Haviland,[36] Lanham,[37] and Leininger[38] are a few examples of work by scholars about ethics of different cultures. These researchers have identified how cultures learn, establish, and maintain certain ethical and moral rules, norms, rights, and legal sanctions related to the prevention of illnesses and death and ways to prevent cultural conflicts in health care practices. For example, most cultures such as Native Americans and Canadians have explicit legal and ethical rights and ways to protect their health, lives, land, food, property, and children. Anthropological knowledge of how cultures handle ethical problems and when their rights are violated awaits full use in transcultural nursing and general nursing. Cultures will fight to defend their ethical rights, even at the cost of human lives and property damage. In general, *ethical, moral, and legal rights are powerful areas to understand and value in cultures worldwide.* Human beings generally live by ethical and cultural values, moral rights, legal justice buttressed by religious and spiritual beliefs and historical facts.

Transcultural nurse researchers continue to study cultural and ethical values and beliefs and how they influence clients, nurses, nursing education, and health care systems.[39–45] For example, Luna found that Arab Lebanese Muslim women held that it was unethical for Anglo-American nurses to press for bonding between a newborn infant and the father in a hospital nursing context as it was counter to their cultural values.[46] Among the Old Order Amish, Wenger found it was unethical to take pictures and use them for public purposes or to use high technologies in hospital nursing care without appropriate family consent.[47] Leininger discovered that the Gadsup people of New Guinea would consider a female nurse unethical if she revealed sex secrets to males in the village.[48] She also found that Arab Muslim clients make their own decisions when a loved one is dead. These beliefs must be respected by health personnel to avoid ethical imposition practices. Such examples and many others are found in transcultural nursing research studies and these findings need to be respected and understood.

Transcultural nurses and anthropologists who study moral, ethical, and legal values of specific cultures try to make this knowledge known to outsiders who attempt to violate the ethical rights of cultures. This protective stance is important when health professionals are unaware of culture-specific rights related to death, birth, marriage, abortions, circumcisions, gender, and even community property rights of cultures living in specific geographic areas. Ethical values about abortion, assisted suicide, and euthanasia practices are all sensitive issues in many cultures. For example, the author found the Gadsup villagers of New Guinea were stunned to learn that some Western women requested abortions. This was a cultural shock because the Gadsup people greatly value children and actively protect their newborns. Gadsup mothers and their kinswomen do everything possible to have healthy infants and consider it wrong to kill any fetus within or outside the womb. Also, consider the Eskimos who do not view a fetus as human until it is named, and so their ethical position is different about being a human. Many Catholics and other Christians believe that a fetus is human being from the time of conception and support the culture of life. Such ethical positions sharply contrast with "pro-abortion" and "pro-choice" supporters in the world.

There are also major ethical problems that nurses may experience in functioning in the Middle East or in Indonesian Arab Muslim cultures such as the removal of body organs for an organ transplant. This violates body integrity and religious beliefs. For Arab Muslims, the ethical principle is to keep the entire body (including all organs) intact and in their natural position. The whole body must be buried at death for their beliefs in afterlife. Arab Muslims also believe that it is unethical for physicians and nurses to tell an Arab client with cancer about the client's malignancy or impending death. It is Allah who knows and is guiding the Arab client's destiny, not health professionals.

As nurses study different cultures with focus on ethics and legal aspects, it is important to search for *both* universal (common features) with the diversities among and between cultures. This provides a comparative view and helps nurses to learn different ethical values of cultures. It is the shared universal ethical and moral values that help to promote peace, harmony, and general cultural understandings. The nurse will find the theory of Culture Care Diversity and Universality provides a valuable framework to discover transcultural ethical care differences and similarities.[49] With the use of the theory, the nurse will be able to search for explanations as found in the worldview, religious, kinship, education, historical, legal, cultural values, and professional experiences or in other areas that influence ethical and moral behaviors. The theory also helps nurses to contrast emic client data with nurses etic views about the sources of ethical, moral, and legal conflicts and taboos.

Another challenge for nurses is to study Western and non-Western philosophies, religion, and worldviews of the ways cultures explain or give meaning to their ethical, moral, and legal beliefs and actions. Nurses will find that in the Western cultures, there are generally *normative, descriptive, utilitarian, and deontological ways* to interpret or explain ethical behavior, but the nurse should *not* assume these are universal ethical principles and typologies. In many non-Western cultures ethical and moral behaviors are embedded in principles about the philosophy of life, spirituality, religion, kinship, and politics and in relation to culturally specific contextual situations. For example, the Gadsup of New Guinea rely on *distributive values* that are context-based and those based on ancestral norm directives that have been passed on intergenerationally as ethical guides of what to do or avoid.[50] In other non-Western cultures such as in Southeast Asia, there are multiple "spirits" that guide the ethical behavior such

as the Vietnamese Buddhists who are guided by many spirits. Hence, ethical and moral guides to behavior tend to vary considerably in Western and non-Western cultures.

Another related and major concern in nursing is the problem of *cultural imposition* nursing practices, which can influence the nurse's ethical decisions with clients and nursing outcomes. As defined earlier, cultural imposition refers to the tendency to impose one's own values, beliefs, and practices on another culture because of the belief that they are superior to or better than those of another person or group.[51] If nurses are not knowledgeable about the different ethical values of a culture, one can anticipate that cultural imposition practices will occur. Such imposition practices can lead to unethical acts, client dissatisfaction, noncompliance, stresses, and a host of other problems, including legal problems and counter-revenge terrorist practices.

Currently, one can identify several examples of cultural imposition practices in different nursing care contexts. To reduce or prevent such problems and negative consequences, the nurse needs to consider these self-examination questions:

1. What are my ethical beliefs and practices, and how can they influence the client's health and well-being?
2. How can nurses with strong ethnocentric values, biases, and actions prevent ethical dilemmas that lead to cultural imposition practices and ethical conflicts?
3. In what kinds of clinical illnesses or contexts do nurses tend to impose their professional and personal ethical beliefs or values on clients, families, or groups?
4. In what ways can nurses prevent cultural imposition or pain and best handle ethical or moral dilemmas?
5. What are the potential legal consequences associated with the nurse who violates a client's ethical values?

If the nurse begins with these questions and then tries to remain sensitive to clients with an open learning attitude toward the client and culture, many weighty ethical problems can be avoided, resolved, or reduced.

Today, many nurses are traveling to and working in unfamiliar cultures or with "cultural strangers."

Understanding the world of strangers who have different ethical and moral values and beliefs can be unsettling to nurses who like to be confident of their knowledge and skills. Nurses who do their homework before traveling to foreign countries and who are prepared in transcultural nursing can respond appropriately to ethical values and lifeways of the cultures. Cultural knowledge can reduce ethical stresses, conflicts, and imposition practices and prevent cultural problems and offensive acts. Since ethical values are seldom written down in explicit ways, the nurse has to study a culture's religious beliefs, values, and lifeways in advance and in-depth or should be mentored by transcultural specialists.

Interestingly, cultural strangers often show signs of being annoyed when they are refused help or are avoided by professional health personnel. Potential ethical conflicts and cultural offenses often exist and can be reduced by listening attentively to the clients' explanations and interpretations of *why* they avoid or are annoyed with personnel. The nurse can facilitate positive ethical relationships. Most importantly, the nurse searches to understand specific ethical values, cultural sanctions, cultural taboos, and specific religious conflicts. Some clients may also be very candid and explain their reasons for refusing certain nursing practices. The nurse's attitude of showing genuine respect, a caring interest, and sincerity with clients is most valuable in ethical nursing care practices.

Discovering the specific emic reasons underlying the client's unusual behavior often opens a whole new world of knowing. However, the nurse's knowledgeable responses can be most helpful to prevent premature judgments about the client's behavior. Imposing professional ethical values onto the client or the family may occur unintentionally or because the nurse does not know the client's cultural and ethical values. Nurses must be aware that some clients will be most hesitant to share some ethical and other cultural values because they fear that health professionals may misinterpret, demean, or devalue them, or that they may even deprive them of nursing care. For example, the nurse's ethical beliefs about abortion, AIDS, blood transfusions, folk remedies, gay or lesbian behavior, and other areas may lead to major conflicts with the client if the nurse expresses strong views about these matters and expects the client to accept the nurse's views.

In providing health teaching to a client, the nurse often discovers the client's ethical and moral views. The client may "test" the nurses ideas to see if they match. Cultural secrets are usually only shared if the client *trusts* the nurse or has moved from a stranger to friend role.[52] Since some ethical values and beliefs are complex and seemingly ambiguous, they may require some examples to be understood. Clients generally like to tell stories and give examples of their ethical beliefs and situations. Listening to stories takes patience, time, and focused attention along with the nurse's genuine interest in the story teller. The nurse should always recheck with the client to be sure of understandings and accurate interpretations of the clients' views, beliefs, or stories.

Selected Culture-Specific Ethical and Moral Research Care Values and Considerations

In transcultural nursing, it is essential to know cultural, ethical, and moral values and their potential transmission to offspring over time by identifing intergenerational enculturation and acculturation practices with clients. Rewards are often given to children and adults when they learn acceptable moral and ethical culture behaviors. Traditional cultures are quite conscientious in teaching and monitoring ethical behavior to their children throughout the life cycle, such as the Old Order Amish, Orthodox Jewish Americans, Hutterites, and others. Some cultures such as Anglo-Americans tend to be less conscientious in teaching ethical and moral values intergenerationally with their offspring. In contrast, Japanese tend to teach ethics and moral values in quite explicit ways and for longer periods than most parents in the United States. Japanese have a course called *Dotoku* (referring to ethics) and Japanese students receive ethical and moral instruction related to it. Values such as group perseverance, diligence, quietness, patience, respect for elders, and teamwork are emphasized.[53] The Japanese ethical values are mainly derived from their social structure and worldview, but especially from their religious beliefs and kinship relationships. Their ethical values have guided the Japanese for many years and many generations in decision making and actions, which shows a tenacity and consistency in teaching ethical values and principles to promote cultural identity and explicit enculturation practices.

The author has studied care expressions of Japanese and American individuals and families in different nursing contexts and has found contrastive behaviors. *Ethical care values* of *deference to* and *respect for the elderly, reciprocal kindness to one another, benevolence,* and *a tendency to forgive easily* were documented with the Japanese-American clients.[54] A dominant ethical care value of Japanese families is to *show respect for the elderly*, which is expected with Japanese clients. In fact, the Japanese care values of deference to and respect for the elderly were held as moral imperatives and responsibilities for family caregivers to be maintained with first, second, and third generations. While there have been some intergenerational variations over time, still these values remain fairly dominant ones. With the influence of United States exchanges and acculturation, the Japanese say there is "slippage" in ethical and cultural behaviors from their traditional values.

In a big industrial context, the ethical care values of *respect* and *deference* were identified by the author as important to recent Japanese employees in a large manufacturing plant in the midwestern area of the United States. These employees had recently come directly from Hiroshima and Tokyo, Japan, in 1989. They showed markedly deferent behaviors toward one another, but especially toward older employees in authority or in responsible positions. There was also strong reciprocal loyalty toward each other as "one big corporate family." These ethical values were evident among Japanese employees, but especially deference for the Japanese managers. The Japanese president of the company was greatly respected for his benevolent and responsible role with his employees, and they showed reciprocal deference to him. In this action-based research study of Japanese who recently came to the United States, it was clear that explicit institutional goals of the plant were made known and were expected to be followed. There were only a few Anglo-American employees in the plant. They had great difficulty adjusting to these Japanese ethical care values because the Anglo-Americans valued individualism, competition, self-reliance, autonomy, and less respect for the elderly and those in authority.[55] These Anglo-American cultural values were in direct conflict with the Japanese care values and gave rise to institutional tensions and conflicts. As a consequence, the Anglo-American em-

ployees were greatly concerned about their individual rights and ways to change the Japanese to *their* ethical norms and values. Through transcultural nursing consultation, the Anglo-American employees began to recognize cultural differences, their ethnocentric ideas, and how to accommodate and respect differences in a corporate institution. It took time, patience, and understanding for intercultural care accommodations to occur successfully in this large corporate industrial institution.

Another research study of the meanings and expressions of ethical care was discovered with Luna's study of Arab Lebanese Muslims in three urban culture contexts.[56] Luna's ethnonursing study covered a 3-year research project focused on identifying the meanings and expressions of culture care with Arab Lebanese Muslims, including their moral and ethical care behaviors. The researcher identified that their ethical and moral decisions were clearly derived from the Qur'an, which is the holy scripture containing the tenets of Islamic religious beliefs and practices. The Qur'an guides Arab Muslims in their ethical care practices. Luna found that *care* was viewed as an *ethical responsibility and a moral family obligation*. For example, male Arab Lebanese Muslims were expected to honor, protect, and be the economic provider and protector of the Lebanese family. Female Lebanese Arab Muslims emphasized and practiced ethical care as *family honor, unity, and social and domestic family responsibility*. These ethical care responsibilities with gender differences were clearly embedded and related to their religious, kinship, civil law, and social responsibilities. Accordingly, Arab Lebanese children were taught at an early age to learn these ethical and moral care values to protect themselves and to guide them appropriately in their daily relationships as Arab Muslims. These ethical care values needed to be respected as nurses cared for the Arab Lebanese Muslims in the home and hospital.

Prior to Luna's research, hospital and clinic nurses, as well as physicians and social workers, were unaware of how much Arab Lebanese used these culture-based ethical care values while in the hospital. Some nursing staff had been frustrated trying to get Arab Lebanese clients to cooperate, comply, or to understand what the staff wanted them to do, and so cultural imposition practices were apparent in client/nurse relationships. It was also clear that the Arab Lebanese could not change their dominant, ethically based behavior overnight, nor were they willing to do so. As a consequence, mutual avoidance was evident between nurses and clients. Other ethical care expectations of many Arab clients made them uncomfortable with nurses, particularly when nurses gave medications to them with the left hand rather than the right hand, as the left hand is unclean and the right hand is clean. By respecting ethical care proscriptions derived from religious beliefs, nurses could give congruent care to Arab Lebanese, which they valued and appreciated. When the nursing staff learned of Arab Muslim ethical values and rights, the clients responded in a cooperative and appreciative manner. It is this important body of transcultural nursing research knowledge that helps nurses to provide culture-specific and congruent ethical care decisions and actions. Transcultural nurses realize the importance of ethical, moral, and legal cultural expectations and that there is intracultural variability that must be identified and respected.

In the author's search for *universals* or *commonalities* of shared ethical care knowledge, there was evidence from the 1983 to 1989 research study with Mexican Americans, a few Native American groups, Chinese Americans, Arab Lebanese, and Vietnamese Americans that they shared some similar ethical care values.[57] The *commonly held values were filial respect, obedience*, and *deference to their elderly* but with slight *variations* in the cultural care expressions and meanings. It was of interest that Chinese Americans who had been in America for 5 years retained very strong ethical care practices with moral obligations as being obedient to authority, compliant, and deferent to their elderly but especially older Chinese government official in the United States. From the five cultures cited above, there were explicit ethical prescriptions for what *ought to be* or should be ethical caring behaviors and with moral commitments of what made their actions right or wrong. These cultural informants were pleased to identify and explain the meanings of such care expectations from their religious beliefs, kinship practices, and explicit cultural values that supported *filial respect* and *obedience* as care essentials for the elderly. These ethical and moral care values are still evident today to guide nurses in giving culture-specific and ethically congruent nursing care to clients of these five cultures in the United States.

In studying these cultures in the hospital context, the author's research findings revealed that Anglo-American nurses showed less overt respect for clients of the five above cultures, and especially with Anglo-American elderly. For Anglo-American hospital nurses, care of the elderly was often viewed as a duty or task, and nurses often expressed a preference to care for young or middle-aged hospitalized clients. Anglo-American nurses encouraged the elderly to be self-reliant and independent, which was in contrast to the above non-Anglo cultures. Self-care was important to Anglo-American nurses. They followed Orem's Self-Care Deficit Theory that nurses had been encouraged to use in their professional nursing education. In contrast, the Mexican and Vietnamese elderly clients did not like self-care practices as they were not congruent with their traditional emic cultural values and ethical expectations. It was also observed that Anglo-American nurses would avoid Vietnamese and Chinese clients who could not speak English. These clients, therefore, felt neglected and that they were not respected and requested that their extended family care for them in the hospital. In general, Anglo-American professional nurses were uncomfortable and not confident in giving care to elderly clients of non-Anglo background and who were not acculturated to Anglo-American lifeways and values.

In the American (ANA) nursing literature and in the Code of Ethics of Nursing there are ethical guides for patient care.[58] Some of these ethical statements pose problems as some do *not* fit all Western and non-Western cultures and some are inappropriate transcultural principles. These "social values," however, are viewed as "essential professional ethical values" and as a code to guide all nurses and cultures. Cultural ignorance of diverse ethical values of different cultures and lack of comparative ethical and moral values of Western and non-Western cultures need to be understood to provide professional and congruent care. A critical and urgent need remains for nurses to discover transcultural ethical and moral values of Western and non-Western cultures and to use available transcultural nursing research-based culture care concepts, principles, and practices. Such culturally based knowledge is essential for culturally competent and ethical code principles. Nurses need to shift from relying mainly on their *own ethnocentric personal or cultural values* to consider and use specific *emic values* and practices with clients of a designated culture. The use of *culture-specific ethical values* can greatly reduce cultural imposition practices, can decrease ethical conflicts and legal suits, and can ensure beneficial, satisfying, and culturally congruent nursing practices. Transcultural nursing education on ethical values remains imperative today for all nurses worldwide to prepare a new generation of nurses to be ethically knowledgeable, competent, flexible, and reliable in a transcultural nursing world. Keeping an open and flexible mind with diverse cultures is essential, as well as being able to learn from other cultures how to provide ethically based care. At the same time nurses' ethical and moral values need to be respected and upheld, but not imposed on clients.

 ## Contextual Spheres of Ethical Culture Care and Conflict Areas

In this last section *five* contextual spheres of ethical and moral culture care will be briefly discussed from different perspectives: 1) *personal or individual*; 2) *professional or group*; 3) *institutional or community*; 4) *national, cultural, or societal; and* 5) *worldwide human culture.*[59] These five spheres can be viewed as different contexts that give meaning to and influence ethical, moral, and legal decisions or actions. They are the reality contexts or perspectives in which nurses and clients function and that provide a basis to understand and accurately assess ethical behavior. The five contextual spheres of knowing and understanding can also be used to guide nursing decisions and actions related to ethical and moral decisions.

As nurses consider the five contextual spheres of ethical, moral, and legal behavior, they will recognize the author's principle that cultural *understanding and making appropriate responses to different contexts are essential for therapeutic nursing care practices.* Since the spheres reflect different cultural frames of reference for meaningful ethical nursing care decisions and actions, an example of the United States with its dominant focus on *individual personal views*, rights, beliefs, and actions is clearly evident. Ethical decisions for Anglo-Americans are strongly focused on *individualism* as essential. Such high emphasis on individualism contrasts with the People's Republic of China in

which the dominant value is for "*the collective societal good.*" Decisions in China are societal rights and *communal obligations with communal rights and duty to the central government.* These rights are made known and explicitly used as normative Chinese cultural rules and regulations. Today, more young Chinese are seeking democratic rights in their homeland; still, the authoritative dominant norm prevails as some individuals struggle or protest to the societal collective or the mandates of the Chinese society. These dominant Chinese culture care values of *obedience* and *compliance* also support the collective work group norms in the People's Republic of China. Traditional Chinese immigrants to the United States follow these norms.[60] These same cultural values of obedience and compliance were clearly evident during the June 1989 prodemocratic student's movement in China. The central political committee of the communist government (Politburo) denied all individual or personal wishes of students as they actively rallied for a democratic society and government in the 1989 event. These strong collective central government norms were of deep concern to many Americans who greatly value individual freedom, the right to be heard, human rights, and religious rights. For Anglo-American students, the Chinese cultural norms and ethical values of obedience, compliance, and deference to authority were difficult to accept along with the brutal killings in the government square and religious oppression. Interestingly, Chinese American students who had come from China since 1980 and who were studying at a Midwestern university told the author that they felt obligated to value obedience and deference to their government to prevent being killed or kept in prison if they returned for a visit to China.

In the Western world of nursing, especially in the United States, the nurse's individual and professional *etic* values and perceived personal rights are dominant ethical values governing what nurses should or ought to do. Therefore, United States and Canadian nurses often become upset, protest, or march if their perceived individual or professional rights are violated. Institutional or group ethical norms or values are often questioned and viewed with suspicion if leaders are too authoritative or threaten individual's human rights, autonomy, and decisions.

Most nurses deal with at least three major sets of ethical spheres of rights. First, there are the *personal (emic) cultural ethical values* that the nurse has learned in the family culture context in the early and ongoing life with the family. Second, there are *professional (etic) cultural values* that the nurse learns while in schools of nursing. Third, the nurse is expected to live by and value the *societal or dominant cultural values* such as the American cultural lifeways and ethical expectations.[61] This latter set of values cannot be ignored as nurses and nursing profession members are expected to serve society as public citizens in hospitals and agencies or wherever they are employed. In addition, nurses belong to a *global human culture* in which there are certain obligations, and they are expected to be sensitive and to respond to worldwide human caring needs of people. This global or worldwide sphere of ethical values has yet to be fully studied and adopted, but is being pursued by transcultural nurse researchers with the theory of Culture Care and in transcultural discussions.

As the professional nurse travels, reads, and functions in a global nursing context, many diverse ethical and moral values become evident. Transcultural nurses can play a major role in helping nurses extend their knowledge beyond their local or professional cultures to consider global ethical, moral, and legal viewpoints. When this goal is accomplished, nurses will be better prepared to respect diverse cultural values and beliefs and to function competently and knowingly in different cultures. Nurses will learn how to accommodate and sometimes restructure human values to meet cultural needs of specific individuals. Nurses learn about different contextual and global ethical spheres of knowing and experiencing as important for understanding and functioning professionally in a multicultural world. Transcultural perspectives of ethical knowledge and the use of appropriate culture care ethical practices are essential for nurses to become culturally competent. When these expectation are reached, one can predict less cultural burnout, cultural imposition practices, ethical offenses, and a decrease in legal problems and conflicts. Clients and nurses can become coparticipants to provide culturally congruent nursing care with nurses respecting and using transcultural ethical knowledge in informed, sensitive, and meaningful ways. Nurses will also know how to meet JCAHO standards and those of different nursing cultures, as well as specific client cultural care rights and values.[62]

Reflecting on the author's extensive research and that of other transcultural nurses over the past four decades (1960 to 2002), there remains a great need for the client's and nurse's ethical and cultural values to be known, respected, and acted on sensitively.[63] Clients are becoming astute to assess the nurse's cultural values and institution's norms to govern their actions accordingly. However, today, the client's ethical cultural care beliefs and values still get limited attention by nurses because of lack of knowledge about them. When clients acquiesce to nurses', physicians', or institutional ethical norms, or if clients' cultural actions fail to fit or comply with the values of the professional staff, one can find signs of cultural tension and conflicts. Nurses and physicians need help to understand and respect the clients' cultural values and arrive at appropriate cultural decisions. In the hospital context, clients may accept the professional staff's ethical values and choices to get care, the treatment desired, or funds. Clients who are strangers to the staff often feel vulnerable to assert their own rights and especially to "save face" or to be submissive to authority of physicians and nurses. Such ethical issues need to be dealt with by nurses and other personnel to prevent legal action.

Currently, with acute and chronic illnesses, the high cost of health services, and managed care practices, American clients may feel their human rights are violated with limited voice of their needs. Clients, especially those from non-Western cultures, may find that staying in modern Western hospitals with managed care policies and practices is offensive because of the short hospital stay, the high costs, and no time to fit treatments and care practices to their values and needs. Again, clients may feel that if they do not comply, they will not receive care or treatments. Hence, clients may remain silent and not make their ethical values and expectations known to nurses and other health personnel.

The author has also discovered that with some cultures such as the Philippine, Korean, and mainland Chinese, clients want and expect the physician and nurse to *make decisions for them.* This is especially evident when they are in the hospital and, because of their cultural value beliefs, are deferent and obedient to those in authority. This contrasts with Anglo-American clients who value *making and asserting their own independent decisions* "as their American cultural and ethical right of freedom." Middle- and upper-class

Americans are becoming more active not only in choosing their hospitals, physicians, nurses, and other therapists, but also in trying to reform or change the health care systems and medical practices that are offensive. The "Patient's Bill of Rights" is a document in the United States that reflects the client's growing rights to protect their individual ethical rights and freedoms. In the future such major ethical and cultural value differences must be anticipated and known for congruent nursing care and ethical obligations in health systems.

Critical Questions and Research Areas

Given these above five differential contextual spheres that influence the nurse's ethical decisions, the nurse should consider what ethical decisions are appropriate or inappropriate in these different contextual spheres of functioning. Is there a hierarchical ordering in which one sphere supersedes the other in different cultures? What happens if the "traveling nurse" follows Western personal or national types of universal-like ethics in an unknown non-Western culture such as the Republic of South Africa? How will the nurse know what is ethically or morally desired for the client, or for the common good in the strange cultures where the nurse is employed? Or, if the nurse makes an ethical care decision from a deontological stance, how congruent will this decision be with what is *best or fair for the individual* unless the nurse knows the cultural values, beliefs, and practices? What ethical or philosophical actions violate the ethical values of non-Western cultures? These are important transcultural ethical and moral issues and research questions that merit systematic study in this 21st century.

As more nurses become prepared in transcultural nursing and ethics courses, ethical theoretical knowledge, research findings, principles, codes, and covenants, it will enable nurses to use transcultural ethical knowledge appropriately. *Nurse ethicists also need to be prepared in transcultural nursing or comparative ethics to be effective teachers, researchers, and consultants in this specialty area.* An encouraging development is that qualitative paradigmatic research methods such as phenomenology, ethnonursing, and use of metaphors, narratives, and life histories will continue to be extremely valuable to discover embedded and covert ethical, moral, and legal values that exist in

human cultures.[64] Subjective, intuitive, spiritual, and nonverbal ethical and moral meanings and expressions are also important to discover ethical and moral cultural phenomena. Ethical behavior remains extremely difficult to measure or be treated as empirical data, but in-depth descriptive and interpretive data findings are valuable to use in care practices. Most assuredly, transcultural ethical, moral, and legal research studies with education must increase markedly in nursing in this new century along with religious and spiritual knowledge that buttresses ethical and moral actions.

Transcultural Nursing and Health Care Principles

From observing and studying many cultures the past four decades, I have formulated several ethical, moral, and legal principles for comparative transcultural nursing and health care. These principles can be used in Western and non-Western cultures as common or more universal ways to understand and help cultures. They are as follows:

1. The *principle of moral justice* to redress the gap between the rich and the poor worldwide
2. The *principle of cultural respect and human rights* to preserve human cultural heritage, values, beliefs, and lifeways
3. The *principle of benefits of the common good* to justify and support shared resources for the betterment of human beings and sociocultural justice
4. The principle to *serve and protect others* from destructive acts
5. The principle of frequent ethical and moral assessments to strengthen ethical and moral decisions in beneficial ways in diverse and similar cultures

These principles when fully understood and applied could increase quality care services.

It is also important to restate that transcultural nurses are interested in discovering both *universal* and *diverse* ethical and moral principles. Contrary to some nurses' views, transcultural nurses do not hold that all ethical values and beliefs are *relative* to each culture or that there are no universal ethical and moral truths or beliefs guiding human beings. Nor is transcultural nursing all based on *cultural relativism* or that all cultures are totally unique. Cultures worldwide have some shared and common values and beliefs of what is "right and wrong" among diverse cultures. It is these philosophical, ontological, and epistemic views that are important to the discipline. I hold there are some universal values and "truths" grounded in moral theology, philosophy of life, and supernatural beliefs that are powerful influencers of ethical, moral, and legal thinking and decisions. Such epistemic, religious, and ontological knowledge sources must become known and used for ethical and moral guides to decision making with cultures. If nurse ethicists fail to become knowledgeable in transcultural nursing and anthropology research findings with diverse and universal ethical and moral perspectives, they will continue to be handicapped in their endeavors. Recently, some nurse ethicists have begun to realize the importance of transcultural nursing research and ethical-moral care practices. Some ethicists' work provides some intraprofessional dialogue to advance transcultural ethical and moral knowledge development such as work by Davis, Silva and Donnelly, and a few others.[65-67]

Summary

In this chapter the author has discussed that transcultural ethical, moral, and legal knowledge remains very important in human caring, but still limitedly explored to advance transcultural and general nursing research, education, and practice. Western nurses tend to rely on their own personal and professional (etic) ethical values as guides to care for clients. Likewise, non-Western nurses have their own ethical and often emic cultural values to guide their ethical practices. The theory of Culture Care and use of qualitative research methods with findings have been a major source for helping nurses discover ethical, moral, and legal aspects of human care. Understanding and appropriately responding to people of diverse ethical and moral expectations requires in-depth knowledge of cultures and general ethical philosophies and use of relevant research findings for specific cultures. A major challenge remains to discover diverse and common universal ethical, moral, and legal culture care values worldwide in this 21st century. Several transcultural principles were presented along with research findings to guide cultural, specific

and universal care practices. While transcultural nurses have opened the doors to the importance of transcultural ethical, moral, and legal practices, considerably more research and education of nurses is needed to advance the knowledge and practice base worldwide.

References

1. Leininger, M., "Culture: The Conspicuous Missing Link to Understand Ethical and Moral Dimensions of Human Care," in *Ethical and Moral Dimensions of Care*, M. Leininger, ed., Detroit: Wayne State University Press, 1988, pp. 50–51.

2. *Webster's New World Dictionary of the American Language*, college ed., New York: The World Publishing Company, 1981.

3. Aroskar, M., "The Interface of Ethics and Politics in Nursing," *Nursing Outlook*, v. 35, no. 6, 1987, pp. 268–272.

4. Carper, Barbara, "The Ethics of Caring," *Advances in Nursing Science*, v. 1, no. 3, 1979, pp. 1–19.

5. Curtin, L. and J. Flaherty, *Nursing Ethics: Theories and Pragmatics*, Bowie, MD: Robert J. Brady Co., 1982.

6. Davis, A.J., "Compassion, Suffering, Morality: Ethical Dilemmas in Caring," *Nursing Law and Ethics*, v. 2, no. 6, 1981, p. 8.

7. Fowler, M., "Ethics Without Virtue," *Heart and Lung*, v. 15, no. 5, 1986, pp. 528–530.

8. Fry, S., "Moral Decisions and Ethical Decisions in a Constrained Economic Environment," *Nursing Economics*, v. 4, no. 4, 1986, pp. 160–163.

9. Fry, S., "The Ethics of Caring: Can It Survive in Nursing?" *Nursing Outlook*, v. 36, no. 1, 1988, p. 48.

10. Gadow, S., *Existential Advocacy: Philosophical Foundation for Nursing*, San Francisco: Image Ideas Publication, 1980.

11. Leininger, op. cit., 1988, pp. 37–61.

12. Ibid.

13. Leininger, M., *Care: The Essence of Nursing and Health*, Thorofare, NJ: Charles B. Slack, 1984 (Reprinted Detroit: Wayne State University Press, 1988.)

14. Ray, M.A., "Health Care Economics and Human Caring in Nursing: Why the Moral Conflict Must be Resolved," *Family Community Health*, v. 10, no. 1, 1987, pp. 35–43.

15. Ray, M.A., "Discussion Group Summary: Ethical Dilemmas in the Clinical Setting — Time

Constraints, Conflicts in Interprofessional Decision Making," in *The Ethics of Care and the Ethics of Cure: Synthesis in Chronicity*, J. Watson and M.A. Ray, eds., New York: National League for Nursing, 1988, pp. 37–39.

16. Veach, R. and S. Fry, *Case Studies in Nursing Ethics*, Philadelphia: J.B. Lippincott, 1987.

17. Watson, J., *Nursing: Human Science and Human Care. A Theory of Nursing*, Norwalk, CT: Appleton-Century-Crofts, 1985.

18. Watson, J. and M.A. Ray, *The Ethics of Care and the Ethics of Cure: Synthesis in Chronicity*, New York: National League for Nursing, 1988.

19. Beauchamp, T. and J. Childress, *Principles of Biomedical Ethics*, 2nd ed., New York: Oxford University Press, 1983.

20. Callahan, D., "Autonomy: A Moral Good, Not a Moral Obsession," *Hastings Center Report*, v. 14, no. 5, 1980, pp. 40–42.

21. Gilligan, C., *In a Different Voice: Psychological Theory and Women's Development*, Cambridge: Harvard University Press, 1982.

22. MacIntyre, A., *After Virtue*, Notre Dame, IN: University of Notre Dame Press, 1981.

23. Noddings, M., *Caring: A Feminine Approach to Ethics and Moral Education*, Berkeley: University of California Press, 1984.

24. Pellegrino, E., P. Mazzarella, and P. Corsi, *Transcultural Dimensions in Medical Ethics*, Frederick, MD: University Publishing Group, Inc., 1992.

25. Toulmin, S., "The Tyranny of Principles," *Hastings Center Report*, v. 11, no. 6, 1987, pp. 31–39.

26. Leininger, M., *Culture Care Diversity and Universality: A Theory of Nursing*, New York: National League for Nursing Press, 1991.

27. Leininger, op. cit., 1988, pp. 49–66.

28. Leininger, M., "Culture Care: An Essential Goal for Nursing and Health Care," *American Association of Nephrology Nurses and Technicians*, v. 10, no. 5, 1983, pp. 11–17.

29. Leininger, M., *Care: Discovery and Uses in Clinical and Community Nursing*, Detroit: Wayne State University Press, 1988.

30. Leininger, op. cit., 1991, pp. 1–45.

31. Leininger, M., "Issues, Questions, and Concerns Related to the Nursing Diagnosis Cultural Movement from a Transcultural Nursing Perspective," *Journal of Transcultural Nursing*, v. 2, no. 1, Summer, 1990, pp. 23–32.

32. Boas, F., *Race, Language and Culture*, New York: Free Press, 1966.

33. Herskovits, M., *Cultural Dynamics*, New York: Knopf, 1964.

34. Kluckhohn, C., *Mirror for Man*, Greenwich, CT: Fawcett Press, 1970.

35. Downing, T. and G. Kushner, *Human Rights and Anthropology*, Cambridge, MA: Cultural Survival, 1988.

36. Haviland, W.A., *Cultural Anthropology*, 5th ed., New York: Holt, Rinehart, and Winston, 1987.

37. Lanham, Betty B., "Ethics and Moral Precepts Taught in Schools of Japan and the United States," *Japanese Culture Behavior: Selected Readings*, J. Libra and W. Libra, eds., Honolulu: University of Hawaii Press, 1986, pp. 280–296.

38. Leininger, op. cit., 1988, pp. 49–66.

39. Ibid.

40. Leininger, M., *Transcultural Nursing: Concepts, Theories, and Practices*, New York: John Wiley & Sons, 1978.

41. Stitzlein, D., "The Phenomena of Moral Care/Caring Conceptualized within Leininger's Culture Care Theory," Ph.D. dissertation, Detroit: Wayne State University, 1999.

42. Leininger, op. cit., 1991.

43. Horn, B., "Transcultural Nursing and Childrearing of the Muckleshoot People," *Transcultural Nursing: Concepts, Theories, and Practices*, M. Leininger, ed., New York: John Wiley & Sons, 1978, pp. 223–239.

44. Luna, L., *Care and Cultural Context of Lebanese Muslims in an Urban US Community: An Ethnographic and Ethnonursing Study Conceptualized within Leininger's Theory*, Ph.D. dissertation, Detroit: Wayne State University, 1989.

45. Wenger, A., *The Phenomenon of Care in a High Context Culture: The Old Order Amish*, Ph.D. dissertation, Detroit: Wayne State University, 1988.

46. Luna, op. cit., 1989.

47. Wenger, op. cit., 1988.

48. Leininger, M., "Transcultural Care Principles, Human Rights, and Ethical Considerations," *Journal of Transcultural Nursing*, v. 3, no. 1, 1991, pp. 21–24.

49. Leininger, op. cit., 1991, pp. 345–372.

50. Leininger, M., "Culture Care of the Gadsup Akuna of the Eastern Highlands of New Guinea," in

Culture Care Diversity and Universality: A Theory of Nursing, New York: National League for Nursing Press, 1991, pp. 231–238.

51. Leininger, M., "Becoming Aware of Types of Health Practitioners and Cultural Imposition," *Journal of Transcultural Nursing*, v. 2, no. 2, 1991, pp. 32–39.

52. Leininger, op. cit., 1991, pp. 91–93.

53. Lanham, op. cit., 1986, pp. 284–296.

54. Leininger, op. cit., 1991, p. 359.

55. Ibid.

56. Luna, op. cit., 1989.

57. Leininger, op. cit., 1991a, p. 355.

58. Viens, D., "A History of Nursing's Code of Ethics," *Nursing Outlook*, v. 37, no. 1, 1989, pp. 45–49.

59. Leininger, op. cit., 1988, pp. 61–64.

60. Leininger, op. cit., 1991, p. 361.

61. Leininger, M. "Transcultural Ethnonursing and Ethnographic Studies in Urban Community Contexts," unpublished research report, Detroit: Wayne State University, 1960–1993.

62. Joint Commission on Accreditation of Health Care Organizations, *Comprehensive Accreditations Manual for Hospitals: The Office Handbook*, Oakbrook Terrace, IL: August 1997.

63. Leininger, op. cit., 1991, pp. 21–24.

64. Bandman, B., and B.C. Bandman, *Nursing Ethics Through the Life Span*. Norwalk, CT: Appleton & Lange, 1995.

65. Davis, A.J., "Global Influence of American Nursing: Some Ethical Issues," *Nursing Ethics: An International Journal for Health Care Professions*, v. 6, no. 2, 1999, pp. 118–125.

66. Silva, M.C., *Ethical Decision-Making in Nursing Administration*, Norwalk, CT: Appleton & Lange, 1990, pp. 40–80.

67. Donnelly, P.L., "Ethics and Cross-Cultural Nursing," *Journal of Transcultural Nursing*, v. 11, no. 2, 2000, pp. 119–126.

III

Culture Care Theory, Research, and Practice in Diverse Cultures

15

Anglo-American (United States) Culture Care Values, Beliefs, and Lifeways*

Madeleine Leininger

To work effectively with people of diverse cultures, one must first understand their own cultural heritage as a means to understand other cultures. This understanding should reflect differences and similarities in order to know and appropriately respond to the wonderful gift of diversity among human beings. LEININGER, 1970

The Anglo-American way of life tends to become obscure because many contend that if one lives in the United States that "all Americans are alike and there are no differences among them." This is a myth as there are cultural differences and variations among Americans by virtue of their diverse cultural heritage, specific values, and cultural lifeways. Within the American culture are the dominant Anglo-Americans who are mainly Caucasian immigrants from European countries whose lifeways reflect their cultural beliefs, values, and practices. The United States remains a land of immigrants except for Native Americans who are the first national original people. Thousands of immigrants, refugees, and migrants continue to settle each year in the United States. Attracted by democracy, freedom of speech, and many economic opportunities, Anglo-American beliefs and lifeways are so pervasive that one assumes all Americans are alike, but cultural diversity exists among Anglo-Americans because of the specific cultural heritages

from many places in the world. Some contend America is a "melting pot," a "tossed salad," or a "stew." Others speak of dominant cultures in a specific geographic area. The purpose of this chapter is to present the Anglo-American cultural values and lifeways that have become known as "Anglo-American" in the United States. Such knowledge is important to understand Anglo-Americans and to distinguish them from other cultures who have different health care needs or expectations. Since Anglo-American nurses are currently the largest health care providers in the United States, it is important to understand this dominant culture with its variations and similarities.

Importance of Understanding Historical and General Features of Anglo-Americans

The original term *Anglo* is derived from Latin and refers to one of the four Germanic peoples together with the Saxons, Frisians, and Jutes who invaded England from the third to the sixth century as the Romans retreated. These Germanic tribes displaced the native Celts who eventually referred to all their Germanic conquerors as Anglo-Saxons.[1,2] When the colonists immigrated to America from England beginning in the 1600s, they brought English cultural values, language, and many beliefs to the United States. Gradually,

---

* In this chapter the term Anglo-American refers mainly to people of Caucasian ancestry who have lived in the United States and have been fully acculturated. It does not include new or recent immigrants or refugees who are now living in the United States but who are not acculturated or not citizens of the country. This is an updated chapter from a previous writing on Anglo-American culture beginning in 1970 until the present time.

these Anglo-Saxons or English people became known as Caucasians; Anglo-Americans are often referred to as "WASPs," that is, White, Anglo-Saxon, Protestants.[3-5] This large cultural group, along with other immigrants such as the Irish and Polish who were not Protestant, has for many centuries profoundly influenced and shaped the legal, economic, health care, educational, religious, political, and cultural values of the United States of America.

The genetic and physical features of Anglo-Saxons are quite heterogeneous with Mediterranean, Alpine, and Nordic racial features and influences of the Celtic, Teutonic, and Scandinavian peoples. The Anglo-Saxon culture prevailed over successive waves of immigration to America, much as the Anglo-Saxon world of early England absorbed Celts, Norse, Danes, and Frenchmen.[6] Arsenberg and Niehoff maintain that the United States has several streams of culture flowing side by side, but assert there is a national, white middle-class with its origins from Western European cultures. They state the following:

> The language is English, the legal system derived from English common law, the political system of democratic elections comes from France and England, the technology is solidly from Europe, and even more subtle social values such as egalitarianism (though modified) seem to be European derived. Anglo-Saxon civil rights, the rule of law, and representative institutions were inherited from the English background.[7]

Essentially, the English were the first Europeans to colonize the Americas in large numbers even though they were preceded in the Southwest by smaller numbers of Spaniards. The English gave the Anglo-Saxon label to Anglo-Americans in that their origins were derived from the original inhabitants of the British Islands who were subdued by the Celts.[8] The latter ancestors first appeared in central Europe and later moved to northern France, southern Britain, and finally Ireland. However, as these people immigrated to the United States, they still became known as "Anglo-Americans." Arsenberg and Niehoff, and McGill and Pearce say that Anglo-Americans had British roots that led to cultural values such as the nuclear family that were largely derived from pre-industrial Britain. These cultural values and others became Anglo-American values in the United States.[9,10]

For several decades many anthropologists and sociologists have been studying Anglo-American core values.[11-21] These scholars with their rich descriptions, theories, and narrative accounts have been extremely helpful to grasp the general features of the Anglo-American culture and to identify differences among other cultures in the United States and elsewhere such as the Japanese, Chinese, and Russians. Understanding the overt or subtle differences about Anglo-Americans can help nurses to prevent cultural clashes, imposition practices, cultural stresses, and other problems that may arise between nursing staff and clients. In addition, knowledge of the history of Anglo-Americans has been extremely valuable to facilitate communication, to guide decision making, and to prevent gross misunderstandings between cultures within and outside the United States.

It is strange but true that often Anglo-American cultural values and patterns of thinking and acting are usually not studied until outsiders comment or raise questions about "Anglo ways." Most Anglo-Americans take their culture for granted as a part of their lifeways and may fail to recognize its unique features. Sometimes, people from very different backgrounds speak of Anglo-American behavior as strange, peculiar, or even bizarre. Becoming aware of such differences of Anglo-Americans in relation to other cultures is important so that not all people in America are assumed to be the same. For example, the author has often heard outsiders say that Anglo-Americans tend to be so individualistic and autonomous that they have difficulty valuing or conforming to group norms and other ways of living when outside the United States. Some non–Anglo-Americans view Anglo-Americans as highly materialistic and competitive and too technologically oriented. Other outsiders or visitors find that "Anglos" tend to take many kinds of pills to avoid physical pain or suffering and keep them healthy. Anglo-Americans who travel to very different cultures in the world also discover that other cultural groups dress, speak, and act differently. Such differences noted by outsiders about the Anglo-American culture makes one pause to understand the *why* of the intercultural differences within and between cultures worldwide. Knowledge and understanding of one's own culture and that of others remain the hallmark of professional nurses and scholars, but especially of transcultural nurses as they work today with people of many different cultures in any typical health care context and remain attentive to acculturation, assimilation, and enculturation processes.

Since the mid 1950s, the author has been studying and observing Anglo-Americans and changes in their values, beliefs, and communication modes to advance transcultural nursing knowledge and improve nursing care practices.[22,23] Identifying differences and similarities of Anglo-American and other cultures is helping to dispel the "all alike American syndrome" in nursing and helping nurses to be attentive to subtle or gross differential client care practices. Some of the greatest problems of Anglo-American nurses have been *ethnocentrism* and *cultural blindness* in which nurses fail to recognize cultural variations among Americans and between other cultures. Of course, nurses in other cultures also have this problem. Anglo-Americans tend to be "lumped and dumped together as all alike" without awareness of subtle and major differences. Such tendencies have led to cultural clashes, stereotyping, racism, legal suits, and inadequate care. Cultural awareness of Anglo-Americans is essential for cultural care competencies. It is difficult to be knowledgeable or to care for others without understanding one's own and other cultural values. Nurses learn about themselves and others through education and people contacts.[24]

Through the study of transcultural nursing, nurses are realizing that most United States hospitals, clinics, community agencies, and corporate institutions have historically been largely established and maintained with dominant and largely unicultural Anglo-American values and practices. This is evident in nursing education and practices in hospitals, health care agencies, and most organizational structures dealing with health care. However, among these Anglo-American values, there are specific cultures that need to be recognized such as Swedish, Danish, Finnish, German, Italian, Greek, and many other immigrant, native, and minority cultures. These cultures live and function in the United States and need to be understood in client care and staff relationships. Transcending specific cultures are some common Anglo-American values, beliefs, and practices that are shared and have been passed on to succeeding generations as *dominant* Anglo-American values as cited above by many scientists and writers of Anglo-American culture. Knowledge of the dominant or overriding Anglo-American culture, values,

beliefs, and lifeways are important along with other immigrant cultures living in the United States. Nurses need to understand the Anglo-American cultural values and lifeways to be effective, competent, and sensitive to this culture and many others. Let us turn to some of these *dominant* Anglo-American cultural values in the United States, remembering that there will be some individual differences among the dominant values.

■ Dominant Anglo-American Cultural Values

Since cultural values are the powerful directive forces that give meaning and direction to human action and decisions, Anglo-American cultural values identified below are held to be essential to understanding and use in practices. The values identified below came from decades of research on Anglo-Americans with a focus on culture care meanings and actions using the Culture Care Theory. These values are also generally reaffirmed from anthropological and sociological research and writings such as those by DuBois, Fried, Gorer, Hall, Kluckholn and Kluckholn, Mead, Nash, and Stewart and Bennett.[25–32] In this chapter, the following Anglo-American middle- and upper-class cultural values are identified and discussed with a focus on transcultural nursing care meanings and practices, largely from transcultural nursing research and practice.[33–35]

1. Individualism and self-reliance
2. Independence and freedom
3. Competition, assertiveness, and achievements
4. Materialism
5. Dependence on technology
6. Equal gender roles and rights
7. Instant time and action (doing)
8. Youth and beauty
9. Reliance on "scientific facts" and numbers
10. Generosity and helpfulness in crises

Individualism, Freedom, and Competition

Unquestionably, most Anglo-Americans value *individualism*, *self-reliance*, and being quite *autonomous in thinking and actions*. They value their individualistic freedom to speak, act, and be on their own and generally dislike being treated as a collectivity or group. Personal identity and uniqueness as individuals are important to most Anglo-Americans. Nash contends that Americans are the most individualistic people in the world, which he holds comes from their traditional English pre-industrial norms and from American industrialism.[36] Anglo-Americans want to be recognized as individuals and as being self-reliant, independent, and self-determining persons. They also value privacy and having their own material goods and possessions. Most adult middle- and upper-class Anglo-Americans are socialized and rewarded and promote themselves with the idea of being unique and having their own things, name, and of being self-reliant and focused on oneself. Such values are taught at home at an early age and reinforced in schools and work. For example, Anglo-American children are taught at a very early age to feed themselves, brush their teeth, dress themselves, make decisions, and talk independently in their unique and individualistic ways. Children learn early what belongs to them as their material possessions and about their owner's rights. Such child-rearing enculturation practices and others are related to individualism, self-reliance, freedom of speech, and autonomy. These values are sharply different from Chinese, Vietnamese, and many other non-Western children who are taught to value being part of a group (often large families), living communally, and sharing material goods.

Anglo-Americans dislike being constrained or having their freedom infringed on by others, especially by government and institutional policies or practices. Speaking openly about almost any matter is valued, defended, and protected by Anglo-Americans. Hence, policies or decrees that limit such expressions are often resisted, avoided, or responded to negatively. Political ideologies and practices such as Marxism or working for the collective good tend to be questioned by most older Anglo-Americans. Accordingly, Anglo-American nurses usually resent autocratic or oppressive leaders that suppress their individual rights, autonomy, freedom, or special ways of doing their professional work.

The Anglo-American cultural values of *competition, achievement, and assertiveness* are visibly part of everyday living. Competition and achieving measurable outcomes are supported. Likewise Anglo-American nurses have become more competitive in recent years and like to show their achievements, worth, and measurable gains in "products" or money. Most women's rights and goals are professionally upward bound at home, outside work, college, or in public arenas. Anglo-American nurses pursue their competitive and assertive efforts to achieve by tapping available rewards and by competing with other individuals and groups in the workplace. "Playing the game" and gaining access to key people, positions, and awards have become important to Anglo-American nurses in recent decades or in the "new" culture of nursing.

The Anglo-American values of achieving, being competitive, and getting key positions, honors, or rewards may be directly at odds with nurses and clients of other cultures who do not value these attributes. For example, traditional Native Americans in the United States and Canada generally do not promote competition and achievement because they believe these values lead to disharmony with others and their environment. Being aware of such differences among cultures can prevent major cultural clashes, offensive acts, noncompliance, and negative nursing experiences. These values are also important in nursing education and administration, especially when nurse leaders are promoting competition and achievement activities between students, staff, and others. Nurses from non-Western cultures that value cooperation, interdependence, and avoiding open competition often experience cultural strain, conflicts, and dislike for their work. Transcultural nurses can be helpful to bring an awareness and understanding of these cultural value differences to nursing staff, to educators, and to others who are not knowledgeable of such cultural differences. There are many incidences and unfavorable outcomes that can be identified in schools of nursing and in health services today where competitive actions and fierce competition behaviors fail to be recognized, let alone dealt with in nursing situations.

Materialism and Technologies

Other dominant Anglo-American middle- and upper-class values are *materialism and reliance on technological goods and equipment*. Anglo-Americans value having material goods and a great variety of high-technology products as conspicuous items in their homes and work environments. Many Anglo-Americans feverishly work to get money and often possess many different material items, technologies, and electrical products that are obtained to make their work easier and more efficient. Several cars, television sets, freezers, computers, and a great variety of electrical or mechanical appliances can be found in middle- and upper-class Anglo-American homes. High-tech gadgets are viewed today as essential and justified in work and play, and Anglo-Americans may buy several varieties of small technologies to be sure there is always one to replace the other. Moreover, as new technologies come on the market, the old one (which is often still functional) tends to be discarded. Cultural anthropologists have been studying this behavior and found that most Anglo-Americans dispose of more material and technological goods than any other culture or country in the world.[37] Future archaeological digs will undoubtedly reveal lots of technologies, aluminum cans, plastic products, and other materials as belonging to the 20th and 21st century Anglo-Americans. Being modern, progressive, and possessing material goods are often associated with success and status; hence, money for the newest and latest products on the market is valued.

The concept of *conspicuous consumption* of middle- and upper-class Anglo-Americans is evident as wasteful and as a "throw away" culture. Having the newest, latest, and most efficient technologies in Anglo-American middle- and upper-class homes, offices, and places of leisure is highly desired. Such vast amounts of materials, goods, and electronic equipment contrast sharply with Anglo-American poor (lower class) and minorities, refugees, and new immigrants into the United States who have limited material goods, money, and modern technologies. In fact, many of these cultures could live for months or years from what is thrown away by wealthy upper-class Anglo-Americans in material goods and foods. Still today, the poor, homeless, and others may be found scrounging in garbage cans and other places for food and clothing to survive. Living on "toss aways" is a way of daily and nightly life for these people in America and with other cultures where conspicuous material goods are absent or limited. Today, many different electronic and technological products and large and beautiful homes and cars have become a dominant hallmark of upper-class

Americans, which contrasts sharply with the poor and lower class.

Many kinds of technologies in hospitals, clinics, and more recently in homes can be found in health facilities. Modern computers, x-ray machines, special instruments, and a great variety of powerful technologies are evident to assess and promote medical and nursing treatments. Health care systems have become technology centers with health personnel depending on such equipment for professional services. Nurses and physicians have become technologically dependent for health care services in hospitals and homes by requiring effective and safe technologies. Hospitals continue to buy the latest and most effective technologies as their budgets permit. Similar purchases can be found in wealthy homes today for their own private health uses and for instant self-diagnostic and treatment purposes. However, in America not all cultures believe in and use such technologies. For example, the Old Order Amish do not value the use of high technologies unless for very specific reasons. If an Amish member is threatened by illness and death, they may refuse to use some hospital services that have high technologies. Generally, such considerations are weighed very carefully so that the use of technologies does not violate Amish religious beliefs and caring values. Nurses prepared in transcultural nursing teach and alert other nurses to these areas of cultural conflict so that the Amish client and the family are not offended or demeaned for not using high technologies and other hospital or health products.[38] Moreover, if such technologies are used with ignorance or inappropriately, this may influence their total well-being or may threaten their survival according to Amish beliefs and values.

Gender Roles and Rights

Another dominant Anglo-American middle- and upper-class value is that *males and females should be treated with equal respect, rights, and role opportunities in the home, work place, or anywhere.* Equal gender rights and opportunities are promoted and defended for Anglo-American women if their rights are violated, neglected, or oppressed.[39] During the past two decades with the feminist movement in the United States there has been an active pursuit of equal rights for women in different education and service centers. Anglo-American women have been active to obtain salaries comparable to their male counterparts and to seek some of the top positions traditionally held by men in diverse organizational settings. Anglo-American nurse leaders have been especially active in making men and women aware of their behaviors, especially to reduce acts and decisions that are offensive and oppressive to women. Most female nurses have worked hard to free themselves from being dominated by male physicians and other patriarchal and power control practices.[40] Some progress has been made as there are more signs of nurses moving into some top leadership positions, gaining access to better employment environments, and getting salaries fairly equal to men. There are, however, still gender gaps in salaries with women doing the same kind of work but receiving less pay and less recognition.

This gender struggle of Anglo-American women and nurses may be an enigma for women and men in non-Western cultures.[41] For some non–Anglo-Americans the push by women for equal rights with men is frightening as some gender role differences are important in their cultures. Non-Western nurses are sometimes surprised to find Western nurses imposing and pushing for equal rights when they do not know the culture and consequences when women drastically change their traditional cultural roles and behaviors. Abuse and severe battering of women may occur when male spouses in some cultures learn about wives' drastic changes in their roles. There are, however, women today in non-Western cultures who are interested to change traditional oppressive gender practices and will seek Anglo-American nurses to help them make changes. Transcultural nurses are extremely important to help women from diverse cultures because they know that some changes can lead to harmful consequences.

Transcultural nurses have ethical and moral responsibilities to protect men and women who may not fully understand using Anglo-American values, beliefs, and practices. Assisting clients and staff who have different gender values than Anglo-Americans is, therefore, an ethical responsibility so that culturally congruent, safe, and meaningful practices can occur. Some Anglo-American feminist nurse leaders who have not been prepared in transcultural nursing may impose their gender role expectations onto other cultures as a result of cultural ignorance and strong feminine interests worldwide. It should also be noted that males in the United States and overseas may be changing some of their traditional values and practices to protect their rights and to prevent feminine discrimination practices in homes, health institutions, and society. Male cultural rights organizations are found in the United States. There are also current and unresolved philosophical, religious, legal, and biosocial controversies about gays, lesbians, and changing gender identities in the United States and other places in the world. Male and female nurses are actively involved in these issues today.[42]

Time Value and Doing

Turning to another Anglo-American value, the metaphors "time is money" and "time must not be wasted" reveal that *time* is a dominant value in the American culture. If time is not appropriately used and respected, Anglo-Americans often become angry, frustrated, restless, and upset. Moreover, maintaining time schedules and meeting time expectations are linked to being seen as competent, successful, and efficient in America. Anglo-Americans want technologies as "time savers" or "extenders" to help them to use time to be successful or to have leisure time. Figuratively, time dictates where one should be day and night. Many Americans today are *born into the world by the clock, work by the clock, get married by the clock, and can die by the clock.* Time truly pervades most Anglo-American lifeways. Transculturally, the power of time and its uses regulates Americans considerably more than in most cultures in the world.

Reflecting on time, a contrast example with the Papua New Guinea (non-Western culture) whom I lived with and studied for nearly 2 years was clearly different from Western time values. The Gadsup had no mechanical or electronic timepieces in the 1960s. They had no sense of Western clock time in the 1960s in their daily and nightly activities, and only very recently do a few men have watches. The Gadsup, however, did have a general concept of time based on daily activities of living such as the rising and setting of the sun, changes in plant growth, and changes in their village activities, physical environment, life-death, and historical events.[43] There are a few other cultures in the world in which time is not the central focus for living and well-being, but this may change in time. Such awareness of time differences is extremely important for nurses to gain cooperation and to provide culturally congruent and satisfying care. Accommodating and adjusting to the rhythm of other cultural lifeways based on their concept of time, their values, and their lifeways are very important in transcultural nursing.[44]

Western nurses are keenly aware of differential time concepts. In many hospital contexts, Anglo-Americans consider that they receive "good care" when nurses respond quickly to their calls, whereas clients from another culture believe time means "the nurse will come later and will be more compassionate and caring when they come." Some Anglo-American clients, if delayed more than 10 minutes with the nurse, may become very impatient and angry, and some may want to leave the hospital.

The concept of time is also closely related to another Anglo-American value, namely *that of doing*.[45] Being active and doing something have been strong normative expectations for most Anglo-Americans, especially nurses and other health personnel. People are evaluated today on "production outcomes." How much one produces or what activities have been completed with numbered outcomes are important. Producing and doing are again related to Anglo-American success, promotion, and rewards. Quantifiable data, measurable (empirical) outcomes, and cost savings are emphasized and rewarded. Anglo-American nurses feel very compelled to "produce" and show what they have done or how much they have completed in their clinical work and with clients, students, and others. This Anglo-American value of *doing* and *measuring outcomes* often comes into noticeable conflicts with non-Western nurses in which doing and measuring outcomes are often not valued such as with many groups in South Africa, Mexico, and Indonesia. Transcultural nurses who value and practice caring by listening to, giving time, and offering care as presence to clients, takes time, but sometimes there is "no time allowed" by supervisors and others for whom time must show measurable outcomes.

With respect to doing and producing, *managed care practices* in the United States have become a critical problem for professional nurses who deeply value human caring and quality services to clients. With managed care, the goal is to get clients in and out of the hospital (or any official health care service) as quickly as possible to *reduce costs* whether healed or not. Outcome in numbers of clients served is also valued by insurance companies and hospital managers as essential to managed care philosophy, goals, and cost savings. Often, the short client time in the hospital and rapid health services by different professionals leads to nurse and client frustrations and sometimes unfavorable client outcomes. *Time, doing and cost saving are clearly evident with managed care* and often counter to some clients needs and professional nursing care practices.[46] Indeed, clients are often dismissed within 1 to 3 days, and transcultural nurses and others who know the therapeutic value of human caring often see negative outcomes with managed care operations. Cultural differences among clients in relation to the meaning of doing and caring, especially with Vietnamese, Mexican-Americans, and Native Americans, are very important in healing and client care satisfactions and are often limitedly considered in managed care.

Space and Environment Values

Another Anglo-American value is *space* and *territory*, especially with middle- and upper-class Americans. Anglo-Americans seek ways to increase their space at home and at work. Space is viewed as money and necessary to handle material goods they have bought and possess as essential to their style of living. The more square footage, extra bedrooms, bathrooms, office, storage, and garage space the better for Anglo-Americans. Wealthy Anglo-Americans in United States have additional space for physical exercise rooms, televisions, and computer rooms, as well as space for large kitchens and entertaining areas. Considerable money is needed to purchase large homes, hospitals, and other territorial areas. Most new hospitals and clinics are built today to accommodate new technologies, equipment, treatment facilities, client comforts, grief rooms, research and laboratory space, and many other space needs. Anglo-American nurses in the hospital and clinics value space in comparison to earlier days when nurses usually had very small nursing stations and areas to care for clients. Nurses working in the community and homes look for space with home care practices today with new modern health care technologies and other equipment in the home. Non-Western nurses in remote, less developed and economically poor areas often have limited space and learn to use whatever is available in their immediate environments. Nurses from non-Western cultures often experience cultural shock when they come to the United States and other Western countries to practice hospital nursing. They are overwhelmed to see so much space with modern equipment and beautiful patient rooms.

Youth and Beauty Values

Youth and *beauty* are two other dominant cultural values of Anglo-Americans. These values can be noted in the public media, television, Internet and other electronic modes, and in the performing arts. Beauty and youth usually bring attention, praise, and rewards such as with annual beauty queens. These values may get transmitted to nurses' preference to care for youths and attractive clients, with less interest in the elderly who appear less attractive in body appearance and dress. Some American nurses enjoy caring for the elderly. Unfortunately, elder abuse with families is of concern in some United States nursing homes. Such practices to elders are quite very different from how the elderly are treated in non-Western cultures. For example, in non-Western cultures such as the Philippine, Japanese, Korean, Thai, and others, the elderly are generally revered, deeply respected, valued, and shown much kindness and affection by caretakers and families. These elderly are especially valued for their wisdom and advanced years by their families, groups, communities, and organizations. The Anglo-American emphasis on "good looking, young, and beautiful" often leads nurses wanting to make the elderly appear younger than their chronological age by offering youthful hairstyles, younger-age clothing, and special facial cosmetics. Anglo-Americans like to keep people young, beautiful, active, and vibrant and to prevent aging. These values become a dominant part of nurses' norms, attitudes, and practices. There are many immigrants in the United States who value the elderly

and care for them by integrating their kinship, religious, and desired cultural values into elder care. The Korean, Philippine Americans, Arab-Americans, Old Order Amish, and Japanese Americans expect respectful caring to their elderly.[47] In general, youthfulness, beauty, and old age are *culturally constituted*, defined, valued, and expressed in the Anglo-American culture. Transcultural nurses help other nurses to understand and provide care that fits the culture.

Reliance on Facts and Numbers

Still another dominant Anglo-American value is to rely on *scientific facts and numbers gleaned from television, radio, research studies, newspaper articles, and reports as "the scientific truths."* Facts that are quantifiable or statistical figures are greatly valued by Anglo-Americans as "hard" empirical data. Only recently some Americans are beginning to value nonquantifiable data and listening to faith and life stories, events, and rich narratives as credible information. Subjective, symbolic, nonnumerical, spiritual, or religious information tend to be viewed as less reliable, less accurate, or not the "real facts" to use. The United States public media extols and holds "scientific facts," statistics, or measurable indicators as the most credible truths. The realization that scientific facts can be manipulated and altered to fit certain motives or goals is often hard to accept by many number and statistical advocates. Transculturally, people of different cultures have many different ways of knowing what is "true" and how they know the truth as science.[48] Life experiences and quality of life and living may be more important than statistical facts in some cultures. Quality indicators of health maintenance and healing care will be emphasized, discovered, and valued more in this century by consumers. Accordingly, nurses will discover that client cultural values of caring, well-being, and spirituality cannot usually be reduced to measurable numbers or finite outcomes but are powerful in healing. Letting clients tell what they know and how they experience life and arrive at *their healing facts* are important. Eastern cultural philosophers were early to discuss quality lifeways and nonreality (spiritual) ideas as different ways of knowing people and the world. Transcultural nurses learn these qualitative cultural values to promote quality of life, healing, and well-being.

American Generosity and Helping

A highly positive feature of Anglo-Americans is their *generosity to others and especially in times of crisis, suffering, gross neglect, disabilities, or tragic situations.* Americans generally take pride in being generous by giving money, direct help, and sharing resources to those in need, especially when called on or when they know about major natural or other kinds of catastrophes such as tornadoes, floods, storms, explosions, mass killings, and accidents. Most wealthy, middle-class, and even poor Anglo-Americans are quick to respond to worthy causes and crises, as shown during and after the terrorist attacks on the World Trade Center and the Pentagon on September 11, 2001. Indeed, many Americans have helped poor and oppressed cultures who have experienced war, famine, destruction, and other obvious needs. The Honduras crisis with the terrible hurricanes in 1998, the droughts and tornadoes in the Midwest, large forest areas burnings, and loss of property are a few examples of American generosity giving money, prayers, and direct help. Religious beliefs and being charitable in giving to others are motivating factors for many Christian and Jewish Americans to share their wealth or resources. Clothing, money, and other items are generously given by Americans through local, religious, and community organizations. These are very positive values that give Anglo-Americans an altruistic and charitable image. Sometimes, Anglo-Americans may be less generous in countries such as those in Africa or South America if they do not understand the culture, the people's history, and human needs. Television and the internet are powerful means today to learn about distant and unknown cultures, especially the poor, oppressed, and neglected.

United States Rural and Urban Comparative Cultural Values and Care

Other important areas to study are dominant rural and urban cultural values and care expectations that characterize the United States. Understanding recurrent and comparative patterns of how rural and urban people live in America with their dominant care meanings and expectations are important and different knowledge areas for transcultural practitioners. The author, with graduate students and faculty, has studied United States rural and urban lifeways over several decades and has identified and documented dominant themes as presented in Table 15.1. Using the qualitative (emic and etic) ethnonursing research method with the Culture Care theory, the domain of inquiry studied was focused on major, recurrent rural and urban American cultural values and care meanings with actions across different areas of the United States. This domain of inquiry was important to guide nurses in practicing nursing care in rural and urban America to provide culturally congruent and specific care to these cultures. As people move from rural to urban lifeways, acculturation factors need to be assessed, as well as environmental and ecological community resources.[49] As one studies Table 15.1, several contrastive or different dominant themes become evident with rural and urban Americans. These differential cultural values and care meanings of mainly Anglo-American middle-class and some poor cultures are important reflective research-based knowledge for nurses to use in care practices.

Historically, it is important to know that many immigrants and those born in the United States in the late 19th and early 20th century began their lives living on American farms to earn a modest living and to survive with large families. However, with the industrial revolution and with periods of drought leading to economic farm depression, rural people gradually moved to urban community areas for new job opportunities to survive.[50] The shift from rural to urban or suburban lifeways was a major cultural change and cultural shock for many rural people. Much later, urban Americans moved to the rural areas, and they experienced cultural differences from their urban lifeways with both desired and less desired features. Urban nurses may encounter cultural differences and culture shock when they begin to provide care to rural people in an urban context often because of different cultural beliefs, values, and lifeways.[51] The lack of nursing research-based knowledge of cultural values and care meanings often leads to cultural clashes, cultural conflicts, and cultural imposition problems as nurses help rural and urban clients in different cultural and environmental contexts. Unfortunately, there has been limited transcultural nursing research-based knowledge to guide the nurses using rural-urban care meanings and values.

Table 15.1   United States Comparative Rural and Urban Major Cultural Values and Care Meanings* (Mainly Middle Class and Diverse Cultures)

Rural Culture	**Urban Culture**
Dominant Cultural Values Focused on:	*Dominant Cultural Values Focused on:*
1. Family and community interdependence	1. Less family and community orientation dependent
2. Living in isolated (geographic) areas	2. Living close to people
3. Conservative views ("let's wait and see")	3. Many politically active with assertive views
4. Question drastic changes and distrust of "city folks"	4. Changes and problems resolve quickly
5. Low context communication modes	5. High context communications modes
6. Limited access to health services and costly	6. Access to diverse health services with costs
7. Reliance on folk (generic) care	7. Reliance on latest professional services
Caring Means	*Caring Means*
1. Active concern for others (family and "my neighbors")	1. More concern for self or group
2. Helping others as "good neighbors"	2. Getting experts to quickly help
3. Reciprocity in relationships over time	3. Friendship with social ties
4. Knowing how to improvise and "to use what you have"	4. Knowing latest or best professional care services
5. To remain practical and "use good common sense"	5. Use medical media facts and popular care modes
6. Rely on known family (folk) care remedies and treatments (good tolerance for pain)	6. Rely on known medical facts, pills, surgery and professional treatments (less tolerance for pain)
7. Overcome handicaps & inconveniences	7. Get help to deal with handicaps
8. Direct help and assistance within family or from friends	8. Get specialized services soon as possible

* Leininger's research with colleagues (1985–1999).

Transcultural nursing research findings shown in Table 15.1 provide important holding information about dominant differences between rural and urban clients to guide nurses caring for individuals and families in rural and urban communities. Essentially, this is knowledge for transcultural community nurses, which should gradually replace traditional community or public health nursing knowledge to focus on care meanings and value differences between rural and urban cultures as shown in Table 15.1. For example, some major *cultural value* contrasts from *rural* to *urban* are as follows:

1. Limited versus good access to rural health care
2. Rural conservative views compared to active political urban views
3. Dependence on generic (emic) folk practices versus professional urban (etic) practices
4. High versus low context communication modes
5. Rural family and community focus versus urban individualism

With *caring* meanings there are also major contrasts from rural to urban such as the following:

1. Concern for others versus concern for self
2. Reciprocal care versus friendship care
3. Being "practical" versus using medical facts
4. Improvising to give care with limited equipment
5. Reliance on *home* remedies versus professional medicines and treatments
6. Family help versus help from strangers or professionals

These scientific findings on the rural and urban cultures are essential to increase cultural competencies and favorable caring outcomes. Other countries also need to study and share their rural-urban dominant cultural values and care practices to arrive at what are universal and diverse features for culturally competent practices.

In worldwide societies, there are other kinds of cultures and subcultures that need to be studied transculturally such as the drug, alcohol, elderly, adolescent, gay and lesbian, and the homeless subcultures, as well as the cultures of poverty and affluence. These cultures should be studied with specific criteria that differentiate subcultures from cultures (see definitions earlier in the book on these concepts). Subcultures have unique and distinct values that reflect differences from the dominant culture; hence, specific criteria must be used by the researcher as shown in the chapter on the subculture of the homeless to identify differences in certain areas within the larger culture. Subcultures are difficult to study because they reflect embedded, covert, and often subtle features within the dominant cultures.[52] Recently, gay and lesbian subcultures are being studied as shown in the work of Eliason.[53]

Culture of Death and Life

Finally, in this chapter it is important to discuss briefly the *Culture of Death* and the *Culture of Life*. These two cultures are presently popular topics in the United States but also in other places in the world today. Health personnel, religious leaders, ethicists, social scientists, and lay consumers frequently discuss these two cultures. It is of interest that in 1968, Pope Pius VI first addressed the Culture of Life as he spoke about preserving life of newborns and preventing the unjustified killing of human beings.[54] Since then, Pope John Paul II and other Catholic moral theologians have frequently addressed these cultures in religious and public arenas. It has, however, been Pope John Paul II who has made the concepts of the "Culture of Life" and the "Culture of Death" meaningful and explicit.[55] The Jewish, Muslims, and other Christians are also speaking about the culture of life and death and human rights.

The *Culture of Life* focuses on the prevention of killing newborns, the elderly, the deformed, or the handicapped as moral, ethical, and God-given rights of human beings by moral theologians, religious leaders, and some ethicists. In contrast, the *Culture of Death* promotes values, beliefs, and practices that lead to ending the life of individuals or groups for a great variety of reasons such as personal inconveniences, cost factors, overpopulation fears, poor quality of life, undue suffering, and absence of caretakers. The pro-choice and pro-abortionists, euthanusiasts, and neo-Nazi killers are some groups who ascribe to the Culture of Death. Individuals facing death penalties for heinous criminal offenses are also discussed with different views about rights to death and to life.

In some states in the United States such as Oregon and in other countries such as the Netherlands laws have been passed to support the Culture of Death by assisting the elderly to die. The terminally ill, as well as deformed humans and heinous criminals, are also prescribed to die. Major ethical and moral decisions are ongoing about the right to take life and especially that of innocent human beings who have been given life by God. Catholic moral theologians and other Christian, Jewish, and Muslim groups are also active discussants holding to the position that a human life is sacred and no other human has a right to kill another human being such as killing the unborn or taking the life of the elderly, handicapped, and others. This philosophy and the actions related to the Culture of Life and the Culture of Death have many implications as transcultural nurses work with different cultures who have different views about life-death matters. There are presently many ethical and moral personal dilemmas with nurses who are caught personally and professionally with decisions and participation in the Cultures of Life and Death.

Transcultural nurses who are knowledgeable about cultural value and belief differences need to discuss ideas with staff and clients as fundamental human rights of cultures. Nurses are expected to uphold their own beliefs and practices, educate clients but not impose their values on clients who may espouse different beliefs than the nurse. With the growing interest to integrate spiritual and religious values, moral and ethical principles, beliefs, and truths into healthcare, one can anticipate that the Cultures of Life and Death will remain important discussion areas.

■ Summary

In this chapter Anglo-American middle and urban culture care values, beliefs, and lifeways in the United States have been presented. While individual and group cultural variabilities exist among all Anglo-Americans, still there are *dominant cultural patterns* and *care meanings* that have been identified from transcultural nursing in-depth emic and etic research studies as presented in this chapter. These research findings serve as holding or reflective knowledge for nurses. Rural and urban Anglo-American research cultural values and care meanings were also presented using the Culture Care theory with the ethnonursing research method. These dominant values and care meanings serve as valuable holding research-based knowledge to help nurses provide culturally congruent care practices or for teaching and research purposes. Subcultures and the Culture of Life and Death were presented. Most importantly, this chapter emphasized that nurses and others need to be knowledgeable about Anglo-American cultural values and action modes to be helpful in providing therapeutic and responsible transcultural care practices. Transcultural nursing research findings need to be incorporated into all areas of nursing and especially with Anglo-American nurses as they care for other cultures to prevent cultural clashes, pain, and destructive outcomes. It is also important to remember that the roots of culture are deep and seldom change quickly, and therefore culture care practices are predictable and can be used effectively to respect client variabilities.

▓ References

1. Blair, P.H., *An Introduction to Anglo-Saxon England*, 2nd ed., New York: Cambridge University Press, 1977.
2. Baugh, A.C. and T. Cable, *A History of the English Language*, 3rd ed., Englewood Cliffs, NJ: Prentice Hall, 1978.
3. Anderson, C.H., *White Protestant Americans: From National Origins to Religious Groups*, Englewood Cliffs, NJ: Prentice Hall, Inc., 1970.
4. Baugh and Cable, op. cit., 1978.
5. Winawer-Steiner, H. and N.A. Wetzel, "German Families," in *Ethnicity and Family Therapy*, M. McGoldrick, J.K. Pearce, and J. Guidrano, eds., New York: The Guilford Press, 1982, pp. 247–268.
6. Anderson, op. cit., 1970.
7. Arsenberg, C.M. and A.H. Niehoff, "American Cultural Values," in *The Nacirema: Readings on American Culture*, J.P. Spradley and M.A. Rynkiewich, eds., Boston: Little, Brown, 1975, pp. 363–378.
8. Anderson, op. cit., 1970.
9. Arsenberg and Niehoff, op. cit., 1975.
10. McGill, D. and J.K. Pearce, "British Families," in *Ethnicity and Family Therapy*, M. McGoldrick, J.K. Pearce, and J. Giordano, eds., New York: The Guildford Press, 1982, pp. 457–482.
11. Boorstin, D., *The Americans: The Colonial Experience*, Vol. 1, New York: Random House, 1958.
12. Boorstin, D., *The Americans: The National Experience*, Vol. 2, New York: Random House, 1965.
13. Cohen, M., *American Thought: A Critical Sketch*, New York: Collier Books, 1954.
14. DeBois, C., "The Dominant Value Profile of the American Culture," *American Anthropologists*, v. 57, Part 1, December 1955, pp. 1232–1239.
15. Gorer, G., *The American People: A Study in National Character*, New York: W.W. Norton, 1948.
16. Goodenough, W.H., *Cooperation in Change*, New York: Russell Sage Foundation, 1963.
17. Hall, E., *Beyond Culture*, New York: Anchor/Doubleday, 1976.
18. Hsu, F., *Americans and Chinese: The Two Ways of Life*, New York: Schuman, 1953.
19. Kluckholn, C., "American Culture: A General Description," in *Human Factors in Military Operations*, Chevy Chase, MD: John Hopkins University, 1954.
20. Kluckholn, C., "The Evolution of Contemporary American Values," *Daedalus*, no. 2, 1958, pp. 78–109, 1954.
21. Leininger, M., "The Traditional Culture of Nursing and the Emerging New One," in *Nursing and Anthropology: Two Worlds to Blend*, M. Leininger, ed., New York: John Wiley & Sons, 1970, pp. 63–82.
22. Ibid.
23. Leininger, M., *Transcultural Nursing, Theories, Concepts, and Practices*, New York: John Wiley & Sons, 1978.
24. Leininger, M., *Transcultural Nursing, Concepts, Theories, Research and Practice*, Blacklick, OH: McGraw-Hill, 1995.
25. Fried, M., *Readings in Anthropology, Vol. II: Readings in Cultural Anthropology*, New York: Thomas Y. Cromwell, 1959.
26. Gorer, op. cit., 1948.
27. Hall, op. cit., 1976.
28. Kluckholn, C. and F. Kluckholn, "American Culture: Generalized Orientations and Class Patterns," in *Conflicts of Power in Modern Culture: Seventh Symposium*, New York: Harper and Bros., 1947.
29. Mead, M., *Sex and Temperament in Three Primitive Societies*, New York: William Morrow and Co., 1963.

30. Mead, M., *And Keep Your Power Dry*, New York: William Morrow and Co., 1965.
31. Nash, D., *A Little Anthropology*, Englewood Cliffs, NJ: Prentice Hall Press, 1989.
32. Stewart, E. and M. Bennett, *American Cultural Patterns: A Cross Cultural Perspective*, Yarmouth, MN: Intercultural Press, Inc., 1991.
33. Leininger, M., *Nursing and Anthropology: Two Worlds to Blend*, New York: John Wiley & Sons, 1970, pp. 45–62.
34. Leininger, M., *Care: The Essence of Nursing and Health*, Detroit: Wayne State University Press, 1988. (Originally published, Thorofare, NJ: C. Slack, Inc., 1984).
35. Leininger, M., *Culture Care Diversity and Universality: A Theory of Nursing*, New York: National League for Nursing Press, 1991, p. 355.
36. Nash, op. cit., 1989.
37. Rathje, W. and C. Murphy, *Rubbish: The Archaeology of Garbage*, New York: Harper Collins Publications, 1992.
38. Wenger, A.F., "The Culture Care Theory and the Old Order Amish," in *Culture Care Diversity and Universality: A Theory of Nursing*, M. Leininger, ed., New York: National League for Nursing Press, 1991, pp. 147–178.
39. Bird, C. and P. Ricker, "Gender Matters: An Integrated Model for Understanding Men's and Women's Health," *Social Science and Medicine*, v. 48, 1999, pp. 745–755.
40. Leininger, op. cit., 1970.
41. Ibid.
42. Leininger, op. cit., 1995.
43. Ibid.
44. Ibid.
45. Leininger, op. cit., 1970.
46. Leininger, Personal communication with hospital nursing staffs. Detroit and Omaha 1995–2000.
47. Wenger, op. cit., 1991.
48. Leininger, M., "Types of Science and Transcultural Nursing," *Journal of Transcultural Nursing*, October 2001, p. 423.
49. Leininger, M., "Transcultural Nursing Care in the Community, in *Community Health Nursing: Caring for the Public Health*, K. Lundy and S. Janes, eds., Sudbury, MA: Jones and Bartlett, 2000, pp. 218–234.
50. *World Almanac and Book of Facts*, Mahwah, NJ: Premedia World Almanac Books Reference Inc., 2000.
51. Wenger, A.F., "Cultural Context, Health and Healthcare Decision-Making," *Journal of Transcultural Nursing*, v. 7, no. 1, 1995, pp. 3–14.
52. Leininger, op. cit., 1995.
53. Eliason, M.J., "Cultural Diversity in Nursing Care: The Lesbian, Gay or Bisexual Client," *Journal of Transcultural Nursing*, v. 5, no. 1, 1993, pp. 14–20.
54. *Pope John Paul II*, encyclical given Vatican City, March 25, 1995.
55. "Pope John Paul II", in *Evangelium Vitae*, English Translation, Vatican City Press, 1995.

CHAPTER 16

Arab Muslims and Culture Care

Linda J. Luna

Caring for Arab Muslims poses a real challenge to most nurses today since Western awareness of their unique cultural beliefs, values, and lifeways is just beginning to develop. Muslim religious values and the worldview of Islam are markedly different from the values that underpin life in the Western world. Understanding these values requires that nurses learn about the religious and cultural factors, social structure features, and health care features, as well as their own cultural background. The central and important goal of transcultural nursing necessitates learning about the culture and then developing care practices that are culturally congruent with the values of the people. Delivering culturally congruent care further requires becoming aware of one's own culturally learned assumptions. To be unaware of our culturally learned assumptions is not consistent with the notion of culturally competent care and transcultural nursing practices.

Today, more nurses are beginning to recognize the importance of transcultural nursing and the evolving body of knowledge about the influence of cultural factors on health and care behaviors and lifeways. Such knowledge is extremely imperative in professional practice to bridge the gap between the experiences and worldview of the nurse and that of the client or the family whose cultural values, lifeways, and worldview may be quite different from those of the nurse.

In this chapter some fundamental transcultural concepts and ethnonursing insights will be presented to help nurses understand and care for Arab Muslim clients. Leininger's Culture Care Theory with a focus on worldview, ethnohistory, social structure (especially religion and kinship), language, cultural values and beliefs, and environment will be presented.[1,2] Transcultural nursing care guidelines and practical applications to support ways to provide culturally congruent

care will be offered as derived from the literature, from the author's research of Middle Eastern people, and from direct field experience with several Arab cultural groups in a large community in the United States.[3-5] These experiences, as well as almost 15 years' residence in the Middle East, have been most valuable in understanding the importance of transcultural nursing knowledge and in developing clinical skills to care for and communicate with Arab Muslim clients.

Leininger's Theory of Culture Care Diversity and Universality provided the theoretical frame of reference for this chapter and the author's research.[6] The theory was used to discover and understand cultural values and lifeways of the Arab Muslims through an analysis of social structure, worldview, language, and environmental features. With the theory, Leininger holds that care is essential to human health and well-being and is the major feature that distinguishes nursing from other disciplines.[7] The goal of the theory is to provide culturally congruent care to individuals, families, and cultural groups. While the concept of care is central to Leininger's theory, the concept of health is also studied in relation to care to discover the relationship of health (well-being) to care. Health and care behaviors are held by Leininger to vary transculturally and to take on different meanings in different cultures.[8,9] Leininger postulates that if one understands the meanings and forms of care, one can predict the health or well-being of human beings.

Culturally congruent nursing care requires in-depth knowledge and direct experiences with cultural groups. Congruent and effective nursing care needs to be grounded in transcultural knowledge to achieve care congruence and health. The three nursing care decisions or actions that Leininger holds to provide culturally congruent care for clients and that were studied by the author were 1) culture care preservation and/or maintenance, 2) culture care accommodation and/or negotiation, and 3) culture care repatterning and/or restructuring. These three modes or patterns of care are helpful to consider as the nurse uses knowledge from Arab Muslim clients to plan and give nursing care. If these modes of action are used, Leininger predicts there will be fewer signs of cultural conflict and stress between the nurse and client and fewer negative responses from clients in nursing care practices. Culturally congruent care will reflect the nurse's knowledge of and sensitivity to clients' cultural lifeways. Clients will find nursing care more acceptable and satisfying. Accordingly, the nurse will feel more satisfied and rewarded in her or his care practices.[10]

Learning About Arab Muslims

At the outset it is important to state that a review of nursing care literature reveals limited research related specifically to the Arab Muslim culture and to nursing care phenomena. Islam is the fastest growing religion in the world with an interesting and important ethnohistory. Yet many misunderstandings and myths continue to exist in the West about Islam and the Arab culture.

It is important to realize that considerable variability exists within the Arab Muslim culture as Arabs come from a number of countries throughout the Middle East and North Africa. Because of such variability, some ideas may not be directly applicable or relate specifically to all Arab Muslim groups in the world. In this chapter only some knowledge about Arab Muslims in the United States will be discussed, rather than focusing on all Arab Muslim cultures and their variabilities worldwide.

To begin, the nurse needs to know which groups are represented by the term "Arab Muslim." Frequently, the terms "Arab" and "Muslim" are used as being synonymous, which is not accurate. Not all Arabs are Muslim, and not all Muslims are Arab. To understand this statement, let us explore further the differences and some ethnohistorical facts.

Most Arab scholars view the Arab world as stretching from Morocco to the Arabian Gulf. Although reference is made to the "Arab world," there exists no single Arab nation, but rather a number of separate Arab states. Countries that make up the Arab world are the countries of North Africa, including Morocco, Algeria, Tunisia, Libya, Egypt, Somalia, Sudan, Djibouti, and Mauritania; the Middle Eastern countries of Lebanon, Syria, Iraq, Jordan, and Saudi Arabia; and the states and territories bordering the southern and eastern edge of the Arabian peninsula such as Yemen, Bahrain, Kuwait, and the United Arab Emirates.[11] Although most inhabitants of these Arab countries are Muslim, there are several million Christian Arabs who reside within these boundaries, including Maronites of Lebanon and the Chaldeans of Iraq. A commonly accepted meaning for the term "Arab" is "any person who resides in the area stretching from Morocco to the Arabian Gulf, who speaks Arabic, and who takes pride in the Arab culture and the Arabs' historical accomplishments."[12]

In contrast, a Muslim is a practitioner of the faith of Islam. Most Muslims, however, are not Arab.[13] With the expansion of Islam in the 7th century, the religious culture moved out of the Arabian peninsula in all directions to embrace many cultural groups. Today, the largest Muslim states are situated outside the Middle East in Indonesia and the Indian subcontinent.[14] Pakistani and Indonesian Muslims, however, are not Arab Muslims. Arab Muslims are Muslims who originate from any of the previously mentioned countries that comprise the Arab world, that is, Lebanese Muslims, Saudi Muslims, Egyptian Muslims, etcetera. Actually, Arabs constitute only 25% of the world's Muslim population, a fact that surprises most people.[15]

Muslims are divided into two major and legitimate religious orthodoxies, the Sunni and the Shi'a, plus a number of smaller orders. The Sunni constitute the largest group of Muslims, whereas the Shi'a are a minority. With regard to the major beliefs and practices of Islam, there are similarities and differences. The points of divergence revolve around the issue of early leadership following the death of the Prophet Muhammad. The nursing concepts and research findings addressed in this chapter apply to both groups of Arab Muslims, the Sunni and the Shi'a, as well as to the smaller groups.

Ethnohistorical Aspects of Arab Muslim Immigration

There are currently no reliable statistics on the number of Arab Muslims in the United States. Various sources give estimates on the number of Arabs as a whole, while others approximate the total number of Muslims. Naff attempts to separate the two by citing the approximate number of Arabs in the United States to be roughly two million, 10% (or 200,000) of whom are Muslim.[16] There appears to be a consensus among Arab writers that such figures are a conservative estimate, since several regional wars in the Arab world during the past decade have motivated many Arab Muslims to migrate.

Early Arab immigrants to the United States were primarily Christian. Haddad contends that the first major influx of Arab Muslims to the United States occurred between 1875 and 1912.[17] The incentive for migration at this time was to achieve financial success similar to that reported by the earlier arriving Christians. Most of the early Muslim immigrants were single males who planned to return to their homeland after accumulating a certain amount of wealth. Many of these early arriving Muslim males did return home; however, a significant number stayed on in America and were instrumental in establishing institutions and organizations to preserve the Islamic faith. A second wave of Muslims came to the United States before World War II, followed by a third wave from 1947 to 1960 and a fourth from 1967 to the present.[18] During these periods various political and economic factors in the Arab world such as wars and coups d'etat, as well as an expanding American economy and changes in the United States immigration laws, provided incentives for Arab Muslims to migrate.[19]

Many Arab Muslim scholars tend to emphasize a distinction between early arriving immigrants and those who came in later years, with the latter identified as better educated and with greater numbers from the professional class. Haddad notes that such a distinction may be exaggerated, since many later immigrants were not professionals, but rather were part of the flow of "chain immigration" of relatives joining other family members in the United States.[20] Chain migration continues to characterize the migration patterns of most Arab Muslims with the exception of the Yemenis, who are primarily men who come to work, save money, and return to Yemen.[21]

The early growth of Islam in America showed an adaptation of traditional practices to a new environment. As the presence of more and more Muslims in urban American communities grew, mosques, Islamic centers, and other educational institutions developed to teach and perpetuate the faith to the next generation.[22] Since the early 1970s, events in the Middle East have precipitated a strong tendency among many Muslims to return to the essential teachings of Islam. There has been a movement in many Muslim communities in the United States toward reform or reviving traditional Islamic practices. Many new immigrants, as well as an increasing number of earlier arrivals, are reaffirming their total commitment to Islam as a way of life. To provide effective nursing care, nurses need to be aware of these changes and the increased religious awareness on the part of many Arab Muslims.

The World View of Islamic Culture and Nursing Considerations

To care for Arab Muslim clients effectively, nurses need to be aware of the worldview of Islam as a cultural influence on the daily life of the people. The worldview of a cultural group is their way of looking at reality and the world around them. One aspect of worldview is the role of religion, as it gives meaning to living, dying, and the maintenance of health and care practices.

The religion of Islam began in the center of Arabia during the 7th century and is a monotheistic religion— to associate other gods with Allah (God) is a capital crime. The term "Islam" is an Arabic word meaning "the act of submission or resignation to God."[23] For the Muslim believer, the Qur'an (or holy book of Islam) is the absolute authority of the word of God, and understanding this tenet is essential to understanding Arab Muslim clients. To Muslims, "the Qur'an is the actual word of God transmitted by the angel of prophecy, Gabriel, to the Prophet Muhammad, who transmitted it to the people."[24] As such, it lacks any tampering or changing by human leaders. Muslims resent reference to Islam as Muhammadanism, since the term implies divinity to Muhammad. According to Muslim belief, Muhammad was merely a man and the messenger of God, but he was in no sense divine.

The single most important feature of the worldview of Islam is the concept of *tawhid. Tawhid*, a verbal noun derived from the root *wahada*, carries the meaning of "unity" or "intense unification."[25] The idea of unity refers to the unity of the Supreme Being (Allah) and the subsequent unity of nature. *Tawhid*, or the doctrine of absolute unity, affirms that "there is only One Creator who deserves our praise and gratitude and whose guidance needs to be followed."[26] The existence of God is not in isolation; rather, all the world is united in God. *Tawhid* is the fundamental principle of Islam from which all other principles are derived. The obedient Muslim lives his life in a way that reflects *tawhid* in the unity of mind and body, a tenet that is essential to grasp in planning nursing care interventions.

Tawhid implies that all Muslim believers are a single brotherhood, the *ummah*, which knows no superiority in terms of color or ethnicity. Prayer and recitation of the Qur'an are said daily by Muslims all over the world in the Arabic language, even though Arabic is not the mother-tongue of most Muslims. An Arab Muslim, however, has no superiority over a non-Arab Muslim; rather, all are members of a universal community of Islam, the *ummah*. This "unity in diversity" is a distinctive feature of the permeating world view of tawhid and is the major reason many people from minority cultures are attracted to the religion of Islam.

The moral and ritual obligations that help Muslims lead a disciplined life are summed up in five main duties known as the pillars or foundations of Islam.[27]

1. The first is a confession of faith: "There is no God but God, and Muhammad is the Prophet of God." The confession of faith is uttered on a number of occasions such as birth and death.
2. Prayer is the second duty of Muslims and is said at five specified times each day.
3. The third pillar is the obligation of almsgiving, or giving to the needy. The Qur'an stipulates that one should share with the less fortunate the blessings of wealth that God has given.
4. The fourth duty required of Muslims is fasting during the holy month of Ramadan, during which no food or drink is taken during daylight hours. Many Muslims extend this to oral medications, although according to Islamic law, the ill are exempt from the obligation of fasting as are travelers or others whose health could be at risk from fasting.
5. The pilgrimage to Mecca, the holy city of Islam, is the fifth duty that every pious Muslim strives for at least once in a lifetime.

The above duties for Muslims produce a sense of fulfillment, well-being, and health and are a source of guidance in today's perplexing world.

Within Islam, the concepts of *halal* and *haram* are important to understanding Muslim culture. Halal describes those things that are permissible or lawful according to the tenets of Islam, and haram describes those things that are forbidden.[28] For example, the code of halal applies to the manner in which meat is slaughtered. To be considered halal and lawful for consumption, an animal must be slaughtered in accordance with certain Muslim prescriptions, that is, the use of a sharp knife to spare the animal unnecessary pain, recitation of verses from the Qur'an, and facing toward Mecca. However, the code of halal is demanded in other activities also such as in manner of dress. According to Islamic doctrine, clothing and adornment must take into consideration the principles of decency, modesty, and chastity for both men and women.

There are many nursing implications related to the worldview of Arab Muslims that should be kept in mind as nurses care for patients of this faith. Like members of any religious group, the intensity of an individual's belief and faith will vary. For example, the devout Arab Muslim who has a diabetic condition may find the sense of spiritual health and well-being brought about during the fast of Ramadan equally as important as maintaining a diet that balances insulin requirements. Maintaining spiritual health and well-being is important since the concept of *tawhid* implies that physical health is not separate from the spiritual dimension; that is, there is mind-body unity. The Arab Muslim view of health, therefore, correlates with the worldview concept of unity reflected in tawhid. In working with an Arab Muslim client who has a diabetic condition and who wishes to fast during Ramadan, the nurse could use Leininger's decision-action mode of culture care accommodation/negotiation in an effort to allow the client to retain his beliefs and practices, but could negotiate ways in which dietary and metabolic needs can be met to prevent insulin imbalances and maintain holistic health.

Still another nursing consideration centers around the performance of prayer. Before entering into obligatory prayer, the Muslim believer carries out ritual cleansing according to Islamic tradition. This ritual cleansing includes washing the feet up to the ankles, washing the arms to the elbows, and washing the face and the inside of the ears.[29] A part of the worship ritual includes removing the shoes and facing toward Mecca. For women, covering the hair is also required. Some Muslims may not feel the need for daily prayer, while others may see this practice as essential to recovery or maintenance of health and well-being. During the culturological assessment, the nurse should assess the client's wishes regarding prayer and the desired frequency. If prayer is desired, the nurse may provide assistance with the ritual cleansing or allow a family member to assist, especially if the client is of the opposite sex. Providing a basin of water and finding a quiet place for the client to perform the religious duty supports culture care accommodation as in important nursing intervention. Religious articles such as prayer rug or a copy of the Qur'an are often brought from home for the Arab Muslim client to the hospital or clinic. These articles should be treated with respect, and nothing should ever be placed on top of the Qur'an, as it is a sacred object.

For many Arab Muslims, observing the fast of Ramadan and performing the religious obligations of prayer are important cultural expressions for maintaining health and preventing illness. The nurse should attempt to assess the meaning and importance to the client of these rituals, since for many Arab Muslims they function as more than simple acts of worship. Fasting and prayer help to maintain a pure heart, a sound mind, and a clean, healthy body.

The culturally knowledgeable and sensitive nurse will realize the concern of many Arab Muslim females for modesty. Taking measures to provide culture care accommodation and culture preservation by respecting the female's modesty should be an integral part of nursing care. The traditionally oriented female usually expects to have female caregivers.[30] The nurse should remain with the female client during any type of examination or procedure and give special attention to draping and preventing unnecessary exposure of the body. The Muslim female may desire to have another female relative present, and, occasionally, she may wish to have her husband present during a health examination, especially if the health provider is a man. Culture care accommodation is an important transcultural nursing mode of caring for Arab Muslims.[31]

 ## Language Significance, Symbolism, and Nursing Care

In caring for Arab Muslim clients, language expression and use can serve to facilitate care. Language is more than simply a medium of communication. It is a means to understand the cultural values and beliefs, worldview, and perceptions of health and care. To Arab Muslims, Arabic is regarded as the most perfect of all languages, since it was the vehicle through which the message of Islam was revealed. Inherent in the religious significance of Arabic is the conviction that the Holy Qur'an cannot be translated into other languages without losing a great deal of meaning. For this reason, Muslims, regardless of their native tongue, pray and recite the Qur'an in Arabic. Knowledge of the Arabic language brings a great deal of prestige to the Muslim who can speak and read it.

The Arabic language has developed in three forms. There is a distinction between various regional dialects of Arabic; a modern standard Arabic utilized by radio, television, and press media; and the classical written Arabic of the Qur'an. All spoken dialects are considered inferior to the classical form, which is regarded as ideal and complete, being the revealed word of God. Although Arabic is a relatively difficult language to learn, the Arab Muslim client who speaks no English appreciates, respects, and is influenced by the nurse who makes an effort to communicate in Arabic. Besides using the language for exchanging ideas, facility in Arabic creates a positive atmosphere of acceptance that is conducive to constructive communication and caring modes. For many clients, language poses a tremendous barrier when attempting to enter the Western health care system. For this reason, many available community services are frequently unused by Arab Muslim clients. Bilingual staff and translators are helpful in dealing with the non-English speaking client; however, learning a few simple phrases and greetings in Arabic will facilitate establishing and maintaining a caring relationship with the client and the family.

Every culture and religion has its own set of symbols that give insight into underlying cultural norms and values. By assessing the client's symbolic construction of reality, the nurse can get close to thoughts, actions, and feelings of the client and can deal with barriers that might otherwise interfere with effective nursing care. A variety of symbolic icons, objects, and forms of human expression provide support in the life of Arab Muslims. As mentioned earlier, religion is all-pervasive. Seldom does an Arab Muslim make a promise or plan of action without uttering the term *Inshallah* (if God wills).[32] The utterance reflects the Muslim belief in divine authority for all intended actions. Prayer beads are a common symbol of Islam used by both males and females. Similar to a rosary, the string usually consists of thirty-three beads and is used in private worship to recall the ninety-nine attributes of Allah listed in the Qur'an. The use of prayer beads is a reminder to Muslim clients of the nearness of God and thereby serves to reduce anxiety and provides a sense of peace and well-being.

From the very beginning of Islam, there has been a reluctance among Muslim artists to render reality in human or anthropomorphic form. Any symbolic representation of the Prophet Muhammad or his family is avoided; instead, reality is depicted through abstract art and calligraphy. Again, the concept of tawhid is inherent in the geometric patterns known as arabesque, which have no beginning and no end, thus giving the impression of infinity. The purpose of such art for Muslims is to direct one toward the remembrance of Allah.[33] A variety of cultural values are inherent in the above concepts of language use and symbolism. The nurse should be attentive to Arab Muslim clients when giving care or treatments or when carrying out actions that conflict with the clients' cultural values, symbols, and language meanings.

Social Structure Factors and Nursing Care

To comprehend fully any culture, but especially Arab Muslim culture, social structure factors are very important to understand. Religion is a major factor of social structure for the Arab Muslim client. Another important factor is family and kinship ties. The nurse needs to have holding knowledge of the importance of the family as the major unit of the social organization of the Arab Muslim culture. The Arab Muslim is born into an extended family that fashions and uses kinship ties to achieve various daily activities, values, and goals throughout life. It is largely within the family that a person derives his or her sense of identity. In all

matters an Arab Muslim is expected to place family or group concerns before any individual concerns.[34] This often means making great personal sacrifices to put the good of the family foremost. However, certain advantages are inherent in such a system. Bashshur points out that an extended family provides multiple role models for children who vary in age, sex, and other personal and social attributes.[35] Furthermore, the extended family serves many of the naturalistic caring functions that are delegated to institutions in Western cultures (money lender, job placement center, and nursing home), as discovered by the author's research.[36]

Age commands a great deal of authority in an extended Arab Muslim household. Elderly Arab Muslims are treated with a great deal of respect.[37] Aged parents usually live with their oldest son because it is considered disrespectful for old parents to live alone. According to the Qur'an, taking care of one's family is as important as other religious duties.

Until recently, nursing homes or homes for the aged were unknown in the Arab world. Even though a few such institutions now exist, for example, in Egypt, the idea of sending one's parents to a nursing home is still undesirable and counter to cultural norms. Elkholy notes that senility among the aged appears to be a rare occurrence in the Middle East, since the elderly gain status with age rather than experiencing loss of self-esteem and self-worth, as is often the case with the elderly in the Western cultures.[38]

Islam and the teachings of the Qur'an provide cultural rules that guide family living and influence care practices. The nurse should be aware of these cultural norms and function within their orientation. The Arab Muslim culture strongly upholds the married state, which is reinforced by the Qur'an teaching that "men and women are created mates, a pair, to treat each other with affection and compassion within the bonds of matrimony."[39] Celibacy, for the purpose of dedicating one's life totally to God's service, is not highly regarded in Islam. Instead, Muslims are encouraged to marry, since the single state is considered unnatural and potentially leads to sin.[40]

Arab Muslims value and have a strong procreation orientation that is supported by Islamic beliefs. Children are regarded as God's greatest gift since they bring continuation of life. Although the Qur'an makes no reference to contraception, birth control and family planning are traditionally sensitive topics since there tends to be a strong belief that the number of children to be born is determined by Allah. It is usually not within the traditional role of the Muslim woman to decide alone on a family planning method. The husband is generally consulted, but the attitude toward birth control and family planning will vary with acculturation, education, and according to the country of origin. Abortion is not allowed under Islamic law.

 ## Cultural Food Values and Care Considerations

Cultural values and beliefs regarding food and nutrition are important factors to consider in nursing care. Functions, beliefs, and practices of food-use vary cross-culturally.[41,42] The nurse assesses the use and function of food as an important dimension in understanding Arab behavior and health outcomes. As with other religious groups, Arab Muslims subscribe to a number to dietary rules and taboos derived from religious law. Under Islamic law the consumption of pork, alcohol, and improperly slaughtered meat (meat that is not halal) is forbidden. Since few hospitals provide halal meat on the menu, the Muslim who observes strict dietary regulations may select a vegetarian diet when hospitalized. Furthermore, many American processed foods use pork products such as lard, which poses a problem for the Muslim client. Using Leininger's culture care accommodation mode of decision-action, the nurse should first assess with the client the extent to which dietary restrictions are observed, and then take steps to accommodate the client in the choice of food. Most Muslims when hospitalized expect and appreciate accommodation to their dietary laws, even though they may be less diligent in other religious practices.

Food and diet vary considerably throughout the Arab world; however, in all Arab Muslim cultures, food is closely associated with hospitality and quality of care. The traditional sign of Middle Eastern hospitality is the serving of a small cup of Arabic coffee to visitors, regardless of the time of day. Certain rules of etiquette govern the serving of coffee. The elderly are served first and generally men before women, although this may vary throughout the Arab world. To refuse a cup of coffee from one's host is considered disrespectful and uncaring.

Bread is a major staple of diet of most Arab Muslims. While many families purchase bread daily from an Arab bakery, many Muslim women in the United States continue to make bread at home in the traditional fashion. Bread is generally eaten at every meal and symbolizes the abundance of God's blessings. Should a piece of bread accidentally fall to the floor, the Arab Muslim may pick it up and touch it to the lips and forehead while uttering praise to God for giving bread to eat.

A field study conducted by the writer with Lebanese Muslims in a large, urban United States city revealed diet to be the area of least acculturation, in that the people have maintained the food habits of their native country.[43,44] Neither frozen nor canned foods were eaten with any regularity. Instead, foods were cooked fresh daily and a variety of spices and herbs (e.g., *za'atar, yansoun, na'ana*) are used for both cooking and medicinal purposes. Meleis notes that "American food is thought to be too bland for Arab patients," and therefore food is often brought into the hospital from home.[45] Hospitals that provide services to a large Arab population need to consider employing a transcultural nutritionist or transcultural nurse to facilitate effective caring practices, since food is closely linked to care, health and well-being.

Health, Illness, and Care Beliefs and Practices

According to Leininger, health, illness, and care are largely cultural phenomena with meanings that vary significantly according to cultural background.[46] Care is seen as influencing the health state of individuals, families, and groups, whereas health tends to be congruent with and reflect many care practices and philosophical orientations.[47] Health includes more than just physical and psychological dimensions; it encompasses important social and cultural aspects of well-being as well. Understanding health, illness, and care from a cultural frame of reference is important according to Leininger,[48] since culture provides the framework for human behaviors, including health and care practices. Prior to initiating a plan of care, it is imperative that nurses assess the clients' perceptions of their health-illness state in light of their cultural values, beliefs, and patterned lifeways. These emic interpretations are important for guiding the modes of nursing interventions.

Several traditional beliefs regarding health and illness still prevail among many Arab Muslims. One example is the phenomenon of the "evil eye" (*ain al-hasud*), as one of several supernatural origins of disease or misfortune. Referred to in the Qur'an, central to the phenomenon is the belief that one can project harm or misfortune on another by admiring that person's possessions with jealousy or envy. Any form of admiration thus becomes suspect as a potential vehicle for casting the evil eye, and blue-eyed persons and women without children are particularly thought to have evil-eye power.[49] Aswad, based on anthropological fieldwork in a Muslim village in Turkey, identified that the evil eye is often attributed to the in-marrying female who has access to family secrets on marriage but who retains a strong bond to her natal family.[50] To avert the evil eye such things as blue beads or charms with verses from the Qur'an are worn. These should not be removed in the caring process unless it is unavoidable since the client may then consider himself or herself particularly vulnerable to evil forces within the environment. The nurse can avoid contributing to any suspicions of casting the evil eye by refraining from overt expressions of admiration for an infant and by uttering the term "Bis-mallah" (God's blessings) and touching the infant.

Visiting patterns in Arab culture have been recognized by a number of anthropologists as constituting important social and political functions.[51–53] Through ethnonursing research with Arab Muslims in the United States, the writer discovered that visiting, as an important sign and reflection of caring behaviors, was expressed in a variety of beliefs and actions.[54] For example, traditional practices in the Middle East necessitate the visiting of the sick by relatives, neighbors, and friends. These visits constitute a social caring obligation to the point that illness often becomes a social gathering—a time when family and friends come together and social ties are renewed. When an individual is hospitalized, there is a more deeply felt obligation of family and friends to visit. Islam teaches that visiting a sick person, along with other good deeds, is an act through which a believer obtains nearness to Allah.[55] To fail to visit at the time of illness is considered damaging to the social relationship and may result in a complete severing of social ties. Although visiting is expected on other occasions such as marriage or birth, failure to do so at these times may affect the relationship, but it usually does not result in complete severing of relations.[56]

Rather than label the Arab Muslim family problematic because large numbers of visitors show up at visiting hours, a culture care accommodation of cultural and religious obligations to visit the sick should be kept in mind by the nurse along with the inherent therapeutic benefits to the client. The nurse should anticipate this critical cultural need and provide a comfortable location in the hospital setting that would accommodate several visitors. Attention to these essential, indigenous acts of care/caring by family and friends should be anticipated, recognized, and accommodated rather that criticized if the goal of culture care congruence is to be attained.

Attitudes toward death and dying and the cultural expression of grief are other important areas that the nurse needs to consider in providing culturally sensitive care to Arab Muslim clients. Traditional Muslim beliefs support the deterministic position that whatever happens in life is a result of destiny, or God's will. Therefore, a traditionally oriented Muslim may believe that the time of death is predetermined; when death is to occur, there is nothing that can change it.[57] However, a sense of hope always remains, since it is believed that only God knows when death will occur. The nurse can assist Arab Muslim clients in maintaining a sense of hope by avoiding the utterance of a potentially fatal outcome or avoiding the communication of a terminal diagnosis to a client or the family.[58] The subject of death is usually avoided, since there is a belief among some that to "speak of death is to bring it about."[59] For this reason the nurse should be extremely cautious in counseling Arab Muslim clients with terminal cancer or other fatal illnesses. Western models, which encourage terminal clients to talk about approaching death, may be inappropriate in the context of Arab Muslim culture.

Death in the Arab Muslim culture is another occasion that enhances the solidarity of family and social relationships and allows for the expression of grief.[60] Traditional rituals of grief differ among urban and village residents throughout the Arab world. In the past, the death of a villager was traditionally accompanied by loud wailing, crying, and moaning of female members and often tearing of the hair and clothing. Although this tradition is undergoing change, visiting by family and friends for several days after death remains an expectation and, as with illness, is a social obligation. Another custom that continues is the wearing of dark colors by female relatives during mourning. Ceremonies and mourning for the deceased may extend for a period of 40 days up to 1 year following death.

According to Islamic law, a Muslim who dies does not own his body; therefore, organ donation or transplantation is usually not considered, nor are post-mortem examinations.[61] Burial, rather than cremation, is considered the only lawful means of disposing of the body. The nurse may discover that a Muslim family may prefer a family member or friend to carry out the task of preparing the body after death, since special rituals of washing the body and wrapping it in a special cloth shroud are part of Islamic belief.

Summary

Transcultural nursing care of Arab Muslim clients can be extremely rewarding if the nurse is knowledgeable about their culture care and health meanings and lifeways. Knowledge of the complex social structure features, worldview, language, and cultural values are critical in promoting and maintaining care for Arab Muslim clients. The centrality of religion and the family are closely interrelated and reflect many aspects of health and care. This chapter has presented an overview of some of these major features. The importance of culturalogical health care assessment for each client and family cannot be overemphasized, since cultural background, education, and degree of acculturation influence variation in cultural patterns. Although this chapter has focused on the Arab Muslim client, it should be kept in mind that some cultural similarities exist among Arabs and apply also to patterns of Arab Christians. The use of Leininger's Culture Care theory with the Sunrise Model for modes of nursing action are most valuable to assess and make decisions regarding care that is culturally specific and congruent to the Arab Muslim client. Only through the use of transcultural nursing care knowledge and sensitivity to clients can nurses be effective in providing culturally congruent and meaningful healthcare. The Culture Care theory has been most useful to this research for over a decade for discovering transcultural knowledge and for understanding the Arab Muslims' worldview and social structure factors, as well as their language, history, and the environmental context in which health and well-being are expressed and become known.

References

1. Leininger, M., "Leininger's Theory of Culture Care Diversity and Universality: A Theory of Nursing," *Nursing Science Quarterly*, 1988, v. 1, no. 4, pp. 152–160.
2. Leininger, M., *Culture Care Diversity and Universality: A Theory of Nursing*. New York: National League for Nursing Press, 1991.
3. Luna, L., *Care and Cultural Context of Lebanese Muslims in an Urban US Community: An Ethnographic and Ethnonursing Study Conceptualized Within Leininger's Theory*, doctoral dissertation: Ann Arbor, MI: UMI Dissertation Services (order number 9022423), 1989.
4. Luna, L., "Care and Cultural Context of Lebanese Muslim Immigrants with Leininger's Theory," *Journal of Transcultural Nursing*, 1994, v. 5, no. 2, pp. 12–20.
5. Luna, L., "Culturally Competent Health Care: A Challenge for Nurses in Saudi Arabia," *Journal of Transcultural Nursing*, 1998, v. 9, no. 2, pp. 8–14.
6. Leininger, op. cit., 1991.
7. Leininger, M., "The Phenomenon of Caring: Importance, Research Questions and Theoretical Considerations," *Caring: An Essential Human Need*, M. Leininger, ed., Thorofare, NJ: Charles B. Slack, 1981.
8. Leininger, op. cit., 1988.
9. Leininger, op. cit., 1991.
10. Ibid.
11. Arab Information Center, *Who Are the Arabs?* New York: The League of Arab States, 1986.
12. Almaney, A. and A. Alwan, *Communicating with Arabs*, Prospect Heights, IL: Waveland Press, 1982.
13. Adams, C., "Islamic Faith," in *Introduction to Islamic Civilization*, R. Savory, ed., New York: Cambridge University Press, 1979.
14. Fry, G. and J. King, *Islam: A Survey of the Muslim Faith*, Grand Rapids, MI: Baker Book House, 1980.
15. Martin, R., *Islam: A Cultural Perspective*, Upper Saddle River, NJ: Prentice-Hall, 1982.
16. Naff, A., "Arabs in America: A Historical Overview," *Arabs in the New World*, S. Abraham

and N. Abraham, eds., Detroit: Wayne State University Center for Urban Studies, 1983.

17. Haddad, Y., "Muslims in the United States," *Islam: The Religious and Political Life of a World Community*, M. Kelly, ed., New York: Praeger, 1984.
18. Ibid.
19. Abraham, S., "Detroit's Arab-American Community: A Survey of Diversity and Commonality," *Arabs in the New World*, S. Abraham and N. Abraham, eds., Detroit: Wayne State University Center for Urban Studies, 1983.
20. Haddad, Y., "Arab Muslims and Islamic Institutions in America: Adaptation and Reform," *Arabs in the New World*, S. Abraham and N. Abraham, eds., Detroit: Wayne State University Center for Urban Studies, 1983.
21. Aswad, B., *Arabic Speaking Communities in American Cities*, New York: Center for Migration Studies, 1974.
22. Haddad, Y., *The Muslims of America*, New York: Oxford University Press, 1991.
23. Ahmad, K., *Islam: Its Meaning and Message*, London: Redwood Burn Limited, 1975.
24. Hassan, R., "Peace and Islamic World View," *Occasional Papers: Proceedings of International Conference—The Quest for Peace Beyond Ideology*, M. Max, ed., Detroit: Wayne State University, 1981.
25. Al Faruqi, L., "Unity and Variety in the Music of Islamic Culture," *The Islamic Impact*, Y. Haddad, B. Haines, and E. Findly, eds., New York: Syracuse University Press, 1981.
26. Hamid, A., *Islam: The Natural Way*, London: MELS Publishing Company, 1996.
27. Bates, D. and A. Rassam, *Peoples and Cultures of the Middle East*, Englewood Cliffs, NJ: Prentice Hall, 1983.
28. Ibid.
29. Fry and King, op. cit., 1980.
30. Luna, op. cit., 1998.
31. Leininger, op. cit., 1991.
32. Weekes, R., *Muslim Peoples: A World Ethnographic Survey*, London: Greenwood Press, 1978.
33. Al Faruqi, op. cit., 1981.
34. Barakat, H., "The Arab Family and the Challenge of Social Transformation," *Women and the Family in the Middle East: New Voices of Change*, E. Fernea, ed., Austin, TX: University of Texas Press, 1985.
35. Bashshur, R., "Aspects of Family Organization and Personal Adjustment in Arab Society: Contrasts

Between Traditional and Western Models," unpublished paper, 1986.
36. Luna, op. cit., 1994.
37. Kulwicki, A., "Health Issues Among Arab Muslim Families," *Family and Gender Among American Muslims*, B. Aswad and B. Bilge, eds., Philadelphia: Temple University Press, 1996.
38. Elkholy, A., "The Arab American Family," *Ethnic Families in America: Patterns and Variations*, C. Mindel and R. Habenstein, eds., New York: Elsevier, 1981.
39. Marsot, A., "The Changing Arab Muslim Family," *Islam: The Religion and Political Life of a World Community*, M. Kelly, ed., New York: Praeger, 1984.
40. Ibid.
41. Leininger, M., *Transcultural Nursing: Concepts, Theories, and Practices*, New York: John Wiley & Sons, 1978.
42. Leininger, M., *Transcultural Nursing: Concepts, Theories, Research, and Practice*, Columbus, OH: McGraw-Hill College Custom Series, 1995.
43. Luna, L., "Health and Care Phenomena Among Lebanese-American Muslims," unpublished field study, Detroit: Wayne State University, 1986.
44. Luna, op. cit., 1994.
45. Meleis, A., "The Arab-American in the Health Care System," *American Journal of Nursing*, 1981, v. 81, pp. 1180–1183.
46. Leininger, op. cit., 1978.
47. Leininger, op. cit., 1991.
48. Ibid.
49. Spooner, B., "The Evil Eye in the Middle East," *The Evil Eye*, C. Maloney, ed., New York: Columbia University Press, 1976.
50. Aswad, B., "Key and Peripheral Roles of Noble Women in a Middle Eastern Plains Village," *Anthropological Quarterly*, 1974a, v. 47, pp. 9–27.
51. Altorki, S., *Women in Saudi Arabia: Ideology and Behavior Among the Elite*, New York: Columbia University Press, 1986.
52. Aswad, B., "Visiting Patterns Among Women of the Elite in a Small Turkish City," *Anthropological Quarterly*, 1974b, v. 47, pp. 9–27.
53. Joseph, S., "Women and the Neighborhood Street in Borj Hammoud, Lebanon," *Women in the Muslim World*, I. Beck and N. Keddie, eds., Cambridge: Harvard University Press, 1978.
54. Luna, op. cit., 1994.

55. Al Muzaffar, *The Faith of Shi'a Islam*, Great Britain: The Muhammadi Trust, 1982.

56. Altorki, op. cit., 1986.

57. Baqui, M., "Muslim Teachings Concerning Death," *Nursing Times*, 1979, v. 75, no. 14, pp. 44–45.

58. Meleis, A. and A. Jonsen, "Ethical Crises and Cultural Differences," *The Western Journal of Medicine*, 1983, v. 138, no. 6.

59. Racy, J., "Death in an Arab Culture," *Annals of the New York Academy of Science*, 1969, v. 164, pp. 871–880.

60. Fakhouri, J., *Kafr El-Elow: An Egyptian Village in Transition*, Prospect Heights, IL: Waveland Press, 1972.

61. Henley, A. and J. Clayton, "Religion of the Muslims," *Health and Social Service Journal*, 1982, v. 97, pp. 918–919.

17

African Americans and Culture Care

Marjorie G. Morgan

One of the largest minority groups living in the United States today is that of the African Americans. It is important that professional nurses understand this culture to provide culturally congruent nursing care. Because of the variability among African Americans living in different places in the United States, the nurse needs to take into account both the diverse and the common beliefs, values, and lifeways of the people when planning nursing care for them.

The worldview of African Americans comes from their cultural heritage and their experiences in the United States. The worldview of most nurses comes mainly from living in this country, but also from nursing education and clinical practice. When an African American seeks professional services, the nurse and client may have difficulty understanding each other unless the nurse has knowledge of the African American culture. Differences in culture care values, beliefs, and practices between the nurse and client may lead to cultural conflicts and less beneficial care for the client. If the nurse does not understand and accept the cultural characteristics of the client, the client may decide to reject the nursing care that is offered.

In this chapter, Leininger's Theory of Culture Care Diversity and Universality[1] will be used to identify patterns of care through beliefs, values, and practices of African Americans. This theory is useful to help nurses learn about care that can contribute to the health and well-being of African Americans. While using the theory, an understanding is awakened that the lifeways and beliefs of the people tend to be embedded in the religious, political, economic, and other aspects of the social structure of the people. In addition to social structures, the language and environmental context of the

African Americans have to be considered to get an accurate picture.

In the use of Leininger's theory, the generic folk care and health beliefs are contrasted with professional health beliefs of nurses and other professional health care providers. Understanding these contrasting folk care and health beliefs, values, and practices enables nurses to use this knowledge to make nursing care decisions. Through the use of culture care knowledge, the nurse can provide practices that facilitate three different modes of action or decisions. The three modes from the Culture Care Theory are nursing care preservation/maintenance, accommodation/negotiation, and repatterning/restructuring. Using these modes of care, the nurse can provide culturally congruent and culture-specific care to African American clients.[2]

Ethnohistory and the African American Caring and Health Ways

Nurses who practice transcultural nursing consider that it is important to know the history of a people to understand the way in which the people view their world and their health care. For example, many of the folk remedies of the African Americans came from the time that they spent in slavery in the United States. Since there were often no physicians and nurses available to the slaves, they had to depend on remedies that they brought with them from Africa.[3,4] This system of folk healing was then passed down from generation to generation until the present time, when many of the same remedies are still in use.[5]

The history of African slavery began in 1444 when Henry the Navigator took 165 Africans to Portugal on a slave ship.[6] The practice of moving people from West

Africa in slave trade lasted for approximately four centuries. As Masrui has stated, "No people in history have been forcibly exported in such large numbers as Africans. And the Americas were the largest recipients of these reluctant exiles."[7] About ten million Africans were removed from Africa and brought to the Americas by slave ship, crossing the Atlantic Ocean in a 6- to 10-week sea voyage known as the Middle Passage.[8] Africans were brought to the New World where they were held as slaves in North and South America and the Caribbean. At the same time, many European countries were involved in the colonization of these same areas. Osborne refers to Sherlock who stated that the three institutions of African slavery, European colonization, and a plantation economy gave impetus to the Creole society, which was common to the Caribbean, southern United States, and Central and South America.[9,10]

From this history and from the Creole society grew the belief and value systems of many African Americans. Snow found that the elements of their health belief system come from a variety of sources, including European folklore, Greek classical medicine, the cultures of West Africa, and modern scientific medicine.[11] Plantation owners and overseers came from Europe, so the slaves combined the European folklore, which they learned from their masters, with their African remedies to deal with injury and illness. Often the European methods included the Greek classical remedies since most Europeans had education in the Greek and Roman traditions. Years later, as African Americans left the rural areas of the South to find work in the urban North and the West, reliance on the biomedicine system began to be seen as the people became more acculturated to the dominant American way of health. However, many of the folk practices from the rural South are still found wherever African Americans live.

After the Civil War in 1870, the Fifteenth Amendment to the United States Bill of Rights gave former slaves the right to vote. Civil rights legislation of 1875 opened public accommodations and jury duty to the same people. However, ways were found by the white majority of Americans to deny these rights.

The rise of the automobile industry in Detroit and other industries in the North provided employment opportunities bringing many African Americans North from the South. Bailey[12] states that, indeed, over one million people moved from the South to the North between 1910 and 1930. Bailey sees the migration as happening from "push-pull factors," as the people were "pushed out of the South because of the boll weevil, flooding, disenfranchishement, and the effect of the Jim Crow acts." They were at the same time pulled to the North "by increased demand for their labor."[13] Dr. Martin Luther King and the Civil Rights movement were instrumental in getting the 1964 Civil Rights Bill passed by Congress. This legislation banned discrimination in jobs, schools, public accommodations, and voting. While racism is still found in the United States, African Americans have carved out a niche in the society through the exercise of their rights. Today, many elected officials are African American. Better educational opportunities have enabled more African Americans to reach their dreams of professional life. However, as an African American colleague stated, "many" still does not translate into "the majority."

More recent history of African Americans has included a rise in Afrocentric awareness as the concepts of plurality and cultural heritage consistency have begun to gain prominence in the United States. The old American belief in the "melting pot" as being the proper means to enfold new and different cultures into the fabric of the land has been questioned. Nathan Glazer and Daniel Patrick Moynihan in 1963 asserted that "negroes" were Americans with no African beliefs and practices left to value.[14] Masrui, writing in 1986, saw a new pride rising and re-Africanization occurring after years of attempts by the Western world to dis-Africanize Black Americans.[15] More African Americans are now learning about their cultural heritage in schools and colleges throughout America, but all too often the history of African Americans is usually limited to that provided during "Black History" month or that taught to African American students who have the time and money to fit such a course into a plan of study. Black history often has been poorly integrated into formal American history courses.

Nurses who understand the care, health, and illness beliefs, values, and practices that rise from the ethnohistory of the African Americans can plan and provide better nursing care. Knowledge of social structure, worldview, and environmental context also help the nurse to identify and understand the beliefs, practices, and values. These factors will be considered next.

▪ Social Structures, Worldview, Health, and Care

Studying human care with reference to the African American worldview and social structure can be a challenging yet most stimulating learning endeavor in light of the diversity that exists among African Americans in the United States. Bloch has stated that factors such as social class, age, sex roles, region or location in the United States, socialization patterns, individual life experiences or circumstances, and ongoing changes in the cultural environment all contribute to variation in the African American group of people.[16] However, among these variations some common characteristics in beliefs, values, and practices prevail.

In the United States there are over 33 million African Americans who make up 17% of the American population. The majority live in industrial Midwestern and Northeastern cities of the United States and in the rural South. About 53% live in the southern states where in-migration is equal to out-migration.[17]

No matter where in the United States African Americans live, one of the most important social structure features in this group is the extended family and its kinship ties. The extended family is one that includes not only people related *by blood*, but also those who are brought into it as fictive kin, such as boyfriends, preachers, family friends, and many others. Close friends from organizations such as sororities, fraternities, and church are considered *brothers* and *sisters* or *aunts* and *uncles*.[18] The concept of "my brothers and sisters" and "my aunts and uncles" must therefore be considered to include many who may not be related by biological ties. A review of pertinent literature shows that this African American family closeness often goes beyond geographical, legal, political, and economic borders. Members of the extended family lend support to one another by gifts, child care, financial help, home repairs, and advice for personal problems.[19-22]

Stack[23] and Twining[24] discovered in their studies that families in an indigent African American community practiced cooperative sharing and swapping of goods and services within the kinship system as strategies for survival. Families that have been separated because of members moving from one geographical area to another find that family reunions, marriages, and funerals are valuable times to maintain the family.[25]

These celebrations and rituals also reinforce bonds of solidarity and closeness in caring for each other in the African American community.

Many researchers have explored and debated the basis for the strength of the extended family in the African American community. Some classic writers argue that the African American family has its roots in Africa,[26,27] while others view the influence of the American political, economic, and social struggles as contributing to the values and characteristics of the family.[28-30] Aschenbrenner found that the values related to the family were "1) a high value placed on children; 2) the approval of strong, protective mothers; 3) the emphasis on strict discipline and respect for elders; 4) the strength of the family bonds; and 5) the ideal of an independent spirit."[31] There is evidence of a caring ethos among extended family members that strengthens many African Americans in times of crisis and that enables them to face daily living and survival.[32,33]

Specific statements related to the family and health care were given in articles by African American nurses Bloch[34] and Thomas.[35] When a member of a family is ill, the family is less likely than in some other cultural groups to see this as a personal burden, but will instead view the problem as a family illness. Both authors state that there is a strong tradition of having kinfolks "sit up" with a family member who is ill. The family in the African American community usually has one person who is given the duty to make the major decisions for other family members, including those related to care and health concerns. Sometimes, health decisions are refused until this person is consulted.

Religion is another important factor of the social structure that influences the care and health values, beliefs, and practices of African Americans. A belief in a higher power extends to every facet of life, including health. Many African Americans believe that without the power of God no one can be healed or saved from death. Gospel and African American folk music reflect this belief in God's or Jesus' healing power.[36] The moral teachings from the church can lead to good caring and health practices. Health is attributed to "living right." For example, by not doing too much "partying" and by doing good deeds, health will come as a "blessing from God."[37]

The belief that God, health, and illness are closely connected can be found in the work of several researchers. Leininger reported statements from her informants such as "If you follow what is in the Bible, you will be well and stay well," "The Bible teaches you how to keep well and avoid evil thoughts and actions that could make you ill," and "One has to let Jesus be the healer.... People who are not working with Jesus have to use other people to heal them."[38] Roberson stated that Bible passages were frequently cited as sources for particular health beliefs by her informants. One of the key beliefs that she found was that God does nothing bad to people, but that he can turn a person over to the devil who can then cause malevolent illnesses.[39] The ability for God to give relief from illness is found in William's ethnography about members of a Black Pentecostal Church.[40] He quoted several of his informants about God and illness. One person testified, "When my bronchial tubes were stopped up and I could not breathe for myself, I needed an artificial respirator and God got in them tubes." Another person said, "I got a sore throat yesterday. God is a throat specialist."

African American churches are not only places of worship, they often function as "an escape mechanism from the harsh realities of daily life."[41] Church activities furnish opportunities for many African Americans to have roles of respect such as preacher, deacon, usher, choir leader or member, or Sunday School leader. The minister, along with deacons, members of missionary circles, choir members, Sunday School teachers, and others, will often expect and be expected to visit a member of their congregation who is ill. These people offer encouragement and meet the spiritual needs of the person and the family in stressful situations such as an illness.[42,43]

There is, however, diversity in the religious beliefs of African Americans, and nurses should not assume that all clients are Christian. Some African Americans are followers of Islam, some embrace the Jewish faith, and others belong to various other groups with diverse beliefs.[44] Getting information from clients about their religious beliefs is part of the culturalogical assessment.

Education is another aspect of social structure that is extremely important to African Americans. Older members of the group have a great desire for their children to obtain a good education as a means for advancement in society. During the past three decades the illiteracy rate in the United States has dropped appreciably, and college enrollment has increased. Still, there is great discrepancy in the different races when education is taken into consideration. For example, while 20% of white Americans have bachelor degrees, only 10% of black Americans achieve this higher education.[45] This increased opportunity for education has not translated into an equitable situation in the job market for African Americans. According to Sidell, only 47% of African American college graduates earn the same income that Anglo-Americans earn with high school education.[46]

Many authors have advanced the idea that economic factors have a major effect on the lifeways of the African Americans and on their health.[47–49] During a 20-year period between 1962 and 1982, the percentage of African Americans living below the poverty level was twice that of Anglo-Americans.[50] Rather than improving, recent figures based on the 1994 census show a wider disparity, with 9% of Caucasians living below the poverty level, while 30% of African Americans do so.[51] As Sidel stated, "If you're poor, you're more likely to be sick, less likely to receive adequate medical care, and more likely to die at an early age. The effects of poverty on health and general well-being are clear-cut and profound."[52]

Studies have shown that the inability of many African Americans to get health care within the professional system is caused by their impoverished economic state.[53] While many factors may be related to the high morbidity and mortality rates in the African American population, lack of professional care resulting from poverty contributes to the high rates of heart disease, cancer, hypertension, tuberculosis, and infant deaths in this group.[54]

The author has found in both her research and her practice of nurse-midwifery that many pregnant African American mothers do not receive needed prenatal care because of a lack of medical insurance, money, transportation, and other factors associated with poverty.[55] A study in the Morbidity and Mortality Weekly Report,[56] based on research from 1987 to 1996, reported that while the morbidity-mortality rate for white women fell from 5.5 to 5.0 per 100,000 live births, the rate for African American women rose from 18.8 to 20.3.

Poverty also contributes to concern with the present rather than with the future. Living with poverty forces many African Americans to think about the day-to-day necessities of life, rather than about what might happen in the future. The nurse will soon learn that for some African Americans taking time off from work for nursing care or medical treatment is not considered important when money has to be earned for food, shelter, and other basics for the extended family, especially for those needs of the children and the elderly. Sometimes, health care has to receive less attention.

The cultural philosophy of being present oriented, rather than future oriented, is sometimes combined with a fatalistic view about illness and pain. Considering these values and philosophical beliefs, the positive effects of preventive and continuing health care, as taught by some nurses and other health care providers, are often difficult for the African American client to understand.

 African Americans and Their Folk Health Care System

The inability of some African Americans to get professional health care does not mean that the people do not get any health care. Instead, the African Americans have long had a folk or generic health care system. This folk system is the traditional way of caring and healing. Most people seek out extended family members, friends, and neighbors for advice on illness, caring, and curing. There is also use of folk health practices and healing ways brought originally from Africa. Herbs and nonprescription drugs are often used. Assistance may be sought from folk practitioners and faith healers, with reliance on the professional health system only during extreme injury or illness.[57] Bailey,[58] in a study in an urban community, discovered a cultural pattern of seeking health care. He found six steps were taken by African Americans when faced with illness:[59]

1. The illness appears.
2. Individual waits for a certain period of days.
3. The body is allowed to heal itself while the individual uses prayer or traditional, generic healing regimens.
4. Individual evaluates daily activities and may try to reduce work or stress.

5. Individual seeks advice from a family member or some friend (church leader and/or traditional, generic healer included).
6. Individual finally attends health clinic or sees family physician.

Research by Capers also found that many African American people use their religious beliefs, friends and neighbors, root doctors, spiritual healers, and magic vendors before they seek professional health care.[60] She reported that her informants felt that the treatments provided by generic or folk healers seemed to "lie closer to the everyday experiences and worldviews of the clients than the more esoteric explanations based on a biomedical model of health and illness."[61] Mothers and grandmothers are often consulted, especially in health care related to babies. For example, advice is frequently sought for such things as colic.[62]

Leininger stated that the informants she interviewed in the southern part of the United States gave several cognitive reasons for beliefs related to professional health care. She reported that the people did not trust such care because they felt that it was dangerous, unfriendly, slow, costly, and strange and that they were not treated as "whole" people. They preferred to trust generic, traditional care and used many folk care practices to maintain well-being and health.[63]

To identify ways in which African Americans remain well or become ill, Leininger's theory of studying care values, practices, and beliefs is important. Some of the beliefs and practices within the African American folk or generic system of health care and curing came to the United States from Africa and have been passed down from generation to generation as part of the transmission of culture.

For African Americans good care can lead to good health. Good care and good health depend on being in tune with nature and its forces. Illnesses are classified as natural ones when they have natural causes. For example, illnesses are caused by such things as exposure to cold air, rain, heat, impurities in the air, or bad food or water without adequate protection.[64] An example of a natural illness is arthritis-type pain. The cause of the pain is seen as exposure to cold air or to rain. Prevention is to bundle up with heavy clothes, carry an umbrella, or stay indoors during inclement weather. When one is exposed to the elements, illness may be revealed much later in life. A close African American friend of the author was told by older women that she was running a risk of getting arthritis when she did not remain in the house for 6 weeks after her child was born.[65] In this author's clinical practice with postnatal clients, if a new mother calls to report a complication and is told to come to the clinic, she will often reply that she cannot go out yet, because her mother or grandmother told her she could not. Respect for the opinion of the elder is paramount.

In the face of illness brought on by natural forces, books may also be consulted by African Americans such as the *Farmer's Almanac*, which contains information on the position of planets, the phases of the moon, and weather forecasts. These natural forces are seen as important factors that can affect the health and well-being of people.[66]

This writer also found in her own research that many books written by and for African Americans that relate to holistic health care are being sold in African American bookstores. These books contain instructions for herbal remedies and ways to use heat and cold, crystals, massage, and meditation in generic health care. These can be considered as generic care modalities to improve the health and well-being of African Americans.[67]

The opposite of natural illness is unnatural illness. Unnatural illnesses are caused by evil influences on the person in the form of witchcraft, hoodoo, voodoo, or rootwork. While the professional health care personnel work to treat and possibly cure natural illnesses, they usually have limited effect on unnatural ones. For these illnesses, generic or traditional healers must be consulted.[68,69]

Traditional healers use roots, herbs, potions, oils, powders, tokens, rites, and ceremonies in their healing practices. These healers will often combine secular and religious rituals in their care and curing of African Americans. The patient is sometimes told to go to a candle store to get oils, incense, candles, soaps, and aerosol room sprays to repel evil forces.[70] In the Southern part of the United States where this writer practiced nursing, the doors, window frames, and sills are painted light blue on many houses in the African American community. This is also to keep out the "haunts," "haints," or evil spirits that can cause unnatural illnesses.[71]

When African Americans enter the professional health care system, they often bring these beliefs with them. Bloch suggested that when an African American goes to a professional health care provider, the nurse or doctor should assume that the client has already tried some generic healing methods. The professional needs to ask what treatments have been used to be sure that there will be no conflict or incompatibility with the professional modes of helping the person.[72]

■ Language and the Power of Words

Language is an important aspect to be considered in studying any culture. Specific words and nonverbal expressions related to African American health beliefs, practices, and values are often expressed in nurse-client situations in the cultural context. Many can be heard and observed by nurses in the home, hospital, and clinic. There are diverse patterns of thinking and expressing ideas about care, health, and illness in the African-American culture. There are sometimes differences between the Anglo-American and African American languages that the nurse needs to recognize. Smitherman wrote that the language is particularly important in the African American culture. According to the same author, Anglo-Americans depend on the written word to shape their lives, while African Americans uses a spoken mode that is based on the African "orally oriented background." Smitherman continued that the power of life itself in Africa came from the concept of *Nommo* or the "magic power of the word." The power of *Nommo* can be seen from the traditional African culture where ". . . a newborn child is a mere thing until his father gives and speaks his name."[73] This same importance of naming a baby can be seen in American hospitals' newborn nurseries. Distinctive names that reflect the African cultural background of the parents are often given to their new boys or girls by their mothers, fathers, or grandparents.

In American hospitals and clinics many nurses and physicians report that they are too busy to spend more time to get to know, to understand, and to explain illnesses and care to their clients. For many African American clients, who come from an oral tradition, time spent for conversation is seen as more important than nursing care, medical treatments, or recordkeeping. African American patients think that the nurse does not care if she has not talked and listened to them. As Smitherman stated, "No medicine, potion, or magic of any sort is considered effective without accompanying words."[74] The nurse needs to be aware of the value of oral stories, legends, and personal experiences in caring for African American clients. These oral accounts enable the nurse to understand ways to link folk and professional care together for culturally competent care practices.

Some African American clients in the health care settings may use a style of communication that is cultural in nature but foreign to the health care providers. The use of Black English, a distinctive language that reflects African heritage combined with historical factors of American life, may lead to misunderstandings in a health care setting and a lack of sensitive modes of caring. Smitherman wrote that 80% to 90% of African Americans use Black English some or all of the time.[75] This varies with the geographical area in which the client lives and the age and educational background of the person.[76] Black English is a highly oral, stylized, rhythmic, spontaneous language with the meaning of words dependent on the environmental context in which they are said.[77] If the nurse does not understand what is being said, it is important to clarify ideas with the patient and the family.

A particular problem can arise in treating African American clients related to their health and illness expressions. For example, the nurse needs to understand the various ways in which the term *blood* is used by some African Americans. Blood can be called high or low, rich or poor, thick or thin, up or down, clean or defiled, sweet or sour, and new or used. Since the terms are used in so many different ways, with, for example, "low blood," "low blood pressure," and "low blood count" being considered equivalent, the nurse needs to clarify what is meant when blood is referred to by the client.[78]

The nurse can confuse many clients of any cultural group with the use of highly technical health terms. This may result in the client not understanding, but pretending that he or she knows what is going on. Another reaction of the client may be anger and suspicion of the nurse who is trying to communicate. The patient may get frustrated when the nurse does not understand what the client is saying. Unfortunate, embarrassing situations can arise from not understanding terms such

as "I've got to make water" indicating the need for urination. Another complaint of a client went untreated because the nurse did not realize that the client had a swollen gland, when the patient complained of having a "kernel."

From the above study of the worldview, social structure, language, and environmental context of African Americans, one can find patterns and expressions of care that contribute to health and well-being or that lead to illness. For example, the extended family has many caring ways such as being concerned about or for one's brothers and sisters. These attitudes and actions can lead to health and well-being as predicted in Leininger's theory. In addition, transcultural nurses have studied and discovered specific care meanings, which will be discussed next.

The Meaning of Care

Several researchers have done ethnographic and ethnonursing studies of African Americans and have determined the meanings and actions that express care in that culture. In Leininger's theory culture and care are directly linked and must be considered in the planning and delivering of culturally congruent care. Leininger studied care phenomena among African Americans living in a rural area of the southern United States. She found that one manifestation of care came from "concern for others." Within this construct were patterns of providing for the needs of *brothers* and *sisters*, being aware of others' needs, and helping others obtain these needs. Other expressions of caring were seen in "being present" in the community and of being "involved with" family and neighbors. She discovered that "touching" others within the community, particularly in times of sorrow and loss, was important to demonstrate care and caring. Finally, "sharing" showed care in the African American group that she studied. This had such diverse meanings as the sharing of food, sharing religious experiences, sharing as a survival strategy, and the responsibility of family members to share.[79]

In an indigent urban area, Stack[80] reported that care was demonstrated by her African American informants by sharing of goods and services but with the added activities of *swapping*. As she points out, sharing generally implies the giving of something to another person without obligation, and swapping entails an exchange relationship with the obligation to eventually return an item or activity of equal value to the giver. Both sharing and swapping care activities provided what the author calls a "... steady source of cooperative support to survive."[81]

In her research with extended families in Chicago, Aschenbrenner reported that both men and women agreed that it is of *supreme importance* to care for and bring children up properly. Care for the young ones involved strict discipline and teaching them to have love and respect for their elders.[82]

Osborne found that this respect for the elderly extends well into adulthood.[83] The extended family often is multigenerational. In a study in 1988 Flaherty[84] reported on caring functions of grandmothers who took care of the infants of their adolescent daughters. Four of these caring functions were, "... managing activities to meet family needs, caretaking of the infant activities, coaching or role-modeling the maternal role, and nurturing and loving the mother and the grandchild."[85] Care was also shown to the daughter by assessing the new mother's attitude about mothering, assigning with expressions the mother's ownership of the baby, and patrolling the new mother's lifestyle and life goals.[86]

In this author's research, four main themes emerged from the data related to African American women and prenatal care. These were 1) cultural care meant protection, presence, and sharing; 2) social structural factors that greatly influenced the health and well-being were spirituality, kinship, and economics; 3) professional prenatal care was seen by the women as necessary and essential, but there was distrust of noncaring professionals and other barriers to care; and 4) folk health beliefs and practices and indigenous health care providers were widely used by pregnant women in the African American community.[87]

A study by Mann et al., describing the personal experiences of pregnant African American women, outlined some of the provisions of practice that contributed to the care and well-being of the women. Recognition by nurses of the meaning of pregnancy as a transitional period from childhood to adulthood to motherhood was an important theme. Further, stresses as experienced by the women included a lack of material things and emotional support. Finally, the heightened need for interpersonal support with other significant people such as other women, mothers, and partners was put forth in interviews with the women.[88]

 ## Culturally Congruent Nursing Care

To plan for and provide culturally congruent professional nursing care, the nurse bases decisions on a culturalogical assessment to see if the clients's health beliefs and practices should be maintained, accepted, or changed in some manner. From this assessment of the cultural beliefs, values, and practices of the client, the nurse uses Leininger's three care modes of nursing decisions and actions. As stated earlier, these three modes are culture care maintenance/preservation, accommodation/negotiation, and restructuring/repatterning. If current health care beliefs and activities are beneficial, then the nurse will use culture care maintenance or preservation. If there is need for change in the care of a client, a decision must be made regarding whether and how the care can be modified with cultural care accommodation or negotiation or whether it needs to be changed by cultural care restructuring or repatterning. A few examples of these modes for planning and carrying out nursing care will be presented.

In caring for the African American client, nurses should consider the cultural values of extended family and religious beliefs. The nurse should preserve the right of the client to draw on these resources for strength and support. Culture care maintenance and preservation would be used to ensure that the family and church members could stay with the client to express their "concern for" and "involvement with" the client. Sometimes, nurses have to use several modes to provide culturally congruent care. In the case of family and others visiting in the hospital, more than just culture care preservation may be needed. Accommodation to these caring needs may entail the nurse's using his or her skills to negotiate with physicians or case managers in the health care institution. This is particularly true if the client is an in-patient where there are hospital rules against visitors at certain times of the day or night. The nurse's knowledge of the cultural importance of family and religion to the African American client's well-being should strengthen her ability to teach the hospital authorities and other practitioners about this and to then use cultural care negotiation effectively.

The cultural value in the African American community in relation to time needs to be considered in planning or providing nursing care. Nurses have been taught that being on time and paying attention to the clock is a fine value and attribute in the Anglo-American culture and in the nursing subculture. The African American patient may be inclined to adhere to a less rigid or more flexible time orientation.[89] Nurses may maintain the cultural value of flexible time for their client by accommodating or negotiating with him or her about when a bath is desired or what time a tray should be served. On the other hand, this flexibility might not be therapeutic in regard to when a medicine or treatment is given. Here the nurse would discuss the matter and then develop a specific negotiation or repatterning care plan.

The trend for short-term hospital care has meant that many nurses are moving into the community to care for patients. This has made transcultural nursing care even more important as clients are less likely to change their usual folk or generic health care practices in their homes than they are in a strange and frightening environment such as the hospital. Evidence of the folk health system of African Americans is often more apparent when nurses go to the homes of their clients. Such things as religious statues, candles, oils, incense, and ointments may be seen at the bedside of clients. Some professional healthcare practitioners find humor in and may ridicule clients about objects of this sort or about generic healthcare practices and practitioners. The transcultural nurse, however, will recognize the importance of incorporating the folk healthcare practices and traditional healers of their clients into the planning and delivery of professional health care.

When giving care in the home, the nurse will often find multigenerational extended family living under one roof. Health care interventions may be ineffective and ignored if the key members of the family are not consulted and included in the planning and delivery of care. Attention to the family and their beliefs, particularly the elders in the group, can lead to culturally congruent care that is meaningful and accepted more readily.

Most nurses realize that using derogatory, offensive, and discriminatory words to describe members of cultural groups will hinder the provision of culturally based care. However, a second form of giving offense, which is sometimes not as apparent, is stereotyping. To stereotype is to assign a trait or belief to all members of a group, rather than realizing that people are individuals and that cultural variabilities exist. Some of the stereotypical beliefs about African Americans are that they all eat watermelon and soul food, that all of the men play or favor basketball as a sport, that all live in dysfunctional families with no concern for their own or others' property, and that "they" all love gospel music.

A striking example of stereotyping was given by one of the members of the Harlem Boys' Choir on television recently. He said that when the group travels, many Anglo-Americans ask the African American boys if they are a basketball team. The young man told his questioner that instead they are members of a choir that sings the works of many composers, including Mozart, Bach, and others.

A culturalogical assessment regarding the individual and family, performed by a transculturally prepared nurse who is mindful of the cultural beliefs, practices, and values, can help prevent rigid stereotyping and profiling and can increase awareness of cultural variability that prevails among African Americans.

While many nurses in the United States place high value on independence, technology, and legal factors in the society, the African Americans view family, religion, and economic factors as being more important. Nurses must realize this difference in worldview and cultural values and use their transcultural nursing skills to meet the needs of their African American clients.

Putting Transcultural Nursing Research Findings into Practice

With the finding that the African American elderly are respected authorities in their culture and that credence is given for their wisdom, an outreach program was devised based on this knowledge in the public health district where this author works as a nurse-midwife and transcultural nursing specialists. She and a colleague went to African American churches to present diverse viewpoints of pregnancy to the elder members in the churches. The elders would then relay the information to their daughters and granddaughters. The program was called *Yesterday, Today, and Tomorrow* and consisted of a discussion between the two nurses. The author presented the folk or generic ideas of pregnancy and childbirth, while her colleague gave the newer more scientific and professional information. This method demonstrated culture care preservation and culture care accommodation by showing respect for the generic ideas, while at the same time teaching current pregnancy practices. The program was considered to be a success. At the churches the presenters felt well received and had the opportunity to respond to many questions from their audience.

Summary

The purpose of this chapter was to discuss some of the transcultural care, health, and illness beliefs, practices, and values that are found among African Americans in the United States. Because of the wide diversity of beliefs and practices in this culture, nurses need to learn about the value of transcultural concepts, principles, and practices, as well as to recognize the importance of using a culturalogical assessment when planning care for clients. The cultural beliefs, values, and practices of African Americans are many and varied. The dominant cultural values are the extended family, religious beliefs, and education. Care beliefs and practices include concern for, respect for, involvement with, presence with, nurturing of, touching of, and sharing with other people, particularly those in the extended family, in the African American community. Transcultural nurses are prepared to incorporate these caring values, beliefs, and practices into professional nursing care with the generic folk care practices and beliefs.

Sawyer, in her summary of a research study, says that her data demonstrate the importance of nurses and other health care providers recognizing the impact of racism on the lives of African American women, confronting the common assumptions that all African Americans are alike, and assessing each woman individually to provide respectful, effective, and stress-reducing care.[90]

Transcultural nurse specialists can be helpful in guiding other nurses in these important ways of caring for African Americans. This chapter demonstrated the discovery of care values and practices through the use of the Theory of Culture Care Diversity and Universality. Discovery of the care, health, and illness beliefs embedded within social structure, worldview, language, and cultural context of African Americans provides a sound and reliable basis to understand this culture. Several modes of action can be used to provide nursing care such as culture care maintenance/preservation, accommodation/negotiation, and repatterning/restructuring. These modes are used to plan and provide culturally specific congruent care. This is the goal of Leininger's theory and the goal of transcultural nurses so that African American clients can receive quality care that helps them recover from illness and maintain their caring lifeways in society.

References

1. Leininger, M.M., *Culture Care Diversity and Universality: A Theory of Nursing*, New York: National League for Nursing Press, 1991.
2. Ibid.
3. Bailey, E.J., *Urban African American Health Care*, Lanham, MD: University Press of America, 1991.
4. Spector, R.E., *Cultural Diversity in Health and Illness*, 3rd ed., Norwalk, CT: Appleton & Lange, 1991.
5. Savitt, T.L., *Medicine and Slavery: The Diseases and Health Care of Blacks in Antebellum Virginia*, Urbana, IL: University of Illinois Press, 1978.
6. Osborne, O.H., "Aging and the Black Diaspora: The African, Caribbean, and African American Experience," in *Transcultural Nursing: Concepts, Theories, and Practices*, M. Leininger, ed., New York: John Wiley & Sons, 1978, pp. 317–333.
7. Masrui, A.A., *The Africans: A Triple Heritage*, Boston: Little Brown & Co., 1986.
8. Rotberg, R.I., "Exploitation," in *The Africans: A Reader*, A.A. Masrui and T.K. Levine, eds., New York: Praeger, 1986, pp. 108–132.
9. Osborne, op. cit., 1978.
10. Sherlock, D., *West Indies*, London: Thames & Hudson, 1960.
11. Snow, L.F., "Popular Medicine in a Black Neighborhood," in *Ethnic Medicine in the Southwest*, E. Spicer, ed., Tucson: University of Arizona Press, 1977, pp. 19–95.
12. Bailey, op. cit., 1991.
13. Ibid.
14. Glazer, N. and D.P. Moynihan, *Beyond the Melting Pot*, 2nd ed., Cambridge, MA: M.I.T. Press, 1970.
15. Masrui, op. cit., 1986.
16. Bloch, B., "Nursing Care of Black Patients," in *Ethnic Nursing Care: A Multicultural Approach*,

M.S. Orgue, B. Bloch, and L.S.A. Monroy, eds., St. Louis: C.V. Mosby, 1983, pp. 82–109.

17. U.S. Department of Commerce, Economics and Statistics Administration, Bureau of the Census, 1999.

18. Bloch, op. cit., 1983, pp. 82–109.

19. Aschenbrenner, J., *Lifeline: Black Families in Chicago*, Prospect Heights, IL: Waveland Press, 1975.

20. Billingsley, A., *Black Families in White America*, New York: Simon & Schuster, 1968.

21. Leininger, M.M., "Southern Rural Afro American and White American Folkways with Focus on Care and Health Phenomena," in *Care: The Essence of Nursing and Health*, M. Leininger, ed., Detroit: Wayne State University Press, 1988, pp. 133–159.

22. Stack, C., *All Our Kin: Strategies for Survival in a Black Community*, New York: Harper and Row, 1974.

23. Ibid.

24. Twining, M.A., "Time is Like a River," in *Sea Island Roots: African Presence in the Carolinas and Georgia*, M.A. Twining and K.E. Baird, eds., Trenton, NJ: Africa World Press, Inc., 1991, pp. 89–94.

25. Aschenbrenner, op. cit., 1975.

26. Stack, op. cit., 1974.

27. McAdoo, H.P., "Black Kinships," *Psychology Today*, 1979, v. 12, pp. 67–79.

28. Glazer and Moynihan, op. cit., 1970.

29. Aschenbrenner, op. cit., 1975.

30. Herkovits, M.J., *The Myth of the Negro Past*, Boston: Beacon Press, 1958.

31. Aschenbrenner, op. cit., 1975.

32. McFarland, M., "Use of Culture Care Theory with Anglo- and African American Elders in a Long-Term Care Setting," *Nursing Science Quarterly*, 1997, v. 10, no. 4, pp. 186–192.

33. Morgan, M.G., "Prenatal Care of African-American Women in Selected USA Urban and Rural Cultural Contexts," *Journal of Transcultural Nursing*, 1996, v. 7, no. 2, pp. 3–9.

34. Bloch, op. cit., 1983, pp. 82–109.

35. Thomas, D.N., "Black American Patient Care," in *Transcultural Health Care*, G. Henderson and M. Prideaux, eds., Menlo Park, CA: Addison-Wesley Publishing Co., 1981, pp. 209–223.

36. Snow, L.F., *Walkin Over Medicine*, Boulder, CO: Westview Press, 1993.

37. Wicks, M.N., personal communication, 1990.

38. Leininger, op. cit., 1988, pp. 133–159.

39. Roberson, M.H.B., "The Influence of Religious Beliefs on Health Choices of Afro-Americans," *Topics in Clinical Nursing*, 1985, v. 7, no. 3, pp. 43–49.

40. Williams, M.D., *Community in a Black Pentecostal Church*, Prospect Heights, IL: Waveland Press, 1974.

41. Martin, E.P. and Martin, J.M., *The Black Extended Family*, Chicago: The University of Chicago Press, 1978.

42. Bloch, op. cit., 1983, pp. 82–109.

43. Aschenbrenner, op. cit., 1975.

44. Morgan, M., "Prenatal Care of African American Women in Selected USA Urban and Rural Cultural Contexts Conceptualized Within Leininger's Cultural Care Theory," unpublished doctoral dissertation, Wayne State University, Detroit, MI, 1994.

45. U.S. Department of Commerce, Economics and Statistics Administration, Bureau of the Census, 1999.

46. Sidell, R., *Women and Children Last: The Plight of Poor Women in Affluent America*, New York: Viking Press, 1986.

47. Stack, op. cit., 1974.

48. Bloch, op. cit., 1983, pp. 82–109.

49. Thomas, op. cit., 1981.

50. Sidell, op. cit., 1986.

51. U.S. Department of Commerce, Economics and Statistics Administration, Bureau of the Census, 1999.

52. Sidell, op. cit., 1986.

53. Spector, op. cit., 1991.

54. Ibid.

55. Morgan, op. cit., 1994.

56. "State-Specific Maternal Mortality Among Black and White Women—United States, 1987–1996," *Morbidity and Mortality Report 48*, Centers for Disease Control and Prevention, 1999, pp. 492–496.

57. Snow, op. cit., 1993.

58. Bailey, op. cit. 1991.

59. Ibid.

60. Capers, C.F., "Nursing and the Afro-American Client," *Topics in Clinical Nursing*, 1985, v. 7, no. 3, pp. 11–17.

61. Ibid.

62. Snow, op. cit., 1993.

63. Leininger, op. cit., 1988, pp. 133–159.

64. Snow, op. cit., 1993.

65. Wicks, op. cit., 1990.

66. Snow, op. cit., 1993.
67. Morgan, op. cit., 1994.
68. Snow, op. cit., 1977.
69. Leininger, op. cit., 1988, pp. 133–159.
70. Morgan, op. cit., 1994.
71. Ibid.
72. Bloch, op. cit., 1983, pp. 82–109.
73. Smitherman, G., *Talkin and Testifyin*, Detroit: Wayne State University Press, 1977.
74. Ibid.
75. Ibid.
76. Ibid.
77. Bloch, op. cit., 1983, pp. 82–109.
78. Snow, op. cit., 1993.
79. Leininger, op. cit., 1988, pp. 133–159.
80. Stack, op. cit., 1974.
81. Ibid.
82. Aschenbrenner, op. cit., 1975.

83. Osborne, op. cit., 1978, pp. 317–333.
84. Flaherty, M.J., "Seven Caring Functions of Black Grandmothers in Adolescent Mothering," *Maternal-Child Nursing Journal, 1988*, v. 17, pp. 191–207.
85. Ibid.
86. Ibid.
87. Morgan, op. cit., 1994.
88. Mann, R.J., P.D. Abercrombie, J. DeJoseph, et al., "The Personal Experience of Pregnancy for African-American Women," *Journal of Transcultural Nursing, 1999*, v. 10, no. 4, pp. 297–305.
89. Twining, op. cit., 1991, pp. 89–94.
90. Sawyer, L.M., "Engaged Mothering: The Transition to Motherhood for a Group of African American Women," *Journal of Transcultural Nursing, 1999*, v. 10, no. 1, pp. 14–21.

18

South African Culturally Based Health-Illness Patterns and Humanistic Care Practices

Grace Mashaba*

Knowing and respecting the culture of one's clients is a major factor in providing congruent and effective health care in any country, including South Africa. This country is not culturally homogeneous, but reflects cultural diversities. With multiracial and tribal differences in South Africa, cultural diversity exists with many generations of Western influences by whites. Health care personnel need to consider the possibility of their indifference to distinct cultural values being a barrier to healthy communication, understanding, and mutual acceptance between the health care provider and the recipient of care. Such indifference reflects a lack of caring, which can leave the client wounded inwardly, even with the best nurses and the best technologies. Barker, a medical practitioner for many years at Charles Johnson Hospital, Nqutu, sounds this warning:

> We should cease from scorning those who pass our hospitals to the care of the traditional medicine man, or seeing this movement as necessarily retrogressive. It is nothing of the kind, but rather a barometer of our failure to satisfy that part of a sick man's consciousness which he reserves for himself.[1]

The purpose of this chapter is to present, explain, and introduce the reader to those aspects of traditional cultural practices of Africans of South Africa that pertain to health and illness. This is to highlight those humanistic nursing care practices that are based on tran-

scultural nursing theory with the goal to improve health care to people in South Africa. This is especially important for nurses in South Africa, but also for nurses coming to this country desirous to understand and work with the people with a transcultural nursing perspective.

South Africa and Its People

South Africa refers to the area that lies south of the Limpopo River. This includes the Republic of South Africa and its independent and self-governing states of Transkei, Ciskei, KwaZulu, Venda, Gazankulu, Bophuthatswana, Lebowa, Qwaqwa, and Kangwane, as well as the countries that were previously British protectorates and are therefore outside the borders of the Republic. These are Swaziland, Lesotho, and Botswana. There continues to be a marked intermingling of populations of these countries. Swazis, Basothos, and Batswanas cross their borders to seek work primarily in the mining industry in the Republic of South Africa. Health and nursing services of the Republic must, of necessity, serve all these cultures.

South Africa's major cultures are indigenous Africans (who can be further subdivided into Sotho, Tswana, Shona, Zulu, Xhosa, Venda, Swazi, and others); Coloreds (who are a culture that developed from marriages between Anglo-Caucasians and Africans); Anglo-Caucasians, or Anglo-Europeans who immigrated from European countries; and Asians who came from the Middle and Far East. Although Anglo-Europeans are the political majority, Africans are the numerical majority. The total population of the

---

* Dr. Mashaba died in 1998, but this chapter remains her important contribution to transcultural nursing.

Republic of South Africa in 2000 was about forty-four million. Africans were thirty-three million; Coloreds, about four million; Anglo-Europeans, about six million; and Asians a little more than a million.[2]

If the country's goal of "health for all" is to be realized, nurses need to make an effort to reach the numerical majority by getting to know the African folk traditions, beliefs, and values to meet their health care needs. Providing culturally congruent care should improve nursing care and reduce illness, especially in the light of Gumede's statement that "... over 80% of African patients visit the traditional healer before coming to the doctor and to the hospital."[3]

The Cultural Background of African Healers

From anthropological data, Africa is one of the oldest countries in the world. Archaeological data attest to finding hominids back millions of years. Many people, however, have come into the country. Since the 18th century, when British and Dutch missionaries and settlers came to Africa, there has been an ongoing movement to Westernize the indigenous African people who long inhabited the continent. To date, cultures are mixed, but the more dominant culture of South Africa has become Westernized. However, health-illness beliefs and values vary within and between the cultural groups with respect to traditional and Western practices. In light of this reality, nurses need to assess the extent to which the health practices and behaviors of patients conforms to the Western model or to generic folk ways.

Spector maintains that values exist on a continuum and that a person can possess value characteristics of both a consistent heritage (traditional) and an inconsistent heritage (acculturated).[4] African values, beliefs, and practices have a tight grip on their practitioners, more than appears on the surface. Gumede maintains that his informant, a teacher, said it is a disgrace for a teacher, a graduate, or a nurse to say that he or she *once* used traditional medicinal practices such as *ukuncinda* (to lick); *ukubhema* (to inhale medicine like snuff); and *ukugcaba* (to be incised and have medicine rubbed into the incisions). These folk treatments are, however, practiced by affluent Africans, as well as by the less affluent, to achieve their desired goals.[5]

Further, Gumede gives many examples to illustrate that neither living in the rural areas nor in the urban area of the city of Johannesburg shakes the African's belief in witchcraft as "one of those things which belong to the childhood of our race."[6] Gqomfa, a senior professional psychiatric nurse speaking at a National Convention on Holistic Health and Healing testifies as follows:

> Customs, rites, rituals, and ancestral spirits make up a culture whose complexities are bewildering to the Western orientated person; yet these traditions have been carried on from generation to generation without the benefit of the written word. I, as a Xhosa tribesman in my own right, have attended and assisted at rites and rituals never for a moment doubting their importance within the Xhosa cosmology.[7]

As a way of reducing the cutting edge from the competition between African traditional doctors and Western medical practitioners in South Africa, there are rumblings of a movement to have dialogue with traditional healers and to even bring them within the fold of health services. A bold, positive step in this direction has been taken through passing the KwaZulu Act No. 6 of 1981, providing for the practice of African medicinemen, herbalists, and midwives. Gumede studied, presented, and explained a list of the inyanga's (traditional herbalist) pharmaceutical medicines or healing modes,[8] which was an improvement on earlier, similar work by Bryant.[9] These statements support the fact that nurses need to know and understand the established cultural lifeways and values of Africans and others of diverse color and creed. Such knowledge will enable nurses to help clients and to win their confidence and cooperation in a genuine and competent way. Both generic folk and new health (Western) practices need to be understood.

The African Tradition of Health, Illness, and Healing

Literature shows that the worldview of African nations across the continent have much in common. Diversity is largely limited to the use of different terminology because of differences in languages. According to Ngubane, it is possible for a Zulu traditional medicine practitioner to operate in a Sotho, Xhosa, Shona, and Thonga society.[10] This is reflected in the works of Kenyatta,[11] Krige,[12] Lienhardt,[13] Bryant,[14] Vilakazi,[15] Kuper,[16] and Gumede.[17] Accordingly, the health-illness status of Africans becomes a major area for nurses to understand.

In the African lifestyle there are ceremonies, customs, and rituals for every stage of human development, from birth to death at an old age, which, if observed, bring about a normal steady state of individuals and families. Traditionally, for an African health and healthy living are interwoven with religion, which is a way of life and of daily living. It is not confined to worship on one particular day. Africans believe in the existence of God or a supreme being, but each nation gives Him a different name. Zulus call Him *Mvelinggangi*; Sothos, *Modimo;* Xhosas, *Tixo;* Shonas, *Mwari;* and Tsongas, *Tilo*.[18] Traditionally, this supreme being is not approached directly through individual prayers. He is approached through the ancestors or spirits of dead relatives (*amadlozi* or *abaphansi*). A bond exists between the living and the ancestral spirits in that the latter not only safeguard the living and make them successful in their undertakings, but they also intercede for the living people to the unseen God. When a relative dies, a beast is slaughtered and a ceremony is made to bring back the spirit of the dead relative from the grave to the family house, so that this spirit can be with other ancestral spirits and look after the living family members. Regular sacrifices must be made to the ancestors to retain the well-being, health, and welfare of the family.[19]

When misfortune or illness strikes in the family, when an illness is not responding to treatments, or if a newly wed bride does not conceive, it is interpreted to mean that the ancestors are angry. The head of the family or the afflicted person then slaughters a goat, brews beer, and pleads with ancestors (*ukushweleza*). In response, the ancestors reverse the situation or problem. At times, the ancestors decide to pay a visible visit to the family, and so they become a particular kind of harmless snake that enters the house. Family members do not chase or kill such a snake, because it is symbolically a visitation by ancestors. A story is told of a woman who once found and kept a puff adder in her clay pot for weeks believing that it was the ancestors. Ancestors also communicate messages to the living members through dreams. Therefore, being in harmony with ancestors and keeping the ancestors appeased promotes

health and prosperity. For this reason, nurses are often faced by a patient who fails to improve after being hospitalized for weeks and requests to go home. The client may or may not explain the reason for this request to the nurse and other health personnel. Members of the family or the client become convinced that his or her illness is caused by the anger of the ancestors (*ulaka lwabaphansi*). A sacrifice is needed to appease them. At times, leaving the hospital against medical advice is because of the realization that one's illness cannot be cured by the white man's medicine and caring modes because it is the disease of the African people (*ukufa kwabantu*). It can be cured and cared for *only* by traditional healers, and it is thus culture-bound.

There are also cultural belief practices and taboos that are observed and, if maintained, lead to a state of health and protection against evil forces. Some customs are no longer kept, and several taboos have been abandoned as superstition. For some people failure to observe these culturally based taboos affects the whole person physically, psychologically, and in sociocultural relationships. Some of the customs that are still observed are paying *ilobolo*, or paying bride money or giving cattle to the parents of the girl that one intends to marry. Burial of the dead, mourning in a traditional way, and circumcision of boys carried out in the mountains accompanied by a certain ceremony are often customs that can be identified in African lifeways. In the process of circumcision, occasionally some of the boys develop an infection and come to the hospital.[20]

Most importantly, to retain a healthy state Africans must try to maintain a balance with their environmental surroundings and between people. People often go to the extent of using medicine to maintain this balance. It is alleged that using such medicine not only ensures protection against evil spells, but also ensures a positive reaction and relationships with other people. Employers and authorities do favors or even promote one even if one does not deserve promotion. When an individual is the accused in a court case, such medicines are used to help the person win the case, even if this individual is actually guilty. If the individual uses very strong medicine for maintaining balance, this can adversely affect other people with whom one associates and they can fall ill as a result of such influences. This is called *ukweleka ngesithunzi*, meaning to overpower or overshadow other people. For this reason people who live together are strengthened at the same time to keep this balance among them.[21] Transcultural nurses functioning in South Africa would need to understand these indigenous beliefs and practices to be effective and practice what Leininger refers to as *culturally congruent* care.[22]

Traditional Cure of Illnesses

Apart from accidents and animal bites, diseases are believed to take one of the following forms. There are those diseases that are natural such as flu, diarrhea, and others. These are cured by herbs, most of which are commonly known by most people and can be found in one's surroundings. There also are indigenous or culture-specific diseases or illnesses that are caused by the anger of the ancestors. There is also a group of illnesses that is related to *witchcraft*. Witchcraft practices can bring about illness through eating food or drinking a beverage with medicine that has been deliberately added to the food to harm the victim. Pulmonary tuberculosis is one such illness. It is called *idliso* because the victim ingested poisonous food. At times, a person falls acutely ill from "walking over medicine" that has been deliberately put in the path, with the intention to harm this person. This is called *umego*, meaning "jumped over medicine." There are times when an evil spell is cast to make one ill.

Witches also magically use lightning to kill people. Some illnesses are caused by dreaming, seeing, or being sent "familiars," which can be a snake, baboon, river dwarf, owl, tiger, or other animal. Witches or night sorcerers use charms to cast a spell on the above-named animals. Thereafter, the animal is under the sorcerer's control and carries out his instructions entirely. Victims of these familiars get very ill.[23] At other times, people are possessed by wandering evil spirits or spirits of the ancestors, which leads to serious illness. It is believed that most of the above-stated diseases and illnesses cannot be cured by Western medical practitioners. However, some illnesses such as *umego*, which can lead to cellulitis of the leg; *idliso*, which is known as pulmonary tuberculosis; and other illnesses can get cured through Western treatments and medications if used by the people.

Traditionally and in Africa's long history, it is a popular practice to go to a diviner or diagnostician

(*isangoma*) to find out who bewitched the sick person. This is done regardless of whether the sick person dies, recovers, or remains chronically ill. In most instances of witchcraft-induced illnesses when the patient is acutely ill, wastes away, or can be mentally deranged, medical tests and investigations will show nothing abnormal. At times, it could only be an elevated temperature. Knowledge about the African traditional beliefs and practices is essential to understanding African behavior, which seems strange or baffling to Western health personnel. The healer (*inyanga*) uses one or more of the following methods to heal the afflicted person. Use is made of emetics (*ukuhlanza*); enemas (*ukuchatha*); inhaling medicine (*ukubhema*); steaming (*ukugguma*); licking medicine (*ukukhotha* or *ukuncinda*); making small razor incisions on different parts of the body and rubbing in medicine (*ukugcaba*); and chewing a root or bark and then spraying this in the air from the mouth (*ukukhwifa*).[24]

With the advent of Christianity there came a new breed of healers called *African spiritual healers*. They heal using the same means as traditional healers such as emetics, enemas, and steaming, but instead of using medicine they use candles and water. Spiritual healers take ordinary water, pray for it to have medicinal properties, and then give it to patients. Patients are instructed to either drink it, wash with it, or use it for steaming, enemas, and so on. They communicate with ancestors, but give them the name of *izidalwa* or *izithunywa*. Spiritual healers have prophetic powers and pray to God and to Jesus Christ. "Saved Christians" refer to this phenomena as spiritualism to differentiate the works of spiritual healers from the miracles of God and the Holy Spirit.

These brief accounts are essential holding knowledge for the transcultural nurse. They are very important to know, interpret, and understand African traditional values, beliefs, and lifeways. The nurse should not impose these practices on African patients because some Africans may be acculturated and have accepted other beliefs as the Islamic religion and others. Some are committed, saved, and born-again Christians. Many people in these groups have tried to distance themselves completely from the *inyanga-sangoma* syndrome, for they use methods within their religion to fight magic spells and evil spirits. There are also some people in South Africa who have become indifferent or deny such traditional practices. Today, however, most Africans essentially hold a firm belief in the magicoreligious aspects of their traditional culture and use some Western caring and curing practices. Indeed, traditional folk (generic) care and cures are some of the oldest and most complex in the world, and the nurse needs to learn about them.

Looking to the Future

In the future, South Africa will be a fundamentally different society from what it is today. This means that nurses need to be prepared and open-minded to cultivate an atmosphere of mutual respect and trust between themselves and the people. In support of this, Gumede maintains that "As we learn more about other people's cultures and values, as our understanding and our humility grow, as our prejudices erode . . . (we can) have much to learn from each other."[25]

Leininger, our transcultural leader and founder, has also held to this view for many decades. Trying to relate to clients in terms of identifying and respecting their culture is not meant to create stereotypes or to divide people. On the contrary, it purports to enable the nurse to forge links across people of different cultures. In fact, according to Leininger, "Nurses will have to learn about their own cultural background and how their cultural values facilitate or serve as barriers in helping people of different cultural orientations."[26] This statement serves to clarify and explain the intention of this presentation lest we fall into the trap described by Nakagawa who warns, "Too often we are drawn to the colorful or exotic aspects of cultural manifestations and inadvertently lead students to strengthening rather than reducing stereotyping."[27] Most of all, cultures are not static. On the whole, South African people align themselves with more than one culture and can be described as culturally multifaceted. The nurse needs to capitalize on commonalities while being mindful of diversities.[28] This is especially important with Africans seeking democratic lifeways and less oppression and racism.

Humanistic Caring Practices

The foregoing information should enable culture-sensitive and knowledgeable nurses to develop nursing care plans and practices that promote culturally congruent care with Leininger's three action modes. During the assessment phase of the nursing process nurses can accumulate facts and information that lead not only to a nursing assessment, but also to understanding of client's fears and anxiety about particular health problems. A client may dream of a baboon and thereafter wake up with a severe headache. When talking to a client, the nurse will discover that the client is anxious and worried more about the dream than the headache. In other words, being a victim of a familiar requires, besides taking headache pills, a traditional healer's treatment to remove the evil spell. A client may refuse surgical removal of a tumor if this tumor is perceived to be the result of the anger of the ancestors and surgical removal therefore amounts to defying or disregarding the ancestors. This may be difficult for Western nurses to understand, especially medical-surgical nurse specialists.

Knowledge of African health-illness cultural practices can help nurses understand and interpret culture-specific terms accurately. In this way proper communication can be fostered even with a traditionally oriented African patient. If the client reports that his swollen painful leg is due to *umego*, the nurse will understand this to mean that the client "jumped over medicine." Another patient may explain the cause of his chest pains as being *idliso*, meaning that he ate poisoned food or drink. This implies that, in addition to assisting the patient to recover from tuberculosis chest pains, the nurse has to deal with the client's cultural belief, which may cause him to abandon hospital care and go for traditional healing.

Culture Care Preservation and Maintenance

At this stage of nursing assessment, patients' responses can be analyzed using Leininger's Acculturation Health Care Assessment Enabler for Cultural Patterns in Traditional and Nontraditional Lifeways. This Enabler provides criteria that are gradated from 1 (mainly traditional) to 5 (mainly nontraditional).[29] Such ratings will show the position of the particular client on the traditional and nontraditional continuum. Nurses can then make decisions on nursing action using Leininger's Culture Care theoretical model. This model focuses on culture care preservation and maintenance, culture care accommodation, and negotiation and culture care repatterning and restructuring.[30]

There are aspects of this culture that could be preserved and maintained by the nurse in the process of giving nursing care. The African belief in a supreme being could be strengthened. In daily contact with the client, the nurse can discuss how this supreme being is the creator, giver, and taker of life and that this being is actually superior to forms of magic and to any force. Strong reliance on this being should enable the patient to be resilient to the influence of evil forces and magic spells. As this reliance grows, patients will become less likely to yield to the notion that their fate is in the hands or at the mercy of witches and ancestors. Guidance and support can be given to patients to talk or relate regularly to this supreme being to build a stronger person-to-God relationship. However, ancestor respect needs to be understood.

Kinship ties can be preserved and maintained through involvement of the family in care practices. The family support and cooperation that is evident in making decisions about traditional healing practices needs to be used by nurses. Nurses can get information from relatives to either support or refute the client's statements. Relatives can be consulted, especially if the patient is unable to answer questions properly. They can be involved in a decision to give consent for a surgical operation when the client is hesitant. Members of the family can be asked to take on roles to facilitate recovery of their sick relative. They can remind and assist the client to take pills or treatment, watch for signs of bleeding, assist with ambulation, or assist the patient with exercises for a limb to return to its normal functioning. Nurses may identify other aspects that can be maintained to the advantage of specific therapeutic and humanistic caring practices.

Culture Care Accommodation and Negotiation

With respect to culture care accommodation and negotiation, an example of the client's reliance on herbs can be used. Nurses need to be familiar with medicinal herbs that are commonly used by African people. Gumede's list of herbs will give guidance and explain the pharmacological action of these herbs, as well as their side effects.[31] Clients using these herbs are usually not aware of other actions and effects of herbs apart from what the traditional healer prescribes. The nurse can establish the nature, action, and effect of medicinal herbs that a client insists on using. Based on the nurse's professional knowledge of the medicine, discretion can be used to accommodate continued use of the medicine while the client is undergoing hospital care. This should be the case if the medicinal herb will not interfere with prescribed care. On the contrary, if the herb causes vomiting when the patient is supposed to rest the gastrointestinal tract, depress appetite when the patient needs to have regular meals and a nourishing diet, or cause mental alertness when the patient must relax and sleep, then the nurse should negotiate with the patient for suspension of use of the herb, at least, pending the outcome of hospital care.

Traditional healers could be allowed to visit their clients while hospitalized or at home. This opportunity could be used by nurses to secure the cooperation of the healers and promote holistic well-being. The nurse can negotiate for a compromise on the traditional healer's part for suspending and omitting some of the healer's prescriptions using the principle discussed in the previous paragraph. The traditional healers could also be encouraged to refer to nurses those clients that appear to be problematic. If the traditional healer is taught about healthy habits such as eating a balanced diet and cleanliness of people, houses, and the environment, the traditional healer may be persuaded to use these ideas and practices with clients.

Culture Care Repatterning and Restructuring

African clients could be taught ways to perform minor skin incisions (*ukugcaba*) and circumcisions through hygienic means to reduce the risk of infection and to do these common folk home practices properly. The nurse could negotiate with physicians, if necessary, to have these surgical operations done by health personnel or under their supervision. Client education as part of nursing care plans is an essential means for repatterning and restructuring aspects of traditional culture and caring modes. In the case of pulmonary tuberculosis, alleged to be *idliso*, clients can be assisted to focus attention on what causes the illness instead of consulting the *isangoma* to establish who is responsible for inflicting the disease. Other patients with a similar diagnosis can be used as a reference and support group.

The idea of maintaining balance in the traditional sense could be repatterned around the prevention of spreading an infectious disease to other members of the family. Nurses could emphasize to patients that the microbes that caused the disease from which the clients are suffering should be prevented through immunization and/or certain precautions against spreading them to other people and disturbing balance. Susceptibility to diseases caused by microorganisms can be structured and patterned around the idea of susceptibility to magic and evil spells. Clients can be helped to understand that poor nourishment, lack of fresh air, dirt, and uncleanliness raise the level of susceptibility not only to microorganisms but also possibly to evil spirits and magic spells. In this way nurses can repattern for meaningful and acceptable care. In evaluating nursing care, the nurses could consult and involve the client and relatives to get their opinion on the effectiveness of care given and suggestions for improvement.

Summary Considerations

Africans, like members of other cultures, are proud of their cultural identity and heritage. There are practices and beliefs that may need to be considered rather than dismissed as myths or superstition in view of the fact that strong traditional healing has been part of African culture for years and some aspects should be protected.[32] For the African these beliefs are real because they have been handed down by their foreparents or ancestors, and they are firmly held to be important and efficacious. Nurses should not ridicule these beliefs because in doing so it may antagonize and repel the client from the nurses. This will defeat the goal of quality nursing care and health for all.

Respect for other people's culture has implications also for nonclinical nursing areas. Nurse administrators and nurse educators should serve as role models by resisting the tendency to be ethnocentric in their dealings with colleagues and students. The nurse administrator has to recognize culturally constituted situational variations in role expectations of the staff. Through staff development the nurse administrator should assist a colleague in resolving conflicts between the passive traditional role of a woman and the assertive pro-

fessional role of a client's advocate. The professional nurse needs to take the initiative to negotiate, restructure, and repattern activities discussed earlier to help patients take responsibility for their own health and to attain culturally congruent care.[33]

The nurse educator who has African students in her class should be careful of sole reliance on unicultural educational practices. Students will probably imitate the nurse educator and adopt unicultural approaches in caring for clients. The educator needs to be flexible and transculturally knowledgeable to support culturally congruent care and practices known in the student's environment and culture. There will be organizations and social groups in the community with which students can establish contact for mutual education and information toward enabling more and more people to be health conscious within and outside of their culture.

Clinical nurse researchers need to discover and respect the adherence by clients to their traditional lifeways and to establish credibility of African subjective experiences and thinking. In view of the fact that South Africans are in a state of great cultural transitions and that transcultural nursing research focuses on subjective and objective experiential humanistic inquiry, research studies can help generate some new and traditional knowledge about South Africans in terms of who they are, what they do, and where they want to go. A cultural analysis of different people of all cultures with variations is essential rather than to assume that all Africans in the country share the same beliefs about health, illness, and healing.

Transcultural nursing remains essential and meaningful today in South Africa as the people continue to assess and use the best of indigenous (folk), traditional, and their rich, cultural heritage with that of different Western cultures. Professional nurses, however, need to maintain an open discovery attitude using transcultural nursing theories and concepts to develop creative ways to practice nursing. This will enable them to provide meaningful care to their people and to others in the country.

This paper was written in 1991 before the National Election in April, 1994. The traditional health-illness conditions and care practices are still an integral part of the culture with some Western practices. It was also written before the democratization era began in recent years with Mandela and other African and non-African leaders under great stresses and conflicts. Most important, it was written before the current pandemic AIDS/HIV conditions, but those are covered by O'Neil in Chapter 12 in this book.

References

1. Barker, A., "The Social Fabric," *The Leech*, 1974, v. 44, no. 2, p. 32.
2. *The World Almanac: A Book of Facts*, Mahwah, NJ: Primedia Reference Inc., 2001.
3. Gumede, M.M., *Traditional Healers*, Johannesburg: Skotaville, 1990.
4. Spector, R., *Cultural Diversity in Health and Illness*, Norwalk: Appleton-Century-Crofts, 1985.
5. Gumede, op. cit.
6. Ibid.
7. Gqomfa, J., "Tradition and Transition," *Odyssey*, 1987, v. 12, no. 4, p. 29.
8. Gumede, op. cit.
9. Bryant, A.T., *Zulu Medicine and Medicine Men*, Cape Town: C. Struik, 1970.
10. Ngubane, J., *Body and Mind in Zulu Medicine*, London: Academic Press, 1977.
11. Kenyatta, J., *Facing Mount Kenya*, New York: Vintage Books, 1965.
12. Krige, E.J., *The Social System of the Zulus*, Pietermaritzburg: Shuter and Shooter, 1957.
13. Lienhardt, G., *Divinity and Experience: The Religion of the Dinka*, Oxford: The Clarendon Press, 1970.
14. Bryant, op. cit.
15. Vilakazi, A., *Zulu Transformation*, Pietermaritzburg: University of Natal Press, 1962.
16. Kuper, H., *An African Aristocracy*, London: Oxford University Press, 1969.
17. Gumede, op. cit.
18. Ibid.
19. Ibid.
20. Funani, S.L., *Circumcision Among the Ama-Xhosa*, Johannesburg: Skotaville, 1990, p. 37.
21. Ngubane, op. cit.
22. Leininger, M., *Culture Care Diversity and Universality: A Theory of Nursing*, New York: National League for Nursing, 1991, pp. 5–68.
23. Gumede, op. cit.
24. Ngubane, op. cit.
25. Gumede, op. cit.
26. Leininger, M., "Transcultural Nursing for Tomorrow's Nurse," unpublished paper, Detroit: Wayne State University, 1986.
27. Nakagawa, M., "Multicultural Education," *Transcultural Nursing Newsletter*, 1991, v. 1, no. 1, p. 2.
28. Leininger, M., op. cit., 1991.
29. Leininger, M., "Leininger's Acculturation Health Care Assessment Tool for Cultural Patterns in Traditional and Non-Traditional Lifeways," *Journal of Transcultural Nursing*, 1991, v. 2, no. 2, p. 40.
30. Leininger, M., "Leininger's Theory of Nursing: Cultural Diversity and Universality," *Nursing Science Quarterly*, 1988, v. 1, no. 4, pp. 152–160.
31. Gumede, op. cit.
32. "Traditional Healers in Health Care in South Africa: A Proposal," Johannesburg: The Center for Health Policy, 1991, p. 1.
33. Leininger, op. cit., pp. 5–65.

19

Family Violence and Culture Care with African and Euro-American Cultures in the United States

Joanne T. Ehrmin

Violence is a complex phenomenon affecting people in diverse cultural groups. In the United States, violence has continued to occur in almost epidemic ways within and between cultures as it has in many other places worldwide. In the United States, many clients have come into health care facilities for physical, emotional, and cultural care related to violence. Victims of stabbings; gunshot wounds; infant, child, and adult abuse (physical, sexual, cultural, and emotional) are but a few of the people health care professionals treat. Frequently, the first people outside the family to care for these victims of abuse and violent acts are nurses. Cultural care factors related to intergenerational meanings, expressions, and practices of family violence remain limitedly documented, studied, or understood. This chapter is a contribution to meet this important need.

Leininger[1] hypothesized that throughout the history of Homo sapiens, caring for self and others was a critical factor for human survival but that the caring dimension had been limitedly investigated. This researcher was interested in discovering the meaning, source, and general knowledge about violence in families from an intergenerational perspective. Such research was needed for new knowledge and practices in the nursing discipline and for all health service providers. Transcultural nursing knowledge about violence would help to reveal values, beliefs, and expressions from informants or victims of violence and from their emic (insider) perspective rather than an etic (outsider) perspective. The researcher was particularly interested in studying African and European American

(Euro-American) violence intergenerationally. This knowledge seemed imperative for understanding violence from a cultural perspective with a focus on culture care meanings, expressions, and practices.

Purposes and Domain of Inquiry

The purposes of this transcultural ethnonursing research study were 1) to discover expressions of violence with African and Euro-Americans in the United States intergenerationally, 2) to discover cultural differences and universalities or commonalties with African and Euro-Americans related to violence intergenerationally, and 3) to discover culture care practices that African and Euro-Americans in the United States could use to reduce intergenerational conflicts and maintain peaceful and healthy lifeways. The researcher held that family violence was culturally learned, expressed, and transmitted intergenerationally and that the theory of Culture Care would be useful to study this domain. The domain was focused on intergenerational meanings, expressions, and practices of family violence and culture care with African and Euro-American cultures in the United States. The theory of Culture Care became most helpful to systematically discover the culture care practices and ways to prevent violence and to maintain peaceful and healthy lifeways intergenerationally in a culturally congruent manner.

Significance of Study

With the alarming rise in violence today, nurses in hospitals, clients' homes, local communities, and other nursing centers are increasingly caring for clients and families who have experienced noncaring or violent acts. The researcher was interested to discover transcultural nursing knowledge about comparative cultural family violence meanings, expressions, and practices of African and Euro-Americans in the United States. The manner in which families express conflicts or are able to experience peaceful caring relationships was of interest, as well as how families use caring to prevent or control violence. These seemed to be important knowledge areas for nurses and other health care providers. Leininger predicted the expressions of violence and intercultural conflicts are "... often based on intergenerational breaking of normative cultural values and practices" and that "... an understanding of transcultural caring patterns of potential violence within and between cultural groups could help nurses to work effectively and knowingly with cultures to prevent serious acts of violence and to promote health caring behaviors."[2]

Research Questions

In keeping with the qualitative research paradigm, several broad-based research questions were used as a guide to study the domain of intergenerational meanings, expressions, and practices of family violence and culture care with selected African and Euro-American cultures in the United States. The following questions were used with this ethnonursing research study:

1. What are the meanings, expressions, and practices of intergenerational family violence among African and Euro-American cultures, as well as, how is violence prevented or controlled?
2. What are the comparative social structure factors influencing covert and overt expressions of family conflicts, violence, and/or peaceful ways of African and Euro-Americans?
3. What are the family caring or noncaring meanings, expressions, and practices related to violence from an intergenerational perspective among African and Euro-Americans?
4. How do worldview, social structure factors, environmental context, language expressions, ethnohistory, and cultural care values and beliefs influence family violence with consideration of enculturation and socialization processes?

Theoretical and Conceptual Framework

The theory of Culture Care Diversity and Universality was chosen for this investigation because it is a theory to discover holistic dimensions related to family violence.[3,4] This broad, open, and comprehensive in-depth theory was held as essential to explicate complex and multiple factors such as the worldview, social structure, environmental context, and cultural care values and beliefs influencing intergenerational family violence. According to Gordon, theoretical perspectives must be developed "... which allow for a movement away from a locked-in application of models and paradigms developed for a Eurocentric society to Afrocentric beliefs and lifestyles."[5] Leininger's Sunrise Model depicting the components of the Culture Care Theory served as an important guide to conceptualize and guide the researcher to study the domain of inquiry.[6,7] Since human care with a transcultural comparative focus was held by the theorist to be the essence and dominant domain of nursing, this theory was relevant to this investigation focusing on family care and violence.

Orientational Definitions

In keeping with the philosophical underpinnings of the qualitative research paradigm, the following orientational definitions were used in this study to maintain an open inquiry research approach to discovery. Definitions such as care, culture, and culture care were derived directly from Leininger's Culture Care Theory. They are not presented here, as they have been presented in other chapters in this book and are found in other sources, but the following definitions were important to this study:[8,9]

African American: Refers to people of African ancestry who identify themselves as African American.

European American: Refers to people of European ancestry who identify themselves as European American.

Intergenerational: Informants with families having three generations (two descending and one ascending) of the designated cultures.

Family Violence: Refers to the action of one or more individuals that is intended to lead to physical and cultural harm to another family member.

Review of the Literature

Since this was the first documented transcultural qualitative in-depth nursing research study on family violence intergenerationally with a focus on culture care and noncare beliefs, values, practices, and experiences within Culture Care theory, only literature closely related to this domain of inquiry is presented. In her initial study of "Culture Care of the Gadsup Akuna of the Eastern Highlands of New Guinea," Leininger discovered from several key informants that cultural beliefs and values of peace as health promoting, included "...having a peaceful and caring social world if we (Gadsup) are to maintain good kinship ties, share foods, and perform our work ... we must also follow the ways of our good ancestors."[10] Leininger discovered care and noncare beliefs, actions, cultural values, and practices among the Gadsup Akunans. She stated the following:[11]

> Violence behaviors were evident when kinship and social expectations were violated, cultural taboos overlooked, and role responsibilities neglected. Noncaring manifestations were usually altered by physical punishment to children, strong negative verbal responses to adults by the villagers, and open talks to those who violated cultural practices.[12]

Hence, cultural taboos and violations of values and daily practices were clearly identified and dealt with by the Gadsup related to violent behaviors. Moreover, desired behaviors and values related to violence were explicitly taught, largely through role modeling and enculturation socialization processes. Several generations over many years were considered in dealing with values or noncaring actions.

In Rosenbaum's study on cultural care with Greek Canadian widows, most informants spoke about "great mutual respect and shared love," but a few widows discussed "...unhappy marriages related to alcohol abuse."[13] Rosenbaum reported that cultural conflicts sometimes led to violence, which were linked to neglected or violated care values of "reciprocation,

concern, love, companionship, family protection, and helping."[14]

Although violence has been described as a major public health issue in the United States, few studies specific to culture, culture care, and violence have been documented in the literature.[15–17] Malone identified the importance of conducting nursing research on violence in the United States, particularly in "Black" communities where "Black-on-Black homicide is the leading cause of death for adolescent and young adult males, rendering them an endangered species."[18] She likened the experience for children growing up in violent communities to that of "living in a war zone."[19] Increasingly, nurses will be required to recognize and deal with the emotional distress of child and adolescent victims who have either witnessed or have directly experienced violence in their communities.[20]

Ethnohistory

In this section a brief ethnohistorical account of the African and European American cultures in the United States will be presented, focused on meanings, expressions, and practices of violence but with recognition that a full history is beyond the space limitations. However, ethnohistory is essential to understand the people with their patterns and practices related to violence.

Ethnohistory of African Americans

An ethnohistorical account of African Americans cannot be isolated from the context of slavery and its long historical roots. The African Diaspora began in 1444 when Henry the Navigator took 165 Africans to Portugal. Following the abolition of slavery, racism and segregation were rampant in the southern United States. In 1875 Tennessee adopted the "Jim Crow" law, separating Blacks and Whites on trains, depots, hotels, restaurants, and theaters, and other southern states quickly followed. White supremacy was established with lynchings becoming commonplace practices and clashes between the races routinely occurring on a daily basis.[21,22]

Although African Americans had occupied the lowest rung on a rigid caste system in the southern United States, labor recruiters had misrepresented the North as "the promised land." The people frequently found themselves competing for scarce jobs leading to hostile and racist sentiments between the diverse cultural groups in the North.[23] African Americans, out of necessity, were forced to a strange and often cruel land, and they were exploited and constrained at the bottom of a social class system. Baer and Singer stated that African Americans, "...cling to cultural patterns that by their existence challenged the naturalness and certitude of day-to-day subordination."[24] The African American ethnohistorical background reflects strong evidence of segregation, hardships, suffering, discrimination, and other unfavorable human experiences in their long history.

Leininger's recent research findings with the African American culture and the additional ethnonursing data have served as a guide for nurses caring for clients from diverse cultures.[25] Reflecting on the research and care findings for the African American culture, Leininger identified the following cultural values: "extended family networks, religion valued with many Baptists, interdependence with 'Blacks,' daily survival, technology valued, folk (soul) foods, folk healing modes, and music and physical activities."[26–28]

Ethnohistory of Euro-Americans

European immigration into the United States began on a large-scale basis in the early 1800s because of discontent with existing European conditions and a heightened awareness of many American opportunities.[29] The Ellis Island Immigrant Station was used to process large numbers of immigrants into the United States.[30] Interestingly, many United States citizens who live in the land of immigrants have had some hostile views about immigrant groups, while at the same time proudly professing to be a "land of refuge" and "an asylum for the oppressed."[31]

Early 17th century patterns of family life in the United States were fairly consistent with fathers as the identified head of the household, with women as wives and helpmates who were clearly subordinate, and with children trained to be obedient and respectful to others. Cultural family values of discipline, orderliness, and productivity were held in high regard. Paternal authority began to decline in the mid 18th century. Fathers no longer had control or influence to select their children's mates, occupations, or residence. The influence of kin such as grandparents, aunts, and uncles diminished, and "...the nuclear family became increasingly autonomous."[32]

Ethnohistorical and transcultural nursing research findings for the European/Anglo American culture identified by Leininger included the following dominant cultural values prevailing today: "...individualism with a focus on a self-reliant person, independence and freedom, competition and achievement, materialism (things and money), technology dependent, instant time and actions, youth and beauty, equal sex rights, leisure time, reliance on scientific facts and numbers, less respect for authority and the elderly, and generosity in time of crisis."[33] Hence, ethnohistorical factors differed considerably between African American and Euro-Americans, especially regarding their history, attitudes, and lifeways.

▪ Research Design

Ethnonursing Research Method

The ethnonursing qualitative research method developed by Leininger, which was designed to systematically study the theory of Culture Care, was chosen for this study.[34–36] The researcher held that to gain an in-depth understanding of intergenerational meanings, expressions, and practices of family violence and culture care with African and Euro-Americans, the ethnonursing qualitative research method was appropriate and essential to study the domain. A major part of the ethnonursing method is to tease out covert and complex data with the use of enablers. The major enablers used in this ethnonursing study were: 1) The Leininger Stranger to Trusted Friend Enabler to facilitate obtaining data as the researcher moved from a distrusted stranger to a trusted friend; 2) The Leininger Observation-Participation-Reflection (O-P-R) Enabler used to facilitate and guide the researcher to gain in-depth knowledge about culture care and noncare, meanings, expressions, and practices related to family violence; 3) A Semi-Structured Inquiry Enabler was developed by the researcher to obtain culture-specific data related to the domain; and 4) Short Family History Narratives, or comfortable talkouts, were used to obtain intergenerational, culturally based family care and value patterns.[37,38] Acculturation factors were assessed related to the extent that informants focused on traditional or nontraditional lifeways.

Criteria for Selection of Informants

The following criteria were used for selection of key informants in this study: 1) Middle-class African American and Euro-American families who were born and lived in the United States for at least 10 years; 2) Informants currently living in a large urban community in the United States; 3) Informants with families having three living generations of the designated cultures (eldest or first generation, middle or second generation, and youngest or third generation); and 4) Informants who spoke English and volunteered to participate in the study. Four key African American families (12 informants) and three Euro-American families (9 informants) were included in this study. Key informants are most knowledgeable about the domain of inquiry and are held to reflect the norms and values of the culture under study.[39] General informants in this study included eight African Americans and seven Euro-Americans. General informants met the above identified criteria (1, 2, and 4), but were not required to currently have three living generations within their family. General informants are not as fully knowledgeable about the domain, but have general ideas about the domain and culture under study.[40] Although Leininger generally recommends a ratio of 1:2 key to general informants in an ethnonursing research study, the researcher was able to reach saturation with the data collected from the key and general informants in this study.[41]

Data Collection, Entry, Coding, and Analysis

Data obtained from this ethnonursing qualitative research study were entered and managed using the Leininger-Templin-Thompson (LTT) Ethnoscript Qualitative Software.[42] Data entries included a wealth of detailed raw emic data from African American and Euro-American informants that included verbatim statements and many hours of observational data

collection. Two to three interviews were conducted with key informants lasting approximately 2 to 3 hours; one to two interviews were conducted with general informants lasting approximately 1 to 2 hours. Researcher dialogue, theoretical speculations, feelings, and environmental contextual data were also included for a full and detailed account. The coding was done by use of the Coding Data System for the LTT Field Research Ethnoscript, which reflects categories and domains from the Culture Care Theory.[43] Additional codes unique to this study were added as new or unexpected data was collected from informants. Data were analyzed using Leininger's Four Phases of Ethnonursing Data Analysis guide, which can be found in other chapters in this book.[44]

▮ Research Study Findings

In this section findings are presented from the enablers used, including the Observation-Participation-Reflection Enabler and the Stranger-Friend Enabler, which focused on the domain of inquiry and the theory of Culture Care. Patterns and themes were identified related to intergenerational meanings, expressions, and practices of family violence and culture care of the African American and Euro-American informants. African American themes will first be presented followed by the Euro-American themes, followed by a brief discussion of each major theme.

African American Culture

Four universal African American cultural themes were discovered in this study from the raw data, descriptors, and patterns. The first African American theme was as follows:

> *For African Americans, teaching respect was identified as a parental responsibility necessary for survival care and influenced by traditional family, religious, spiritual, and cultural lifeways.*

Respect was considered an important cultural care value, particularly by the elder or first generation informants to prevent violence and other unfavorable behaviours. Informants talked about the young, especially males, as increasingly involved with the criminal justice system and frequently being incarcerated for violent crimes. Teaching the children early in life through the enculturation process about care as respect for elders, including those in authority, was a valued cultural care belief and practice to prevent violence and to survive. The first generation of grandparents believed that some children today had not been taught to respect their elders as they themselves had learned as children and, in turn, had taught their own children. Moreover, the older generation believed that the young today had not learned a sense of fear and respect for others, which they believed was responsible for an increase in African American children becoming involved in gangs and legal problems. One key informant stated:

> The problem today is people don't have that fear. People always have to know the lines not to cross. I always knew the lines and avoided crossing them. They also don't have respect for others or even for themselves.

Respect was identified as a twofold reciprocal care practice for children, namely, to have respect for their elders and for adults to respect their children. One key informant said: "The kids feel bad, they're bad and they're angry. And they'll say any inappropriate word to their mother, because they don't care anything about respecting her if she hasn't held respect for them."

Ten African American key informants talked about physical punishment as "whoopings," and maintained whoopings were not physical or psychological violence, but a parental responsibility as a disciplinary measure for the child. One key informant said: "I don't believe whoopings are violence. Had to do that as a part of the parent's responsibility in raising kids." Another key informant stated: "We got whoopings . . . but I was never punished unjustly where it was abuse or anything. I believe violence is murdering and rapings." The practice of whoopings as "disciplining" was viewed as a means to set limits and teach respect to the child beginning in their early years and was not viewed as abusive or punitive in nature.

All three of the third-generation grandparents spoke about differences in child-rearing practices today. Past care practices were to teach children respect and responsibility, but in their view this was not being done today with the present young generation. An elder, first-generation key informant stated: "I gave the teachers permission to whoop the kids, then they got a second whooping when they got home, 'cause they shouldn't have gotten the first. Those teachers aren't allowed to do that stuff today."

A third-generation key informant identified the word "whooping," but reflected her educational preparation in psychology and used the word "hitting." This reflected a change in cultural values and beliefs based on a socialization process within the mainstream American educational system. This informant said: "My mother never believed in hitting. So even before it was popular not to hit kids, my mother never believed in it." A sense of frustration and a tendency to leave the responsibility of raising children to the parents was reflected as an important parental enculturation process. Another key informant stated:

> My grandson is about 16 years old. I have some problems with him. Kids today aren't like they used to be. They don't mind. They don't do what you tell them, and they don't respect their elders, like I did, and like my kids did. I tell him to go out and do snow shoveling, and he says no way. I don't talk to him anymore because if he didn't do what I asked him to, I'd have to ask him to leave. To avoid having to ask him to leave, I don't ask him to do anything anymore. Now I talk to him through his mother.

From the above data, teaching respect to the young was held as an essential and almost imperative parental responsibility in raising children. First-generation grandparents identified the necessity of teaching the young to respect others as a means to decrease violence and noncaring lifeways. The reciprocal nature of respect, with adults also respecting children, was discovered as an important intergenerational care practice. Elder informants expressed a concern for differing child-rearing practices today and believed this reflected a parental, or second-generation, enculturation process.

The second major theme discovered was as follows:

For African Americans, conflicting culture care values and societal values lead to changes in patterns of communication, diminished parental responsibility, and a general lack of direction in the home and increased violence and substance abuse as influenced by kinship, religious, spiritual, and cultural values and lifeways.

Changing societal values were held by all African American informants to be in conflict with culture care values and were considered to have a major influence on violence today. Parents, especially mothers, who had an increase in responsibilities outside the home and no one at home to "teach" the children were identified as the major concerns. Key informants talked about parental role conflicts, especially with mothers participating in mainstream societal beliefs and practices of working outside the home and maintaining busy schedules. Several informants talked about these changing societal patterns conflicting with traditional culture care values, beliefs, and practices. Such changes were held to lead to noncaring child-rearing practices in the home.

Inadequate communication and "not taking responsibility" for problems were also identified by the youngest generations of African Americans to have influenced an increase in violence. One key informant stated: "I don't believe violence would happen if parents would communicate with their kids. A good way to talk about things that happen during the day to everyone in the family is at dinner. Parents aren't there to take care of their kids anymore." Although another key informant did not believe there were patterns of violence in her own family, she described a broader cultural pattern of ". . . decreased communication and not caring enough to be parents. Parents are taking too little responsibility . . ." She believed this had led to an increase in violence within her own culture.

Nine key informants maintained that parental use of drugs and alcohol in the home led to an escalated use of drugs and alcohol by the children with increased signs of violence. Noncaring, which was held as "not taking responsibility" in the parental role, was associated with the rise in violence today. Although "parents" were discussed in general terms, more specifically the "mother" was blamed for problems with the children. One key informant stated:

Where the parent's problems are coming from right now are the mother not using her intelligence around her kids, not using a basic thing like up and up livin', and being sober minded. You can't smoke and drink and lie around talking all type of garbage around your kids.

Another key informant stated:

We're always told the way you behave is a reflection of your parents, or the way they teach you your values and stuff, but it doesn't seem that it's like that any more. Some of the parents behave the same way or worse than the children.

From the above statements conflicts in traditional cultural care values and beliefs about parental role responsibilities with mainstream societal values and beliefs, particularly with the mother and the increasing demands outside of the home and away from her children, were identified as related to an increase in violence today. The importance of communication within the family to decrease noncaring lifeways was expressed by the youngest generation. Parental use of drugs and alcohol in the home was associated with an increase in violence and noncaring practices and attributed to a rise in the use of drugs and alcohol by children.

The third major theme was as follows:

For African Americans, caring for oneself and others was believed to reflect a loving connection to God, as influenced by their religious, spiritual, and cultural values and lifeways.

Belief in God was held by all key informants as essential to maintain caring lifeways and to prevent violence. One key informant stated: "The reason for so much violence today is because people don't have faith in the Lord. Loving the Lord helps people love and respect themselves and others." Informants talked about respecting and caring for "others," as well as "oneself," which came through a loving connection to God. Another key informant stated: "You need to respect and take care of yourself. You learn this through loving the Lord."

African American informants described care as a sense of "group spirit" and "brotherly/sisterly" love and support derived from their religious/spiritual and cultural values and lifeways of doing good on this earth. It was not a goal or end result in and of itself, but rather that positive benefits would come to those who gave freely of themselves to their brothers and sisters with the Lord's love. One key informant said: "I value helping others who can't help themselves, or need to show them the way. You can't do it to get something in return. But God always sees you. You get back the positive or negative you dish out." Respect was held as a major cultural care value associated with maintaining caring and nonviolent lifeways, which were deeply embedded in the religious values and beliefs of African Americans. One informant stated: "Respecting yourself and your fellow brothers and sisters, you have to do that if you don't want violent ways."

These informants' statements reaffirmed the importance of religious beliefs and their close relationship to caring practices to prevent violence and to become "other" directed. The concept of respect was strongly equated with promoting caring and nonviolent lifeways and practices and was largely embedded in the informant's religious/spiritual and cultural values and beliefs. Although informants talked about the importance of "self respect," a strong regard for promoting the value of "other respect" was repeatedly noted. The "Lord's love" was bestowed on those who demonstrated love and respect for their "brothers" and "sisters," which led to other caring modalities and nonviolent lifeways and practices.

The fourth major theme was as follows:

For African Americans, a diminished sense of "we-ness," viewed as care, was believed to have led to an increase in violence.

All 12 African American key informants talked about the significance of helping their "brothers" and "sisters," referred to as an act of "we-ness," and caring. The "we-ness" concept was viewed as maintaining caring and nonviolent cultural lifeways in the past since the days of slavery. One key informant stated: "Being loyal to each other was caring. I always believed in togetherness. That's my talk. When you have togetherness, you can live."

Several elder key informants expressed a sense of loss in changing societal and cultural values today and a strong regard for values of "times past." They believed the cultural value their generation had placed on helping one another had been lost with the younger generation. One key informant added: "Used to be we could always depend on each other." A general informant spoke about the African American cultural value in helping one's brothers and sisters with this comment: "I believe the Black culture helps their own, more than Whites do." Yet, this same informant talked about the increasing commonality of violence among all cultures: "Today though, I'm starting to see decreased differences between cultures in violence," demonstrating a need to extend care and positive regard to all our "brothers" and "sisters," regardless of one's cultural identity.

From the above key and general informant statements, theme four substantiates the close connection of caring and nonviolent lifeways. Informants repeatedly described the concept of "we-ness" as a caring mode and essential today to prevent violence. An underlying sense of loss was expressed by the first or older generation with respect to the cultural care values of helping others, particularly in times of need. The prevalence of violence as a societal trend was repeatedly noted, and informants stressed the importance of "helping others" as a means to return to caring lifeways and decrease acts of violence.

In summary, four universal themes were abstracted from African American key and general informants from descriptors and patterns. Similarities and differences were systematically identified among intergenerational informants. Many repeated patterns from observations and interviews confirmed and substantiated meanings-in-context. Unquestionably, the influence of religious/spiritual and cultural values and lifeways and other social structure factors on intergenerational meanings, expressions, and practices of family violence and culture care for African Americans was discovered.

Euro-American Culture

Three Euro-American universal culture care themes were discovered from the raw data, descriptors, and patterns. The first Euro-American universal theme was as follows:

For Euro-Americans, misplaced anger, violent family expressions, and ineffective patterns of communication were associated with noncaring practices and lifeways.

Eight key informants and five general informants, from all generations, spoke about noncaring practices they had experienced with other family members.

They spoke of problems in expressing their anger appropriately to others and that noncare practices had been learned and passed on intergenerationally. Informants talked about "silence" as a cultural noncare practice to communicate anger. One key informant said: "When my mom gets mad at me, she won't talk to me. One time she didn't talk to me for four days. Her mother used to do that with her too."

They also talked about misplaced anger with children and spouses, described as the inability to communicate their anger with the appropriate individual(s). Informants spoke about "hitting" their children or being "hit" as children. One key informant stated: "My mom used to hit me. I was afraid of her. I wouldn't call it abuse, because it didn't happen all the time, but my mom used to get mad at me, for no reason, and she would start slapping me." Three key informants talked about learning to communicate in this manner from a family member, usually a mother or father. In talking with three generations within the same family, the researcher was told about the noncaring practices of expressing one's misplaced anger as learned cultural values and lifeways. One first-generation key informant, a grandmother, stated:

I didn't drive and I was home all the time, and that was kind of rough. I took in ironing. I'd have to do all that after the kids were in bed. So then I was up to about 3:00 in the morning, ironing and cleaning. Spanking a child is not child abuse, it didn't harm us. I just spanked my kids when they were little if they did something. I think a lot of the reason I did it was being tired, and I might have taken it out on the kids.

The daughter (second generation) talked about learning to express anger from her mother. She said: "My mom was the same way. If she was angry at Dad, she used to take it out on us kids, and I'm the same way." The granddaughter (third generation) in this family said:

With my mom, if she's angry, she'll hit one of us, and I feel that that's how I learned how to deal with anger. I just get afraid of that. When I get angry, I just want to hit. I don't care what I hit or who I hit. I'm just afraid one of these days I won't be able to control myself.

In talking with three generations within one family, noncaring expressions and ineffective communication was learned and passed on intergenerationally. The researcher observed the difficulty for several informants in talking about personal experiences with violence, yet they were able to talk about violence with respect to the "other" (brother, neighbor, etc.). One key informant stated:

There was never violence with us, not like with my older brother and his kids. That was violence. He would be really violent with his kids. We would get after him sometimes, because even when the kids were little, he would get angry about something and then take it out on the kids and really beat 'em. The older boy is a little slow today, and we thought maybe it was from getting hit in the head or something. The oldest boy ended up in jail.

Another key informant spoke about the violence she had witnessed at a neighbor's home. The concept of misplaced anger as noncaring and violence passed on intergenerationally is well delineated in this informant's comment: "My one neighbor takes a belt to her kids. But I think she had a horrible home life. I think it happened to her a lot. I think she's angry, and I think her kids are going to be the same way. I think it's a vicious cycle. I think her kids will do that too."

In Theme 1, Euro-Americans identified noncaring as learned cultural values and practices with ineffective patterns of communication frequently expressed as misplaced anger that led to violent family expressions. Noncaring and ineffective patterns of communication, described as misplaced anger, were associated with violent family expressions. These patterns were culturally learned and passed on intergenerationally.

The second Euro-American theme was as follows:

Euro-Americans believed noncaring role modeling led to an increase in societal violence, particularly among children.

Caring and nonviolent role modeling was believed to be an important responsibility of parents, yet these Euro-American informants (from three generations) felt it was "somehow missing today." All key and general informants were concerned about a general lack of caring role models with the "younger generation." Violence on television, noncaring parents, and rapidly changing societal and cultural care values were "blamed" for the increase in American violence today. Informants believed "care" was needed in the home and was held to be a parental responsibility by instilling caring attitudes in their children through socialization and enculturation processes. One key informant said: "A lot of the violence is coming from families who don't care what their children are doing." One key informant spoke about the abuse she had experienced from her mother: "I know with my mom, the way she would spank me, like grandma did it with her. A lot of it is passed on." This same informant did not believe she was noncaring or violent with her children; yet, her 16-year-old daughter said: "I'm afraid of my mother."

Care was identified as a learned cultural value passed on intergenerationally with one diversity view. One informant stated: "Caring comes naturally. You're either born with it or you're not. Caring has to come from within." All other informants identified that care was influenced by what was taught in the home. As one key informant stated: "Caring is something we learn at home, it's either there or it isn't." Changing cultural values and beliefs, particularly those related to social structure factors, were associated with an increase in violence in American society today. Several key informants who had "chosen" to stay home and raise their children recognized that their children were "doing things different today." One key informant stated: "I think the answer to all this violence is that mothers should be home with their kids, because too many kids are left on their own."

From Theme 2 the data substantiated that role modeling was an essential means to instill caring meanings, expressions, and practices in children. First-generation informants believed constructive role modeling had been lost with the young generation, but was held to be the responsibility of the parents to help children learn and practice caring through socialization and enculturation. Violence was associated with noncaring and/or absent role models for children within society and most importantly within the home environmental context.

The third major theme was as follows:

For Euro-Americans, an increase in substance abuse was associated with an increase in expressions and practices of noncaring and violence within the family and in society in general.

Substance abuse was repeatedly identified to have a major influence on the increase in family and societal violence. It was often referred to by key informants as a "culture of alcohol and drugs" in America. Several informants spoke about personal experiences with alcohol and drugs, particularly in their own family. Key and general informants frequently identified a connection to alcohol and drug use with violence in the home. One key informant talked about her own experiences with witnessing violence as a child because of her father's alcoholism in the following verbatim descriptor:

> There were a lot of violent times with my mom and dad in our younger years, cause my dad was an alcoholic. He drank a lot. I can remember him beating her, kicking her, throwing her on the floor, things like that. My oldest brother, who's the black sheep of the family, also drinks a lot. Maybe he saw a lot of stuff. He holds a lot against mom and dad.

Seven key and five general informants also talked about the use of drugs and alcohol today, particularly with the youngest (third) generation. One second-generation general informant talked about the difficulty to raise a child today with the increase in use and availability of alcohol and drugs: "With teenagers today and the drugs. I wouldn't want to raise a teenager today. I mean you've got the drugs and the drinking. It's too easy for them to get." Euro-Americans linked the rise in intergenerational family and societal violence with an increase in the use of alcohol and drugs. Both key and general informants talked about the likelihood of violence and noncaring practices in homes in which parents were using alcohol and drugs. First- and second-generation informants expressed concerns about changing societal and cultural values with respect to instilling caring values in the young.

In summary, three universal themes were abstracted from Euro-American informant descriptors and patterns with similarities and differences among informants. Observations and interviews with key and general informants revealed the extent to which their cultural values and lifeways and other social structure factors influenced intergenerational meanings, expressions, and practices of family violence and culture care for Euro-Americans.

Table 19.1 presents a succinct overview of the findings for both groups related to the four universal themes for the African American informants and three universal themes for the Euro-American informants.

Table 19.1   Comparative African and Euro-American Care/Noncare Meanings, Expressions, and Practices

African Americans	Euro-Americans
Tend to talk about "whoopings"	Tend to talk about violence with the "other," i.e., brother, parents, neighbors, but not in the present personal, married, or significant relationships
Do not believe it is violence	
Physical punishment done to "teach" children to "respect" elders and those in authority and thought of as teaching "survival care"	Physical punishment done out of "frustration," "exhaustion," and misplaced anger
Mother more likely to use physical versus verbal punishment	In addition to physical punishment, mothers tend to withdraw love and will not interact or talk to child when angry with child (mothers also frequently experienced this from their own mothers)
Mother and/or grandmother is responsible in the family to promote care	Mother is responsible in the family to promote care
Responsibility of increase in violence is attributed to no one being at home to "teach" the children to care	Responsibility for an increase in violence is attributed to mothers working outside of the home and not being available to care

Discussion of Findings

Culture Care Nursing Judgments, Decisions, and Actions

With the Theory of Culture Care Diversity and Universality, Leininger predicted three major modalities to guide nursing judgments, decisions, or actions to help nurses provide culturally congruent care.[45,46] The three modes are 1) cultural care preservation and/or maintenance, 2) cultural care accommodation and/or negotiation, and 3) cultural care repatterning or restructuring. Based on the findings in this study, the three modes of cultural care nursing judgments, decisions, and actions will be discussed next in relation to the domain of inquiry.

Cultural Care Preservation/Maintenance   Cultural care preservation/maintenance would be used by nurses to strengthen the cultural values and beliefs of extended family, neighborhood, and community systems for members of both cultures. It would be especially important to draw on religious/spiritual factors with African Americans. The nurse would encourage preservation/maintenance of caring relationships with extended family members to facilitate a meaningful understanding of child rearing and intergenerational caring practices to prevent family violence. He or she needs to recognize noncaring expressions and practices of African American family violence patterns and then draw on local community resources such as mental health agencies or family parenting classes or discussion groups to preserve and maintain caring modes among family members.

The church setting would be important to strengthening, maintaining, and preserving community bonds of togetherness or the "we-ness" valued by African Americans. Local church groups could promote the cultural care value of respect for self and others, or one's brothers and sisters, and especially the elderly. Nurses should focus on maintaining family support and respect for individuals within African American families, groups, and communities. Knowledge is essential to preserve "we-ness" through verbal and nonverbal communication modes. Cultural identity roots and values need to be preserved and maintained with pride. Local library, educational, community, and church centers with African American heritage activities would also be encouraged and maintained.

The Euro-American value of inspiring the young to embrace cultural meanings, expressions, and practices of care through the use of positive role models needs to be preserved and maintained. Personal expressions of care that parents, spouses, and children want to pass on to first and second generations could be taught and maintained as model caring practices for the young or third generation in diverse environmental contexts to prevent violence and destructive conflicts.

Cultural Care Accommodation or Negotiation

For African Americans, cultural care accommodation or negotiation means accommodating their lifeways with family, church, and local community interests to prevent or lessen violence tendencies or acts. This means referring clients to parenting classes in local churches and to counseling agencies that have support groups for parents dealing with life stresses experienced by single and/or working parents. Since all third-generation informants identified care as the need to have time to communicate with parents, family members are encouraged to identify strategies to accommodate this need with their children to prevent violent acts. Religious and spirituality needs are accommodated along with family kinship ties to promote caring and nonviolent lifeways.

With the Euro-Americans desire for "self-improvement" and new "life skills," transcultural nurses would accommodate this need by guiding them to self-help and lifeway groups to improve skills to deal with misplaced anger. Families might attend support groups on anger management and/or Alcoholics Anonymous and Al-Anon groups for families having difficulties with substance abuse. Euro-Americans with family violence difficulties require culture care accommodation and negotiation modes to reduce violence through educational home and community programs.

Nurses' judgments need to be held in abeyance, and they need to avoid blaming, accusing, or other modes of noncaring practices with both African American and Euro-American cultures. Intergenerational family violence needs to be discussed by nurses in family and community group sessions. Nurses need to assess African Americans and Euro-Americans for substance abuse, and they need to accommodate and negotiate culturally congruent treatment for clients. African Americans could be encouraged to seek care for substance abuse within their local church and community groups and with professional care service agencies. Nurses might also have Euro-Americans "focus on care of self" through individual therapy referrals, which may require culture care accommodation and/or negotiation practices.

Cultural Care Repatterning and Restructuring

Cultural care repatterning and restructuring for African American parents would include helping them learn to take responsibility for teaching caring and nonviolent lifeways to children. Whooping as generic care may have short-term benefits to control violence, but it always necessitates repatterning and restructuring to maintain nonviolent caring practices. The youngest generation of both African Americans and Euro-Americans were being influenced by American socialization processes of not using physical forms of punishment with children, but the elder generations of both cultural groups and some second-generation informants held to their respective cultural values and beliefs that there are indications and benefits for some "whooping" and mild hitting when children need it. Second and third generations need to understand that care, as respect, is a reciprocal practice with children. Local churches and community groups need to be assessed to help the young or third generation in survival care and to avoid becoming involved in gangs and legal systems.

Euro-American noncaring patterns of family violence need to be repatterned and restructured, especially to deal with misplaced anger and taking anger out on family members. Therapeutic patterns of communication such as learning to appropriately express feelings, particularly anger, with family members needs to be taught to children and adults throughout the life cycle. Providing ways to assist clients in repatterning anger without resorting to noncaring and violent practices is important. Such an action mode might well break the cycle of family violence. Repatterning by use of role modeling with Euro-Americans could improve parent-child relationships. Nurses might role model caring communication patterns with children and make referrals to community agencies such as "Big Brother" and "Big Sister" organizations to develop caring positive role models for culturally congruent lifeways that are health promoting.

Repatterning and restructuring preconceived negative judgments about violence that are not viewed as caring nursing modes need to be made with African Americans and Euro-Americans in co-informant ways. Blaming or passing other negative beliefs to clients was found to be noncaring and nonbeneficial. If blaming and/or judgmental attitudes were used by nurses, it could be a major barrier to helping clients in culturally congruent ways and clients may avoid discussing or seeking help for noncaring and violent lifeways and practices from disapproving and critical nurses.

In-depth understanding of intergenerational violence is essential nursing knowledge to alter a noncaring cycle that is passed on from one generation to the next. The nurse needs to seek appropriate time to discuss such an issue with clients in a co-informant way as advocated by Leininger and should work to repattern destructive and noncaring patterns of violence. Noncaring and culturally incongruent modes of working with clients that alienate and/or silence clients and perpetuate a cycle of violence intergenerationally need to be consciously avoided by nurses.

The author recommends the following "TCN CARE Repatterning Guideline" based on Leininger's major TCN concepts and principles, which could facilitate ways to provide culturally congruent care.[47,48] The research findings from this study also need to be used within the Theory of Culture Care and the domain of inquiry investigated in this study on intergenerational family violence for African Americans and Euro-Americans.

Take the time to learn specific cultural values, beliefs, and practices about care.

Communicate and maintain care modes to clients within a culturally congruent manner.

Negotiate, accommodate, and nurture cultural values, beliefs, and practices that facilitate caring.

Coordinate family and community referrals for clients to facilitate intergenerational caring values, beliefs, practices, and expressions of care.

Accommodate, preserve, and maintain cultural care values, beliefs, and practices of clients.

Restructure lifeways that are noncaring or violent intergenerationally.

Empathize with clients and avoid judgmental nursing decisions and actions by providing culturally congruent care that leads to health and well-being.

The reader can use this "TCN CARE Repatterning Guideline" with other transcultural nursing concepts and principles along with research findings from other cultures related to violence.

Summary

This study, conceptualized within Leininger's Theory of Culture Care Diversity and Universality, demonstrates the importance of nurses caring for clients experiencing difficulties with intergenerational family violence within a culturally congruent manner. Leininger's Theory of Culture Care was essential to discover social structure factors regarding intergenerational family violence within the African American and Euro-American cultures. This study further demonstrates the potential role of the transcultural nurse to discover, alleviate, or diminish intergenerational violence that is widely prevalent in the United States. Transcultural nursing research studies on violence such as this study can assist nurses who are practicing within a similar context to care for clients experiencing violence within a culturally congruent manner. The use of Leininger's Theory of Culture Care with concomitant research findings contributes to the growing body of transcultural nursing knowledge, and the findings need to be used to provide culturally congruent care—the goal of the theory and a worldwide human need.

References

1. Leininger, M.M., "The Phenomenon of Caring: The Essence and Central Focus of Nursing," *American Nurses' Foundation (Nursing Research Report)*, v. 12, no. 1, 1977, p. 2, 14.

2. Leininger, M.M., *Transcultural Nursing: Concepts, Theories, Research and Practice*, 2nd ed., Columbus, OH: McGraw-Hill & Greyden Press, 1995.

3. Leininger, M.M., "Philosophic, Epistemic, and Other Dimensions of the Theory," *Culture Care*

Diversity and Universality: A Theory of Nursing,
New York: National League for Nursing, 1991a.

4. Leininger, op. cit., 1995.

5. Gordon, A.J., "Alcoholism Treatment Services to
Hispanics: An Ethnographic Examination of a
Community's Services," *Family Community Health,*
v. 13, no. 4, 1987, pp. 12–24.

6. Leininger, op. cit., 1991a.

7. Leininger, op. cit., 1995.

8. Leininger, op. cit., 1991a.

9. Leininger, op. cit., 1995.

10. Leininger, M.M., "Culture Care of the Gadsup
Akuna of the Eastern Highlands of New Guinea," in
*Culture Care Diversity & Universality: A Theory of
Nursing,* M.M. Leininger, ed., New York: National
League for Nursing Press, 1991, pp. 231–280.

11. Ibid.

12. Ibid.

13. Rosenbaum, J., "Culture Care Theory and Greek
Canadian Widows," in *Culture Care Diversity and
Universality: A Theory of Nursing,* M.M. Leininger,
ed., New York: National League for Nursing Press,
1991, pp. 305–339.

14. Ibid.

15. Janvier, K.A., "Family Violence: A Public Health
Concern," *DNA Reporter,* v. 23, no. 4, 1998,
pp. 5–6.

16. Leininger, op. cit., 1995.

17. Malone, S.B., "Black Violence in American:
Implications for Nursing Research," *Journal of
Nursing Science,* v. 2, no. 1–6, 1997, pp. 107–116.

18. Ibid.

19. Ibid.

20. Jones, F.C., "Community Violence, Children and
Youth: Considerations for Programs, Policy, and
Nursing Roles," *Pediatric Nursing,* v. 23, no. 2,
1997, pp. 131–139.

21. Franklin, J.H., and A.A. Moss, Jr., *From Slavery to
Freedom: A History of Negro Americans,* 6th ed.,
New York: McGraw-Hill Publishing Co., 1988.

22. Osborne, O.H., "Aging and the Black Diaspora: The
African, Caribbean, and African American
Experience," in *Transcultural Nursing: Concepts,
Theories, and Practices,* M.M. Leininger, ed., 1978,
pp. 317–333.

23. Baer, H.A., and M. Singer, *African-American
Religion in the Twentieth Century: Varieties of
Protest and Accommodation,* Knoxville: The
University of Tennessee Press, 1992.

24. Ibid.

25. Leininger, op. cit., 1995.

26. Leininger, M.M., "Southern Rural Black and White
American Lifeways with Focus on Care and Health
Phenomena," in *Care: The Essence of Nursing and
Health,* M.M. Leininger, ed., Detroit: Wayne State
University Press, 1988, pp. 133–159.

27. Leininger, M.M., "Selected Culture Care Findings
of Diverse Cultures Using Culture Care Theory and
Ethnomethods," in *Culture Care Diversity and
Universality: A Theory of Nursing,* M.M. Leininger,
ed., New York: National League for Nursing Press,
1991c, pp. 345–371.

28. Leininger, op. cit., 1995.

29. Jones, M.A., *American Immigration,* Chicago: The
University of Chicago Press, 1960.

30. Rips, G.N., *Coming to America: Immigrants from
Southern Europe,* New York: Delacorte Press,
1981.

31. Coppa, F.J., and T.J. Curran, *The Immigrant
Experience in America,* Boston: Twayne Publishers,
1983.

32. Garraty, J.A., *The American Nation,* 5th ed., New
York: Harper and Row Publishers, 1983.

33. Leininger, op. cit., 1991c.

34. Leininger, op. cit., 1977.

35. Leininger, M.M., "Caring: A Central Focus of
Nursing and Health Care Services," *Nursing and
Health Care,* v. 1, no. 3, 1980, pp. 135–143, 176.

36. Leininger, M.M., "Ethnonursing: A Research
Method with Enablers to Study the Theory of
Culture Care," in *Culture Care Diversity and
Universality: A Theory of Nursing,* M.M. Leininger,
ed., New York: National League for Nursing Press,
1991d, pp. 73–117.

37. Leininger, op. cit., 1991b.

38. Leininger, op. cit., 1995.

39. Leininger, op. cit., 1991d.

40. Ibid.

41. Ibid.

42. Ibid.

43. Ibid.

44. Ibid.

45. Leininger, op. cit., 1991a.

46. Leininger, op. cit., 1995.

47. Leininger, M., *Transcultural Nursing,* 1978.
(Reprinted in 1994 by Greyden Press, Columbus,
OH).

48. Leininger, op. cit., 1995.

20 Elder Care in Urban Namibian Families: An Ethnonursing Study

Cheryl J. Leuning, Louis F. Small, and Agnes van Dyk

Overview

Since Namibia's independence in 1990, the population of elders (persons 65 years old and older) in urban communities is growing steadily and requests for home health care, health counseling, respite care, and residential care for aging members of society are overwhelming the health care system. This study expands transcultural nursing knowledge by increasing understanding of *generic* (home-based) patterns of elder care that are practiced and lived by urban Namibian families. Guided by the Culture Care Theory and the ethnonursing research method, *emic* (insider) meanings and expressions of care and caring for elders have been abstracted from data collected through semistructured interviews and observations with selected urban family members and synthesized into five substantive themes. The themes, which depict what caring for elders means to urban families, include the following:

1. Care as nurturing the health of the family
2. Care as trusting in the benevolence of life as lived
3. Care as honoring one's elders
4. Care as sustaining security and purpose for life amid uncertainty
5. Providing care within rapidly changing cultural and social structures

These findings add a voice from the developing world to the body of transcultural nursing knowledge and increase understanding of several culture care constructs, including respect, presence, being connected, and protection. Findings are blended with *professional care* practices to facilitate culturally congruent nursing care for elders and their families in urban Namibia.

To care is to be compassionate and so form a community of people honestly facing the painful realities of our finite existence.   —Henri J.M. Nouwen

The population of the world is growing older. By 2025, one out of every four persons in the developed world (about 25%), and one out of every eight persons in the developing world (about 12%) will be 65 years old or older.[1] This latter percentage constitutes over 70% of the world's elders as developing regions continue to experience burgeoning population growth.[2] Such extensive demographic change will affect the economic, cultural, and social well-being of the entire global community and simultaneously present urgent challenges for health care systems serving persons of all cultures.

Since Namibia's independence in 1990, the elder population in this southwestern African country has grown steadily. Increases in the number of elders have touched all cultures in Namibia. Most Namibian people trace their descent from two aboriginal groups, the Bantu from north central Africa and the hunter-gatherers or San Bushmen from southern Africa. Several cultures have evolved from these original Namibians. Owambo, Herero, and Kvango people speak similar Bantu languages and share common traditions, while the Nama, Damara, Colored, Baster, and San groups speak Khokhoi languages and share somewhat different traditions. European and Afrikaner people in Namibia trace their origins to Germany, the Netherlands, and South Africa, respectively, thus introducing additional cultures and traditions to the country.[3] Although cultural differences exist among Namibians, their common experiences through the centuries and their collective struggle against apartheid have created powerful bonds among people and a national sociocultural identity that emphasizes unity and understanding rather than diversity.

Historically, Namibian families of all cultures have cared for elders at home. Women have assumed major responsibilities of looking after aging family members and those with fragile health, while the entire family has devoted time and resources to elder care. Today, many factors have altered these family traditions. Opportunities for young people, including women, are enticing extended families to migrate from rural homelands to cities where both men and women can pursue education and careers. When younger members of urban families become busy with school or jobs, it is increasingly difficult for them to provide adequate social, cultural, physical, and/or emotional care for their elders. Additionally, the AIDS pandemic in Namibia poses an unprecedented health threat. As the leading cause of death and hospitalization in the country, AIDS is claiming the lives of women and men who constitute the work force — persons between the ages of 20 and 49.[4] What this means for elders is difficult to discern. Will they have any surviving children or grandchildren to care for them? Will elders be the sole support and care providers for their grandchildren?

While AIDS is talking its toll on young people, demographic data suggest that Namibian people are living longer today than they ever have before. About 5.6% of the 1.6 million people in Namibia — 90,100 people — are over 65 years of age, and within this age group, 60% are over 75 years old, and 20% are over 80 years old.[5] Like elderly individuals in other parts of the world, the frail oldest of the old in Namibia require a great deal of assistance and supportive care to remain at home. Chronic illnesses, including arthritis, hypertension, recurring respiratory infections, cancer, and diabetes are associated with increasing age in Namibia. When families are not able to care for elders at home, other options are limited. Often the elders simply do not get the attention they need, or they are moved into one of the few old age homes in the country where families are still expected to assist residents with daily needs, including clothing and food. As Namibian nurses begin developing models of assistance and support for families and elders in urban communities, it is critical to know and understand culturally valued patterns of care within the family.

 ## Domain of Inquiry and Purpose of the Study

Emic (insider) cultural meanings and expressions of care and caring for elders in selected urban Namibian families was the domain of inquiry for this study. The purpose of the study was to increase transcultural nursing knowledge and understanding of *generic* (home-based) patterns of elder care within urban Namibian families. The study identified culturally congruent community-focused nursing care for elders and their families by combining *generic* care and *professional* nursing care.

 ## Theoretical Framework

Leininger's theory of Culture Care Diversity and Universality with the ethnonursing research method was used to guide this study within the philosophy and science of human caring.[6–12] The major premise of Culture Care Theory is that care is the essence of nursing and a universal human experience with diverse meanings and unique patterns of expressions in different cultures.[13,14] Culture, the gestalt of human experience and knowledge, includes the "...values, beliefs, norms, patterns, and practices that are learned, shared, and transmitted intergenerationally" that influence care meanings and expressions.[15,16] Differences (diversities) and similarities (universals) in care knowledge and practices among persons, families, groups, and communities were predicted by the theorist to be shaped or influenced by the worldview, environmental context, language, and cultural and social dimensions (including kinship, religion, cultural values, political, legal, technology, economics, and education) of cultures. Furthermore, the theorist predicted that care meanings and expressions greatly influence and explain the health or well-being of individuals, families, groups, and communities.[17–19] Health is constructed by persons and communities as they live in harmony with their cultural and physical environment, including their own biology, and the totality of their human experience.

The theory of Culture Care has been designed by the theorist with a rigorous qualitative method of discovery and analysis, namely, the ethnonursing research method. This method brings forth explicit diverse and universal culturally based care meanings and expressions from *emic* (insider) and *etic* (outsider) perspectives related to health, illness, and dying patterns. The ethnonursing research method is a systematic way of exploring, knowing, and confirming culturally based individual and group knowledge about care and health in the discipline of transcultural nursing.[20–24] Philosophically and epistemologically, ethnonursing data are grounded with people as knowers. Researchers learn from people (culture care informants) how they define, experience, express, and value health and care. With the theory, the research is guided through the research process toward discovering *generic care* (learned at home and within the family and community) and *professional care* (formally taught and transmitted through professional institutions, such as the university) patterns and perspectives.[25,26] Thus the Culture Care Theory facilitates discoveries and possibilities of bringing together generic and professional care knowledge that can lead to providing culturally congruent nursing care to individuals, families, groups, and communities with their full participation and input. This is ultimately the goal of the Culture Care Theory.

The assumptions in this study were derived and modified from Leininger's work[27,28] and include the following:

1. Care is the essence of nursing and a distinct, dominant, central, and unifying focus of the discipline.
2. Caring for elders within the family is a universal human experience with specific meanings and expressions that are culturally and socially determined.
3. Urban Namibian families face unique experiences and challenges as they care for elders.
4. Urban Namibian families have developed culturally specific meanings and expressions of care and caring for elders that are essential for individual and family health and survival.
5. Those members of the family who are primarily responsible for the care and well-being of elders will identify themselves and/or be identified by other family members.
6. Family members who have primary responsibility for the care of elders will discuss their caring activities and the meaning they ascribe to caring.
7. Culturally congruent nursing care is essential to the health of elders, their families, and the communities in which they live.

8. Culturally congruent care occurs when the nurse knows and can participate in *emic* and *generic* meanings and expressions of care.[29–33]

The following orientational definitions were based on the theory of Culture Care Diversity and Universality, but were formulated to focus on the domain of inquiry of this study:

- *Health*—a dynamic experience of well-being that is culturally defined and that enables persons to live and die with dignity.
- *Culture care (noun) / caring (gerund)*—learned ways of valuing, supporting, and fostering one's own or another's health and well-being.
- *Urban family with elders*—a group of people related by marriage and/or kinship that identify themselves as a family, have lived in an urban community for more than one year with at least one member of the family who is over 65 and who relies on the family for care related to activities of daily living, finances, and/or other health needs.
- *Urban community*—a community of over 20,000 inhabitants and with an industrial, business, and retail center.
- *Key culture care informant*—a person who identifies her or himself (or is identified by others) as the primary care provider for an elder and is knowledgeable about care.
- *General culture care informant*—a member of the family (other than the primary care provider) who has experience living with and caring for an elder; a person who is frail and elderly and dependent on family for care; and/or members of the nursing profession or other health professions who have experience caring for elders and have general viewpoints about culturally based care.

Research Questions

Questions relevant to the domain of inquiry included the following:

1. What are the care practices, beliefs, and values related to caring for elders in urban Namibian families?

2. What are the *emic* meanings and expressions of care and caring?

3. How does the cultural context of the urban community influence meanings and expressions of care for the elderly?

4. Which family members assume primary caring roles?

5. What cultural differences and/or similarities exist in care meanings and expressions among urban Namibian families?

6. In what ways do worldview, cultural and social dimensions, ethnohistory, and environmental context influence care practices of the Namibian elders?

■ Literature Review on the Care of Elders

Aging is a transcultural phenomenon influenced by multiple factors in human communities throughout the world. Since the early 1980s, family care for elderly members has been the subject of extensive study in nursing, gerontology, social work, and anthropology. Most studies have investigated the psychosocial and physical aspects of family care giving such as personal burden,[34–39] economic gains and losses to the family,[40,41] general health of caregivers,[42–45] and care giving competence.[46] Other studies have noted that elderly individuals themselves experience overwhelming fears of abandonment,[47] and that families who face the necessity of caring for an elder need a great deal of support from the health professions, including information and education.[48,49] Lack of appropriate instruments to study care phenomena and health relative to elders has also been documented.[50] Studies of elder care within institutions have described *generic* and *professional* care patterns among Anglo- and African-American residents,[51] and personal control as a determinant of elder well-being.[52]

Anthropologists who study aging among diverse cultural groups tend to focus on age as a structural feature of society,[53,54] on the life experiences of elders,[55,56] and/or on understanding and interpreting human behavior relative to aging.[57] These studies identify valuable information about the meanings of age in different sociocultural settings and the status and

treatment of elders, but they do not specifically connect cultural meanings and practices to patterns of care and health within the family.

Studies of elder health done in southern Africa focus on the exponential growth rate of the elderly population,[58] changes in the extended (traditional) family system, rural to urban migrations,[59] the AIDS pandemic,[60] limited financial resources available to support elders in communities throughout Africa,[61–64] and institutional care as a "last resort" for elders.[65,66] Like studies done in other parts of the world, these studies are not generalizable to Namibian society. Additionally, the dominant paradigm undergirding most elder care research is logical positivism, in which phenomena are explained with a set of variables that can be "measured" by objective observation.[67–69] Elder care research within a human science[70–74] or a naturalistic[75] paradigm that seeks to understand, describe, and explain the meaning of care and health as lived and experienced is also a valuable, and still underrepresented, perspective in the accumulating body of nursing knowledge.

■ Research Method and Design

Leininger's[76–78] ethnonursing qualitative research method was used to examine systematically the domain of inquiry. Several enablers were used as part of the method: the *Stranger to Trusted Friend* and *Observation-Participation-Reflection* enablers,[79] along with three specific enablers designed for study of the domain of inquiry. These enablers included the systematic and respectful ways the researchers entered into the communities and lives of informants; the ways of engaging informants in meaningful dialogue, namely, the semistructured interview guides and processes of language translation; and the ways of leaving informants with appreciation for their contributions to *emic* and *etic* understandings of elder care within the family. The *Observation-Participation-Reflection* enabler directed the focus of the research to in-depth observations followed by semistructured dialogue that was guided by informants' knowledge and experiences. The opportunities to "get close to people, study the total context, and obtain accurate *emic* data from the people"[80] were important and woven into the entire research process.

Inviting Participation and Respecting Informants' Rights

Persons from urban communities in a large metropolitan area were invited in a purposive manner to participate in this study. Community health nurses and members of the research team identified most of the informants (Color Insert 11). Key and general informants were selected according to criteria in the orientational definitions cited earlier. Eleven women between 21 and 71 years of age who had cared for an elder member of the family at home for two to 15 years comprised the pool of key informants. Key informants had lived in the city for 6 or more years, and all but one was single. Two were widows, five had never been married, and three were divorced or separated from their partners. Additionally, there were 18 general informants in the study, including elder members of the community, frail elders who were dependent on a family member for care, professional nurses, other family members, and members of the community who were responsible for elder care. The most common kinship relationships between key informants (primary caregivers) and elders (care receivers) were parent-child and grandparent-grandchild, or more specifically, parent-daughter and grandparent-granddaughter.

Two institutional review boards for the protection of human rights in research approved this study. The review boards represented the institutions with which the team of researchers were associated. An Informed Consent Statement was read to each informant in the language of her/his preference (Afrikaans or English) prior to the first meeting with them.[81,82] Each informant signed or made her/his mark on the statement. Several informants preferred that their names remain unchanged in the study, as the stories told are their stories and they wanted to be identified with their stories and experiences.

Collecting, Describing, and Documenting Raw Data

Observation-participation and data collection were based on the following ethnonursing philosophic, epistemic, and ontological principles: 1) Maintaining a perspective of open discovery, active listening, and genuine learning in the total context of the informant's world, 2) being active and curious about the "why" of whatever is seen, heard, or experienced, and being appreciative of what informants shared (reflecting on local, *emic*, and professional, *etic*, points of view), and 3) recording whatever is shared in a careful and conscientious way to preserve full meanings and informant's ideas.[83] Specific inquiry enablers took the form of meetings with informants in their homes, conducting the meetings in a language informants were most comfortable speaking, and designing and using a semistructured interview guide to facilitate conversations about *emic* meanings and expression of care focused on the domain of inquiry. The interview guide included, but was not limited to, the following examples of questions and statements: Tell us what is it like for you to care for _____. How did it happen that you begin caring for _____? From childhood, what do you remember about elders in your family?

All conversations were translated into English during the discussion. English is the official language in Namibia. However, most informants' mother tongue was one of the African languages or Afrikaans. Therefore, not all informants were comfortable expressing complex ideas and experiences in English. Two of the three researchers fluently speak and write both Afrikaans and English. Detailed notes were taken and transcribed into Word Perfect 8.0 for ease of coding, analysis, and transmission via e-mail between the United States and Namibia. Guided by the phases of the ethnonursing method, raw data (transcriptions of verbatim interviews/conversations with informants and detailed observations made in informant's homes and communities) were read and re-read by the researchers.

Analysis of meaning followed contemplative processes where hunches about contextual meanings and symbols were identified and preliminary interpretations were made in the form of notes that attempted to answer the questions, "What's happening here?" and "What does this mean?" When categories and groupings of data began to emerge, descriptive codes were assigned to data groupings based on the domain of inquiry and research questions. Codes and categories were continuously compared to determine patterns and recurrent patterns were studied for their meaning. Patterns were the researchers' best statements that reflected the meanings and experiences of the informants. Patterns were eventually scrutinized to discover saturation of ideas and to identify similar or different meanings,

Cultural Care Descriptors	Cultural Care Patterns	Themes
· We must respect the elder's dignity and keep them clean and never leave them alone. · I try to preserve the dignity of my father always. Like wiping the saliva away from his mouth if he drools. · I had worked outside the home, but I resigned from work to look after my mother. · My caring for Oupa (Grandfather) allows my family to live their lives freely. · My children are happy I am doing this, they would not like to see their grandfather in an old age home · Caring to me is physical and spiritual, you cannot separate the two.	← Being physically present & available to the elder ← Making commitment to care "full-time" ← Attending to physical and spiritual needs of the elder	← Care as nurturing the health of the family by preserving the integrity and dignity of the elder
· I am an only daughter. Caring for my Pa is my responsibility. No one in the family is as able as I. · I love Ouma, that is why I care for her. · We are her children, that is why we care for her. · I know they will look after me. I don't even think about it (elderly participant). · I do not plan for tomorrow or the future. Why? We live from day to day. · I ask people to pray for me and for my father. · All my worries, I pray about. What good is worry. God will provide. · Praying for an elder is very important. They appreciate it very much	← Accepting the care giver role without deliberation ← Living from day to day ← Praying ← Letting go of worries	← Care as trusting in the benevolence of life as lived moment by moment
· We must respect our elder's and keep them clean and never leave them alone. They should always be seen in dignified dress. · My family respects me and listens to me (frail elderly participant.) · I must look after my mother. If I don't she will be unhappy until she dies. · When Pa is very quiet, I tell him to smile. Also, I ask him if he is sick. He says that if he doesn't talk to me, he can talk to God. · I talk to children and elderly alike. I tell them not to abuse alcohol and to look after the elders so they do not suffer. · Caring for an elder means you have a protecting role. · I pick up his pension...it is hardly enough to steal...but it would be very unsafe for him.	← Being respectful ← Keeping elders from despair and loneliness ← Warning elders and family members about destructive life style choices ← Protecting elders from theft, harm, and/or wrong-doing	← Care as honoring one's elders
· This is my father's house, I will inherit it someday. · The nicest thing about caring for my mother is love. This is the most rewarding and I feel happy. · The nicest thing about caring for Ouma is that she is always friendly. · Both the old and young give and receive. The elderly are sometimes giving advice. · Caring for a parent is giving and taking. They mostly give appreciation. · My religious beliefs are deep. Caring for elderly is what we should do. I cannot live if I do not care. · Caring for my father means I will receive a reward from God. This is one of my goals in life.	← Reciprocal sharing of material resources, skills and self ← Giving and receiving non-material gifts ← Fulfilling the Biblical calling to care for one's parent/elders	← Care as sustaining security and purpose for life amid uncertainty
· Young people do not see caring for the elderly as their responsibility so much any more. · I have very little time to think about, or care about myself. · I don't know why some people care and some don't. Maybe it has to do with poverty and the financial limits of people. If it were not for my son and his wife, Pa and I could not live on his pension. So they help us. · I am only human and some days it is very difficult and I'm short tempered with Pa. I'm lonely and I'm not working. This is my life right now to look after him. After I get angry, I feel sorry. But I'm alone and no one is here to help me. · Living in the city, people are close together so there are opportunities for the community to care for elderly, but the city also has problems of drugs and people have very little money. · Times are changing. It used to be cheaper to buy food and clothes.	← Balancing traditional gender roles and responsibilities in the family with individual desires to take advantage of opportunities available to all people, including women ← "Making do" with limited economic resources in a society where everything costs more	← Providing care within rapidly changing cultural and social structures in urban Namibian society

Figure 20.1

Cultural care descriptors, patterns, and themes.

expressions, structural forms, interpretations, or explanations related to the domain of inquiry. Informants were asked to clarify and explicate findings at all stages in the analysis. In this way, patterns of care were examined and confirmed in the context of the informants' experiences.

During the final phase of the ethnonursing analysis, substantive concepts, or themes, were abstracted from the patterns and relationships between and among patterns and themes were identified. The substantive themes depict what care and caring for elders means within urban Namibian families and how care is expressed. Figure 20.1 presents raw data (*emic* verbal descriptors), patterns, and substantive themes that were discovered from data analysis. These statements give evidence of data to support the sociocultural dimensions of the theory, especially the kinship, religion, spirituality, cultural values and lifeways, technology, and economics within the context of the Namibian environment.

Rigor, or trustworthiness of the study, was demonstrated by being attentive to qualitative criteria of credibility, confirmability, meaning-in-context, recurrent patterning, saturation, and transferability.[84-86] That is, the "truth," accuracy, or believability of findings were mutually established among the researchers and informants; direct observations and repeated documentation were reaffirmed by informants and researchers continuously. Situations, settings, and experiences of informants and researchers became meaningful in context as the symbols and activities were explained within the specific and total contexts in which they occurred. Repeated instances and sequences of events and experiences were documented for saturation evidence over the 2 years while the study was in process. The culture care categories and meanings became apparent as information about care meanings and expressions became redundant, and no further data or insights were generated. Transferability of this study's findings to different contexts is contingent on similarities of the cultural contexts and other similarities such as the research purpose, domain of inquiry, and research design.

◼ Findings with Discussion

Figure 20.1 presents the major themes with patterns, descriptors, and raw data. Each theme will be discussed in this section. First, however, it is important to note that women clearly were the primary caregivers for elders in urban Namibian families, and they were most able to describe in detail their caring experiences. Although men were supportive of women's efforts, they knew very little about what women did for elderly family members and seemed generally uninterested. One young man said, "Sure, I admire what my sister does for our *Ouma* (grandmother), but I don't know a thing about taking care of someone. We leave that up to women." The literature supported the near universal tendency for women to assume the primary care giving role for frail elders and other family members among cultural groups throughout the world.[87-95]

Findings showed more cultural similarities than differences. Subtle differences in culture care patterns were noted between Herero families and Nama, Damara, Colored, and Baster families. These differences were associated with cultural norms and values related to kinship structures and will be discussed as substantive themes are presented. The other research questions are answered in the discussion of the substantive themes.

Substantive Theme One: Care As Nurturing the Health of the Family

Nurturing the health of the family was supported by the cultural and social structure dimensions of kinship, religion, and spiritual beliefs. Informants explained that "family members are expected to look after one another" in Namibian society. The care patterns embedded in this theme were being physically present and available to elders, making a commitment to care "full-time," and attending to the physical and spiritual needs of elders. A 54-year-old woman who cared for her 88-year-old father stated, "I never leave Pa alone." Likewise, the elders expected to always have someone in the family close by them. When one person in the family assumed a primary caring role, this freed other family members to pursue their own dreams and ambitions. It also kept the family members' feelings of pride about the family intact. An informant said, "The children are happy I am doing this [caring for her father]; they would not like to see their grandfather in an old age home." Other studies have noted that a family's emotional well-being and ability to function is influenced by successfully providing care for elders.[96,97]

Key informants also spoke of caring as a commitment: "When you make a commitment to care, you make a promise and you must carry it out." Caregivers said that caring for an elderly parent or grandparent was something one did "full-time." The "full-time" commitment to care was demonstrated in a variety of ways. Only two of the eleven key informants worked outside their homes. Most caregivers elected to forgo education or employment, explaining that "caring is my life now." A young woman (key informant) said that when she began caring for her mother she resigned from a job. In their study of caregiver hardiness, Piccinato and Rosenbaum also found that the commitment of a caregiver was critical to their being able to carry on the caregiving role.[98]

The care pattern of attending to the physical and spiritual needs of the elder also *nurtured the health of the family.* Informants believed that caring was both a physical and a spiritual activity. One key informant explained, "You cannot separate the physical from the spiritual; caring to me is both and the same." All key informants spoke of a deep and fundamental faith in God. Living that faith by praying for each other and helping people in need, beginning with members of their own families, were consistent practices in Namibian society. In addition to feeding, bathing, and giving elders "tablets," caregivers said they also walked with the elder to church or took them via a taxi or car, prayed with them and for them, and read the Bible together. Chang et al. documented that caregivers of disabled elders who relied on religious or spiritual beliefs to cope with caregiving had a better relationship with care recipients and lower levels of depression and role submersion.[99] Key informants in this study said that their faith in God helped them to keep going from day to day. One caregiver stated, "Praying on your knees and reading the Bible is where you get your strength. The Lord doesn't get tired."

Substantive Theme Two: Care As Trusting in the Benevolence of Life

Caring for an elder also meant *trusting in the benevolence of life as lived moment by moment.* Reflected in this theme was a confidence that all of life was unfold-

ing and becoming what it was meant to be. Key and general informants believed that "things were the way they should be" and that their day-to-day security would continue because "God's providence would never fail." The cultural and social dimensions of religion, kinship, and life experiences influenced this theme. Key informants spoke of a strong faith in God "to provide for everyday needs," as well as a persistent certainty in the adage that "your kin will take care of you." An elder said, "I know they will look after me. I don't even think about it."

Four patterns of caring supported the theme of *trusting in the benevolence of life.* One pattern was accepting the caregiver role without deliberation. Key informants viewed themselves as the most capable of taking on the role of caring for an elder within their family. One caregiver said she assumed the role of caregiver because her brother and her sister could not provide a stable home for the mother. Another said, "She's my mother and I'm the youngest. All my brothers and sisters are out working and I must do this." All caregivers felt that they were doing what they were meant to do. Caring for an elder was described as a "gift from God that brings joy and meaning to my life." A key informant declared, "My power comes from caring. I care with thanksgiving, joyfulness, and high spiritedness."

Living from day to day, praying in times of difficulty, and letting go of worries were three additional care patterns that supported persons' trust in the overall benevolence of life. A key informant summarized, "I do not plan for tomorrow or the future. Why? We live life from day to day. All my worries, I pray about. What good is worry? God will provide. I believe this because it is my experience."

Substantive Theme Three: Care As Honoring One's Elders

Honoring one's elders was a significant expression of caring in urban Namibian families (Color Insert 12). Care patterns of being respectful; keeping elders from despair and loneliness; warning elders and family members about destructive lifestyle choices; and protecting elders from theft, harm, and/or wrongdoing supported this theme. Listening, doing what the elder asks, keeping them clean, never leaving them alone, and dressing them in dignified clothing were all important ways of expressing care as respect. Generally, these care practices were similar among the cultures rather than diverse. However, an Herero informant explained that in the extended Herero family the eldest man or woman is the "head of the family." Family members cannot do anything without consulting this elder. She or he gives permission for persons to marry, sell cattle, go to school, and to do just about anything. Anthropological accounts of aging in Herero society support the Herero informants' stories about older people receiving care as deference and respect.[99a] Key informants, representing Nama, Damara, Colored, and Baster cultures, did not share this formalized kinship care practice with the Herero. Nevertheless, all informants spoke of the importance of care as respecting an elder for their life and the care contributions they have made and continue to make for the health of the entire family.

Appreciating an elder's care contribution to the household, and in many cases relying on their contributions, kept elders from despair and loneliness. For example, several elders explained how they cared for children by watching them and making meals. Other elders were able to bathe themselves and do some of the lighter housekeeping. One elder talked about what being appreciated meant to her: "When you are old you feel you're only in the way . . . but they [the children] like me and they listen to me and I want to be with them." Several transcultural nursing studies report that reciprocal caring practices enhance within the family.[100–103]

Caregivers in this study also felt that poverty contributed to the destructive lifestyle choices prevalent in Namibian society and escalated the potential for harm and wrongdoing. One caregiver said, "I am worried about the poorness of the elders, and the children do not always support them. I talk to the children about how to look after the elders. I tell them not to abuse alcohol and to look after the elders so families do not suffer." Key informants said caring for an elder meant that families and caregivers in particular had to protect their elders. In the sociocultural context of limited resources in Namibia, harm was described as "being robbed of a pension check," or "having things taken from you." Other transcultural nursing studies cite care as protection from harm. Wenger noted, in her study of health care issues in urban and rural contexts, that urban families were often more concerned with care as safety and

prevention of violence than rural families.[104] Morgan, in her study of prenatal care among African American women, found that care as protection was viewed to be essential to the health and well-being of mothers and infants.[105] Morgan also documented the effects of poverty on health and well-being in her study of care patterns among African Americans.[106] Caregivers in this study were diligent about caring for elders by protecting them from violent experiences. For example, caregivers went with elders to pick up their pension checks each month, or they had made arrangements so that they could pick up the pension check themselves to avoid an elder being robbed.

Because of limited access, few elders had bank accounts in Namibia, and pension checks were usually distributed in the form of cash. This demonstrated protective care was a primary care practice undertaken by the caregiver to ensure the physical safety and well-being of an elder.

Susan's story (Figure 20.2) illustrates the protective care patterns in *honoring one's elders* and it summarizes other features of this theme.

The cultural social structure dimensions of technology and economics influence this theme. Widespread poverty and high unemployment contribute to the limited access to technology in Namibia, including limited access to checking accounts and cars. Nevertheless, the spiritual philosophy of the Judeo-Christian commandment to "honor your father and your mother that their days may be long upon the land that the Lord God gives them" is a strong influence on culture care of elders.

Substantive Theme Four: Care As Sustaining Security and Purpose for Life

Having a place to live and a reason for living was important to all informants in the study — caregivers and elders. *Care as sustaining security and purpose for life in the midst of uncertainty* was a mutual process where the elder and the caregiver both provided care to enhance each other's security and sense of purpose. Many of the homes in which the elder and primary caregiver were living were owned by the elder, and all but one elder shared her/his pension check ($N160 per month or $US30) with the caregiver and the household. Many elders expressed care as "working for the

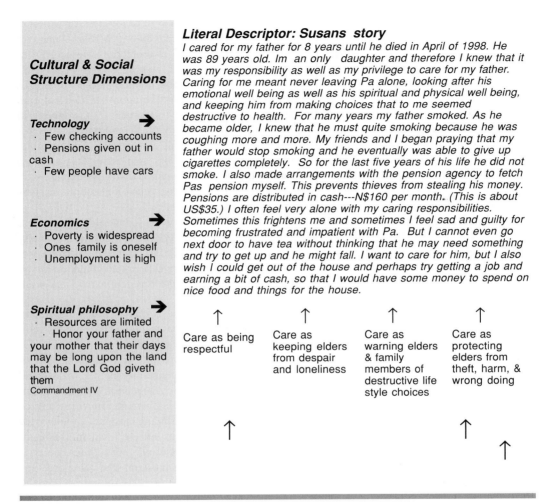

Cultural & Social Structure Dimensions

Technology →
· Few checking accounts
· Pensions given out in cash
· Few people have cars

Economics →
· Poverty is widespread
· Ones family is oneself
· Unemployment is high

Spiritual philosophy →
· Resources are limited
· Honor your father and your mother that their days may be long upon the land that the Lord God giveth them
Commandment IV

Literal Descriptor: Susans story

I cared for my father for 8 years until he died in April of 1998. He was 89 years old. Im an only daughter and therefore I knew that it was my responsibility as well as my privilege to care for my father. Caring for me meant never leaving Pa alone, looking after his emotional well being as well as his spiritual and physical well being, and keeping him from making choices that to me seemed destructive to health. For many years my father smoked. As he became older, I knew that he must quite smoking because he was coughing more and more. My friends and I began praying that my father would stop smoking and he eventually was able to give up cigarettes completely. So for the last five years of his life he did not smoke. I also made arrangements with the pension agency to fetch Pas pension myself. This prevents thieves from stealing his money. Pensions are distributed in cash---N$160 per month. (This is about US$35.) I often feel very alone with my caring responsibilities. Sometimes this frightens me and sometimes I feel sad and guilty for becoming frustrated and impatient with Pa. But I cannot even go next door to have tea without thinking that he may need something and try to get up and he might fall. I want to care for him, but I also wish I could get out of the house and perhaps try getting a job and earning a bit of cash, so that I would have some money to spend on nice food and things for the house.

Care as being respectful

Care as keeping elders from despair and loneliness

Care as warning elders & family members of destructive life style choices

Care as protecting elders from theft, harm, & wrong doing

Figure 20.2
Susan's story and the substantive theme of care as honoring elders.

children, and the children working for the elders." Also, family members often helped the primary caregiver and the elder with money and occasionally with time when they stayed with the elder to relieve the primary caregiver. An informant stated: "The pension of elders is so low in Namibia. If it were not for my son and his wife, Pa and I could not live on his pension. So they help us from time to time with money."

Caregivers did not discourage an elder from participating in household chores if she or he was able. One key informant, who thought she was probably 90 years

old, got up every morning at 7:00 AM and made mealie pop porridge for her great-grandchildren before they went off to school. She was very proud of the ways in which she expressed care by contributing to the smooth running of the household. Also, the relationship between Tane Elie and Fritz depicts the theme of *care as sustaining security and purpose for life*:

Fritz is not Tane Elie's father, but an elder for whom Elie has assumed the role of primary caregiver. Tane Elie began to care for Fritz when she found him homeless and sleeping on the street. Fritz had no family, he was depressed, lonely, and drinking heavily. One of the arrangements Elie made for Fritz was to have him watch over a neighbor's house. In return Fritz could live in this family's back yard and come over to Elie's for meals. Fritz lives (or more accurately sleeps) about three houses away from Elie. "It's not much," Elie explained, "but having his own space is an important way of respecting Fritz's independence." In caring for Fritz, Eli explained that she had to keep him from becoming too lonely because when he was lonely he would get depressed and begin to drink again. Elie warns Fritz about how destructive such a lifestyle is and for the last couple years he's been listening to her. Elie also warns families in the community about drinking and neglecting their parents or grandparents. Elie explains that her strength to care comes from God. She is an active member of her church and prays for people constantly. About caring, Tane Elie said, "Caring is my life — it's me and who I am."

Other informants spoke of fulfilling the biblical calling to care for their aging parents. This gave them peace of mind and the purpose of living out their Christian calling. Caring within this perspective resulted in blessings or spiritual rewards. The ultimate reward was the security of knowing one had a place in heaven. A caregiver said, "Caring for my father means that I will receive a reward from God. This is one of my goals in life."

Substantive Theme Five: Providing Care Within Rapidly Changing Cultural and Social Structures

As cultural change sweeps through Namibian society, Western values of individualism and personal achievement are being assimilated into Namibian lifeways. Since independence in 1990, educational opportunities, employment, and mobility have touched the lives of all Namibian people. Care patterns of balancing traditional gender roles and responsibilities with individual desires to take advantage of new opportunities and "making do" with less were evident in caregivers' experiences. Key informants who were committed to caring for an elderly relative said that it was becoming increasingly difficult to do so for economic reasons. One caregiver who found it necessary to work outside her home said, "I love my mother . . . but I feel a great deal of stress. It is difficult to cope and I do not really care for my-

self . . . I do not have time." Others who were managing with the elder's small monthly pension check and help from relatives expressed worry that the children were not learning the values of the Namibian culture, particularly the value of caring for elders. Values of making money, getting an education, and acquiring common household items that make life more comfortable were competing with cultural care obligations to remain at home and care for the elders. Elders also expressed concern that young people were not as respectful as they were in the past, and that the future of today's youth was not very secure. One elderly women said, "I worry a lot about the children's children; not so much about my own children. The older children are married, but the grandchildren are still young. How are they going to live?"

Informants all talked about making do with less and less. An informant that was responsible for a family of 10 said that "being poor is the hardest thing for me and for my family . . . we must always live in the shadow of doing without something and it seems our choices are so limited." The realities of moving into an economic system that relies on money as a currency rather than bartering of services, time, and goods has only recently been internalized for many people. Pursuing an education and making a commitment to a career are exciting and difficult choices for they often mean giving up or "doing without" something else. As such, change and shifting values are ever-present paradoxical experiences that influence care practices within Namibians families today.

 ## Three Theoretical Culture Care Modes for Culturally Congruent Care

Culture Care Preservation and Maintenance

Informants thought that the culture care patterns and substantive themes describing and explaining the meanings and expressions of care for elders should be preserved and strengthened. Clearly all informants in the study — elders and their caregivers alike — believed the well-being of the family, as well as the integrity and dignity of elder family members, were maintained when elders were cared for at home. Caring for one's elders at home fostered a sense of security and purpose for life in the midst of change and uncertainty. Widespread poverty, AIDS, sociopolitical controversy, and a rapid explosion of information and technology all heightened the uncertainty in peoples' lives. Having the security of being connected to and cared for by a family in the midst of rapid cultural change was reassuring.

Transcultural nursing actions and decisions associated with culture care maintenance and preservation should focus on working more closely with the private sector. For example, churches have already begun to organize support groups for persons caring for elders at home. The role of nursing in community-oriented care practices as these requires careful exploration. The skilled leadership and competence of transcultural nurses has the greatest potential for strengthening and sustaining community transcultural care practices.

Culture Care Accommodation and Repatterning

Culture care accommodation and repatterning refers to those professional actions and decisions undertaken with persons, families, groups, and/or communities to strengthen health and well-being.[107,108] In Namibia, the community and family are the constant sources of care for elders. Therefore, it is important for nurses to strengthen ways of supporting families and communities, particularly primary caregivers and elders. In this study key informants said they wished nurses knew where all the elders lived in a community and that a nurse would be available for them. In this way the professional care system was viewed as helpful, but not substituting for one-on-one family care giving. Rather, caregivers were asking for a blending of *professional* care and *generic* (home-based) care, a caring approach widely supported in transcultural nursing literature.[109–118] An informant said, "Just having a nurse know me and know that there is an elder in this house would make all the difference." Others reiterated, "I need to have somebody to ask if I'm giving him the right tablet or if I must get something different. Who can I talk to about this? I need a nurse who will care about what I'm doing." Most primary caregivers said, "I really don't know where to turn for help."

Although the "rewards" and satisfaction of caring for an elder were evident, caring was a taxing practice

and required a caregiver's complete devotion to the holistic needs of their elder relative. Comments like, "I do not really care for myself because I do not have time," and "I had to take care completely of him, so I had very little time to think about myself," exemplified the caregiver's experience. Caregivers also experienced guilt. They said, "I didn't care enough," and "Sometimes I become cross and impatient and I felt too terrible." Elders as well expressed guilt and discouragement for keeping their family members from doing other things. These remarks reflect what has been discovered through other research, namely, that the physical, emotional, cultural, and social health of the entire family is altered by caring for an aged family member at home.[119–124]

The findings from this study call for culture care repatterning of community health services available for elders and their families for transcultural nursing practices. First, there is a clear need for more community health nurses with transcultural competencies. Even though nurses would not be expected to take over family care practices, they would be expected to offer health guidance and to monitor and foster the health of elders and family caregivers through community-wide decisions and/or actions. Second, nurses need to become skilled in mobilizing and working with the private sector to develop new programs and models of transcultural community nursing practice. Both of these calls for action are challenging nurses to become vocal and articulate advocates for elders and their families at the policy level, to expand their collaborative leadership skills, and to seek liaisons with new community health partners. Government resources for community health services are not going to increase in the near future. In the wake of the overwhelming acute care needs of a growing HIV-positive population, nurses cannot depend on traditional kinds of support for needed community health services. Culture care repatterning calls for creativity, resourcefulness, and above all a relationship with the community. Informants in this study said that a model of care that is urgently needed is community respite care for elders. This care service would give family members release time from their full-time caring commitments of always being present for the elder. It would bring them peace of mind, as well, because they would not have to be providing protective care 24 hours a day. Elders would also get a break in their routine and have opportunities to socialize with persons beyond their immediate families. Caregivers clearly demonstrated great resourcefulness and commitment when it came to caring for elders at home. Partnering with them would be an excellent beginning to culture care repatterning in urban communities.

 ## Significance of Study and Discussion

Findings from this study are valuable for several reasons. First, data provide nurses and health care providers in Namibia with guidance for developing culturally congruent community health policies and practices for families and elders in urban communities. Second, the meanings and expressions of care and caring contribute special insights to the growing body of transcultural nursing knowledge relative to Namibia. Findings also raise public and professional awareness about the significant contributions Namibian families are making to the health and well-being of elders in their communities. Importantly, the Culture Care Theory substantiates *generic* and *emic* care practices that have been identified and can be blended with professional care, as found in this study. Third, findings provide guidance for nursing curriculum development in transcultural community health care. Medical models of diagnosing and treating health concerns on an individual basis, though helpful and important, are not sufficient to respond to the health concerns of the caregivers and elders in this study. Nurses will need to be knowledgeable and skilled in transcultural community-oriented actions, including political advocacy, collaboration, securing of resources, resource distribution, and outcome assessment as these activities pertain to the health of communities and groups.

The aging of populations in all countries brings on great challenges, as well as great changes. Nurses are the largest group of health care providers in Namibia and worldwide. Well educated in the theory and practice of primary health care,[125] Namibian nurses have demonstrated their ability to make a difference in the health and well-being of communities.[126] Nevertheless, more transcultural nurses are needed in Namibia today, especially nurses who will be persistent in developing new and relevant ways to provide culturally congruent care to meet the community health needs of families with elders. As the diverse population in Namibia ages, persons of all cultures in the country will at some point require nursing's attention. Currently, the oldest living man in Namibia is a San Bushman who is thought to be about 112 years of age. The San culture is not represented in this study. Additionally, the Afrikaner culture, the Ovambo culture, and the German culture, among others, were not represented. What are the meanings and expressions of care for elders defined and lived by these cultural groups? Clearly, additional transcultural nursing research knowledge is needed that is relevant to the culture care needs of elders from all cultures.

Cultural change will continue to sweep through Namibian society as demographic trends shift toward increasing longevity. The 21st century is one of great potential and great apprehension. Never before have young people in Namibia had so many choices and opportunities; and never before have their choices been so limited by the life-threatening HIV infection. Who will care for the elders in the next century? Where will "childless" elders live? Namibians must make conscientious decisions about where to allocate scarce resources and how best to mobilize those resources to provide for the health and well-being of all citizens in this new republic. Transculturally prepared and competent nurses will be crucial in the decision-making process. Guided by Culture Care Theory, nursing education, practice, and research findings offer sound culturally congruent knowledge for better and meaningful care to elders and their families in the 21st century.

References

1. United Nations, *The World's Aging Situation*, New York: United Nations Publication, 1991a.
2. Duffy, J., "Expanding Elderly Populations Perceived as a Health Care Challenge," *Saint Paul Pioneer Press*, November 25, 1998, p. 9A.
3. Santcross, N. and S. Ballard, *Namibia Handbook*, Chicago, IL: Passport Books, 1997.
4. National AIDS Programme, *Background Information on HIV/AIDS in Namibia*, Windhoek: National AIDS Programme Publication, 1998.
5. Ministry of Health and Social Services, *Demographic and Health Survey*, Windhoek, Namibia: Ministry of Health and Social Services (MOHSS) Publication, 1992.

6. Leininger, M., *Qualitative Research Methods in Nursing*, Orlando, FL: Grune & Stratton, 1985.

7. Leininger, M., "Leininger's Theory of Nursing: Culture Care Diversity and Universality," *Nursing Science Quarterly* 1988a, 2(4), pp. 11–20.

8. Leininger, M., *Care: The Essence of Nursing and Health*, Detroit: Wayne State University Press, 1988b.

9. Leininger, M., *Culture Care Diversity and Universality: A Theory of Nursing*, New York: National League for Nursing Press, 1991.

10. Leininger, M., *Transcultural Nursing: Concepts, Theories, Research and Practice*, New York: McGraw-Hill, Inc., 1995.

11. Leininger, M., "Overview of the Theory of Culture Care with the Ethnonursing Research Method," *Journal of Transcultural Nursing*, 1997a, 8 (2), pp. 32–52.

12. Leininger, M., "Transcultural Nursing Research to Transform Nursing Education and Practice: 40 years," *Image: Journal of Nursing Scholarship*, 1997b, 29(4), pp. 341–347.

13. Leininger, op. cit., 1988b.

14. Leininger, op. cit., 1991.

15. Ibid.

16. Leininger, op. cit., 1997a.

17. Leininger, op. cit., 1991.

18. Leininger, op. cit., 1995.

19. Leininger, op. cit., 1997b.

20. Leininger, op. cit., 1988a.

21. Leininger, op. cit., 1981.

22. Leininger, op. cit., 1995.

23. Leininger, op. cit., 1997a.

24. Leininger, op. cit., 1997b.

25. Leininger, op. cit., 1991.

26. Leininger, op. cit., 1997a.

27. Leininger, op. cit., 1991.

28. Leininger, op. cit., 1995.

29. Leininger, op. cit., 1988b.

30. Leininger, op. cit., 1991.

31. Leininger, op. cit., 1995.

32. Leininger, op. cit., 1997a.

33. Leininger, op. cit., 1997b.

34. Almburg, B., M. Grafstron, and B. Winblad, "Caring for a Demented Elderly Person: Burden and Burnout Among Caregiving Relatives," *Journal of Advanced Nursing*, 1997. 25(1), pp. 109–116.

35. Bull, M., "Factors Influencing Family Caregiver Burden and Health," *Western Journal of Nursing Research*, 1990, 12(6), pp. 758–776.

36. Faison, K., S. Faria, and D. Frank, "Caregivers of Chronically Ill Elderly: Perceived Burden," *Journal of Community Health Nursing*, 1999, 16(4), pp. 243–253.

37. Jones, P.S., "Paying Respect: Care of Elderly Parents by Chinese and Filipino American Women," *Health Care for Women International*, 1995, 16(5), pp. 385–398.

38. Loma, L., "Asian American Women Caring for Elderly Parents," *Journal of Family Nursing*, 1996, 2(1), pp. 56–75.

39. O'Neill, G. and M. Ross, "Burden of Care: An Important Concept for Nurses," *Health Care for Women International*, 1991. 12(1), pp. 111–121.

40. Mark, S., "Family Caregiving of the Elderly," *Prairie Rose*, 1997, 66(1), p. 8.

41. Robinson, K., "Family Caregiving: Who Provides the Care, and at What Cost?" *Nursing Economics*, 1997, 15(5), pp. 243–247.

42. Given, B. and C. Given, "Health Promotion for Family Caregivers of Chronically Ill Elders," *Annual Review of Nursing Research*, 1998, 16, pp. 197–217.

43. Holicky, R., "Caring for the Caregivers: The Hidden Victims of Illness and Disability," *Rehabilitation Nursing*, 1996, 21(5), pp. 247–252.

44. Ostwald, S., "Caregiver Exhaustion: Caring for the Hidden Patients," *Advanced Practice Nursing*, 1997, 3(2), pp. 29–35.

45. Schwartz, K., and B. Roberts, "Social Support and Strain of Family Caregivers of Older Adults," *Holistic Nursing Practice*, 2000, 14(2), pp. 77–90.

46. Schumacher, K.B. Steward, and G. Archbold, "Conceptualization and Measurement of Doing Family Caregiving Well," *Image: Journal of Nursing Scholarship*, 1998, 30(1), pp. 63–69.

47. Davidhizar, R. and M. Bowen, "Facing Our Worst Fear . . . Abandonment," *Caring*, 1995, 14(7), pp. 50–54.

48. O'Neill, C. and E. Sorensen, "Home Care of the Elderly: A Family Perspective," *Advances in Nursing Science*, 1991, 13(4), pp. 28–37.

49. Ibid.

50. Burnside, I., S. Preski, and J. Hertz, "Research Instrumentation and Elderly Subjects," *Image: Journal of Nursing Scholarship*, 1998, 30(2), pp. 185–190.

51. McFarland, M., "Use of the Culture Care Theory with Anglo- and African American Elders in a Long-Term Care Setting," *Nursing Science Quarterly*, 1997, 10(4), pp. 186–192.

52. Bowsher, J. and M. Gerlach, "Personal Control and Other Determinants of Psychological Well-Being in Nursing Home Elders," *Scholarly Inquiry for Nursing Practice: An International Journal*, 1990, 4(2), pp. 91–102.

53. Bernardi, B., *Age Class Systems: Social Institutions and Polities Based on Age.* Cambridge, U.K.: Cambridge University Press, 1985.

54. Keith, J, "Age in Social and Cultural Context," in *Handbook of Aging and the Social Sciences*, R. Binstock and L. George, eds., New York: Academic Press, 1990, pp. 99–112.

55. Langness, L. and G. Frank, *Lives: An Anthropological Approach to Biography*, Novato, CA: Chandler & Sharp, 1981.

56. Keith, J., C.L. Fry, and A.P. Glascock, et al., *The Aging Experience: Diversity and Commonality Across Cultures.* Thousand Oaks, CA: Sage Publications, Inc., 1994.

57. Holmes, E. and L. Holmes, *Other Cultures' Elder Years.* Thousand Oaks, CA: Sage Publications, Inc., 1995.

58. Ntshona, M., "Determination of Needs of Black Aged Persons in Port Elizabeth: Direction for Future Intervention," *Curationis*, 1995, 18(4), pp. 20–26.

59. Mavundla, T., "Factors Leading to Black Elderly Persons' Decisions to Seek Institutional Care in a Home in the Eastern Cape," *Curationis*, 1996, 19(3), pp. 47–51.

60. National AIDS Programme, op. cit., 1998.

61. Cillers, S.P., *Developments and Research on Aging in South Africa: An International Handbook.* Westport, CT: Greenwood Press, 1991.

62. Ntshona, op. cit., 1995.

63. Nursing News, "Primary Health Care: Gerontology. Aging Well!" *Nursing News South Africa*, 1996, 20(5), p. 54.

64. Tibbit, L., "Are the Elderly Coping with Rising Health Care Costs?" *Nursing RSA Verpleging*, 1992, 7(11/12), pp. 25–26.

65. Fraser, C., "Pets Meet the Needs of the Lonely Elderly," *Nursing RSA Verpleging,* 1992, 7(6), pp. 16–18, 40.

66. Mavundla, op. cit., 1996.

67. Given and Given, op. cit., 1998.

68. Leininger, op. cit., 1997b.

69. Miller, B., "Family Caregiving: Telling It Like It Is," *The Gerontologist*, 1998, 38(4), pp. 510–514.

70. Leininger, op. cit., 1995.

71. Leininger, op. cit., 1997a.

72. Leininger, op. cit., 1997b.

73. Watson, J., *The Philosophy and Science of Caring.* Denver: University Press of Colorado, 1985.

74. Watson, J., *Postmodern Nursing and Beyond.* New York: Churchill Livingstone, Inc., 1999.

75. Lincoln, Y. and E. Guba, *Naturalistic Inquiry.* London: Sage Publications, Inc., 1985.

76. Leininger, M. "Ethnomethods: The Philosophic and Epistemic Bases to Explicate Transcultural Nursing Knowledge," *Journal of Transcultural Nursing*, 1990, 1(2), pp. 40–51.

77. Leininger, op. cit., 1991.

78. Leininger, op. cit., 1997a.

79. Leininger, op. cit., 1991.

80. Ibid.

81. American Nurses' Association, *Human Rights Guidelines for Nurses in Clinical and Other Research.* Washington, DC: American Nurses' Association, 1985.

82. Munhall, P., "Ethical Considerations in Qualitative Research," *Western Journal of Nursing Research*, 1988, 10(2), pp. 150–162.

83. Leininger, op. cit., 1991.

84. Leininger, op. cit., 1990.

85. Leininger, op. cit., 1991.

86. Leininger, op. cit., 1997a.

87. Given and Given, op. cit., 1998.

88. Jones, op. cit., 1995.

89. Miller, B. and L. Cafasso, "Gender Differences in Caregiving: Fact or Artifact," *The Gerontologist*, 1992, 32(4), pp. 498–507.

90. MacNeil, J., "Use of Culture Care Theory with Baganda Women as AIDS Caregivers," *Journal of Transcultural Nursing*, 1996, 7(2), pp. 14–20.

91. O'Neill and Sorensen, op. cit., 1991.

92. Phillips, L., "Elder-Family Caregiver Relationships: Determining Appropriate Nursing Interventions," *Nursing Clinics of North America,* 1989, 24(3), pp. 795–805.

93. Robinson, op. cit., 1997.

94. Sterritt, P. and M. Pokory, "African-American Caregiving for a Relative with Alzheimer's Disease," *Geriatric Nursing*, 1998, 19(3), pp. 127–128, 133–134.

95. United Nations, *The World's Women 1970-1990: Trends and Statistics.* New York: United Nations Publication, 1991b.

96. Carruth, A., U. Tate, B., Moffett, and K. Hill, "Reciprocity, Emotional Well-Being and Family Functioning as Determinants of Family

Satisfaction in Caregivers of Elderly Parents," *Nursing Research*, 1997, 46(2), pp. 193–100.

97. O'Neill and Sorensen, op. cit., 1991.

98. Piccinato, J. and J. Rosenbaum, "Caregiver Hardiness Explored Within Watson's Theory of Human Caring in Nursing," *Journal of Gerontological Nursing*, 1997, 23(10), pp. 32–39.

99. Chang, B., A. Noonan, and S. Tennstedt, "The Role of Religion/Spirituality in Coping with Caregiving for Disabled Elders," *Gerontologist*, 1998, 38(4): pp. 463–470.

99a. Keith et al., op. cit., 1994.

100. Luna, L., "Care and Cultural Context of Lebanese Muslim Immigrants: Using Leininger's Theory," *Journal of Transcultural Nursing*, 1994, 5(2), pp. 12–20.

101. McFarland, M., "Culture Care Theory and Elderly Polish Americans," in *Transcultural Nursing: Concepts, Theories, Research, and Practices*, M. Leininger, ed., New York: McGraw-Hill, Inc., 1995, pp. 401–426.

102. Omeri, A., "Culture Care of Iranian Immigrants in New South Wales, Australia: Sharing Transcultural Nursing Knowledge," *Journal of Transcultural Nursing*, 1997, 8(2), pp. 5–16.

103. Rosenbaum, J., "Cultural Care of Older Greek Canadian Widows Within Leininger's Theory of Culture Care," *Journal of Transcultural Nursing*, 1990, 2(1), pp. 37–47.

104. Wenger, F., "Transcultural Nursing and Health Care: Issues in Urban and Rural Contexts," *Journal of Transcultural Nursing*, 1992, 4(2), pp. 4–9.

105. Morgan, M., "Prenatal Care of African American Women in Selected USA Urban and Rural Cultural Contexts," *Journal of Transcultural Nursing*, 1997, 7(2), pp. 3–13.

106. Morgan, M., "African Americans and Cultural Care," in *Transcultural Nursing: Concepts, Theories, Research, and Practices,* M. Leininger, ed., New York, NY: McGraw-Hill, Inc., 1995, pp. 383–400.

107. Leininger, op. cit., 1991.

108. Leininger, op. cit., 1995.

109. Leininger, op. cit., 1988b.

110. Leininger, op. cit., 1995.

111. Leininger, op. cit., 1997a.

112. Leininger, op. cit., 1997b.

113. Leininger, M., "Special Research Report: Dominant Culture Care (Emic) Meanings and Practice Findings from Leininger's Theory," *Journal of Transcultural Nursing*, 1998, 9(2), pp. 45–48.

114. McFarland, op. cit., 1997.

115. McKenna, M., "Twice in Need of Care: A Transcultural Nursing Analysis of Elderly Mexican Americans," *Journal of Transcultural Nursing*, 1989, 1(1), pp. 46–52.

116. Morgan, op. cit., 1997.

117. Omeri, op. cit., 1997.

118. Rosenbaum, op. cit., 1990.

119. Bull, op. cit., 1990.

120. Given and Given, op. cit., 1998.

121. Gonzalez, E., "Resourcefulness, Appraisals, and Coping Efforts of Family Caregivers," *Issues in Mental Health Nursing*, 1997, 18(3), pp. 209–227.

122. Holicky, op. cit., 1996.

123. Ostwald, op. cit., 1997.

124. Schwartz and Roberts, op. cit., 2000.

125. World Health Organization, "Report of the International Conference on Primary Health Care," *Health for All*, 1978, Series No. 1, pp. 2–6.

126. Ministry of Health and Social Services, op. cit., 1992.

21
Culture Care of the Mexican American Family

Anita Berry

In the United States the Mexican Americans are a cultural group that is rapidly increasing in numbers.[1] This is particularly evident in the southwestern United States, which is close to the Mexican border. Although some group Mexican Americans with other Hispanics, it is important for nurses to recognize that Puerto Ricans, Cubans, Central Americans, and other Hispanic groups share some cultural similarities, but each have their own distinct culture. Based on the author's research of childbearing families,[2] many years of clinical practice, and a review of the transcultural nursing literature, this chapter will examine the culture care of the Mexican American family in the southwestern United States.

Through the study of transcultural nursing, nurses are becoming increasingly aware of how cultural values, beliefs, and practices can affect health care. Leininger's Theory of Culture Care Diversity and Universality[3] provides a theoretical nursing framework to study the holistic lifeways of a culture to discover and understand how individuals and groups view health care within their cultural contexts. Leininger holds that care is universal, but that the patterns and modes of care vary among cultures with their diverse generic and professional care practices. Care is viewed by Leininger[4] as an essential element throughout people's lives from birth to death; it is the central and dominant focus of nursing. Nurses assist clients from diverse cultural backgrounds in their care practices. Moreover, professional nurses come from many different cultures with their own values, beliefs, and lifeways. Thus, cultural differences often exist between the health care provider and care recipient, which can lead to conflicts, stresses, and cultural imposition phenomena.

With the theory of Culture Care, Leininger holds that cultural factors are important in client care and in providing congruent nursing care to clients. It is culturally based care that is predicted to enhance clients' well-being and health or to face disabilities or death.[5] In developing an in-depth understanding of a culture it is necessary to understand the multiple dimensions of culture in the client's life. The author used Leininger's ethnonursing research method to gain in-depth knowledge of the Mexican American culture.[6] This is an inductive method designed to discover emic (people's) and etic (professional) knowledge about the domain of inquiry. This method was designed to fit with the Culture Care Theory. The Sunrise Model was used to explicate the components of the Culture Care Theory as a means to obtain both breadth and depth of knowledge. The Sunrise Model and the theory focus on the dimensions of worldview, ethnohistory, and language, as well as cultural and social structure factors such as religion, kinship, and cultural values and lifeways. These dimensions, the major tenet of predicting cultural diversities and universalities, and the three modes of nursing care actions and decisions have provided the framework for this chapter, which presents the culture care of the Mexican American family in the southwestern United States.

Ethnohistorical Context of Mexican Americans

It is important to review the historical context of any culture as it aids in an understanding of the culture and its worldview and social structure dimensions that influence health care. Mexico began as part of Mesoamerica, which consisted of what is now central Mexico, Guatemala, El Salvador, and Honduras. Today, Mexico is bordered by Guatemala and Belize to the south and the United States to the north. It is ranked as the third largest in size and second largest in population of all the Latin American countries. The 1990 census estimated that 85 million people live on its 761,000 square miles.[7]

Many sophisticated cultures developed in Mesoamerica, such as the Olmecs, Toltecs, Mayans, and Aztecs.[8,9] The Aztecs dominated central Mexico until their conquest by Spain in 1521. The Spaniards then dominated for 300 years during which time the indigenous people blended many aspects of their lives with the Spaniards. Syncretism of cultural values and beliefs occurred in areas such as religion, language politics, art, family ties, and medicine.[10–13] Syncretism is a process by which people of different cultures blend or adapt various beliefs and practices to form a relationship that has meaning for them.

Spaniards settled in a portion of what is now New Mexico. The Mexican Revolution occurred in 1910, and this led to Mexican independence from Spain in 1921. Mexico invited settlers from the United States into its sparsely populated areas of the northern Mexican territory, particularly in what is now known as Texas.[14] Conflict eventually arose between the Mexican government and the United States settlers in the Texas area. This led to the settlers claiming the areas as the Republic of Texas between 1836–1838.[15] War between the Republic of Texas and Mexico began in 1846, and Mexico ceded to the United States much of what is now considered the southwestern United States in the Treaty of Guadeloupe Hidalgo in 1848.[16] There were approximately 75,000 Spanish speaking inhabitants in that territory, most of whom were of Spanish-Indian heritage. The majority chose to remain as Mexican American residents and were guaranteed certain rights under the treaty. However, through legalistic manipulations many of the Mexican Americans lost their land and rights and became laborers for the *norteamericanos*.[17]

Because of the poor economy in Mexico, immigration across the border to the United States has continued to the present time. In the 20th century immigrants came in three major waves. The first wave arrived by the 1920s following the political upheaval of the Mexican revolution (1910–1929). Free rail transportation was provided by the Mexican government to the border, and an estimated one person in five left Mexico.[18] The majority of the immigrants settled in

Texas as agricultural workers. The second wave in the late 1920s brought craftsmen, as well as laborers. The new immigrants met the need in the United States for additional workers willing to work at low wages. When the depression of the 1930s occurred, Mexicans who were either legal or illegal residents were deported to Mexico.[19] This government deportation action typified the erratic pattern of immigration laws during the 20th century with the United States encouraging entry in times of labor shortages and setting up restrictive policies in times of economic recession.[20,21] The third wave of immigrants occurred in the 1940s when there was a shortage of laborers because of World War II. At this time the *bracero* program was begun in which temporary workers were recruited (without their families) to work in the United States for low pay for 6 months without the legal protection that United States citizens received. The bracero program was terminated in 1964 as a result of growing opposition by organized farm workers who were citizens of the United States since where braceros worked, the prevailing wage dropped.[22] In addition, substandard living and working conditions existed for many of the farm workers.

Once in the United States, the majority of immigrants settled in the southwestern United States or traveled through the Midwest to work in agriculture such as in the sugar beet fields of Michigan.[23] In 1985 the U.S. immigration law was revised to allow for reunification of families.[24] Through the amnesty program of 1986, two million undocumented workers and families received permanent legal status in the United States.[25] The flow of undocumented aliens has not diminished across the common border of the United States and Mexico because of the continued depressed economy in Mexico and the opportunity to earn money in the United States to support their large families.[26] Thirty-nine percent of all undocumented aliens in the United States in 1992 were from Mexico, 43% of whom resided in California.[27]

Worldview and Religion of Mexican Americans

Cultures have a way of viewing the world around them that influences how they respond to life experiences, including generic and professional health care.[28] The Mexican American worldview is tightly woven with the concept of a divine will that has ultimate control over their lives. While intercessions with God may be attempted, there remains a worldview that one must accept what God gives. A classic statement was written by Madsen,[29] "What the Anglo tries to control, the Mexican-American tries to accept."

Religion is an important part of the Mexican American social structure and is embedded in their daily lives. To understand the role of religion one must go back to the Spanish invasion of Mesoamerica. The Aztecs had an elaborate religious system in place before the arrival of the Roman Catholic Spaniards. The Aztecs had a pantheon of deities, and multiple ceremonies were held related to the various deities throughout the year.[30] The Spaniards were determined to impose their religion on the Aztec society.[31] Many of the Aztec temples were destroyed and replaced with Christian structures. The conversion process was greatly facilitated by a vision of a brown-skinned Virgin Mary seen by a native boy who had been converted to Catholicism.[32] This vision of the Virgin of Guadalupe occurred at the site of the shrine to the Aztec goddess Tonantzin who was the mother of all gods.[33] Our Lady of Guadalupe continues to be revered today by Mexican Americans. The Roman Catholic church has many saints and rituals, which may be viewed to be similar to the Aztec worshipping their traditional multiple gods. The Aztecs had a history of respecting and adopting gods from conquered tribes and even maintained a temple for the adopted gods.[34] The Indians were able to syncretize beliefs and practices from the Catholic and Aztec faiths into religious practices that were meaningful for them.

Faith is a major sustainer against the trials of daily life for Mexican Americans. The majority of Mexican Americans are Roman Catholics.[35] Their worldview is evident in statements such as, "I have faith," "God will take care of me," and "It's best to put it in God's hands."[36] Many mothers are concerned for the safety of their children outside of the home. Frequently, they will walk them to school and then rely on God to take care of them during the day. Not all Mexican Americans attend church regularly, but religiosity is evident in their homes in pictures of Jesus or the Virgin Mary, statues, and calendars with a religious theme. Throughout a Mexican American community the markets and other shops carry religious candles with pictures of various saints, Jesus, or the Virgin Mary, which are used for special prayers. When there is an illness in the family, they may go to the church for a special mass. Depending on God leads Mexican Americans toward being more present rather than future oriented, which has important implications for health care.[37] Preventative professional health care is not available in much of Mexico, and many Mexican Americans believe that whatever happens to them is God's will. In the United States, professional nurses can do a culture care assessment to ascertain the Mexican American's beliefs to form a culturally congruent nursing care plan that incorporates preventive health care practices.

■ Mexican American Kinship

One of the most important social structures in the lives of Mexican Americans is family and kinship ties.[38,39] In contrast to the worldview of many North Americans who value individualism and success, Mexican Americans are collectively oriented.[40] To most Mexican Americans the value and sense of obligation to their families surpass their individual needs. Familialism does not diminish with succeeding generations and is just as strong in the third generation as the first.[41]

Mexican American extended families prefer to live near their kin but not necessarily in the same household, which was a prevalent care practice in the past. There is a desire for the family members to reciprocate care through frequent visits or telephone contact because the lack of daily contact makes them feel "all alone."[42] The concept of family extends beyond immediate relatives to include fictive kin or *compadres*.[43] Compadres are friends or consanguinal relatives who are chosen for special occasions such as baptism, confirmation, or first communion.[44] A strong mutual care bond develops and fictive kin are accorded a lifetime family status with reciprocal care practices. Fictive kin are often described in phrases such as, "She's like my mother." In addition to care as emotional support, families and compadres also provide care through succorance to one another with exchange of transportation, baby-sitting, food, material goods, and financial support. When family members immigrate from Mexico to the United States, they frequently receive care from relatives such as financial assistance, housing, and emotional support, even though these relatives have limited resources. These practices are not viewed as an imposition but a family obligation for care.

Mexican American family members have traditionally held certain roles. The elderly are esteemed and respected, and children are expected to obey parents and elders.[45] The elderly are valued for their generic or folk care knowledge and experience, which often takes precedent over professional health care advice. The nurse should be aware what generic care is being given and have respect for the role that family members have in the provision of that care. When there is an illness, members of the family will usually go to the elder mother first as, "She knows what to do." There is a family obligation to care for the parents as they get older. As one young woman said, "She took care of me when I was little, now it's my turn to take care of her."[46] This was deemed a care privilege rather than a care burden.

Mexican American families are often viewed as patriarchal with male dominance (*machismo*) and female passivity.[47] The woman is responsible for care within the household, and the husband provides care as the protector and financial provider. While many woman would like to work outside their homes, the husbands often object. As one husband said, "Who would fix my food? Who can take better care of the children than you?"[48] In Mexican American families the typical role of the female has been reproduction and care of the family. Finkler[49–51] stated that in Mexico the role of women is to suffer. Villarruel's[52] research revealed a cultural obligation to accept pain. The professional nurse should consider this when making care decisions and actions related to pain for Mexican American clients. The expectation of suffering is particularly evident in childbearing and child care. One elderly woman said that in Mexico, "I had 15 children, but three died. I had a baby every year until I stopped. My husband was mad at me for not having more."[53] The average number of children per family in Mexico declined from 6.3 in 1973 to 3.8 in 1990.[54] For economic reasons some Mexican American families in the United States wish to limit the number of children to provide better care for them. However, the final decision regarding use of birth control rests with the husband. It is important for the nurse to keep in mind the role of the husband and religious beliefs when caring for Mexican American women. Some husbands practice care for their wives by agreeing to the use of contraceptives, but are reluctant to agree to the more permanent form of tubal ligation in case the family desires more children. Male vasectomies are not culturally acceptable as they, "Make you less a man." The husband of a mother pregnant with her fourth child reported that there was conflict with his mother who had had 16 children in Mexico. The mother disapproved of the couple's desire not to have more children. He told her, "When I was little, we didn't have shoes and only one meal a day. Do you want me to bring up my children that way?"[55] The father felt that he could be a better care provider for his family by limiting the number of children.

Respect and family honor are important care concepts in the Mexican American culture. Stasiak[56] found that giving respect, protecting family honor, and being with one's family were forms of caring in Mexican American families. In traditional Mexican American families pregnancy outside of marriage is considered noncaring, shameful, and shows a lack of respect because it violates family honor. The woman may be ostracized and, while this usually does not mean physical abandonment, it may mean deprivation of the emotional care support from her family during the pregnancy. As one unwed woman stated, "Mother turned her back on me. She's embarrassed." The father is the ultimate authority in the traditional Mexican family, and sons have responsibility for protective care of their sisters. A second-generation Mexican American woman stated that in Mexico, "If the oldest brother thinks you have done something to shame the parents or is disrespectful he will make you leave. It happens all the time."[57]

Mexican Americans accord professional nurses respect for their health care knowledge. They value the health care instruction that nurses can provide and have made comments such as, "I wish they would have explained more."[58] Mexican Americans view personalization (*personalismo*) of interactions as a form of care as cultural respect.[59] A small social exchange before beginning professional nursing care, inquiring about the family, addressing the person by last name, and showing personal interest increases satisfaction with health care as evidenced by comments such as, "They seemed concerned," and "They ask how I feel, if I have any questions."[60]

Cultural Beliefs of Mexican Americans Related to Health and Illness

The Mexican concept of disease and healing practices are a syncretism (blending) of Aztec and Spanish beliefs.[61] In the Mexican American culture there is a folk belief system regarding cause and cure of illnesses that has been transmitted across generations.[62] These concepts are intricately interwoven with religious beliefs that stress the omnipotence of God, the inevitability of suffering in life, and lack of personal control. Disease is thought to result from either supernatural or natural causes. The mind and body are thought to be one, and achieving balance in all aspects of life is considered important. This is evident in the hot-cold theory, which is based on balance within the body and with the outside elements. Air, water, foods, herbs, and medicines are believed to have hot-cold properties, but there is no uniform consensus within the Hispanic cultures as to which substances are hot and which are cold.[63] An interesting example of the hot-cold concept has been evident during the Mexican American childbearing period when during pregnancy it is believed that a woman has difficulty maintaining heat because of the developing fetus and then again in postpartum when she and the infant are very susceptible to cold entering the body.[64] Generic (folk) care practices attempt to keep the body in balance through certain care prescriptions handed down through the elder women of the family. One belief is that a person should not walk around without some foot covering or subject the feet to cold as this can result in foot pain later in life. As one woman related, "I went near some refrigerators in the store after my last child and now I still have [foot] pain."

During the period of *la cuerentena* (first 40 days after birth), Mexican American women are thought to be particularly susceptible to harm from cold, and so some women avoid taking showers, washing their hair, air drafts, and consuming iced drinks. These beliefs can readily be accommodated in professional nursing care practices after childbirth. Mexican American women gave specific belief examples of physical harm from cold that they had suffered themselves or that they heard of from acquaintances who had been afflicted. Examples include cold air on the back reducing breast-milk production, drinking cold water could "make your teeth fall out," and getting cold could "cause your monthly blood to come all the time."[65] Generic care practices that were considered to be important, especially through la cuerentena, were to keep the infant warm, as well as the mother, by the use of care practices such as providing multiple layers of clothing, head coverings, and blankets regardless of the ambient temperature. During summer months in some climates it may be necessary to educate the mother on thermoregulation of the newborn to repattern this care practice. Many mothers are concerned about air entering the infant's body through the umbilical cord and will use *fajitas* as a preventive care practice. Fajitas are cloth bands applied around the abdomen to cover the umbilicus until the cord dries and falls off. One mother stated that it was not necessary to use the fajita when the infant was lying on his back because, "He won't get air in then, but when he's lifted up it can go in," which was believed to make the infant ill. The major nursing care concern is preventing umbilical cord infection while maintaining this generic culture care practice.

There are Mexican American culture care practices concerning food in pregnancy. In a prenatal context the mothers expressed that, "You can't watch your weight. You have to eat everything for your baby. When you're pregnant, you're suppose to eat even if you're not hungry."[66] As one young Mexican American woman stated, "We Mexicans eat a lot!" The families demonstrated care by preparing food and satisfying any cravings of the mother for the health of the fetus. This may be a health care concern as the traditional diet consists of beans, which are sometimes fried in lard and tortillas made with lard. Also, carbonated beverages have replaced some of the healthier drinks such as fruit juices.

A folk disease of concern of new mothers is *caida de mollera*, or "fallen fontanel," which is thought to occur by pulling the nipple out of an infant's mouth too rapidly or by a fall.[67] This folk belief was traced back to the Aztec belief in the loss of *tonalli* through the fontanel.[68] Tonalli is one of the three souls and is thought to be located in the same area of the fontanel. The symptoms in the infant are depressed fontanels, restlessness, and poor appetite, which correlate to the health care professional's diagnosis of dehydration. The folk cure is to restore the fontanel through gravity or pressure on the palate. This folk belief and related practices are of significant concern to health care providers as the family may delay taking the infant in for professional care while they first attempt traditional care/cure practices that could be life threatening for a young child with dehydration.

Diseases may result from magical thinking, which may or may not have evil intent.[69] *Mal de ojo* (evil eye) is believed to cause illness in children. Some individuals are thought to be born with a strong vision, which can be unintentionally projected when admiring a child. These individuals may not know they have this strong vision, but the effect of it can be prevented by the protective care practice of individuals touching the child, especially when admiring him or her. In contrast, witchcraft always has evil intent. *Brujas* practice noncare by placing hexes on people through the use of image magic with dolls, photographs, or incantations.[70] Hexes may be removed through prayers and religious sacrifices. Some Mexican Americans believed that during pregnancy women should avoid viewing an eclipse as it may cause structural deformities in the fetus, particularly cleft lip. To avoid this, women will wear safety pins or metal keys under their outer clothing to deflect the eclipse. Ortiz de Montellano[71] traced this back to the Aztecs who wore obsidian knives for a similar purpose.

Use of herbal preparations is a common generic/folk care practice among Mexican Americans.[72,73] In Mexico herbalists are available to prescribe the traditionally appropriate medicinal remedies. In the United States it is usually an elderly woman who is considered the expert. In Mexican American communities there are *botanicas* (folk medicine pharmacies) where various combinations of herbs, candles, religious symbols, and other objects are available for purchase to treat disease and to maintain or regain health. Herbal preparations may be administered through bathing in a mixture of herbs, rubbing the herbs on the body, or drinking teas. One of the more common tea herbs is *manzanilla* (chamomile), which is thought to be helpful in gastrointestinal problems for adults, as well as colic in infants. During labor herbal teas may be taken by expectant mothers for warmth and as uterine irritants to facilitate contractions.[74] Knowledge of perceived causes of folk illnesses and generic/folk care therapies can assist the nurse in decisions and actions for culturally congruent care by combining generic and professional care practices.

Economic, Political, and Legal Factors

Economic, political, and legal aspects have a major impact on all the interrelated social structure factors but in particular on family dimensions and those factors facilitating adequate health care in the Mexican American culture. Diminished financial resources frequently impact the ability to access professional health care. Despite Hispanic men having a higher rate of participation in the workforce than other cultural groups, Hispanic families have the highest rate of poverty among all cultural groups.[75] First-generation Mexican Americans are primarily employed in construction, manufacturing, and the service areas, which do not always provide adequate health care benefits, although upward employment mobility is found in subsequent generations. Undocumented workers fare even worse, having low pay and few benefits as job opportunities are limited. Despite their poverty level, Mexican Americans have a low rate of participation in welfare programs.[76] This may be because of their strong work ethic and the major care construct of succorance in the family, which may serve as a buffer when finances are diminished.

There has been increased political pressure in the United States to reduce the cost of professional health care to indigent noncitizens. Leininger[77] identified that generic and professional health care could be influenced by government and political pressures. Because of the high cost of professional health care for the uninsured, political decisions have been made as to the availability of health care and who will receive it.[78] An example was the passage of Proposition 187 in California in 1994, which barred undocumented immigrants from receiving any social services, including health care. Lack of professional health care for undocumented Mexican Americans is a source of concern as they value these services. As stated by one man, "It's better here because in Mexico they just let you go. They don't do nothing. It's God's will. Here . . . they don't let anyone die. When you die, it's because it's your time."[79] The bureaucratic process of obtaining health care can be frustrating for Mexican Americans, especially for first-generation immigrants. Because of their poverty status many are eligible for government assisted health care, which requires completing multiple complex forms. "Here there is so much paperwork" stated one woman.[80] Also, many new immigrants have difficulty with transportation to the various health clinics because of their impoverishment. Reliance on bus transportation can be difficult, particularly when children need to accompany the parent.

Obtaining legal status as a Mexican immigrant is desired, not only for access to professional care services but also to be able to cross the border back into Mexico to visit relatives with whom they have strong family ties. Some families had to leave children with relatives in Mexico when they immigrated. Generic care was given by the relatives by providing for the children until their parents could return. Parents desired to bring their children back from Mexico, but as one undocumented father stated, "It's too hard, and what if we can't get back?"[81] Obtaining legal status can be a challenge as many new immigrants do not understand the legal process and are vulnerable to unscrupulous individuals who purport to be able to assist them in becoming a documented immigrant. This was evidenced by an undocumented individual who stated, "There was a lady who said she could do the papers. We paid her $500. By the time we went to look for her she was gone."[82]

Language, Education, and Technology

The social structure factor of education is influenced in the Mexican American culture by language,[83] which in turn influences both professional and generic health care. Many of the immigrants come to the United States with a limited elementary school education, which is reflective of the normative level in Mexico, not a lack of interest in education.[84] The overall educational levels of Mexican Americans trail behind those of other Hispanics, African Americans, and European Americans.[85] With each subsequent generation the educational level of Hispanic people has risen.[86] While first-generation Mexican Americans are often monolingual in Spanish, the second generation usually has developed some English language skills through attending school, although Spanish may be

spoken at home. As a means to preserve their culture, one young mother stated, "In the house they must speak Spanish. Outside it is okay to speak English with their friends."[87] Lack of ability to speak English can complicate accessing professional health care as not all providers have staff that are bilingual. While some providers may feel that it is the client's obligation to learn English once they are in the United States, it can lead to misunderstandings. Informants have reported that they have encountered bilingual health care providers who, on finding out that the informant spoke some English, would refuse to speak in Spanish to them, which the informants viewed as being disrespectful and a noncaring practice. Even health care literature translated into Spanish may not be helpful for some individuals because of their limited educational level and inability to read.

The United States culture values the use of technology in all aspects of life, which is particularly evident in health care.[88] According to Leininger,[89] high technology in Western nursing practices tends to act as a barrier between client and nurse when the emphasis is put on medical equipment. Jordan[90] provided an example of this distancing in her research on births in four cultures. Videotapes of births in the United States where electronic fetal monitoring was used revealed that during a 5-minute segment the nurse looked at the monitor 19 times. The nurse evaluated the uterine contractions by looking at the monitor rather than the client. Mexican Americans prefer that nurses provide more personalized care. While appreciative of the benefits of advanced technology, new immigrants usually are not accustomed to such sophisticated professional health care in Mexico; consequently, they may need additional explanations from the health care provider. There is a desire on the part of Mexican Americans for the nurse to provide a combination of generic (personalized) and professional health care.

Culture Care of the Mexican American Family

Transcultural nursing knowledge of the values, beliefs, and practices of Mexican Americans can contribute to the provision of nursing care that is culturally congruent with their lifeways. Meanings and expressions of culture care are embedded in the worldview, language, social structure, and environmental context.[91] It is important that nurses providing professional health care to Mexican Americans understand holistic cultural care to avoid ethnocentrism and cultural imposition practices. It is also very important to recognize that all clients are individuals and to avoid cultural stereotyping. A culturalogical assessment can provide the basis for using Leininger's three modes of culture care to develop a nursing care plan with actions and decisions that are congruent with the client's cultural values, beliefs, and lifeways.

Through the culture care preservation or maintenance mode of nursing care the nurse can assist the family to continue those cultural practices that are helpful in attaining or sustaining their health and well-being. When there may be conflict between the client's generic health care beliefs and practices and those of the professional health care provider, the nurse can act as a cultural broker.[92] A cultural broker is a nurse who is knowledgeable about the client's culture and the professional health care system and who mediates between the client and health care professionals to support the client's cultural beliefs by using the nursing care mode of accommodation or negotiation.

In the Mexican American family the nursing modes of culture care preservation or maintenance and accommodation or negotiation are especially important in relation to the areas of kinship, religion, familial roles, respect, and generic folk care practices. There are many culture care beliefs and practices of Mexican Americans' lifeways that are beneficial to their health and well-being and that the nurse can support. A culturalogical assessment will assist the nurse in providing culturally competent care. For instance, spiritual care beliefs and practices are a major source of strength that are woven into the life of the Mexican American family, particularly when there are health care needs. The nurse may notice religious symbols such as medals, rosaries, or pictures when caring for a Mexican American client in the hospital. To preserve this cultural practice the nurse will want to ensure the safety of these articles during hospitalization such as when surgery is required. Since Mexican Americans have a spiritual dependence on God as part of their worldview, it is important to facilitate the presence of spiritual advisors and provide a time for prayer if desired. This will demonstrate care as respect for their spiritual beliefs.

Families are of major importance in the Mexican American lifeways. Wherever a nurse cares for a Mexican American client, there usually will be family members or fictive kin (compadres) involved. Since the family provides major psychological support and succorance as care practices, the nurse needs to consider the importance of family members to the client and how to best incorporate them into professional nursing care. Care as respect for Mexican Americans' generation and gender should be combined with professional care practices. If decisions must be made, the role of men and their authority in the family need to be considered. As family presence is an important culture care practice, when hospital rules limit the number of visitors and visiting hours, the nurse could negotiate with the family, staff, and hospital administration regarding family visits. When family presence is not permitted, the nurse could attempt to be in frequent contact with the client and reassure the client that call lights will be promptly answered as there is often a fear of being alone. Thus, culture care accommodation/negotiation may be an important nursing action when caring for Mexican Americans in the hospital.

A cultural assessment of the generic care that was given to the client prior to coming for professional health care will enable the nurse to determine which culture care modes to use. Respect should be shown toward the role of the elders in the family providing the generic care. If the generic care was beneficial or not harmful, then the nurse may chose to use culture care preservation/maintenance by giving positive feedback on the health benefits of the practice. For example, in pregnancy, generic care precautions about using illicit drugs, alcohol, or tobacco are consistent with professional health care practices. If the pregnant Mexican American woman is found to be wearing metal to ward off the effects of an eclipse, the nurse can show respect for that cultural belief by not removing the pins as it is not a harmful care practice. When mothers want to use *fajitas* on the infant's umbilical cord, the nurse can instruct about frequent cord cleansing and changes of the umbilical band to prevent infection while still preserving this generic culture care practice. Culture care accommodation may be appropriate if, for example, the family wishes to bring certain foods or teas into the hospital when such foods are not incongruent with professional health care practices. If generic care is not beneficial, the nurse may work with the client and family to use the care mode of repatterning/restructuring of generic care. Mexican Americans are very receptive to professional health care education through which repatterning may be accomplished. As a form of respect the Spanish language is generally preferred when bilingual nurses are available. The nurse may find it necessary to construct an educational enabler using pictures and phrases in Spanish and English keeping in mind the level of education of the client to provide culturally congruent care.

Summary

Care of the Mexican American family offers an opportunity for the transcultural nurse to provide culturally congruent care that can be rewarding and beneficial for the family and the nurse. In this chapter some of the Mexican American cultural values, beliefs, and practices related to health care have been discussed. The primary cultural lifeways were presented relative to the involvement of kin, presence, family roles, cultural generic care/folk practices, use of the Spanish language, and respect. Leininger's Theory of Culture Care Diversity and Universality provided a holistic guide to discovering the lifeways of a people. The Sunrise Model was useful as a comprehensive cognitive map for performing a culturalogical assessment, including worldview, language, environmental context, and social structural factors of kinship, religion, cultural vales and lifeways, political and legal, technology, economic, and educational. Through using the ethnonursing research method values and beliefs that are embedded in a culture can be discovered and then made known to transcultural nurses as the basis for their professional nursing care.

It is the goal of the Culture Care Theory that all cultures be cared for by nurses who are knowledgeable and can integrate generic and professional care to provide culturally congruent care that is satisfying and health promoting for clients. Examples of Leininger's three care modes of culture care preservation/maintenance, culture care accommodation/negotiation, and culture care repatterning/restructuring were presented to illustrate how culturaly congruent nursing care can be provided to Mexican American families. After reading this chapter, it is hoped that nurses will have a better understanding of how to incorporate generic cultural aspects into their professional nursing care for Mexican American families.

References

1. 1990 Census Results, *Statistical Bulletin*, 1991, v. 72, no. 4, pp. 21–27.
2. Berry, A.B., "Mexican American Women's Expressions of the Meaning of Culturally Congruent Care," *Journal of Transcultural Nursing*, 1999, v. 10, no. 3, pp. 203–212.
3. Leininger, M., "Overview of Leininger's Culture Care Theory," in *Transcultural Nursing: Concepts, Theories, Research and Practice*, 2nd ed., M. Leininger, ed., New York: McGraw-Hill, 1995, pp. 93–114.
4. Leininger, M., "The Theory of Culture Care Diversity and Universality," in *Culture Care Diversity and Universality: A Theory of Nursing*, M. Leininger, ed., New York: National League for Nursing Press, 1991.
5. Ibid.
6. Berry, op. cit., 1999.
7. Gill, L., "Mexico," *Population Today*, 1991 v. 18, p. 12.
8. Coe, M., *Mexico*, 3rd ed., New York: Thames and Hudson, 1984.
9. Ortiz de Montellano, B.R., *Aztec Health, Medicine, and Nutrition*, New Brunswick, NJ: Rutgers University Press, 1990.
10. Finkler, K., *Women in Pain: Gender and Morbidity in Mexico*, Philadelphia: University of Pennsylvania, 1994.
11. Ortiz de Montellano, B.R., "Aztec Sources of Some Mexican Folk Medicine," in *Folk Medicine*, R.P. Steiver, ed., Washington, DC: American Chemical Society, 1986, pp. 1–22.
12. Ortiz de Montellano, op. cit., 1990.
13. Vigil, J.D., *From Indians to Chicanos*, Prospect Heights, IL: Waveland Press, 1984 (original work published in 1980).
14. Ford Foundation, *Hispanics: Challenges and Opportunities*, New York: Author, 1984.
15. Ibid.
16. McWilliams, C., *North from Mexico*, New York: Greenwood Press, 1990.
17. Melville, M.D., "Ethnicity: An Analysis of Its Dynamism and Variability Focusing on the Mexican/Anglo/Mexican American Interface," *American Ethnologist*, 1983, v. 10, pp. 272–289.

18. Vega, W.A., R.L. Hough and A. Romero, "Family Life Patterns of Mexican-Americans," in *The Psychosocial Development of Minority Children*, J. Yamamoto, A. Romer, and A. Morales, eds., New York: Brunner/Mazel, Inc., 1983, pp. 194–215.

19. Becerra, R.M., "The Mexican American Family," in *Ethnic Families in America, Patterns and Variations*, 3rd ed., C.H. Mendal, R.W. Habenstein, and R. Wright, eds., New York: Elsevier, 1988, pp. 141–159.

20. Bean, F.D. and M. Tienda, *The Hispanic Population of the United States*, New York: Russell Sage Foundation, 1987.

21. Marin, G. and B.V. Marin, *Research with Hispanic Populations*, Newbury Park, CA: Sage Publications, 1991.

22. Melville, op. cit., 1983.

23. Valdez, D.N., *El Pueblo Mexicano En Detroit Y Michigan: A Social History*, Detroit: Wayne State University, 1982.

24. Ortiz, V., "The Diversity of Latino Families," in *Understanding Latino Families: Scholarship, Policy and Practice*, R. Zambrana, ed., Thousand Oaks, CA: Sage Publications, 1985, pp. 18–39.

25. Meier, M.S., "Introduction," in *North from Mexico: The Spanish Speaking People of the United States*, C. McWilliams, ed., New York: Greenwood Press, 1995.

26. Falicov, C.J., "Mexican Families," in *Ethnicity and Family Therapy*, M. McGoldrick, J.K. Pearce, and J. Giordano, eds., New York: Guilford Press, 1982, pp. 134–163.

27. *B-California Immigration*, Associated Press, July 3, 1994.

28. Leininger, M., "Leininger's Theory of Nursing: Cultural Care Diversity and Universality," *Nursing Science Quarterly*, 1988, v. 1, pp. 152–160.

29. Madsen, W., *The Mexican American of South Texas*, New York: Holt, Rinehart, and Winston, 1964, p. 16.

30. Ortiz de Montellano, op. cit., 1990.

31. Vigil, op. cit., 1984.

32. Mirande, A., *The Chicano Experience: An Alternative Perspective*, Notre Dame, IN: University of Notre Dame Press, 1985.

33. Ortiz de Montellano, op. cit., 1990.

34. Ortiz de Montellano, op. cit., 1986.

35. Hurado, A., D.E. Hayes-Bautista, R.B. Valdez and A.C.R. Hernandez, *Redefining California: Latino Social Engagement in a Multicultural Society*, Los Angeles: UCLA Chicano Studies Research Center, 1992.

36. Berry, op. cit., 1999.

37. Leininger, op. cit., 1991.

38. Vega et al., op cit., 1983.

39. Villarreul, A.M. and M. Leininger, "Culture Care of Mexican Americans," in *Transcultural Nursing Concepts, Theories, Research and Practices*, 2nd ed., M. Leininger, ed., New York: McGraw-Hill, Inc., 1995, pp. 365–382.

40. Marin and Marin, op. cit., 1991.

41. Hurtado et al., op. cit., 1992.

42. Berry, op. cit., 1999.

43. Ramirez, O. and C.H. Arce, "The Contemporary Chicano Family: An Empirically Based Review," in *Explorations in Chicano Psychology*, A. Baron, ed., New York: Praeger Publishers, 1981, pp. 3–28.

44. Falicov, op. cit., 1982.

45. Rothman, J., L.M. Gant, and S.A. Hnat, "Mexican American Family Culture," *Social Service Review*, 1985, v. 59, no. 6, pp. 197–215.

46. Berry, op. cit., 1999.

47. Ortiz, op. cit., 1995.

48. Berry, op. cit., 1999.

49. Finkler, op. cit., 1985.

50. Finkler, K., *Physicians at Work, Patients in Pain*, Boulder, CO: Westview Press, 1991.

51. Finkler, op. cit., 1994.

52. Villarreul, A.M., "Cultural Perspective of Pain," in *Transcultural Nursing Concepts, Theories, Research and Practices*, 2nd ed., M. Leininger, ed., New York: McGraw-Hill, 1995, pp. 365–382.

53. Berry, op. cit., 1999.

54. "Survey Report Mexico," *Population Today*, 1990, v. 18, no. 2.

55. Berry, op. cit., 1999.

56. Stasiak, D.B., "Culture Care Theory with Mexican Americans in an Urban Context," in *Culture Care Diversity and Universality: A Theory of Nursing*, M. Leininger, ed., New York: National League for Nursing Press, 1991, pp. 170–201.

57. Ibid.

58. Berry, op. cit., 1999.

59. Ibid.

60. Villarreul and Leininger, op. cit., 1995.

61. Berry, op. cit., 1999.

62. Ortiz de Montellano, op. cit., 1990.

63. Villarreul, A.M., *Mexican American Cultural Meanings, Expressions, Self-Care and Dependent Care Actions Associated with the Experience of Pain*, unpublished doctoral dissertation, Wayne State University, Detroit, 1994.

64. Roeder, B.A., *Chicano Folk Medicine from Los Angeles, California*, Berkeley: University of California Press, 1994.

65. Ortiz de Montellano, B.R. and C.H. Browner, "Chemical Basis for Medicinal Plant Use in Oaxaca, Mexico," *Journal of Ethno-Pharmacology*, 1985, v. 11, pp. 57–88.

66. Berry, op. cit., 1999.

67. Ibid.

68. Ortiz de Montellano, B.R., "Caida De Morella: Aztec Sources for Mesoamerican Disease of Alleged Spanish Origin," *Ethnohistory*, 1987, v. 34, no. 4, pp. 381–395.

69. Ortiz de Montellano, op. cit., 1990.

70. Holland, W.R. "Mexican-American Medical Beliefs: Science of Magic?," in *Hispanic Culture and Health Care*, R.A. Martinez, ed., St. Louis, MO: The C. V. Mosby Co., 1987, pp. 99–119.

71. Ortiz de Montellano, op. cit., 1990.

72. Ortiz de Montellano, op. cit., 1986.

73. Kay, M.A., "The Mexican American," in *Culture, Childbearing, and Health Professionals*, A. Clark, ed., Philadelphia, PA: F.A. Davis and Co., 1979, pp. 88–108.

74. Roeder, op. cit., 1988.

75. Ortiz de Montellano, op. cit., 1985.

76. Hayes-Bautista, D.E., A. Hurtado, R. Burciago Valdez, and A.C.R. Hernandez, *No Longer a Minority: Latinos and Social Policy in California*, Los Angeles: UCLA Chicano Studies Research Center, 1992.

77. Leininger, M., *Transcultural Nursing Concepts, Theories, and Practices*, New York: John Wiley & Sons, 1978.

78. Hurtado et al., op. cit., 1992.

79. Berry, op. cit., 1999.

80. Ibid.

81. Ibid.

82. Ibid.

83. Rothman, op. cit., 1985.

84. Hayes-Baustista, C. et al., op. cit., 1992.

85. Davis, C., D. Hobb, and J. Willette, "U.S. Hispanics: Changing the Face of America," *Population Bulletin*, 1983, v. 38, pp.1–43.

86. Hurado et al., op. cit., 1992.

87. Berry, op. cit., 1999.

88. Leininger, M., "Toward Conceptualization of Transcultural Health Care Systems: Concepts and a Model," *Journal of Transcultural Nursing*, 1983, v. 4, no. 2, pp. 32–34 (original work published in *Health Care Dimensions: Transcultural Health Care Issues and Conditions*).

89. Leininger, op. cit., 1991.

90. Jordan, B., *Birth in Four Cultures*, 4th ed., Prospect Heights, IL: Waveland Press, 1983.

91. Leininger, op. cit., 1991.

92. Leininger, op. cit., 1995.

22
Philippine Americans and Culture Care

Madeleine Leininger

Culture provides intergenerational patterns for living, surviving, and dying.
LEININGER, 1995

The number of Philippine immigrants to the United States has steadily increased since World War II, and among them are Philippine nurses who are one of the largest groups of foreign-born nurses practicing in the United States.[1,2] Philippine nurses have come to this country largely for economic and political reasons, but also to advance themselves through American nursing education and practice experiences.[3,4] With the increase of Philippine nurses in nursing service and educational contexts, there have been some signs of intercultural tensions and conflicts largely related to misunderstandings.[5,6] Differences in cultural beliefs, values, and lifeways between Anglo-American and Philippine nurse immigrants have been frequently identified in hospitals, clinics, and schools of nursing. For example, Anglo-American nurses who are assertive in the work situation and who also value individualism, autonomy, and competitiveness often come in conflict with Philippine nurses who do not value these attributes. Instead, traditionally oriented Philippine nurses tend to value ways to maintain smooth working relationships and be deferent to those in authority. Such cultural differences may prevail in the work situation, but may not always be recognized with the busy daily activities of the nurses. These differences are, however, the source of tension, nurse burnout, distrust, and other problems that limit nurses' effectiveness. Moreover, intercultural staff problems can lead to work dissatisfaction and resignations and reduce the quality of nursing care to clients.

In this chapter the author shares her nursing research findings of the Philippine people living in a large urban Midwestern community and also draws on related nursing and anthropological studies focused on Philippine health and nursing care aspects. There were very few nursing studies of Philippine nurses and client care until the author's study in the mid 1980s and those of her students in recent years. The need, however, for discovering cultural factors in nursing care and the education of Philippine and other nurses has been clearly evident for several decades. This need has been evident with the active recruitment of Philippine nurses to meet nurse shortages in the United States and other countries since Philippine nurses are the largest immigrant group.[7,8] The lack of research in this area has been, in part the result of the tendency to overlook the importance or role of Philippine nurses as immigrants from their homeland to a country such as the United States. Moreover, nurse researchers with no preparation in transcultural nursing have been handicapped in studying Philippine nurses and understanding the meaning of their behavior and needs. With the advent of transcultural nursing, interest in this neglected culture has grown. Spangler's study and that of the author are major studies of importance.[9,10] In this chapter the author will draw on these findings and other available sources (including her consultant visits in the Philippines [beginning in the 1970s], her work as advisor to the Philippine Nurses Association in the United States, and her educational and service experiences) to help nurses understand the Philippine culture to improve client care and intercultural nurse relationships.

 ## Ethnohistorical Dimensions

Philippine nurses who immigrated to the United States came from the Philippine Islands, which are located in the Pacific Ocean near the eastern edge of Southeast Asia. There are 7100 islands in the Philippines, only some of which are inhabitable. Nearly fifty million people live in three main regions of the Philippines, namely, Luzon, Mindanao, and the Visayas.[11] There are eight major language groups and 87 dialects. Manila is the capital of the Philippines and is the industrial and educational center of the country.

The Philippine people were influenced by several groups who immigrated to the islands beginning in the 17th century such as the Indonesians, Malaysians, Chinese, Japanese, Spanish, Europeans, and North Americans.[12] These peoples came to the Philippines for trade, war, exploration, conquest, and many other purposes. Prior to the 1500s little was known about the Philippines until the Spanish and Portuguese reported on them. Magellan claimed the islands for Spain in 1521, and with the Spanish conquest came Christianity and Roman Catholicism. The Philippine Islands were named after Philippe II of Spain, and the islands were initially placed under the administration of the viceroy of Mexico as part of Spain's New World empire.[13] With Spanish control for three decades, trade with China, Japan, and other southeast Asian countries began to increase. Roman Catholicism became the major religion in the Philippines under Spanish rule. The Portuguese, Dutch, and British made attacks on the Philippine Islands and occupied them finally in 1762.

After several revolts by the South American colonies against Spain, the people of the Philippines became critical of Spanish rule, the clergy, and forced labor. This led to the emergence of a nationalist movement under Jose Rizal (1861–1896), and after his execution General Emilio Aguinaldo resigned. Then came the Spanish-American War of 1898, and later the United States gradually passed acts to give the Philippine people more autonomy and freedom. Manuel Quezon was elected the first president of the Commonwealth.[14] Independence, however, was not given to the Philippines until after the end of the wartime occupation of the country by the Japanese (1942–1945). During World War II, nearly 40,000 Philippinos were killed. On July 4, 1946, the Republic of the Philippines was proclaimed and Manuel Roxas became the Republic's first president.[15] Since then, the Philippine people have been threatened by communist guerrillas, rebels, and with autocratic leaders such as Carlos Garcia and Ferdinand Marcos. In 1985 Corazon Aquino became the first woman president of the Philippines and took office with the goal of providing a democratic government. Gloria Macapagal-Arroyo is the current president of this country of 79 million people.

 ## Theory and Research to Discover Philippine Culture Care

The author used the Culture Care Theory and the ethnonursing research method to study twenty key and thirty general Philippine informants living in an urban Midwestern city from 1984 to 1986. Since the theory and method have been presented in earlier chapters, they will not be discussed here. She also studied violence, care, and health from 1993 to 1995 with selected families in Detroit.

Worldview, Religion, and Kinship Factors

The majority of Philippinos have a deep sense of loyalty and pride in their country, language, kinship ties, philosophy of life, and religion. Accordingly, informants in the author's study viewed the world as "a gift from God" that they were to care for and respect and in which to live in harmonious relationships with one another. The majority of Philippinos are Roman Catholic, with nearly 80% belonging to this faith. Approximately 9% are Protestant, 6% Muslim, 3% animist, and 2% of other religious views.[16] It is of interest that when the Spaniards found the Muslims in the southern Philippines, they called them Maros after the Muslim Moors of Spain and Morocco. The Maros fought the Spanish, disliked Americans, and continued to defend the Manila government. Roman Catholicism has greatly influenced the daily lives of Philippinos, and they have many religious ceremonies and feasts. The informants reaffirmed the importance of Catholicism and frequently told the researcher how it helped them deal with political oppression, economic pressures, illnesses, uncertainties, and recurrent stressful life problems. A typical comment was, "I always leave my life in the hands of God, and God will take care of me." The majority of key and general informants (92%) regularly attended church and religious ceremonies. Caring ideas were closely linked to the informant's religious beliefs, especially to be deferent and respectful to authority and to maintain charitable and smooth relationships with others.

Strong kinship ties have always been evident with the Philippinos, and this was true with the key and general informants as they talked about the great importance of extended family members and of depending on each other. The care constructs of mutual *help, kin obligations, compassion*, and *direct care* were expected and discovered norms in daily kinship relationships. This finding also confirmed DeGracia's comment of Philippino families showing 1) unquestioned respect for and deference to authority, 2) strong family unity with social control over its members, and 3) an emphasis on extended family obedience to preserve and give the family a good name.[17] Acts of disloyalty, misconduct, or delinquency were held to bring shame to the extended family members in the author's study. Informants told how family members are obligated to provide assistance to their kin and to show respect for one another, mutual aid, and support in times of crisis and threats of illness. One Philippine American informant, who has lived in the United States for more than 10 years, said, "Our family in the Philippines remains important, and we have many extended family members back home that we help." The informants told how they spent much time together and shared food, advice, and money in their urban homes in the United States as they had when they lived in the Philippines. The study revealed that many elderly family members were being cared for in their homes, and none were reported to be in commercial nursing homes, as this is counter to their beliefs. The informants did not endorse the idea of nursing homes for their elderly because it is the responsibility of the extended family members to care for them in their homes. Most evident was the fact that children were socialized to care for and respect their kin, especially their elders. The informants were proud of and talked enthusiastically about their elders and all family members, as well as about good times together. The Philippino informants were expected to keep close

family ties and maintain a deep sense of loyalty, mutual respect, and obligation to each other. Accordingly, they would share anything they had with one another.

There were several important *culture care values*, which were derived from the Philippine religious kinship and worldview, to support extended family relationships. These caring values were held to be very important to support family well-being, healthy lifeways, and smooth relationships. The major cultural value of *pakikisama* was identified, which refers to maintaining smooth harmonious interpersonal relationships, and to get along with others. The term *pakikisama* is a caring value and means "to go along with." Philippinos are taught how to get along with each other and practice *pakikisama* in all their relationships. Conceding gracefully and without conflicts or disharmonious relationships was important to all key and general informants in the study.

Amor propio was another cultural value identified; it refers to personal esteem, honor, and "saving face." Traditionally, it has been important to preserve social relationships, maintain a sense of self-esteem, and save face. Maintaining Philippine self-esteem and avoiding social shame, or *hiya*, was discussed with the researcher by all informants. Several said, "One must not shame (*hiya*) oneself for others. Shaming or depreciating another Philippino could cause the person to lose face and experience a loss of *amor propio*.

Still another closely related value was *utang na loob*. The term refers to an obligation in which one person is expected to help another by *mutual reciprocity*.[18] The recipient of help is morally bound to repay the helper at some time, and this was known and valued by all families studied. A "give and take" among relatives and other friends was expected as they cared for one another, without expectations of money or instant repayments of any kind. If a monetary debt was incurred, the recipient was not expected to repay the money or kindness until a later time, and then it was like receiving a gift during a time of need. Finally, there was the cultural care value and belief of *bahala na*, or to "leave oneself to the will of God." This value permeated the thinking and explanations given to the researcher by many informants. It referred to accepting the will of God and resigning oneself to His will.[19]

From a political viewpoint, Philippinos have traditionally experienced many different kinds of political leaders and government ideologies with practices of threats, violence, and unexpected actions. Their ethnohistory has reflected past patterns of political conflicts and clashes related to government affairs, and the people have coped with diverse changes.[20] Maintaining respect for those in political roles of authority was difficult when one did not especially like their way of functioning. Several informants expressed their concerns about this matter. Data for this study was collected during the Marcos regime, and most informants were very guarded about sharing any political ideas for fear of retribution to themselves or harm to their families in the Philippines. Indeed, the informants were quite afraid, tense, and very restless about the political condition of their homeland and the political power of the Marcos regime during the 1980s. In fact, 90% of the key and general informants said they came to the United States to avoid political oppression, violence, and killings. In addition, they spoke about their desire for better jobs to improve their economic situation, buy a home in America, and send money back to their Philippine kinsfolk.

Economics and Education

Traditionally, the Philippine people lived in rural communities and depended on a subsistence farming income from small plots of land. The economic pattern of living was valued. Many informants in the study missed this lifeway in the United States while living in a large urban community where only a few had gardens, called their "small farms." Agriculture had also been their traditional means of livelihood by raising crops such as copra, rice, corn, abaca, sugar, fruits, vegetables, and tobacco in the Philippines. Land use was valued, but it was always a major and long-standing problem in their homeland. Key and general urban informants living in the United States said it was difficult to adapt to a complex urban life with high technologies and complex jobs and to work with Americans and their competitive work ethic. Approximately 80% of the informants were middle-class professionals, that is, nurses, engineers, common laborers, and tradesmen, who were pursuing additional education so they could be retained in their professional positions. All the informants said they saved money to buy (or build) a home with modern plumbing, appliances, and other conveniences. They were very pleased with how their frugal lifeway had enabled them to purchase a home and be financially successful in the United States. However, all the informants missed their farms with homegrown vegetables and fruits, which they talked about often, and the elderly especially remembered their vegetable farms "back in the homelands" in the Philippines.

Education has been traditionally valued by most Philippinos in the past and still is valued today in the United States. All the informants talked about their eagerness to go to school or college and become a "good professional." All the informants except those over 65 were or had been recently involved in educational programs or courses. Educational preparation was held to be extremely important for Philippinos to get ahead and to retain good positions in urban society. None of the informants had top administrative positions in the city. Parents were most supportive of their children getting an education and felt it was their responsibility and obligation to educate them. The informants spoke of initial problems with learning English, but they had mastered the language over time. Older Philippinos learning English relied on younger adults or children to learn the new language. Families were very proud and supportive of their children who had earned a degree or received a diploma, and these awards were framed and placed in a prominent place in their living rooms.

 ## Dominant Ethnocare Values, Beliefs, and Practices

From many interviews and observations of the Philippine informants in their natural and familiar home settings and in other life situations, several dominant culture care constructs were discovered and confirmed.[21,22] These care constructs were ideas embedded in the worldview, social structure, environmental context, and language. The informants often shared their ideas about care, health, and illness in their home settings, often while having tea with the researcher. Their warm and gracious hospitality was always evident, and they were pleased to talk about differences and similarities of living in the Philippines and the United States. Care meanings were important to discuss, especially their kinship and religious practices. They also talked about the noncaring political behavior of authoritative and aggressive leaders in the two cultures.

The *first important care construct* of Philippine informants in this study was that caring means to *maintain smooth and harmonious relationships with others, but especially with family members.* One was a caring individual or family member if one could maintain favorable relationships with others at home, in the hospital, at work, or wherever one functioned or lived. To be caring was to avoid unnecessary conflicts, confrontations, and disruptions. The cultural value of *pakikisami*, or "getting along," was a dominant guide of ways to relate to others. The informants held that a caring person would get along with others, be gentle, and be able to control stresses and conflicts to remain well or healthy and to prevent illnesses, tensions, and shame. Philippino caring ways would also support self-esteem and ways to be healthy or remain well. (They used the latter terms interchangeably).

The *second meaning and action mode* about care or caring was to show *respect for others.* All Philippine informants held a strong belief that care meant *showing respect* for those you lived and worked with but especially for families, the elderly, and those in authority. The older informants aged 55 to 65 years gave several examples of respect for the elderly such as being attentive to, giving assistance, and helping older family members. To be a caring person or group member one should be able to anticipate and offer assistance to others. Respect was a positive signal that one could give to others in time of need in a manner that was supportive. Preserving one's self-esteem and that of the family was a desired goal, especially because one respected the person as God's representative.

The *third dominant* care construct by the Philippine informants was that care meant *reciprocity. Care as reciprocity meant giving to others and receiving in time of need or when assistance was evident.* Reciprocity as care was giving help freely without hesitation or reservation and not expecting immediate return. Reciprocity was *giving* and *receiving* between individuals or the family group in a sincere and spontaneous way. Reciprocity as care was like a gift to another that was not expected or requested from the giver. Informants disliked it if they gave Anglo-Americans something and the latter felt they had to pay them back immediately. Reciprocity with a Philippino caring ethos

meant giving in anticipation and without an immediate "give-back." Reciprocal caregiving should always fit the time, occasion, and event. Philippine nurses who perform acts of reciprocity as caring would never expect to return immediately acts of kindness, but rather would wait until a need arose. Moreover, caring acts needed to be given graciously and sincerely by the caregiver. In traditional Philippine lifeways, the caregiver is often obligated to receive help at a later time. The concept of *utang na loob*, or the "give and take" of a relationship, was upheld by all informants. The informants spoke about the qualities they liked about a nurse who showed proper mutual reciprocity and could combine this attribute with respect for others. Several examples were given of the nurse caring for the elderly and providing respect, but also reflecting the "give and take" between the nurse and the older client, whether ill or well. Care as reciprocity was an important means to attain well-being. Unfortunately, in this country, Philippine reciprocity tends to be viewed by Anglo-Americans as a debt to be paid back, which was disliked by Philippine nurses who knew reciprocity from their cultural orientation.

The *fourth dominant meaning of care was preserve one's self-esteem or face (amor propio) and also avoid shame (hiya).* A caring person or family would not demean or threaten the self-esteem of another because one needed to "save face." A caring person was careful not to reprimand another person or group in public situations as this would lead to being a noncaring person and shaming consequences. For example, if a nurse were to reprimand a Philippine nurse in front of other nurses, this would be most hurtful and shameful to the Philippine nurse and a source of conflict and tension. This was often observed between Philippine nurses and Anglo-Americans in the hospital and was identified as noncaring behavior. A caring nurse would be aware of *hiya* and avoid inducing shameful feelings in another. Shaming Philippine individuals and older men and women was always viewed as noncaring behavior that should be avoided at all times, because it decreased one's self-esteem and honor and led to intercultural negative feelings about the persons involved.

Another caring construct discussed by the informants was *the obligation to care by providing physical comfort to those who showed signs of restlessness and discomfort.* Spangler's hospital study clearly showed that Philippine nurses knew how to anticipate and provide physical comfort measures to the sick, helpless, and those experiencing pain as an obligation to care.[23] A variety of thoughtful strategies were evident to provide physical comfort measures to clients in the hospital that led to the clients' well-being, recovery, and relief of pain and other discomforts. Care as providing physical comfort measures was often demonstrated by acts of tenderness as caring. *Physical comfort and tenderness as care* in the author's study reflected a combined skill of using gentle touches to help others with a compassionate and kind attitude. Gentle touches were soft and given in a sustained manner, according to several key women informants. Such touches were contrasted with those given by Anglo-American nurses, who were inclined to touch in a hard or firm manner. Gentle nursing care meant moving in a slow and deliberate touching way with thoughtful consideration of the person. Being quiet, providing privacy, and being pleasant were also viewed as caring and were linked with gentleness and physical comfort measures. Philippine nurses were skilled in providing generic caring modes, which Anglo-American and other nurses could learn from Philippine caring practices.[24]

Culture-Specific Nursing Care

Using the above specific care findings generated from transcultural nursing research, the theorist predicted that such *generic emic care* constructs could lead to professional, culturally congruent care if used in a specific and conscientious way by nurses. The nurse would need to consider ways to use these specific care constructs in relation to the three predicted or advised modes, namely, culture care preservation or maintenance, culture care accommodation or negotiation, and culture care repatterning or restructuring when caring for Philippine American clients.[25] *Culture care preservation* would be important in the use of care related to saving face and self-esteem and thus avoiding shame. The nurse would preserve respect for and deference to Philippine clients in giving culture-specific care. In addition, the care construct of mutual reciprocity or the give and take in nurse-client relationships would be very important. Providing mutual reciprocity and maintaining self-esteem would need to be given full consideration in the care of Philippine clients in this

country or in their homeland. The nurse would need to maintain ways to provide physical comfort measures and tender, gentle touches to Philippine clients in the hospital, home, or elsewhere. Comfort care should be provided in a quiet, gentle, and respectful way without reducing self-esteem or making clients feel shamed. All of these culture care values would need to be considered culture care preservation and maintenance measures by the nurse to provide culturally congruent nursing care practices.

With the above dominant care constructs in mind, the nurse would consider *culture care accommodation or negotiation in caring* for Philippine clients. The nurse could provide culture-specific care with this modality by accommodating the client's expressed desire for fish, rice, vegetables, and other "hot-cold" foods to restore or maintain their health. Sometimes, there may be medical reasons why these foods may not be given, but frequently they can be given as therapeutic healing modes to Philippine clients. Several informants talked about Anglo-American nurses and physicians who were not aware of their folk food preferences and how staff needed to accommodate their food preferences. Some were afraid to mention that they wanted such foods for fear of being shamed or losing self-esteem if their ideas were rejected. Nurses should understand and provide these important culturally based foods. Over 95% of the informants, who had lived in the United States for more than 10 years and were clients in the hospital, said they longed for their native foods, but had difficulty getting the foods, especially rice and fish. They believed their native foods help them to recover and were much more nutritious than many of the American hospital junk foods such as potato chips and fried hamburgers. They felt Americans should eat more native Philippine foods to maintain their health. Culture care accommodation was a recurrent suggestion by informants with foods, folk healing medications, and respect for using all the caring modes described above such as nurses accommodating respect for privacy and comfort measures as needed.

Culture care repatterning or restructuring would be used when new professional treatments and caring patterns needed to be modified or changed in relation to caring for Philippine clients. These would greatly vary with each Philippine client who became ill or who was ill but living at home. If self-esteem had been lost or threatened, the nurse would consider with the client how to reestablish and repattern self-esteem to prevent exposure to shaming incidents in the hospital or home. The nurse would need to be cognitively aware of ways to repattern or restructure any of the dominant care constructs already identified and described above. This would require creative thinking and planning by the nurse with the client's family to provide culturally congruent care. The nurse could develop a plan with the Philippine clients to repattern his life to regain self-esteem or self-respect if there was a strong fear of loss of self-esteem. These factors would be especially important in dealing with pain as Philippine clients do not like to complain, especially about pain. The Philippine elders contended that pain was a gift from God and should be accepted as suffering for God, but if pain was strong, the nurse should offer the client a little pain relief. Philippine clients become discouraged and some depressed if they cannot maintain their self-respect and deal with insults and offensive interpersonal situations.

Some general culture care *principles* to provide culturally congruent care to Philippine clients with traditional cultural values would be the following:

1. Show deference, respect, and kindness to clients, especially the elderly. Consider that the elderly prefer to be cared for in their home by extended family members rather than in a nursing home.
2. Involve and facilitate extended family members in nursing care activities whether at home or in the hospital as essential for the client's wellness or ability to face death.
3. Consider ways to maintain nonaggressive relationships with Philippine clients and avoid open confrontations and the loss of self-esteem.
4. Respect clients who value privacy and quiet time as essential to their recovery or well-being.
5. Accept gifts that reflect mutual reciprocity without feeling compelled to immediately return a gift.
6. Ask clients how they would like to be cared for, what comfort measures they would like to receive.
7. Consider that pain may be viewed as a gift from God, and often the client can endure more pain than most Anglo-Americans or Jewish Americans. However, small doses of medications to relieve postoperative or chronic suffering may be essential to clients.

The above nursing care considerations are important to provide culturally congruent care to many Philippine clients, especially those who value their past lifeways and practices. If the Philippine client is fully acculturated to another lifeway or living patterns, cultural assessment would be needed with changes in care practices.

Folk Health Beliefs and Values for Transcultural Caring

Folk health beliefs and values continue to play an important part in Philippine caring and health ways. Many of these folk values are based on the "hot-cold" theory related to illness and wellness states. Excessive exposure to heat or cold, for example, being out in the sun, taking a hot shower, or exposure to intense anger, fright, violence, or excitement, is believed to be harmful because it leads to imbalances and illnesses. If a client experiences these extremes or imbalances, the nurse needs to consider ways to counteract excessively hot or cold states with the goal of helping the client regain a balance or normal state. Hospitals are often viewed as places where clients are exposed to excessive amounts of heat or cold with food, air, treatments, and noise, which can lead to imbalances and illnesses. Nurses should be aware that air conditioning and excessive temperatures in the clients' room are of concern to some Philippine clients and their relatives.

In Jacano's ethnography of a barrio in the Philippines he found that the people believed that hot air is absorbed through the pores and goes to the brain to produce mental illness.[26] Likewise, key informants in the author's study spoke about excessive heat that makes them ill in the work place, at home, or in the hospital. They also told how the wind was associated with spirits (*ingkanto*) and leads to pains and aches by penetrating the body. These folk beliefs are considered in the nursing care with other care constructs discussed above and with the awareness that some clients have stronger beliefs in folk practices than others. The author's culturalogical assessment guide helps to assess the extent and focus of folk beliefs.

Stern et al. in their study identified several folk beliefs and practices related to pregnancy and childbearing such as the belief in keeping the baby small for an easier delivery, avoidance of dark-skinned fruits and vegetables during pregnancy to prevent darkening the skin, and using chicken soup to stimulate breast milk.[27] Their study provides additional guidelines to consider with mothers during childbirth. Similar folk practices and beliefs were identified by the author along with a variety of folk herbs, medicines, and mother care practices based on traditional or generic folk care. For example, the mothers spoke about "winds hangin" to cause potential mother-infant problems. The importance of family privacy and keeping the mother and child warm and out of drafts after childbirth were also discussed. These informants confirmed that nurses would be giving good care if they knew and acted on these factors.

Several key informants told how they used home remedies to allay stress and pressure problems now that they are living in an urban environment. They compared it with their past living in rural Philippine communities, which were peaceful and quiet. They identified different folk illnesses that are still caused by hot and cold imbalances and threats, and they often use folk home treatments and medicines to counteract these illnesses and restore their health. Many informants talked about cold winds in the winter that caused abdominal cramps, colds, pneumonia, and high fevers. They were combining their generic folk and a few professional healing modes, but still relying on folk ways because of costs, efficiency, and easy access.

Mental Labeling Discomforts

Several Philippine informants in the author's study were deeply concerned about the tendency of some psychiatrists, nurses, and other mental health personnel to view their behavior as "psychotic," "paranoid," or "severely depressed" when they were quiet and uncomplaining. These key informants talked about their quiet manner and reluctance to share ideas with professional strangers, especially psychiatric staff, "because they do not understand our lifeways and often misdiagnose us." Remaining quiet and answering questions from physicians made them uncomfortable as the questions often did not fit their cultural frame of reference. Many disliked referrals to psychiatrists because their statements and the cultural lifeways of their families were misunderstood. This was evident with Philippine informants

who had lived in the United States for more than 20 years. Most nurses and others in the mental health field were unaware of these potential cultural problems and misunderstanding of clients' behaviors that seem strange or different. Being passive and quiet may not be psychotic. Philippine informants said they had to learn how to protect themselves against strangers to remain well and to help outsiders understand their cultural patterns and learned lifeways. Moreover, the professional nurse needs to realize that most non-Western cultures do not believe in treating the mind separately from the body. They have long viewed the person as a cultural and holistic being rather than people having separate mind and body parts. Such a mind-body dichotomy is often very strange to cultural groups such as Philippinos who expect to be viewed as a *total* functioning and whole person.

 ## Transcultural Clinical Nursing Stresses and Conflicts

In this last section, a few common and recurrent problems occurring between Philippine and Anglo-American nurses will be identified from the author's research, other studies, and from direct clinical experiences with clients and nurses.

It is well known that Anglo-American nurses value assertiveness, independence, direct confrontations, competition, autonomy, technological efficiency, and individualism. These cultural values also reflect many of the dominant cultural values of middle- and upper-class Anglo-Americans in the United States. These values, however, may often be in conflict with the values of Philippinos and lead to serious problems between Anglo- and Philippine American nurses. In Spangler's recent comprehensive study of cultural values and practices of Anglo-Americans and Philippine Americans in a hospital context, she identified such concerns and problems.[28] Her study clearly revealed the differences between Anglo-Americans and Philippine Americans, as well as some areas of similarity, with the use of Leininger's Culture Care Theory to focus on cultural values and nursing care practices in the two cultures. (The reader is encouraged to read Spangler's chapter in Leininger's book *Culture Care Diversity and Universality: A Theory of Nursing*, 1991).

Philippine nurses did not espouse all Anglo-American values, but rather relied on maintaining their cultural values discussed above such as *maintaining smooth relationships, indirect communication, respecting authority, remaining quiet at times, avoiding shame, and maintaining self-esteem.* In clinical settings, Anglo-American nurses often expect Philippine nurses to be like them and to know how to be confrontational, efficient, quick, and politically assertive. Anglo-American nurses may not realize how offensive these behaviors may be to Philippine nurses who are new to this country or dislike some American values. Moreover, Anglo-American nurses in clinical settings often do not like Philippine nurses to be passive, quiet, or stay together. Such Philippine behaviors and practices are often viewed by Anglo-American nurses as being clannish, resistant to American ways, and showing a dislike for Anglo-American nurses. When Philippine nurses on a clinical unit speak in their native language and exclude Anglo-American nurses, this often leads to feelings of distrust and interpersonal tensions that may continue and influence staff relationships and influence client care outcomes.

In several nursing service consultations in the United States during the past two decades, the author has identified several recurrent themes of difficulty between Anglo-American and Philippine nurses. Anglo-American nurses often complain about Philippine nurses being "far too passive, quiet, groupish, and dependent on physicians." Philippine nurses complain that Anglo-American nurses are "far too aggressive, confrontational, direct, and noncaring" in their ways. They also feel that sometimes they are given some less than desirable nursing tasks that Anglo-American nurses dislike doing. Many Philippine nurses were aware of intercultural tensions and their struggles to preserve their self-esteem and confidence and to avoid being confronted in public settings or before other nurses in conferences. Philippine nurses often feel powerless to deal with these situations, and some viewed them as signs of discrimination or prejudice. Some Philippine nurses told how depressed they were with such encounters with feelings of loss of self-esteem and respect. Some Philippine nurses had resigned, and others had been dismissed from the nursing unit when tensions or conflicts were excessive. Covert anger

and resentment could be identified between Anglo-American and Philippine American nurses, but these transcultural problems were seldom discussed on the nursing units. The Philippine nurses disliked the fact that they held no top administrative positions such as head nurse or supervisor. This was of concern to some Philippine nurses who had been employed for many years on a unit. In talking with Anglo-American nurses, it was evident that they thought the Philippine nurses' deference to authority (especially physicians), their quiet manner, and passivity was largely related to limited nursing education and preparation in American lifeways. It is also important to remember that if Philippine nurses were excessively shamed or pushed too far when trying to get them to do something they dislike, some would become angry and make their position known in a firm and direct manner.

In sum, understanding transcultural nursing problems, behaviors, and patterns of interaction between Anglo-American and Philippine American nurses is extremely important to facilitate quality nursing care. The transcultural nursing knowledge generated from research with the use of the Culture Care Theory disclosed many valuable and important insights to guide nursing practices. Culture care values, meanings, and actions need to be used to provide congruent care for good health outcomes and to improve nurse and client relationships. Nurses need to be knowledgeable about traditional and changing Philippine cultural values and caring lifeways through culturalogical assessments to improve nursing practices. Both Philippine and Anglo-American nurses have unique contributions to share to advance and improve human caring modalities, but the challenge is to recognize and understand these contributions and to use them appropriately in nursing care contexts as culture care accommodations.

During the past decade with the use of transcultural knowledge and education and clinical mentoring, Philippine and American nurses are sharing and enjoying more of their unique contributions as complementary to client and human relationships. Philippine friendships and hospitality are valued along with their moral values. The Philippine Nurses Organization has grown across the United States and overseas, and this has been a unifying force for all Philippine nurses.

■ References

1. Anderson, J.N., "Health and Illness in Philippine Immigrants," *The Western Journal of Medicine*, 1983, v. 6, no. 139, pp. 811–819.
2. Spangler, Z., "Culture Care of Philippine and Anglo-American Nurses in a Hospital Context," *Culture Care Diversity and Universality: A Theory of Nursing*, M. Leininger, ed., New York: National League for Nursing Press, 1991a, pp. 119–146.
3. Leininger, M., "Ethnocare, Ethnohealth, and Ethnonursing of Arab, Polish, Italian, Greek, Appalachian, Mexican, Philippine, and African Americans," *Transcultural Nursing: Concepts, Principles, and Practices*, New York: John Wiley & Sons, 1978.
4. Cameron, C., "Relationship Between Select Health Beliefs, Values, and Health Practices of Philippine Elderly," post-masters field study, Detroit: Wayne State University, 1986.
5. Spangler, op. cit., 1991.
6. Leininger, M., "Culture Care: An Essential Goal for Nursing and Health Care," *Journal of Nephrology Nursing*, 1983, v. 10, no. 5, pp. 11–17.
7. Spangler, op. cit., 1991.
8. Anderson, op. cit., 1983.
9. Spangler, Z., "Nursing Care Values and Practices of Philippine-American and Anglo-American Nurses Using Leininger's Theory," post-masters field study, Detroit: Wayne State University, 1991b.
10. Leininger, op. cit., 1984.
11. Thernstrom, S., *Harvard Encyclopedia of American Ethnic Groups*, Cambridge: Belknep Press, 1980.
12. Weddel, C.E. and L.A. Kimball, *Introduction to the Peoples and Cultures of Asia*, Englewood Cliffs, NJ: Prentice Hall, Inc., 1985, pp. 304–307.
13. Ibid.
14. Ibid., pp. 305–306.
15. Ibid., p. 306.
16. Ibid., p. 305.
17. DeGracia, R., "Health Care of the American-Asian Patient," *Critical Care Update*, 1982, p. 20.
18. Melendy, H.B., *Asians in America*, Honolulu: University of Hawaii Press, Wayne Publishers, 1977.
19. Ibid.
20. Kroeber, A.L., *Peoples of the Philippines*, Westport, CT: Greenwood Press, 1973.
21. Leininger, op. cit., 1978.
22. Leininger, M., *Culture Care Diversity and Universality: A Theory of Nursing*, M. Leininger, ed., New York: National League for Nursing Press, 1991, p. 358.
23. Spangler, op. cit., 1991a,b.
24. Ibid.
25. Leininger, op. cit., 1991.
26. Jacano, F.L., *Growing Up in the Philippine Barrio*, New York: Holt, Rinehart and Winston, 1969.
27. Stern, P.N., V.P. Tilden, and E.K. Maxwell, "Culturally Induced Stress During Child-Bearing: The Philippino-American Experience," *Issues in Health Care of Women*, 1980, v. 2, pp. 67–81.
28. Spangler, op. cit., 1991a,b.

Additional Suggested Readings

Bello, M. and V. Reyes, "Filipino Americans and the Marcos Overthrow," *Amerasia Journal*, 1986–87, v. 13, pp. 73–83.

Carino, B.V., J.T. Fawcett, R.W. Gardner, and F. Arnold, "The New Filipino Immigrants to the United States: Increasing Diversity and Change," Honolulu: East-West Population Institute, East-West Center, 1990.

McKenzie, J.L. and N.J. Chrisman, "Healing, Herbs, Gods and Magic: Folk Health Beliefs Among Filipino-Americans," *Nursing Outlook*, 1997, v. 25, pp. 326–329.

23
Culture Care Theory and Elderly Polish Americans

Marilyn McFarland

Transcultural nursing research remains essential for nurses to advance knowledge of the elderly from diverse cultural backgrounds. Since the elderly will continually be a major subculture in the world in need of nursing care today and in the future, transcultural nursing research of the elderly remains crucial for quality care services. Understanding elders from their cultural background remains essentially a new area of study and practice for professional nurses.

This study examined care and health perspectives of elderly Polish Americans and how this knowledge can improve health care practices. Nurses who are knowledgeable about culture care and its influence on improving health will be able to see the benefits of providing culturally congruent care to the elderly. This study was based on Leininger's theory of Culture Care Diversity and Universality with use of her conceptual Sunrise Model.[1,2] Several research questions guided this transcultural care study:

1. In what ways do the factors related to the social structure and worldview in Leininger's theory influence the care and health patterns of elderly Polish Americans?
2. What specific cultural care values, beliefs, and practices influence Polish American elderly health?
3. What Polish American care practices and expressions appear to be most congruent with healthy and beneficial lifeways for the elderly of this cultural group?
4. What nursing care implications can be identified from the ethnonursing data to provide culturally congruent care for the Polish American elderly?

■ Research Method

Informants

Data were gathered from extensive observations and in-depth interviews with three key and five general Polish American informants by the investigator along with an extensive literature study about Polish Americans. This study was an ethnonursing qualitative investigation using Leininger's method and enabling guides. The qualitative naturalistic inquiry method was chosen because of the absence of in-depth emic data about Polish American elderly. It was an appropriate way to enter the unknown world of this culture. They key and general informants ranged in age from 58 to 84 years old, and seven of the eight lived in a Polish neighborhood in a northern city in mid-Michigan which has a population of approximately 43,000 persons.[3] The data were collected by the investigator over a two-year period with three to four interviews and observation-participation-reflection times with the key informants. As data were collected, the focus was on theoretical premises, especially studying the worldview, kinship, and social, cultural, political, technological, economic, religious, and educational factors that seemed to influence the care and health of elderly Polish Americans. In addition, the generic and professional systems were studied.

Data Analysis and Evaluation Criteria

The data were analyzed in this study by using Leininger's four phases of data analysis.[4] The analysis began with collecting and documenting the raw data (first phase), then identifying descriptors (second phase), and discovering patterns (third phase), and ended with abstracting major themes (fourth phase).

The Leininger-Templin-Thompson (LTT) computer software was used for coding and classifying the data.[5] Data analysis was an on-going process throughout the study.

The following qualitative criteria were used for analysis of the data: credibility, confirmability, meaning-in-context, recurrent patterning, saturation and redundancy, and transferability.[6] Credibility referred to the believability of the study findings established by the researcher through repeated engagements over a three month period with the informants. Confirmability was achieved by repeated accounts from the informants and by mutual agreement of the findings by the researcher and the informants. Meaning-in-context referred to the lifeways of elderly Polish Americans that reflected a tendency to recur in patterned ways. Saturation referred to evidence of having taken in all that could be known about the phenomena under study. Redundancy was related to saturation and referred to the tendency to get similar and repeated data. Transferability referred to whether the findings might have similar meanings in a similar context, but generalizability was not the goal of this qualitative study.

Orientational Definitions

Since the orientational definitions help the researcher to discover meanings from the informants, the following definitions were used:

1. Culture Care: Those supportive or facilitative acts specific to the Polish American culture which assist elders to improve their health and lifeways.[7]
2. Cultural Health: A state of well-being which is culturally defined and includes the ability to perform daily role activities.[8]
3. Polish American: Refers to any individual whose parents or grandparents were born in Poland and immigrated to the United States and who identifies himself/herself as a Polish American.
4. Culturally Congruent (nursing) Care: Refers to those cognitively based assistive, supportive, facilitative, or enabling acts or decisions that are made to fit with the cultural values, beliefs, and lifeways of elderly Polish Americans in order to provide or support meaningful, beneficial, and satisfying health care or well-being services.[9]

5. Emic: Refers to people's views expressed in their own words and actions.[10]
6. Etic: Refers to the outsider's or researcher's views.[11]

Theoretical Framework

This study was conceptualized within Leininger's theory of Culture Care Diversity and Universality.[12,13] Leininger views care as a universal phenomenon but with some predicted diverse expressions, meanings, and patterns of care in different cultures. She contends that these care expressions, patterns, and meanings may take on different meanings in different contexts. The theory of Culture Care Diversity and Universality has been important to establish nursing knowledge about what is similar (more universal) and different (more diverse) about care within and among cultures. Leininger also predicts in her theory that professional nursing care combined with generic (folk) care would provide care that would be congruent with a particular culture's beliefs, values, and practices. It would lead to maintaining healthy lifeways for people. The goal of her theory is to provide culturally congruent care to clients of diverse cultures that would contribute to their health and well-being.[14,15] For the elderly, this goal would be especially important to maintain their health. The care which is culturally congruent would also be predicted to be satisfying, meaningful, and beneficial to them.

The Leininger conceptual Sunrise Model was developed to depict various aspects of the worldview and social structure dimensions of a culture which influence care and ultimately the health status of people through the contexts of language, ethnohistory, and environment. The Sunrise Model serves as a cognitive map to guide the researcher in studying the theory in relation to these factors: technological, religious, kinship, and social factors, cultural values and lifeways, and political and legal factors.[16,17] According to the theory these factors, as well as ethnohistory and environment, influence care patterns and expressions and, in turn, the health and well-being of individuals and groups. The theory is holistic and helps the researcher examine multiple factors influencing the health and well-being of elderly Polish Americans in relation to human care. This broad theoretical view of the Polish American elderly's lifeways provided a comprehensive and holistic means to understand their total nursing care needs. Most importantly, if care of Polish American elderly is known from their emic point of view, professional nursing care (largely etic) could be predicted to be more congruent with their health and well-being.

Since the theory contributes to the transcultural nursing field, which focuses on comparative studies of cultures and their care patterns, values, and practices, knowledge of the Polish American elderly should contribute to transcultural nursing knowledge. Although this study explored care of the elderly in depth in one cultural group, transferability of the findings from this study with full cognizance of similar context might provide new and different transcultural approaches to nursing care of elders.

Leininger's Culture Care theory rests on several premises which were used in this study and which focus on describing, explaining, predicting, and interpreting nursing phenomena from the people's emic perspective and contrasting data from the etic view. The following premises were used to guide this study.[18]

1. Culturally specific care is essential for elderly Polish Americans for their health, healing, growth, and survival.
2. The Polish American culture has generic (folk) care knowledge and practices that influence professional culture-care practices.
3. Polish American care values, beliefs, and practices are influenced by and embedded in the world view; language; religious, kinship, political, educational, economic, and technological factors; cultural values; ethnohistory; and environmental context of Polish Americans.
4. Culture care meanings and patterns that influence the health and well being of Polish American elders can be used by nurses with Leininger's three modes to provide culturally congruent professional nursing care.

Ethnohistory, Worldview, Language, and Environmental Context of Elderly Polish Americans

To help understand the Polish American elderly of today, an overview of their history and culture is presented first. The history of the culture provides background information to understand people in their past and present environmental contexts. It also gives clues to human care and health.

Two and one half million immigrants came to the United States from Poland during the late nineteenth and early twentieth centuries, and by 1972 between 5.1 and 6 million Americans claimed a Polish heritage.[19] According to the 1980 United States Census, over 8 million people claimed Polish American ancestry and the Polish people made up the eighth largest cultural group in the United States.[20] Most Polish immigrants who came to the United States during the late nineteenth and early twentieth centuries were village peasants, and they came to America primarily for economic and political reasons.[21] In 1600 Poland was the largest country in Europe, but in 1795 Poland was partitioned by the neighboring countries of Russia, Prussia, and Austria and ceased to exist politically. Austria, Russia, and Germany had little regard for the economic welfare of the Polish people under their rule.[22] By the late 1800s there was political discontent and great economic hardship in the three sectors of Poland, and many Polish people decided to emigrate.[23–25] All informants in this study were second- or third-generation Polish Americans whose parents or grandparents had come to the United States during the late nineteenth and early twentieth centuries.

One key informant, a third-generation Polish American woman, explained the hardships in Poland in the late 1800s and early 1900s:

> My grandmother told me how the Poles suffered under Germany; the people had to use German exclusively in the schools and in the churches. They could practice Catholicism but not in Polish. There were strikes because the Polish people were forced to use German in the schools. The Russian sector was even worse, Poles were not educated at all, not even to read and write. In Austrian Poland life was very poor, as it was in all the sectors, but the Austrians were not so oppressive.

A general informant, a sixty-five-year-old woman, reflected on the reasons her family came to the United States:

> In 1880, my grandmother and grandfather and their four children left Poland because things were bad—not enough food and they were poor. My

grandmother told me how her mother held on to the wagon as they left and cried for them not to go. She knew she would never see them again. It had to be really bad there to leave your families and know you would never be back.

Polish immigrants often migrated into Michigan after brief stopovers in other states. Many came to Detroit, Grand Rapids and then smaller cities farther north where they found work as laborers. Even though most Polish people were originally farmers, they eventually sought factory work because it offered year-round employment.[26] A local Polish American priest, Bishop Povish, wrote, "The first occupation of the Poles (in this city) was in the sugar beet fields, then they went into the sawmills, the manufacturing of lumber products, and finally into the factories of the modern industries."[27]

A second-generation, sixty-four-year-old Polish American male general informant who was a retired electrician told the story of how his family eventually settled in the city and made their living:

My mother and father were born in Poland and came to the United States in the 1880s. My dad was sixteen when he came here with his parents . . . first to Chicago, where there was work in the steel mills, and then to this city. He met my mother in Chicago, married her there, and then they came (here) to do farm work in the sugar beet fields. Eventually he went to a factory. Dad was a sheep herder in Poland, but here the factory work in the foundry paid better than farm work.

Polish immigrants typically settled in Polish neighborhoods that insulated new arrivals against the cultural shock of immigration (Color Insert 13). When the Polish arrived in this mid-Michigan city, they chose to live close to a large Polish American church built in 1874 on the southern edge of the city. One sixty-four-year-old female general informant commented on the Polish neighborhood which is still located around the parish church:

Well, everyone says the Polish neighborhood starts south of Columbus Avenue, but I really think it is pure Polish south of Seventeenth Street. We were on the edge of the city, so everyone in the neighborhood could have a garden and a cow. Most Poles who came here were farmers, so even though they

worked in the factories, we did some farming, right here in the city. In the neighborhood we stayed close and lived close. All my aunts and uncles lived either across the street or around the corner.

The fifty-one-year-old daughter of an eighty-four-year-old female general informant commented on the current Polish neighborhood:

A lot of Polish people still live in the neighborhood . . . our church, St. Stan's, has a lot to do with it. The church here is part of the Polish families. We attend St. Stan's and most people in this neighborhood do. My husband and I stayed in this neighborhood so our kids could go to the parochial school. This is why a lot of young families have stayed.

Many people who live in this neighborhood still identify themselves as Polish Americans. According to the 1990 United States Census, of approximately 39,000 people who live within the city limits, 7300 claimed Polish ancestry; 4200 of these Polish Americans live in the traditionally Polish neighborhood within the city limits.[28]

Worldview includes the way people look outward toward others and their world to form a picture about their perspective life.[29] Bukowczyk explained that even though Polish Americans had made economic and political progress by the end of World War II, they tended to think in the passive voice the world acted upon them.[30] Their worldview was fatalistic and focused inward on their family, home and Polish American neighborhood and parish. The elderly Polish Americans in this study have broadened their worldview in recent years and have looked outward from the Polish American neighborhood to the rest of the United States, Poland, and the world. More recently they have viewed themselves as a vital part of the larger world, and they are proud of their Polish American heritage.

Through the 1950s, parish schools taught the Polish language and Polish history. The parish school preserved the Polish language, encouraged students to acquire the cultural traditions of their parents, and developed familiarity with Polish history.[31] Although Polish is no longer taught in parish schools, Polish Studies programs in colleges and universities provide courses in the Polish language and history.[32] All elderly informants in this study spoke at least some conversational Polish and remembered when it became un-American to speak Polish. However, informants have expressed a new pride in the Polish language and in their ability to speak and read the language.

Review of the Literature on Polish Americans

A review of the literature on Polish Americans revealed several historical and ethnographic studies of this culture. There have also been several nursing studies published about this cultural group. The studies confirm that Polish Americans value their culture, traditions, and the Polish language, and are devoted to their Polish families, neighborhoods, and parishes (Color Insert 14).

There have been several historical studies of Polish Americans. In 1927 Thomas and Znaniecki conducted a sociological and historical study of the migration of the Polish people to the United States and the Polish immigrant experiences in the Polish American parishes of the early 1880s.[33] These authors described the Polish parish as much more than a religious association for worship under the leadership of a priest. They stated:

> It [the parish] became the social organ of the community . . . it . . . assumed the care . . . of the group by organizing balls, picnics, and arranges religious services . . . It was the center of information for newcomers and acted as a representative of the Polish American community with other American institutions which tried to ready the Polish community for political or social purposes.[34]

Wytrwal compiled a social history of the Polish people in America.[35] He focused on the economic and political factors in Poland and in the United States that influenced the Polish people to migrate. In the 1880s and early 1900s young Polish men were subjected to conscription into the armies of the three partitioning powers, and peasants were being forced off their land. At the same time, there were jobs available in American industry and the Polish people believed they could earn more money and make a better living in America.

Bukowczyk, after a dozen years of historical research, wrote a book about the Polish experiences in America.[36] He described Polish immigrants as rural people with customs and values oriented toward stability, family, security, and home. He reported that they were Roman Catholics and were fatalistic, prayerful, hopeful for a better afterlife, and they venerated the Virgin Mary, Poland's patroness. They lived in child-centered families and prized steady factory work, saved their money, and gave generously to their nuns, priests, and parishes. They valued a home of their own, their church, and children who would take care of them in their old age. Bukowczyk claimed that second-generation Polish Americans (those Polish Americans who were the first in their families to be born in the United States) were hard to describe as their culture had Polish and American elements. The third and fourth generations, he asserted, were the most difficult to describe. He stated, "Culturally, little about these young men and women was identifiable as Polish or Polish American."[37]

Researchers have recently conducted ethnographies of Polish Americans in various regions of the United States. Obedinski conducted an ethnographic study of Polish Americans in Buffalo, New York, and reported that Polish Americans were increasingly adopting an American style of life while retaining traditional family and religious practices.[38] Wrobel conducted an ethnographic study of Polish Americans in Detroit which focused on day to day life in a Polish American community.[39] He discovered a Polish American culture as a way of life that was distinct from both Polish and American cultures. He found the parish, family and neighborhood still played a significant role in the lives of urban Polish Americans, fulfilling a variety of religious and social needs.

There have been several nursing studies on the care of Polish Americans. Rempusheski, in her ethnographic study of elderly retired Polish Americans in Arizona, found several care expressions related to traditional Polish American cultural values.[40] Ways to express caring described in her study were: 1) stopping by/visiting, 2) inquiring, 3) giving bringing, worrying/concern, 5) consoling, 6) cheering up, 7) listening, 8) remembering someone, 9) missing someone, 10) sharing joy, 11) sharing sickness, 12) thinking about someone, 13) advising/teaching, 14) praying for someone.[41] She found that although these elders had left their homes and retired to Arizona, they recreated the atmosphere of their Polish American neighborhood by forming and joining an Arizona Polish club where they socialized, reminisced, danced the polka, and celebrated Polish holidays.

It is important for nursing to identify the values of a culture, especially those values related to care and health. Leininger summarized the Polish American cultural values and care meanings from several transcultural nursing studies with Midwestern Polish Americans over the past decade.[42] The dominant emic cultural values identified were: 1) upholding Christian beliefs and practices, 2) family and cultural solidarity (other care), 3) frugality, 4) political activity, 5) hard work, 6) persistence, maintaining religious/special days, and 7) valuing fold practices. The culture care meanings identified were: 1) giving to others, 2) self-sacrificing, 3) being concerned about others, 4) working hard, 5) love of others, 6) family concern, 7) community solidarity, 8) health values of eating Polish foods, and 9) folk care practices.[43] In a videotape presentation of a culturological assessment of a third-generation Polish American informant, Stasiak and Leininger demonstrated that many traditional Polish American care values, meanings, and practices have remained a part of Polish American lifeways.[44] The videotape based on Stasiak's Polish intergenerational life history and nursing care of Polish Americans revealed the dominant emic care constructs of three generations of: 1) concern for and giving to others, 2) solidarity of the family or staying close, 3) helping others in need, 4) hard work and sacrifice, 5) eating natural foods, 6) folk care practices, and 7) prayer derived from the Polish American kinship, religious, and cultural beliefs and values. Stasiak's research supported Leininger's research findings with transferability evidence.

The author noted that many findings from the previous studies just reviewed still held true and were confirmed by second and third-generation Polish American informants in her study. Elderly Polish American informants continued to be devoted to their families, neighborhoods, and parishes and to express care in culturally congruent ways. During the data collection period, Poland was freed from Soviet domination, and all eight elderly Polish American informants expressed a renewed pride in Poland and in their Polish culture and a deep concern for the welfare of the Polish people.

 ## Findings as Themes

The data resulted in the formulation of patterns and themes about the care and health of elderly Polish Americans. These themes reflected the findings that addressed the research questions, as well as other findings about Polish American lifeways related to their care and health mainly derived from observation and participation and reflection experiences and interviews with key and general informants. These discovered research themes are important to guide nurses in providing culturally congruent nursing care practices. Qualitative verbatim statements are presented to help the reader grasp the full world view and emic perspective of the informants.

Theme 1

Care was expressed by elderly Polish Americans by *observing Polish customs, searching for their Polish roots, and in the efforts made to use and preserve the Polish language.* These care expressions were derived from the informants' cultural beliefs, religious values, and world view, and were viewed as vital to the survival and well-being of their culture and the Polish American identity. The Polish informants feared that the loss of their customs and language would be detrimental to the health and well-being of themselves and their families. The practice of Polish customs and the celebration of religious holidays were valued by elderly Polish Americans and were often celebrated and sustained within the family and the church. A third-generation sixty-year-old female key informant spoke of the importance of religious holidays:

> The Friends of Polish Culture is our local group of Polish Americans. We just celebrated our harvest festival, *dozynski*. We have another big celebration at Easter, *swienconka* (blessing of the Easter food). At Christmas we have a Christmas Eve dinner, *wigilia* (Vigil).

One informant described the Christmas Eve dinner:

> All of my kids will be home for Christmas. I will buy a large wafer about six inches wide, the *oplatek* [representing the sacred host], from the nuns. On

Christmas Eve I will break off a piece and pass it to my oldest child; then she will pass it to the next one . . . It is an old Polish custom and a lot of Polish people here still do this. When the wafer is passed, you wish them good health.

Elderly Polish American informants in this study expressed care for their families by planning and participating in traditional religious celebrations that included the practice of Polish customs. Elders believed that the practice of these customs and the celebration of religious holidays contributed to the health and well-being of family members and was essential to the survival of their lifeways and culture.

The search for one's history or roots has become a preoccupation for many Polish Americans. Six of the eight informants in this study have traveled to their European Polish homeland within the last ten years to find their relatives. These Polish American informants were raised in a close, tightly knit Polish American neighborhood where they spent most of their earlier lives focused upon their families, churches, parish schools, and making a living in local factories. One second-generation sixty-year-old Polish American female key informant explained to me, "When we were growing up, a lot of us never traveled as far as the next town [eight miles away], and if we did, it was a big deal." World view includes the way people look outward toward others and their world to form a picture about their perspective of life.[45] The elderly Polish Americans in this study have broadened their world view in recent decades and looked outward from their Polish American neighborhood to the rest of the United States, Poland, and the world. Elderly Polish Americans viewed themselves as a vital part of the larger world, and they were proud of their Polish American heritage. One second-generation sixty four-year-old male general informant said with pride. "Most people on this street have Polish names. I wouldn't change my name. I'm proud of being Polish American and proud of Poland." Local second- and third-generation Polish Americans were interested in political events in Poland and were interested in the welfare of the Polish people. One informant read from the local newspaper, "the mayor declared November 12, 1989 Polzan University Day." She explained that

Polzan is the city's sister city in Poland. She described her family's interest in political events in Europe and in Poland:

I want you to know how very proud we are in this house . . . we are so proud of what has taken place in Germany . . . it is a direct result of what took place in Poland with Solidarity . . . Walesa addressed the United States Congress today . . . and met the President.

Polish Americans were interested in the politics of Poland because it influenced the health and well-being of the Polish people. My informant explained, "We have a deep underlying interest in the welfare of the people in Poland . . . as my husband says, 'All Poles are cousins.'"

The metaphor of the American melting pot idea had been firmly rejected by all informants of this study. They knew who they were and they were proud of being Polish Americans. They believed they had a unique contribution to make to their country and were not melting into a non-identifiable culture. They were also interested in and appreciative of the uniqueness of the culture of others as well. This broad world view was a reflection of their view of themselves and the way they saw others. One sixty-four-year-old third-generation female key informant explained:

I attended a multi-ethnic religious service at the park last summer. One of the priests talked about the melting pot theory. I was mad. I told him to look at the contributions of various people . . . I said look at the stained glass window in a church, look at the beauty, the color, and the shape of each piece of glass. They all have something to add to the whole.

This informant valued her own cultural identity but valued the diversity in other cultures as well. This broad world view was reflected in the data from all eight informants and influenced the concern they expressed for the survival of diverse cultures. They recognized that the survival of all cultures, as well as their own, was essential to the health and well-being of all people.

Bigelow, a geographer who has studied ethnic subcultures in the United States, reported that the third and fourth generations of Polish Americans have intermarried with other Catholic nationalities.[46] He maintained that this has been detrimental to the maintenance of Polish-Catholic ethnicity. All the informants in this study reported that some of their children had not married Polish people, and they expressed concern that this has caused them to worry about the survival of Polish customs and the Polish language in their families. One third-generation sixty-three-year-old key informant explained that she had married a Polish man and that helped her maintain Polish ways:

> I'm Polish and married a Polish guy . . . that has helped us preserve our Polish customs. We belong to the local Polish cultural group. I have no children but my sister has three kids, but they have not married Polish . . . they haven't even married Catholics. We both wonder who we are going to pass all this on to . . . all the Polish recipes, the customs, and the things we share as a family at Christmas and Easter.

Elderly Polish Americans were very attached to their language. Most second- and third-generation Polish Americans in this study learned to speak and read some Polish in parochial schools. Polish was spoken fluently by two key and two general informants with the remaining four informants speaking some limited conversational Polish. Some informants remembered when the nuns stopped teaching Polish. A third-generation sixty-four-year-old female key informant explained her experience in learning Polish, and the relationship of her knowledge of Polish to the care practice of helping others:

> I learned Polish in grades one through four; then it was considered un-American to speak Polish so the nuns stopped teaching it . . . we are rethinking that now . . . twenty five years after high school I went to the local college and took several semesters to relearn Polish. I translate letters now back and forth for people who have relatives in Poland, so they can keep in touch; it is my contribution and I take no money.

She viewed this care practice as being beneficial to the health and well-being of Polish families, as well as essential to the survival of the Polish American culture.

The Polish language and Polish history and culture were no longer the focus in local parochial schools in this study. However, local Polish Americans have worked hard since 1972 to establish a Polish Studies program at the local college. The view of Polish life historically presented in parochial schools in Polish neighborhoods was presented in a broader way in the local university. It included not only the Polish language and the views of Poland's past but also included views of life and cultural events in present-day Poland.

This new educational focus was reflected in the views of care and health and well-being expressed by elderly Polish American informants. Polish American elders have been maintaining the traditions of caring for and being concerned about the health and well-being of immediate family members, but they have extended their care and concern for the health and well-being of family members to Polish relatives, to the people of Poland, and to people from other cultures as well. The elderly informants viewed efforts to preserve the Polish language and traditions as essential caring practices to ensure the survival of their cultural lifeways.

Theme 2

Care was expressed and made meaningful by *visiting relatives in Poland, arranging for Polish relatives to visit in the United States, and by sending money, food, and medicine to them.* This theme was mainly derived from kinship and social values and practices. One eighty-four-year-old general informant related that even as late as the 1940s, her family was attempting to arrange immigration of their Polish kin to the United States:

> My husband tried to get his cousin's family to come here right before W.W.II. I remember being told that we would have to share our home because these relatives were coming from Poland . . . it was bad there . . . no meat, coffee, or soap, . . . but then the war came and after it was over, no one could get out.

Today elderly Polish Americans express care for Polish relatives by visiting them in Poland and arranging for their relatives to visit in the United States. The same informant explained, "I kept writing to my husband's cousin and his wife . . . eventually we sent them money to come for a visit." A sixty-four-year-old general informant reported, "My sister traced my dad's relatives . . . she found my dad's brother in Poland about eighteen to twenty years ago. I have been back three times and my wife once." The care practice of visiting relatives in Poland and arranging visits of Polish relatives to the United States enhances the health and well-being of the Polish people and Polish Americans. One second-generation sixty-four-year-old general informant explained, "I found my older brother who had stayed behind in Poland after my mother and father came to the United States. The whole family was so glad I found him. I was glad we met each other before he died."

Polish American elders also expressed care by sending money and material items to relatives in Poland, many of whom they have never met. One informant explained the transfer of goods and money to Poland:

> I have taken thousands of dollars to Poland. When people give me money to take to Poland, it means people really trust you. We have things worked out when we take money over; I have a picture of the person I am to give it to and that person has a picture of me. A lot of relatives send medicines to Poland . . . I sent cortisone ointment to my cousin. At Christmas time, I ship lemons, oranges and bananas. Two days a week we can drop off packages at an office in town here and they are shipped to Poland.

The care that was expressed by Polish Americans through the transfer of food, medicines and money to Poland was done to enhance the health and well-being of their Polish relatives. One third-generation sixty-four-old female informant explained:

> My cousin in Poland had horrible sores around her mouth. Even though health care is free in Poland, there is no medicine. After my cousin got the cortisone, her sores cleared up. She told me she was able to resume a healthy life.

In this study, "giving to others" was an important care meaning and was practiced by Polish American elders. They have extended this care beyond their immediate families to relatives in Poland and even to the Polish people. Many elders raised and donated money for Polish relief. Some members of the Polish American community have acted as couriers to take American dollars to Poland. Second-and third-generation Polish American elders have extended the traditional care practice of giving to immediate family members to giving to relatives and others in Poland in order to improve the health and lifeways of Polish people.

Theme 3

Care meant spending time with, being there, doing for and reciprocating care with children, grandchildren, and other family members. This theme was derived from their cultural and kinship values, beliefs, and practices. Elderly Polish Americans still prize the home, family, stability, and security over the desire to make money or acquire material things. This was expressed by one third-generation sixty-three-year-old female key informant who worked part-time cleaning offices:

> I think people [young Polish Americans] are too eager for money now. Polish people were poor when they came here and they still aren't rich. There are more important things than money. We [she and her sister] married poor men and they worked hard . . . women didn't work in the past; we were home to care for our kids . . . it was important to be home when your kids came home from school. Today, kids are too eager for money . . . they think it is necessary for both a husband and wife to work . . . but a lot of what they buy isn't necessary.

The care practices of spending time with or being there for their children and other family members were more important then than expressing care for one's family by making a great deal of money to buy material things. The elderly informants believed that caring in this manner was beneficial to the health of children and adults.

Elderly Polish Americans relied on their families for care in the past and continue to do so today. One elderly informant explained how Polish families cared for each other in the Polish neighborhood when she was growing up. She explained:

> In the neighborhood, we stayed close and lived close. All my aunts lived either across the street or around the corner. If someone had a baby, then someone just had to come across the street to help . . . if someone was sick it worked the same way.

Two third-generation key informants who are sisters (fifty-eight and sixty-three years old) explained how Polish American families have continued to care for family members:

> I care for my sister and she cares for me. We do a lot of things for each other. We both have sick

husbands so we depend on each other . . . We care for our husbands . . . Polish American wives care for their husbands . . . a nursing home would be only if things were really bad. Husbands also would care for their wives if necessary.

The seven informants (two key and five general) who had children all believed that their children would care for them if they became ill. When nursing home care was discussed, it was acknowledged as a possibility but only as a last resort. Polish American families continued the practice of taking care of elderly family members when they became ill. Polish American elders were confident that family members would be available to give care if their health was threatened or if they became disabled. Nursing home placement of Polish American elderly family members had not been a traditional care practice in the past, and elderly Polish American viewed it as a care practice that would only be used if a family member was very disabled and could not be cared for in their own home or the homes of their children. The confidence elderly Polish Americans felt in the readiness of their families to give care made them feel secure, and they viewed this feeling of security as an essential part of their health.

Theme 4

Polish American *involvement in politics has allowed Polish Americans to care for elderly family members and other Polish elders in the community.* Political factors in the local city government have influenced the lives of second- and third-generation Polish Americans. A daughter of a second generation eighty-one-year-old female general informant commented, "In my mother's day, most people [Polish] were Democrats . . . but now they vote for the best candidate . . . but if all other things were equal between candidates, I'd vote for the Polish American."

Many Polish Americans have moved into political careers. A local historian stated, "Qualified Americans of Polish ancestry have held major posts in local government, including those of mayor, city manager, county executive, school superintendent, county treasurer and several city and county commissionerships."[47] Polish Americans who have held political posts in city government have been able to care for elders by arranging funding for a senior meal site

at the local Polish parish. This site served a noon meal five days a week for senior citizens in the local Polish neighborhood and provided a place for elders to gather for social activities. The daughter of one elderly informant explained that senior meals and activities at the local parish kept elders active and got them out of their houses which she believed enhanced their health and well-being.

Theme 5

Health for elderly Polish Americans meant being comfortable and secure, working hard, keeping active, and eating the right foods. These beliefs and practices were related to their cultural values. All eight informants viewed themselves as being in good health even though most were taking medication for chronic diseases such as heart disease, diabetes and arthritis. Good health meant being active rather than being free of disease. One second-generation informant explained, "I'm very healthy, I'm sixty-four and all I have is a little high blood pressure." His wife commented, "Good health is being mobile and having a clear mind." A third-generation sixty-four-year-old female key informant commented, "My health is pretty good. I take insulin for diabetes. I had back surgery a few years ago. I'm really stiff today . . . but I was out dancing last night . . . I didn't sit out a single dance."

According to Leininger, theoretical definitions of orientation are used in qualitative research rather than operations definitions and " . . . orientational definitions seek emic knowledge derived from the people and environmental contexts as the epistemological and ontological sources of cultural care knowledge."[48] Orientational definitions may be altered to fit the informants' frames of reference as a study progresses. The informants in this study *defined health as feeling well, being secure and comfortable, having a clear mind and being able to do their daily activities.* This definition is consistent with Leininger's theoretical definition of health. Leininger stated, "Health refers to a state of well being that is culturally defined, valued and practiced and which reflects the ability of individuals (or groups) to perform their daily role activities in a culturally satisfactory way."[49] However, no informant used the term well-being when discussing health. On direct questioning about the term well-being several informants reported that they had heard the term mentioned but really could not define it. Health is an emic term that emerges from the data with a meaning that is culturally relevant to the informants, and well-being is an etic term that the informants have heard mentioned by health professionals.

Elderly Polish Americans in this study identified links between their Polish traditions and lifeways and their views of health. The Polish American traditions of hard work, keeping busy, and keeping active were viewed by elderly informants as care practices to ensure or maximize their health. One third-generation sixty-three-year-old female key informant explained:

Keeping busy is important to your health. It isn't good to think too much about your health or being sick. My husband has leukemia but we still go out. My sister's husband stays home and worries about his heart, that isn't good.

Another third-generation female key informant explained a similar view about keeping healthy, "To keep healthy I do housework and I walk. If I can, I park as far away from a store that I can so I will walk." One second-generation sixty-four-year-old general informant who was retired from his job that required physical exertion explained, "I keep healthy now by exercising and working out at the health club."

All Polish American elders in this study discussed food preparation and production in relationship to their health. Attention to the healthy preparation of foods was viewed as an important care practice both for themselves and for their families. There was concern expressed by several elders about the dangers of food additives and the associated negative implications for their health. One sixty-five-year-old general informant explained, "Good food is important. Our folks and grandparents had huge gardens and raised chickens and ducks right here in town. They didn't use all those chemicals and preservatives." A third-generation sixty-three-year-old general informant acknowledged that heredity played a role in her diabetic condition but viewed a good diet and good food as important to her health. She stated, "I have diabetes. I think it is hereditary, but diet is important. Good food is important. I buy all my chickens and ducks from a Polish woman who raises them herself. She doesn't give them any chemicals." A second-generation sixty-four-year-old male

general informant explained, "I really think my good health is due to the foods we grew when we were kids. We had our own cow, grew our own vegetables. My mother canned all her own foods; everything was our own." His wife added, "Let's face it, everything we get now [food] has chemicals in it. We didn't use any chemical fertilizer like they do now." Eating foods that were organically grown and preserved without additives were care practices that elderly Polish Americans viewed as important in maintaining their health and the health of their families. The preparation and eating of tradition foods such as *pierogi* (fried filled noodle), *paczki* (deep fried, filled doughnuts) and *kielbasa i kapusta* (sauerkraut with pork sausage) were still viewed as important care practices to insure the survival of their cultural lifeways. However, all informants recognized that these traditional Polish foods were no longer considered healthy because of the fats and large number of calories they contain. They have limited the preparation and eating of those foods to traditional holidays in order to protect their health.

All eight elderly informants had health insurance and reported that they could afford to utilize local physicians and the one local hospital. Only the oldest informant, an eighty-four-year-old widow, reported she had problems paying for her prescription medicines. She said, "I have Medicare and Blue Shield, I pay both myself. I have to spend eighty dollars a month on medication ... my kids help me with money because I just have my social security." Her family demonstrated the traditional care practice of providing financial assistance for elderly relatives in order to maintain their health.

Theme 6

Elderly Polish American expressed care for their families and neighbors through the organization, support, and participation in church activities. In this community a Catholic-Polish society was formed more than 100 years ago to establish a local parish. The first church was a wooden structure built by the first-generation Polish Americans.[50] It was dedicated in 1874, and the pastor of the Polish parish in 1974 told the story of how a handful of settlers formed the first church with " ... faith, hard work, and cooperation extending over three generations."[51]

The local church has served this Polish community not only as a place of religious worship but also as a center for social activities and a place to practice Polish traditions. One third-generation sixty-three-year-old female key informant stated:

> The church is the center of our Polish activities. I go to church every week with my husband. Every Wednesday during Lent we have Polish literature [readings], we sing Polish songs. We have two Polish priests . . . they both speak Polish . . . that is very important.

The same informant described a meeting of the local Polish cultural group. Her comment demonstrated the use of the church as a site for social gatherings:

> Our Polish culture group meets once a month. We start at 9:00 a.m. on a Sunday with a Polish mass. At noon we have *Paczki* (Polish doughnuts) and coffee. At night we meet at a hall . . . you should have been there last night . . . we danced until 2:00 a.m. We raised money for Polish relief . . . for the children or nuns or maybe to send some local college students to a Polish university. My sister and I wore our Polish costumes.

A third-generation sixty-one-year-old key informant described her support and affection for the parish even though her family has moved out of the old neighborhood:

> We still go to the same church. We are part of the parish family there. In this neighborhood the church is mostly Dutch. We moved out here from the south end [the Polish neighborhood], and we are the only Polish family on the road. We tried the parish out here, but they didn't welcome us, that is why we went back to the old parish.

The same informant described the importance of the Polish parish in the lives of elderly Polish Americans:

> The south end [the Polish neighborhood] has been let down. We need a high rise for the elderly in the neighborhood. Where did they put the last one? Right behind the jail. Who wants to live there? . . . Old people want to stay in the bosom of their families, close to the church.

One second-generation eighty-four-year-old female general informant explained the support that people in the neighborhood give the church. "The people here really care about the church, they help keep it up and are generous . . . We have special collections for flowers at Easter and Christmas. People really contribute, we get almost $1,000 for flowers at Easter." The elderly woman's fifty-one-year-old daughter explained how the church has provided for seniors:

> We have almost 400 people in the senior citizens group . . . We have a senior meal site at the church, and have lots of activities . . . at Christmas time we give a big party for them at parish hall, and they will have a big dance and a meal.

The neighborhood parish served the elderly as a setting for many social activities which often involved the practice of Polish traditions. Elderly Polish Americans expressed care for their families and neighbors through the support, organization, and participation in these activities that were often related to religious holidays. They viewed these activities as essential caring ways that assist them and others in supporting their health and well being and the survival of their culture and lifeways.

Theme 7

Elderly Polish Americans revealed some diversity in their views of the professional health care system especially nursing and nursing care. A third-generation female informant stated.

> Right up until the 1940s and 1950s, older Polish American people went to the hospital as a last resort: it was seen as a place to die . . . I'm sixty-four and as kids we didn't go to the doctor much.

All eight informants in this study reported that they now utilized the local hospital and other professional health care services and recognized their value in treating illnesses and in providing maternity care. Even though the professional services were viewed as beneficial, they were utilized with some reservation and reluctance. One third-generation sixty-five-year-old general informant explained, "I'm healthy and I was only ever in the hospital to have babies . . . I would go there if I needed to. We [she and her husband] both would go, but I hope we don't have to." A third-generation fifty-eight-year-old key informant explained her doubts about the medications a cardiologist had prescribed for her husband, "He takes sixty-five pills a day for his heart condition. Too many for his own good. He goes to a psychiatrist because he worries about his health, but it doesn't help much."

All informants valued professional health care but five informants expressed some reluctance about using the services. Keeping busy and active and not thinking about or worrying about one's health were believed to be as beneficial to their health and well-being as professional care. Leininger defined a folk health system as "traditional or local indigenous health care or cure practices that have special meanings and uses to heal or assist people which are generally offered in familiar home or community environmental contexts with their local practitioners."[52] Polish American elders in this study utilized the professional health care system but also valued their own folk health beliefs and used folk care practices to maintain their health.

There was diversity in the views elderly Polish American informants held about nurses and nursing care. Six of the eight informants had been hospitalized at some time and offered views on nursing care in that setting. Four (one key and three general) informants reported that they had good nursing care in the hospital, but two third-generation female key informants who were sisters and interviewed together (fifty-eight and sixty-three-years-old) felt nurses did not care as much as they used to. One was a licensed practical nurse who had not worked as a nurse in over twenty years. Her sister remarked, "The nurses don't care as much as they used to. Years ago if a nurse wasn't a caring nurse, the hospital didn't keep them." The informant who was an LPN offered her views on nursing:

> The LPNs were more caring the RNs. The RNs had the cap and wouldn't do the dirty work. A nurse shouldn't be afraid to get her hands dirty to give care ... a caring nurse is friendly and has feeling for a person, a caring nurse lives to take care of people.

A third-generation sixty-one-year-old key informant discussed her experience with nurses, "I've never not had a caring nurse. The patient brings it on himself; if you complain, you suffer. You must be considerate; everyone is a human being, even a nurse." This informant though that a considerate attitude on the part of

the patient was essential for nurses to encounter so they could render good care.

Several informants had utilized home health care nursing services. They valued this care because it was provided in their own homes or in the homes of their children rather than in a hospital setting. A second-generation eighty-four-year-old general informant explained how she was able to care for her sister in her home:

> My sister has been with me about two months and has just about recovered from her mastectomy. She just lives a few blocks away. She left the hospital quite soon after her surgery and then she came to stay with me so I could take care of her. We had a home health care nurse to help us. She really cared and even came over one night when I called, just to reassure my sister. She was glad to come even though nothing was really wrong. My sister is almost better now, so she will be going home.

Discussion

The above qualitative research themes help the nurse to gain an understanding and meaning of the Polish culture in their environmental and historic contexts. They will now be discussed in relation to Leininger's Culture Care Theory Predictions. Culture care was found to be essential to preserve the health of Polish American elders and the survival of their lifeways.[53] *The major and dominant care constructs from this study were: giving to others and sacrificing, helping others, being there (staying close to Polish family and friends-solidarity), reciprocating, and visiting.* These care constructs were embedded in the world view and social structure features within the context of the Polish American culture. Care was continually reciprocated between Polish American elders and their Polish family members. Elders felt secure in the readiness of their families to give care and this feeling of security was an essential part of their health. Elderly Polish Americans cared for their family members by spending time with or being there for their children and grandchildren. All generations of family members were involved in many social activities at the local Polish church. Family members reciprocated care for each other by organizing, supporting, and participating in church activities. These care practices were related to their cultural values. Health for all key and general informants meant being comfortable and secure, working hard, keeping active, and eating the right foods. This is supportive of Leininger's definition of health which refers to health being culturally defined, valued, and practiced.[54] The expressions and practices of kinship, and cultural beliefs and values were the major influences on the care patterns of elderly Polish Americans which lead to their health. This is in accord with Leininger's theory about cultural and social structure dimensions influencing care and then the health of individuals, families, and cultural groups.[55]

Elderly Polish American care practices such as observing and practicing Polish customs, searching for their Polish roots, the efforts made to use and preserve the Polish language, visiting with relatives in Poland, and sending food, medicine, and money to Poland were based on their cultural values and beliefs. This is congruent with Leininger's prediction that care is culturally constituted in every culture.[56]

Even though professional health care services were viewed as beneficial, they were utilized with some reluctance by Polish American elders. Often folk care practices such as keeping busy and active were viewed to be as beneficial to their health as professional care practices and were tried before consulting health professionals. These findings regarding care and health are consistent with the finding reported by Leininger from several transcultural nursing studies with Midwestern Polish Americans in the past decade.[57]

There was some *diversity* in the views elderly Polish Americans held about nurses and nursing care. Four informants reported they had good nursing care in the hospital setting but the two youngest informants reported that the nurses "didn't care like they used to." Cultures are dynamic and changing, and the diversity in the views Polish Americans held about nursing care is an area to be considered for further study.

◼ Culturally Congruent Care

In the theory of Culture Care Diversity and Universality, Leininger predicted that for care to be therapeutic and satisfying and to lead to health, it must fit the client's cultural beliefs, values, and lifeways.[58] The data from this study demonstrated that care constructs derived from and embedded in the world view, social structural factors, and cultural values influenced the care of elderly Polish Americans. Leininger has predicted three modes to guide nursing decisions and actions in order to provide culturally congruent nursing care: 1) culture care maintenance or preservation, 2) culture care accommodation or negotiation, and 3) culture care restructuring or repatterning. Nurses can use these modes to design care that is based on the views of care and health held by the elderly in the Polish American culture.[59,60]

Culture care preservation refers to care that preserves cultural values and lifeways and is beneficial to clients.[61] The Roman Catholic Church was important in the daily lives of the Polish American elderly, and their Polish cultural activities were closely tied to the neighborhood parish. Culture care was preserved among elderly Polish Americans who continued to organize and attend benefits for Polish relief through their local Polish culture club and the local Catholic church. These activities promoted and preserved the care pattern of caring for others in the Polish American culture that elders identified as an essential part of their lifeways.

Elderly Polish Americans continue to care for their immediate family members as well as for relatives in Poland. Culture care preservation was sustained and promoted for Polish American elders by the family structure that was organized to provide care for close relatives, and by the extended family structure that was organized to provide care for relatives in Poland. It was a reciprocal care structure that was intergenerational and international in nature. Polish American elders reciprocated care with other elderly family members. Knowledge of traditions and history were passed from the older generation to their children and grandchildren who in turn provided physical care and social and financial support for elders. Polish American elders expressed care by visiting relatives in Poland and arranging for Polish relatives to visit the United States. Polish American elders also expressed care by sending money and material goods to Poland. Polish relatives reciprocated by the transmission of knowledge of contemporary Polish culture to their American kin. Elderly Polish Americans believed this infusion of current knowledge of Polish culture contributed to the survival of their cultural lifeways in the United States and positively influenced their health.

Nurses should strive to preserve the care pattern of promoting and maintaining cultural values and lifeways that are closely tied to the Roman Catholic Church through the neighborhood Polish American parish. The second care pattern to be preserved is that of family care that was reciprocally practiced intergenerationally and intragenerationally, both on a local and international level. These care patterns contributed to the major care theme of caring for others that has emerged from the emic data of this study. The care practices of giving to others, caring for others, or doing for others may be difficult for Anglo-American nurses to understand because many nurses value primarily self-care practices to maintain healthy lifeways. Nurses should make every attempt to preserve this Polish American care pattern of *caring for others*, which elderly Polish Americans have viewed as essential to their health and to the survival of their cultural lifeways.

Culture care accommodation refers to care activities that reflect ways to adapt health care services to benefit people.[62] Home health care services and institutions can modify services to accommodate family involvement in the care of elderly relatives. Polish American families can be supported by community nursing services if they wish to care for elderly family members at home. Polish American elders in this study preferred to receive health services in outpatient settings or in their own homes rather than being admitted to hospitals. As one third-generation key informant explained to the researcher, "Old people want to stay in their own homes in the bosom of their family, close to the church."

The traditional Polish American care practices of keeping busy and active can be modified to fit elderly Polish Americans health care needs. Exercise programs offered by the local hospital may be able to be offered at the local senior center at the Polish American parish. Exercise and activity programs can be designed and supervised by nurses and other health care professionals to meet professional health care goals for elders and at the same time accommodate the traditional care practices of keeping busy and active. The neighborhood setting would be congruent with the elderly Polish Americans desire to avoid going to the hospital to receive care services unless absolutely necessary.

Dietary information could be offered by dietitians and nurses at the local senior center. Diets that professionals consider therapeutic could be modified to allow for traditional Polish foods that are fried and have a high calorie count on special religious holidays that are celebrated by Polish American elders. The care practice of eating food that is naturally grown and prepared could easily be accommodated in most therapeutic diets.

Culture care repatterning refers to altering health or life patterns that are meaningful to them while still respecting their cultural values.[63] This may be difficult for nurses who do not understand the Polish American culture. If placement of an elder in a nursing home is necessary, both the elderly person and the family will need support as they experience this new pattern of care. Even though the Polish American elderly in this study acknowledged that nursing home care for themselves was a possibility, they viewed it as only as a last resort because they preferred to receive care at home or in the homes of their families. If nursing home care becomes necessary, they will be the first generation of Polish American elders not cared for in the homes of their families. It is important for nurses to recognize and help elders and families to understand that care in a nursing home does not indicate an abandonment of elders by their families, but rather a repatterning in the way their families provide care for their elderly family members. However, nurses need to continue to try to accommodate the traditional care pattern of family care in the elders' own homes if at all possible.

◼ Conclusion

This study was conceptualized within Leininger's Culture Care theory which served as a valuable theoretical framework to study the elders' lifeways by exploring their world view and social structure within the context of the Polish American culture. The ethnonursing method was used to systematically document and gain greater understanding of the Polish American elder's daily experiences related to care and health. In this study, the dominant care construct of Polish American elders was caring for others which substantiated the findings from other Polish American transcultural research.[64] Other care meanings and expressions already discussed were also similar to Leininger's previous findings with the Polish American culture.[65] It is the hope of the author that the findings from this study will assist nurses in providing culturally congruent care.

References

1. Leininger, M.M., "Leininger's Theory of Nursing: Cultural Care Diversity and Universality," *Nursing Science Quarterly*, 1988, v. 1(4), 152–160.
2. Leininger, M.M., "Ethnonursing: A Research Method with Enablers to Study the Theory of Culture Care," *Culture Care Diversity and Universality: A Theory of Nursing*, M. Leininger, ed., New York: National League for Nursing Press, 1991b, pp. 73–118.
3. U.S. Department of Commerce, Statistical Abstracts of the United States, Washington, DC: Bureau of the Census, 1990.
4. Leininger, M.M., "Ethnomethods: The Philosophic and Epistemic Bases to Explicate Transcultural Nursing Knowledge," *Journal of Transcultural Nursing*, 1990, v. 1(2), pp. 40–51.
5. Leininger, op. cit., 1991b.
6. Leininger, op. cit., 1990, p. 43.
7. Leininger, op. cit., 1991a, p. 47.
8. Leininger, op. cit., 1991a, p. 48.
9. Leininger, op. cit., 1991a, p. 49.
10. Leininger, op. cit., 1988, p. 153.
11. Leininger, op. cit., 1988, p. 154.
12. Leininger, op. cit., 1988.
13. Leininger, op. cit., 1991a.
14. Leininger, op. cit., 1988.
15. Leininger, op. cit., 1991a.
16. Leininger, op. cit., 1988.
17. Leininger, op. cit., 1991a.
18. Leininger, op. cit., 1991a, pp. 44–45.
19. Bukowczyk, J.J., *And My Children Did Not Know Me: A History of the Polish-Americans*, Indianapolis: Indiana University Press, 1986.
20. U.S. Department of Commerce, op. cit., 1990.
21. Wytrwal, J.A., *America's Polish Heritage: A Social History of the Poles in America*, Detroit: Endurance Press, 1961.
22. Ibid.
23. Buckowczyk, op. cit., 1986.
24. Anderson, J.M. and I.A. Smith, eds., "Poles," The Peoples of Michigan Series, Vol. 2: *Ethnic Groups in Michigan, Michigan Ethnic Heritage Studies Center and University of Michigan Ethnic Studies Program*, Ann Arbor: University of Michigan, 1983, pp. 218–221.
25. Wytrwal, op. cit., 1961.
26. Graff, G., *The People of Michigan: A History and Selected Bibliography of the Races and Nationalities Who Settled Our State*, Occasional Paper No. 1, Lansing, Michigan: Department of Education Bureau of Library Services, 1970.
27. Allison, M., "100 Years of Polish Heritage: St. Stan's Has Left Indelible Mark on City," Bay City Times, 1974 (February 9).
28. U.S. Department of Commerce, op. cit., 1990.
29. Leininger, M.M., Basic Cultural Concepts for Nurses and Other Health Personnel to Understand About Culture (class handout), Detroit: Wayne State University, College of Nursing, 1989.
30. Bukowczyk, op. cit., 1986.
31. Wytrwal, op. cit., 1961.
32. Buckowczyk, op. cit., 1986.
33. Thomas, W.I. and F. Znaniecki, *The Polish Peasant in Europe and America* (rev. ed.), Chicago: University of Illinois Press, 1984.
34. Ibid., p. 248.
35. Wytrwal, op. cit., 1961.
36. Bukowczyk, op. cit., 1986.
37. Ibid., p. 76.
38. Obedinski, E.E., "Ethnic to Status Group: A Study of Polish Americans in Buffalo," Dissertation Abstracts International, 1968, v. 29(2A), p. 686.
39. Wrobel, P., *Our Way: Family, Parish, and Neighborhood in a Polish-American Community*, South Bend: Notre Dame Press, 1979.
40. Rempusheski, V.F., "Caring For Self and Others: Second Generation Polish American Elders in an Ethnic Club," *Journal of Cross-Cultural Gerontology*, 1986, v. 3, pp. 223–271.
41. Ibid., p. 259.
42. Leininger, M.M., "Selected Culture Care Findings of Diverse Cultures Using Culture Care Theory and Ethnomethods," *Culture Care Diversity and Universality: A Theory of Nursing*, M. Leininger, ed., New York: National League for Nursing Press, 1991c, pp. 345–372.
43. Ibid., p. 363.
44. Stasiak, D.B. (Speaker) and M.M. Leininger, (Speaker), *Cultural Care Assessment of American-Polish Informant* (videocassette), Livonia, MI: Madonna University, 1991.
45. Leininger, op. cit., 1989.
46. Bigelow, B., "Marital Assimilation of Polish-Catholic Americans: A Case Study in Syracuse, NY, 1940–1970," *The Professional Geographer*, 1980, v. 32(4), pp. 431–438.
47. Arndt, L.E., *The Bay County Story: From Footpaths to Freeways*, Detroit: Harlo Printing Co., 1982.
48. Leininger, op. cit., 1988, p. 156.
49. Leininger, op. cit., 1988, p. 56.

50. Arndt, op. cit., 1982.
51. Allison, op. cit., 1974.
52. Leininger, op. cit., 1988, p. 156.
53. Leininger, M.M., "The Theory of Culture Care Diversity and Universality," *Culture Care Diversity and Universality: A Theory of Nursing*, M. Leininger, ed., New York: National League for Nursing Press, 1991a, pp. 5–68.
54. Leininger, op. cit., 1991a, p. 48.
55. Leininger, op. cit., 1991a, p. 43.
56. Leininger, op. cit., 1991a, p. 23.
57. Leininger, op. cit., 1991c, p. 363.
58. Leininger, op. cit., 1988.
59. Ibid.
60. Leininger, op. cit., 1991a.
61. Ibid.
62. Ibid.
63. Ibid.
64. Leininger, op. cit., 1991c, p. 363.
65. Leininger, op. cit., 1991c.

24

Finnish Women in Birth: Culture Care Meanings and Practices

Judith Kilmer Lamp

Worldwide, human beings are born into this world in highly favorable or less favorable conditions; transcultural nurses discover factors contributing to these realities. M. LEININGER

For many women, birth in the United States is an experience of professional care management with medical technology perceived to be necessary to ensure a safe, healthy outcome. The ethos of birth has evolved from an experience of trusting a woman's instinctual knowledge and inner folk wisdom to an experience of dependency on the highly trained medical professionals with technical machines to manage the birth for her. Despite all the modern technology, however, the United States continues to fall embarrassingly short of expectations for improved perinatal outcomes, ranking twenty-second among industrialized nations.[1]

In 1992 Finland's perinatal mortality rate was lowest in the world at 6.8 deaths per 1000 live births; the United States rate is almost two-thirds higher.[2] Finland gives high priority to the care and health of its women and children, and the perinatal mortality statistics reflect this. Rajanen[3] states, "To be born in Finland is to have the best chances to survive." The need exists for indepth study of care meanings and practices for women in birth from diverse cultures such as the Finnish culture to explore the underlying reasons for their reproductive health and well-being. This is essential to contribute to transcultural nursing knowledge and for the provision of humanistic care for women in birth that is congruent with their lifeways.

■ Domain of Inquiry

The domain of inquiry for this study was the *generic and professional culture care meanings and practices of Finnish women in birth*. The purpose was to explore and discover the cultural diversities and universalities that exist in the generic and professional care of Finnish women in birth to assist nurses in providing culturally congruent care that will enhance health and well-being of Finnish women and their families.

■ Significance

In the United States the experience of women in birth often reflects a victimization of women with Western medicine's view of birth as a physiological process, but treated as a pathological event. Davis-Floyd[4] has stated that birth in our society is ". . . an experience belonging uniquely to women, yet all too often removed from their control." Women in the United States tend to be viewed as products of the American medical system; moreover, the definition of birth tends to lie within the medical domain. Davis-Floyd further elaborates that ". . . in their well-planned efforts to create an individually satisfying rite of passage, many of these women won battles with doctors on technical and scientific grounds, only to lose in the end to hospital ritual cloaked in scientific guise."[5] These statements attest to the need for this research. The significance of this research for nursing is to provide knowledge of the Finnish culture, to explore and discover the "emic" view of birth from the women of Finland, and to establish for all women a humanistic birth experience that is culturally defined and congruent in meaning. Care for women in birth that reflects and honors Finnish cultural values and beliefs has the potential to assist nurses to provide culturally congruent care that would contribute to the well-being of women worldwide. Moreover, with the advent of transcultural nursing, generic care, as naturalistic and humanistic care, was important to this nurse researcher and clinician in maternal-child health.

Research Questions

The following questions were used to fully explore and discover the domain of inquiry:

1. In what ways do cultural and social structure dimensions influence generic and professional care meanings and practices of Finnish women in birth?
2. What are the generic and professional care meanings and practices of Finnish women in birth?
3. What are the culture care diversities and universalities in the care meanings and practices for Finnish women in birth?
4. What nursing modalities from Leininger's Culture Care Theory can be used to provide culturally congruent care for Finnish women in birth?

Leininger's Culture Care Diversity and Universality Theory of Nursing

The theory that guided this research was the Theory of Culture Care Diversity and Universality by Leininger,[6] who views nursing as a transcultural human care discipline and profession. She states, "Human care is the essence of nursing and a central, dominant, and unifying domain of nursing knowledge and practice."[7] She holds that human care varies transculturally in meanings, expressions, patterns, and symbols and that ultimately discovering the cultural diversities and the universalities about human care worldwide is important if nursing is to serve people as a global profession and discipline.

The theory was used as a framework in this research study to discover the generic and professional culture care meanings and practices of Finnish women in birth. Knowledge gained from this study in Finland can contribute to transcultural nursing as a discipline and profession. Such knowledge can guide nurses in ways to maintain desired practices, to accommodate or negotiate with women in birth, and/or perhaps to repattern or restructure their care to promote women's health and well-being. Only with consideration of these theoretical modes can the goal of culturally congruent care be attained as conceptualized within the Culture Care Theory.

Leininger's[8] Sunrise Model was designed to depict different dimensions of the culture influencing care. It is a cognitive map to discover the influencing dimensions of generic and professional care to arrive at culturally congruent care for the health and well-being of women. Accordingly, each dimension was studied in relation to the stated domain of inquiry and a brief discussion of each follows.

Worldview

In this study, worldview reflected how the Finnish women viewed their world in their homeland, which is linked to geographic and historical features. Iceland, Sweden, Norway, Denmark, and Finland comprise the Nordic countries. These countries have recently taken measures toward consolidation with the European Union (E.U.), a joint European economic arena for the purpose of free exchange of goods and services among its members. Historically, Finland, dominated by other countries and struggling for its own sense of identity and power, voted to become a member of the European Union effective January 1, 1995. The increasing influence of the E.U. can be seen today with the strengthening of the European trade market, the creation of the Euro dollar, and the enhancement of unity among small, diverse cultures. This is the general worldview discussed and held by the informants.

Ethnohistory

The ethnohistory takes into account past to present developments within the country of Finland. Early foreigners who came to the far north considered the Nordic country of Finland a mysterious place. Natural barriers separated Finland from other countries, that is, the sea, the wilderness, and even the language. Finland's isolated position on the periphery of Europe has made Finns a culturally homogenous and socially introspective people.[9]

Sweden occupied parts of western Finland in the 12th century, which led to hostility that continued for over 600 years and was viewed as one endless battle. In twelve major wars in which the eastern border was moved seven times, Sweden fought with Russia over Finland until 1809 when Finland was joined to Russia as an autonomous grand duchy. Under Russian emperor Alexander I (1809–1825), the country was allowed to retain its constitution and Lutheran religion.[10] This later became significant in preserving Finnish cultural values, beliefs, and practices and other social structure features for political independence, which was not gained until 1917.

Language

Finland is a bilingual country with two official languages, Finnish and Swedish. Finnish, which bears no resemblance to any other existing language, is considered the language that reflects the history of social and geographical isolation of the Finns.[11] Even though Finnish and Swedish are considered the first languages of Finland, English is chosen most frequently as a second language and is spoken by a majority of Finns. Today, great emphasis is placed on languages not only because Finland is bilingual but also because it is considered imperative to teach everyone a major world language so that contacts with others in the world are maintained.

Technological Factors

The Finnish people are proud of their highly developed science and technology related to their industries, which have grown tremendously as evidenced by developed enterprise parks that work in close cooperation with the universities to advance their high-level technological products and services.[12] The Finnish company Nokia is Europe's largest and the world's second largest mobile phone manufacturer. Nokia telephone and paging systems are among the best-selling products in the world. These technological advances are an integral component of Finnish health care and have influenced health care practices for Finnish women as well.

Religious and Philosophical Factors

Finland's cultural heritage has deep roots in religion and philosophical factors that influence the people's lives and care even though only 2% of Finns regularly attend church services.[13] Nearly 90% of all Finns are Evangelical-Lutheran; only 2% are Finnish-Orthodox. According to Rajanen,[14] the church in Finland does not depend on Sunday contributions as the church is state supported. Lutheran philosophy supports family planning options and considers human sexuality as an integral and natural component of one's health and well-being. This philosophy was evident with the women in this study.

Kinship and Social Factors

Family life in Finland is highly valued, which was evident in the traditions of family holidays at their cottages in the country. The lifeways of families include active involvement in open-air theaters, festivals, exhibitions, and concerts. Adherence to family customs and traditions is prevalent and strongly upheld, as was evident with the families in this study.

Cultural Values and Lifeways

The Finnish culture has many distinct cultural values rooted in the lifeways of the people. The major cultural values of maintaining Finnish pride and traditionalism was evident in literature, art, entertainment, and sports competitions. Both Finnish theater and music have received international recognition. Finnish art, architecture, and design are world famous, with Alvo Aalto's Finlandia Hall in Helsinki being a good example. The many Olympic achievements have helped contribute to the nation's proud identity.

Cultural value related to the enjoyment of leisure activities such as summer cottages, boats, and saunas are an integral part of the Finnish lifeways. The sauna has been a part of Finnish culture for the past 2000 years and remains as important evidence of the cultural value of maintaining proper rituals and decorum, especially to support the people's belief in folk and modern healing modes. The Finnish sauna and its origins are linked with the cultural value of cleanliness. It is physically and emotionally therapeutic and because of the feeling of euphoria that it elicits, the Finnish people believe in its healthful benefit. It has been practiced as a cultural lifeway for thousands of years as a healing and caring practice for self and others, even as the place of birth for many Finns.[15] The use of the sauna by the Finnish women in this study was especially evident to relieve minor discomforts of pregnancy and promote cleanliness and feelings of well-being.

Political and Legal Factors

Finland is a republic and a multiparty (eight distinct parties), democratic country. Finnish women were the first European women to gain the right to vote in 1906. There are more women in the Finnish Parliament than in any legislative body in the world: 67, (or 34%) of the 200 in the Finnish Parliament are women, six are nurses.[16] Finland has long recognized the equality of women in terms of employment, as well as political participation. Finnish women are held in high esteem having reached success in the professions requiring intellectual skill instead of physical strength.

Having no military alliance, Finland is a neutral country engaged in policy aimed at peaceful coexistence. Although Finland has fought 42 wars with Russia and lost every one, the country remains stoically independent, perhaps attributable to their long-cherished sense of national identity. The nation has been defeated in war, but has never been occupied, and is now one of the most democratic and prosperous nations in the world.

Economic Factors

Finland is one of the richest countries in the world, but it is costly to live there. The forest, wood processing, and metal engineering industries are leading Finnish enterprises. Finland is the world's second largest exporter of paper after Canada.[17] The shipbuilding industry is one of the most successful in the world. Shipping is necessary year round, and Finland is the world's largest manufacturer of icebreakers, which are crucial to keeping frozen harbors open—the people's gates to the world.[18]

Finnish people sustain and value a high standard of living and support comprehensive health care and welfare programs.[19] Income tax is progressive, that is, as earnings rise, so do personal and property taxes. Municipal health centers provide almost free medical care and laboratory tests. Sickness insurance and voluntary insurance plans reimburse a large part of the charges for private health care. The women in this study, all with variable incomes, received comprehensive and free health care services throughout their childbearing years.

Educational Factors

In Finland education is a duty, not a privilege, which supports their marked cultural value of learning and being productive. This philosophy dates back to an old church law of 1686 that forbade marriage to anyone who could not read, thereby forcing those who wanted to marry to seek schooling first. The Finnish people regard education as vital to democracy. More than 18% of the national budget is allocated for education as compared to 8% for health, 6.9% for housing, and 5% for defense.[20] Finland has one of the highest literacy rates in the world at 99%. Education is compulsory and free and is supported by the government with free tuition, books, and school lunches during the first 9 years of comprehensive education.[21] Upper secondary school lasts 3 years and ends with matriculation exams that allow those interested and qualified students entrance to one of the 17 universities in the country. The women in this study all valued education and had at least completed upper secondary schools.

Environmental Context

Finland is a sparsely populated country of 5 million people. Environmentally, Finland is known for it hundreds of thousands of lakes. The landscape varies from plains to a rolling lake district in central and eastern Finland and the fells of Lapland. There are few mountains but many forests, which is Finland's main natural resource. Although Finland lies in the same latitude as Alaska, the climate is similar to the northern United States because of the warming effect of the Gulf Stream. Light is very important to the Finnish people because of its limited time during the winter months; clean air and water are also highly valued. Many Finnish children nap in their prams that are set outside each day through the year, except for days with temperatures below 10 degrees Celsius. Even hospital windows are opened for fresh air and ventilation to aid in physical and emotional healing. The women in this study greatly valued outdoor activities involving their families and young children.

Literature Review

As early as 1955, Dr. Leininger began her pioneering efforts to develop a theoretical foundation for the field of transcultural nursing. As founder and leader of this specialized field of nursing knowledge, she states that the globalization of transcultural nursing has become a moral, human, professional, educational, and practice mandate.[22] Andrews,[23] Andrews and Boyle,[24] and Horn[25] have also emphasized the need for transcultural nursing knowledge and care practices that reflect the dynamic changes that are taking place not only in the United States in terms of health care reform but internationally as well, with new nations emerging and old ones either undergoing evolution or disappearing altogether. These authors, as well as others, support the need for building transcultural nursing knowledge to provide culturally congruent care for all people worldwide.

Jordan,[26] Davis-Floyd,[27] and Michaelson[28] have asserted that cross-cultural investigation of childbirth caring practices would be desirable because the range of human physiological and behavioral variability can be examined. They also hold that appreciation of organized female networks can be improved (since birth in most societies is women's "business") and that a better understanding of the birth process could be gained. Birth in the United States has been increasingly scrutinized, undergoing many changes that are the result of growing recognition of the position, competencies, and caring needs of women.

Brown[29] emphasized the importance of nurses exploring the birth experience cross-culturally in her statement, ". . . when nurses work with women of another culture, it is important to understand their beliefs and value systems . . . there are many benefits to be derived from looking at the similarities and differences between how various cultures view and handle the childbearing cycle." Understanding the beliefs and values of women in birth is a great challenge for transcultural nurses caring for persons from diverse and similar cultural backgrounds.

Emphasis in Morgan's[30] transcultural nursing study was on the culture care values, beliefs, and practices of the American Hare Krishnas related to pregnancy and childbirth. Morgan[31] also completed a comparative study of prenatal care of urban and rural African-American women using the Culture Care Theory. Her findings revealed that culture care included protection, presence, and sharing; the social structure factors of spirituality, kinship, and economics were important; health care in the prenatal period was valued; and their folk health care beliefs and practices influenced well-being.

Bohay's transcultural study[32] was focused on discovering pregnancy and birth care of Ukrainian-Americans within Leininger's Theory of Culture Care. She found that expressions of care were embedded in the social structure factors of religion, worldview, and kinship. Kendall[33] conducted an exploratory, descriptive ethnographic study of socialization practices and family structure that revealed the role of women in the Iranian culture. She studied social structure factors such as historical, religious, economic, political, and familial dimensions that are included in Leininger's Sunrise Model. She found that nurses need to provide nursing care with respect for a cultural group's needs, beliefs, and values.

In Kay's classic anthropological study of human birth,[34] she claimed that it is important for professional caregivers to be aware of not only what the cultural diversities in birth are but also to understand the source of their variation. Finn's transcultural, phenomenological study[35] focused on the discovery of the meanings of care and noncare for European-American women in birth. She discovered generic and professional, caring and noncaring meanings and expressions and found cultural diversities between professional nursing care and generic care.

For Finnish women, the understanding of care meanings and practices is enhanced when examining Finland's quality health care system. Prenatal clinics have been part of Finnish maternity care for decades. Educating the general public regarding the importance of early prenatal care is a priority. Every pregnant woman is entitled to a maternity benefit if she visits maternity health services before the fifth month of the pregnancy. The maternal benefit is granted either in cash or in the form of a maternity pack (worth twice the amount of cash). The amount of maternity, paternity, and parent's governmental allowance is calculated according to the earned income (about 80% of annual earnings). In 1973 a law on child care was enacted that pays an allowance for every child in Finland until the child is 18 years of age.

Child day care is modern and subsidized by the Finnish government. Nearly half of Finland's children are enrolled in public day care centers. Progressive laws guarantee 10 months of fully paid leave for one parent that can be extended for either mother or father, whomever stays home with the baby.[36] These laws allow a new parent to stay at home in the crucial early months of a child's life. These laws and benefits reflect the high value that the culture has for strengthening the new family through quality health care. The general aim of health policy in Finland is to ensure universal access to care so that economic factors do not prevent the appropriate use of health services.[37]

Ethnonursing and Audiovisual Methods

The ethnonursing method was used to discover the care meanings and practices of Finnish women in birth. This is a "... qualitative research method using naturalistic, open discovery, and inductively derived emic modes and processes with diverse strategies, techniques, and enabling guides to document, describe, understand, and interpret the people's meanings, experiences, symbols, and other related aspects bearing on actual or potential nursing phenomena."[38] This method has been developed to fit the Culture Care Theory and permits the discovery of generic and professional dimensions of care in an inductively holistic manner.[39] Professional care meanings and practices of the nurse and generic care meanings and practices of the women in birth were rigorously studied to discover, describe, and analyze holistic care for Finnish women in birth.

With the ethnonursing method, key informants are central to obtain the in-depth, emic, qualitative knowledge of the domain of inquiry. According to Leininger,[40] key informants are "held to reflect the norms, values, beliefs, and general lifeways of the culture and usually are interested in and willing to participate in the study." The selection criteria for the ten key informants were as follows:

1. Identified themselves to be of Finnish heritage
2. Pregnant in their last trimester
3. Had an expected date of delivery within the time frame of the research
4. Planned for the birth at the research study site
5. Voluntarily consented to participate in the study

The selection criteria for the thirty-two general informants, identified as generic caregivers, were as follows:

1. Nonprofessional individual(s) such as family members or significant others who provided direct care to key informants during their birth experiences
2. Professional nurse(s) who provided direct care to key informants
3. Voluntarily consented to participate in the study

Another research method employed was the use of audiovisual media, that is, taking photographs to develop a visual essay of each of the birth experiences, as well as taping informants' verbal expressions. Audiovisual refers to various messages communicated to humans and others in different ways through all the senses. Visual expression through the use of photography was an important means to closely examine the in-depth feelings and emotions communicated by the women in their birth experiences and was used to discover and understand their care meanings and practices.

The advantages of using this method along with the ethnonursing research method were many. This researcher found that the photographs provided highly accurate documentation of not only the physical life event of birth but the psychological, social, and cultural dimensions as well. Complex insights into human care expressions were revealed in recurrent care patterns and practices, which were reflected in the photographs and audiotapes. The reality of the environmental context and its influence on the birth experiences became evident along with the sequence of care actions that were discovered when analyzing the photographs.

Perhaps the greatest advantage of using this method was to document the actual birth experiences in a naturalistic, humanistic way with the human expressions and responses as captured by the photographs. This visual record offered an invaluable means by which care meanings and practices were discovered and studied with the informants. Photographs in transcultural nursing research are valuable to learn about the expressions and the process of human care and lifeways of diverse cultures.[41]

Qualitative criteria to substantiate the findings that were developed and used by Leininger[42] and Lincoln and Guba[43] were essential to use for this qualitative investigation. The qualitative criteria that were used by the researcher were credibility, confirmability, meaning-in-context, recurrent patterning, saturation, and transferability.

 ## Research Method with Enablers

The ethnonursing research method with Enablers was developed with the Theory of Culture Care as a guide to tease out and explicate data from the naturalistic environment of the informants. These Enablers developed by Leininger included the following:

1. Sunrise Model
2. Inquiry Guide for Ethnodemographic Information
3. Sequenced Phases of Observation-Participation-Reflection Enabler
4. Stranger to Trusted Friend Enabler Guide
5. Phases of Ethnonursing Analysis for Qualitative Data
6. Generic and Professional Care Guide

A Coding Data System for the Leininger, Templin, and Thompson Field Research Ethnoscript was used along with the Leininger-Templin-Thompson Ethnoscript Qualitative Software.[44] The researcher also developed her own Enablers: Observation Enabler for Women in Birth, Inquiry Enabler for Women in Birth, and the Ethnodemographic Inquiry Enabler for use with women during and following birth. These guides were essential as part of the rigorous ethnonursing method to study the domain of inquiry and obtain a full and systematic account from the informants about their care meanings and practices related to birth.

 ## Research Findings

Using Leininger's four phases of data analysis,[45] five major themes, four universal and one diverse, were discovered. Two of the themes reflected universal generic care meanings and practices, and two reflected universal professional care meanings and practices. A final theme reflected cultural diversity as found in the Theory of Culture Care. The findings from this study, which follow, are presented with the actual photographs to communicate visual data with the written verbatim.

Universal Theme One   Generic care meanings and practices meant *comfort care with physical presence and touch* from family.

The observational descriptors included holding, kissing, whispering softly, massage of the back and arms, wiping of the face with a cool washcloth, and holding hands (see Color Insert 15).

Comfort Care Patterns:

1. Comfort care meant physical presence, being near, being with the key informant during birth.
2. Comfort care meant touching or stroking, massage, holding, whispering softly to the women during birth.

> "Although it's impossible, it felt like that he takes away some part of the pain."

> "I'm here to take care of you."

Universal Theme Two   Generic care meanings and practices meant *protective care with empathy and trust* from family.

Protective Care Patterns:

1. Protective care meant the support provided to the women in birth by family offering empathy or sympathy (see Color Insert 16)
2. Protective care meant the trust and safety offered to the women in birth by family.

> "That was one thing very good and I think that he was there very helpful . . . I know I can trust him."

> "He was a good help . . . it maybe looked like he didn't do anything but I thought it so that when he is near, it is safer for me and when I can hold him it helps me to bear this pain."

Universal Theme Three   Professional care meanings and practices meant *ritualized care to build respect and trust* with the women in birth.

The observational descriptors included nursing rituals such as orientation, assessment, fetal monitoring, providing pain relief with massage, nutritional support, suggesting position changes, medication, etc. (see Figure 24.1).

Ritualized Care Patterns:

1. Ritualized care by the nurse meant continuous presence with the women during birth.
2. Ritualized care by the nurse meant building respect for and trust with the women during birth.

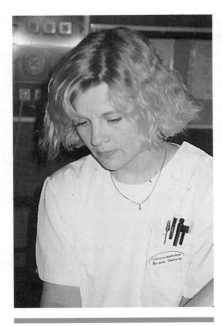

Figure 24.1
Ritualized care with trusted presence:
"It was so beautiful."

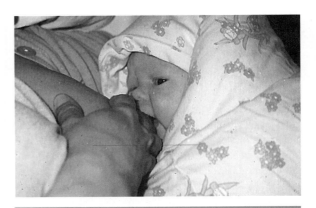

Figure 24.2
Anticipatory care: "It was positive, so they asked me
could I give them roses or branches, and I said roses."

"She was there with me . . . like family . . . all the
things she did, she wasn't hesitating . . . she's
the only nurse and know what happened
beginning to end."

**Universal Theme Four   Professional care meanings
and practices meant *anticipatory care with educational instruction and advocacy* for the women in
birth**.

The observational descriptors included offering instruction on breathing patterns or pushing techniques,
teaching pelvic rock, use of the birth stool, etc. (see
Figure 24.2).

Anticipatory Care Patterns:

1. Anticipatory care meant offering instruction and
explanations in predicting needs of the key informant
during birth.
2. Anticipatory care meant advocating for the key
informant by offering choices in meeting the needs of
the key informant during birth.

"Her suggestions very helped me, please try this
one and if I say that no, no, it doesn't feel good

and I can't be here, she said there's not need to
be, you can do what you want."

**Diverse Theme Five   Cultural care meant respect
for differences in expression of *satisfaction* with the
birth experience**.

Observational descriptors included facial expressions that displayed disappointment from expectations
that were not recognized or joy with the satisfaction
expressed (see Figure 24.3)

Culture Care Diversity Patterns:

1. Culture care is respect for differential expressions.
2. Culture care is expression of satisfaction or
dissatisfaction with the birth experience.

"I don't think that the nurses or doctors failed but
more like on that side . . . none of my wishes are
taken into account."

"I thought that the pain wouldn't be so hard but I
feel it was so awesome and that I am quite
tough."

Discussion of Findings

This study was significant, from a transcultural nursing
perspective, to discover care meanings and practices of
Finnish women in birth and to use this knowledge to
provide culturally congruent care in a competent and

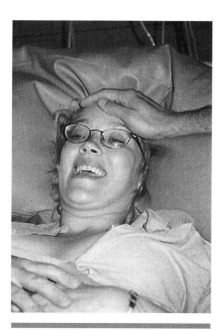

Figure 24.3
Respectful care as satisfaction: "It was
wonderful."

humanistic manner. Although birth is a universal human event, care diversity is often discovered within
the culture itself, which was found in this study. The
generic care constructs of comfort and protection as
care along with the professional care constructs of
ritualized and anticipatory care were evident and meaningful to the Finnish women in birth. An in-depth understanding of the unique qualities of these constructs
was not fully recognized until the Finnish cultural and
social structure dimensions were discovered. Achieving culturally congruent care, based on full and in-depth
understanding of the universalities and diversities of
culture care, enable transcultural nurses to achieve a
greater sense of health and well-being for women in
birth.

In this transcultural nursing study, the ethnonursing research method was used in conjunction with
the audiovisual method to discover in-depth generic
(emic) and professional (etic) care of Finnish women
in birth. Humanistic care was found to be essential for
beneficial, congruent care for Finnish women that respected their cultural care values and needs and that
was reflected in both the generic and professional care

practices. Generic care meanings and practices were
discovered and integrated with the nurses' professional
modes of decisions and actions to achieve care that was
congruent with the culture care values and needs of
Finnish women in birth. Leininger's[46] three care modes
to guide nursing judgement, decisions, and actions of
1) cultural care preservation/maintenance, 2) cultural
care accommodation/negotiation, and/or 3) cultural
care repatterning/restructuring were used in this study.
This researcher's hunches were substantiated that both
generic and professional care would be essential to provide meaningful and culturally congruent nursing care
that would lead to a healthy and satisfying birth with
few cultural conflicts. Specific ways to provide culturally congruent care, and thus contribute to a woman's
sense of health and well-being, are presented.

Culture Care Preservation
and/or Maintenance

Transcultural nurses need to use culture care knowledge for decisions and actions to preserve or maintain
care meanings and practices. Each of the thematic findings of this study is essential to help care for Finnish
women in birth and preserve or maintain generic care
meanings and practices, especially as related to comfort
care and protective care. For example, Finnish women
expressed the value of and need for having generic
or family care providers offering presence, touch, and
massage throughout their birth experiences. The nurse
was also available to facilitate comfort and protective
care expressed by her presence, standing by her side, offering touch and support for the woman throughout the
birth experience. Having a nurse and/or family member or significant other offering care as empathy, trust,
and assurance of safety was found to be valued by the
Finnish women.

Professional nursing care decisions and actions of
the Finnish nurses included ritualized care and anticipatory care. Performing the traditional nursing care rituals provided presence and built trust with the women
and were held to be meaningful and satisfying to them.
The nurses guided the women through their birth experiences, predicting and preparing the women for what
to expect as their labors progressed, which was anticipatory care. In addition, the care practices of nurses
offering information and explanations of procedures,
progress in labor, etc., and allowing the women choices

in anticipation of their needs during their birth experiences were important and should be preserved. Demonstrating advocacy for the women as a care practice encouraged a humanistic birth experience that was respectful of their cultural values.

Transcultural nurses who provide culturally congruent care need to maintain and preserve the women's kinship and family relationships as this is important in the caring process. For example, as discovered in this study, planning care that included family members, and siblings to attend the birth and/or visit soon afterward during the hospital stay is caring, in that their need to be together during this important life event is respected. Since health care in Finland is a social, political, and economic right with concomitant responsibilities, transcultural and other nurses would need to ensure that these rights are upheld in their caring actions and decisions. Social equity and universal access to health care upholds the culture's commitment to improving both the standard and distribution of health care. Finnish nurses need to act politically to eradicate any future disparities in health between different cultural groups as they immigrate to Finland and to preserve the universal and comprehensive health services that their culture values.

Culture Care Accommodation and/or Negotiation

Events occurred during the women's birth experiences that necessitated that the professional caregivers accommodate care practices of generic comfort and protective care. Finnish nurses performed care rituals incorporating the generic caregivers (husbands/significant others) into their professional teaching and care practices. Finnish nurses taught massage and the application of pressure to the husbands to accommodate the women's comfort care needs. In two of the birth experiences, Finnish nurses offered care to the women whose generic caregivers (husbands or family members) were not present. The nurse's care was described by the women as valuable in meeting their needs for comfort and protective care.

Failure to negotiate or accommodate care according to Finnish women's values could lead to cultural conflict and nontherapeutic outcomes. For example, the nurse, with a holding knowledge of the Finnish culture, would understand that Finnish women need to use the sauna to promote relaxation and cleansing during pregnancy. Despite current recommendations to avoid extremely high temperatures during pregnancy, the nurse could negotiate with the woman to adjust her daily ritual by sitting on the lower level of the sauna for shorter periods where temperatures are less extreme. Cultural care knowledge and practices for Finnish women need to be accommodated to provide safe, culturally congruent care that is respectful of Finnish lifeways.

Culture Care Repatterning and/or Restructuring

Another nursing care modality is repatterning and/or restructuring. In this study the Finnish nurses were found to have extensive holding knowledge about the Finnish cultural lifeways to guide them to provide culturally congruent care. The nurses' care demonstrated respect for Finnish women's beliefs regarding Finland and the various cultural and social structure dimensions that influence their care values. Finnish women expect care that is based on social equity and care that is universal for all. Educational, political, and economic dimensions of the Finnish culture support the health care system. Because of Finland's past history of domination and turmoil, Finnish women are proud of their country's independence. They show their pride by being obedient and dutiful to individuals in authority, that is, professional caregivers. Finnish women hold kinship and family relationships in high regard. For example, when Finnish women decide to plan for a family, they expect care that includes their significant others. They expect free prenatal care throughout their pregnancies, which is typical of the socialized health care system and which reflects the Finnish culture's value of universal health care. Finnish women expect to prepare for their birth experiences by participating in classes, tours, and reading resource materials, which reflects the Finnish cultural value of education. They also anticipate their care would be free and accessible. They anticipate their care would be supported economically and politically in their decision to remain home with their young children for a guaranteed 10-month leave. They anticipate the government-subsidized day care with a monthly child allowance and full educational benefits once they choose to return to work. These contribute to health and well-being for families in Finland—one of the healthiest populations in the world.

Many health care systems throughout the world are different and would not offer these care practices. Some care institutions in the United States need to restructure and repattern their health care to provide care that is accessible, meaningful, and beneficial, especially to the women seeking care during their birth experiences. In the United States, in-depth reexamination of priorities in health care that reflect the values of social equity and kinship would be necessary to achieve a similar holistic birth experience for women in the United States. The current health care structure of the United States is problem oriented, focusing on more technology and more specialists to treat disease rather than promote health. Prenatal care that is not only free and accessible, but a human right, would significantly reduce health risks, low birth weight, preterm births, and other problems through early identification and prevention, thereby reducing health care costs and perinatal mortality/morbidity rates. In addition, nursing care in the United States could use the Finnish model of nurse midwifery care, in that, professional care, which includes ritualized care integrated with generic care, could build mutual respect and trust between nurses and women in birth. Anticipatory care with educational instruction and advocacy in the United States could lead to a greater sense of well-being for women in birth. These findings, with the holistic, naturalistic care meanings and practices discovered, could contribute to health and well-being for women and their families and reduce perinatal mortality in the United States. This study demonstrates the value that transcultural nursing comparative studies can have in ongoing and future consideration in health care planning and evaluation.

Conclusion

In general, this study substantiated Leininger's Culture Care Theory and lead to practical outcomes to provide culturally congruent care. The contributions to the discipline of transcultural nursing related to women in birth are growing, including those studies by Bohay (Ukrainian-American), Finn (European-American), Morgan (African-American), Kendall (Iranian), and

others. Contributing to transcultural and other areas of nursing using the ethnonursing and audiovisual methods, this research is essential to advance nursing knowledge and practice. Most importantly, the ethnonursing discovery method, emphasizing the naturalistic approach with the Culture Care Theory, is most significant to tease out covert care meanings and practices of generic and professional care. The theory and methods offer an exciting commitment in building a worldwide body of transcultural nursing knowledge. The need exists to discover and understand women of diverse cultures throughout the world, to explore their experiences of birth, and to know what culture care meanings and practices offer them the greatest sense of health and well-being. An understanding of women and their birth experiences, focusing on their generic and professional care meanings and practices, is essential to guide nurses in discovering new insights, to reaffirm valued care constructs, and to avoid cultural conflict. Far more use of the Culture Care Theory with the ethnonursing and audiovisual methods is needed to discover the universalities and diversities related to care and birth that exist worldwide. This research is crucial to provide for culturally congruent care for women and care that is essential and meaningful in a multicultural world.

References

1. Rice, D., "Health Status and National Health Priorities," in *The Nation's Health*, P. Lee and C. Estes, eds., Boston: Jones and Bartlett Publishers, 1994, pp. 45–58.
2. Ministry of Social Affairs and Health, *Women's Health Profile: Finland* (prepared for the Lifestyles and Health Department, World Health Organization, Regional Office for Europe). Copenhagen: Denmark, 1996.
3. Rajanen, A., *Of Finnish Ways*, New York, NY: Harper & Row Publishers, 1981, p. 95.
4. Davis-Floyd, R., "Pregnancy and Cultural Confusion: Contradictions in Socialization," in *Cultural Constructions of "Woman,"* P. Kolenda, ed., Salem, WI: Sheffield Publishing, 1988, p. 9.
5. Ibid., p. 12.
6. Leininger, M., "Ethnonursing: A Research Method with Enablers to Study the Theory of Culture Care," in *Culture Care Diversity and Universality: A Theory of Nursing*, M. Leininger, ed., New York:

National League for Nursing Press, 1991a, pp. 73–118.

7. Leininger, M., *Culture Care Diversity and Universality: A Theory of Nursing*, New York: National League for Nursing Press, 1991, p. 31.

8. Leininger, op. cit., 1991a.

9. Sauri, S., *Find Out About Finland*, Helsinki: Otava Publishing Company, Ltd., 1992.

10. Ibid.

11. Woolnough, K., "In Defense of Greenness and Finns Who Speak Swedish," in *Finland*, D. Taylor-Wilkie, ed., Boston: Houghton Mifflin Co., 1994, p. 88, 111.

12. Sauri, op. cit., 1992.

13. Rajanen, op. cit., 1981.

14. Ibid.

15. Borjia, L., "Secrets of the Sauna," in *Finland*, D. Taylor-Wilkie, ed., Boston: Houghton Mifflin Co., 1994, p. 223.

16. Central Statistical Office of Finland, *Basic Information on Finland*, 1992, pp. 1–16.

17. Woolnough, op. cit., 1994.

18. Nickels, S., "Intrepid Travel," in *Finland*, D. Taylor-Wilkie, ed., Boston: Houghton Mifflin Co., 1994, p. 117.

19. Lewis, J., "The Two Wars," in *Finland*, D. Taylor-Wilkie, ed., Boston: Houghton Mifflin Co., 1994, p. 51.

20. Rajanen, op. cit., 1981.

21. National Account of the Research Institute of the Finnish Economy, *Basic Information on Finland*, 1992, pp. 1–16.

22. Leininger, M., *Transcultural Nursing: Concepts, Theories, Research, and Practices*, 2nd ed., Columbus, OH: McGraw Hill and Greyden Press, 1995.

23. Andrews, M., "Cultural Perspectives on Nursing in the 21st Century," *Journal of Professional Nursing*, 1992, 8(1), pp. 7–15.

24. Andrews, M. and J. Boyle, *Transcultural Concepts in Nursing Care*, 3rd ed., Philadelphia: Lippincott, 1995.

25. Horn, B., "Cultural Concepts of Postpartal Care," *Journal of Transcultural Nursing*, 1990, 2(1), pp. 48–51. (Reprinted from *Nursing and Health Care*, 1978, 2(3), pp. 516–517, 526–527.)

26. Jordan, B., *Birth in Four Cultures*, Prospect Heights, IL: Waveland Press, Inc., 1993.

27. Davis-Floyd, R., *Birth as an American Rite of Passage*, Berkeley: University of California Press, 1992.

28. Michaelson, K., *Childbirth in America: Anthropological Perspectives*, South Hadley, MA: Bergin & Garvey Publishers, Inc., 1988.

29. Brown, M., "A Cross-Cultural Look at Pregnancy, Labor, and Delivery," *Journal of Obstetrical, Gynecological, and Neonatal Nursing*, September/October 1976, pp. 35–38.

30. Morgan, M., "Pregnancy and Childbirth Beliefs and Practices of American Hare Krishna Devotees Within Transcultural Nursing," *Journal of Transcultural Nursing*, 1992, 4(1), pp. 5–10.

31. Morgan, M., "Prenatal Care of African-American Women in Selected USA Urban and Rural Cultural Contexts Conceptualized Within Leininger's Cultural Care Theory," unpublished doctoral dissertation. Wayne State University: Detroit, MI, 1994.

32. Bohay, I., "Culture Care Meanings and Experiences of Pregnancy and Childbirth of Ukrainians," in *Culture Care Diversity and Universality: A Theory of Nursing*, M. Leininger, ed., New York: National League for Nursing Press, 1991.

33. Kendall, K., "Maternal and Child Nursing in an Iranian Village," in *Transcultural Nursing: Concepts, Theories, and Practices*, M. Leininger, ed., Columbus: Greyden Press, 1994.

34. Kay, M., *Anthropology of Human Birth*, Philadelphia: F.A. Davis Company, 1982.

35. Finn, J., "Caring in Birthing: Experiences of Professional and Generic Care," unpublished doctoral dissertation, Wayne State University: Detroit, MI, 1993.

36. Peltonen, A., "The Welfare State," in *Finland*, D. Taylor-Wilkie, ed., Boston: Houghton Mifflin Co., 1994, p. 67.

37. Ministry of Social Affairs and Health, op. cit., 1996.

38. Leininger, M., *Qualitative Research Methods in Nursing*, Orlando: Grune & Stratton, 1985, p. 79.

39. Leininger, op. cit., 1991a.

40. Leininger, op. cit., 1991, p. 110.

41. Leininger, op. cit., 1985.

42. Leininger, op. cit., 1991.

43. Lincoln, Y. and E. Guba, *Naturalistic Inquiry*, Newbury Park: Sage Publications, 1985.

44. Leininger, op. cit., 1991a.

45. Leininger, M., *Transcultural Nursing: Concepts, Theories, Research, and Practices*, 2nd ed., Columbus, OH: McGraw-Hill and Greyden Press, 1995.

46. Leininger, op. cit., 1991a.

CHAPTER 25

Taiwanese Americans Culture Care Meanings and Expressions

Lenny Chiang-Hanisko

Discovering diverse cultures and their care needs expands nurses knowledge and provides better ways to care for people.[1]

Discovering care meanings and expressions in diverse cultures remains a major research area that has been spearheaded by Leininger since the 1950s. This chapter is focused on the author's research study to discover the care meanings in Taiwan and with Taiwanese living in the United States. As a Taiwanese-American, this area was of great interest to me after being born and living in Taiwan and then coming to live and work in the United States.

Taiwan is different from mainland China in many ways. It is a small island, while China is a large country with a large population. With a history of colonization, Taiwan has been shaped through the centuries by many outside influences, whereas China has remained relatively isolated. Taiwan also has its own native language and is quite advanced industrially and technologically, whereas China remains struggling with its economy and large population. The two countries are historically, linguistically, economically, and culturally different. These facts need to be recognized and understood at the outset by health care providers to provide culturally based care that is congruent with the Taiwanese cultural values, beliefs, and practices.

Domain of Inquiry

The central domain of inquiry of this research study was to describe, analyze, and explain care meanings and expressions of Taiwanese Americans in a large Midwestern city in the United States.

Rationale for the Study

Leininger[2] states that one of the greatest challenges in nursing is to know and understanding people in their familiar or naturalistic living contexts in different places in the world. Each year, thousands of immigrants from all over the world arrive in the United States, and the Taiwanese are one of the large immigrant groups that have come to the United States. These immigrants have brought their homeland values, beliefs, and lifeways, including health and illness practices. Still today, Taiwanese immigrants practice their traditional cultural lifeways after long periods of residing in the United States. Such transcultural practices need to be studied and addressed by transcultural nurses. The ethnonursing method was purposefully chosen to discover largely unknown care and culture knowledge of the Taiwanese who have lived in America.[3] The Theory of Culture Care that fits with the ethnonursing method was also chosen for this study. To date, there has been no transcultural or health study focused on Taiwanese American cultural care meanings and expressions. Hence, this study was important to obtain knowledge about Taiwanese American culture care lifeways.

Research Questions

Four research questions were developed to guide this study:

1. What are the meanings and expressions of care of Taiwanese Americans?

2. What culture care values are held by Taiwanese Americans today?
3. In what ways do social structure factors, environment context, cultural lifeways, and generic (folk) and professional practices influence the care of Taiwanese Americans?
4. What nursing decisions and actions of Leininger's three modalities are important in the care of Taiwanese Americans?

Significance of the Study

This study is important as it can provide largely unknown transcultural nursing knowledge of the Taiwanese culture with Leininger's Culture Care Theory and ethnonursing research method.[4] Nursing in a pluralistic society in the United States and in other countries provides wonderful opportunities to work with culturally different individuals. Because cultural beliefs, values, and lifeways can have a strong influence on human care meanings and desired services, identifying cultural differences and similarities is essential to plan and implement specific, effective, and congruent nursing care practices, which is the goal of the Culture Care Theory.[5] It is also important to assess the extent of the traditional cultural practices by individuals and the groups of a culture to help them preserve or maintain the traditional beliefs and practices that they value.

Theoretical Framework

The Theory of Culture Care Diversity and Universality guided the researcher to discover the culture values and beliefs of Taiwanese people and to analyze the theory with respect to the worldview, social structure, ethnohistory factors, language used, and environmental context of the Taiwanese informants.[6] Leininger's Sunrise Enabler served as a holistic cognitive guide to identify specific and interrelated cultural care dimensions of the people, especially as related to the domain of inquiry. The above social-structure dimensions were important to get a holistic and meaningful picture of Taiwanese as it relates to their care and health. This researcher holds that emic folk and etic professional care knowledge can significantly influence human care and health practice with Taiwanese Americans. Identifying and understanding the meanings and expressions of care

and then using this knowledge were essential to get an accurate and holistic knowledge related to the domain of inquiry. Most importantly, Leininger's theory focuses on three modes of care, which the researcher explored in-depth with the worldviews, language, social structure factors, ethnohistorical aspects, and the environmental context of Taiwanese Americans in data collection and analysis.[7]

Research Method

The ethnonursing research method was used for this in-depth qualitative research study with Taiwanese Americans. The ethnonursing method was selected to obtain specific knowledge about caring, health, and folk and professional care expressions of Taiwanese Americans. The goal of the ethnonursing method is to discover largely unknown nursing phenomena and knowledge about the domain of inquiry under study to arrive at culturally congruent care practices.[8] The method provides a systematic way to carefully document, describe, and explain the care phenomena and their meanings as related to cultural care, health, and well-being or to help in the dying process.

A mini ethnonursing study was chosen because the domain of inquiry is focused specifically on culture care values, meanings, experiences of care, worldview, social structure, cultural values, and environmental factors influencing folk and professional health care among selected Taiwanese Americans. The study was conducted over a 7-month period of data collection in a large urban city in the midwestern United States. This mini study provided the researcher with an opportunity to discover specific care meanings and expressions within a short period compared with a maxi study that often takes considerably longer and covers even more on the social structure factors in depth and breadth.[9]

Selection of Informants

The six key and twelve general informants were purposely selected for this study. They were individuals who were selected according to specific research criteria. The key informants were knowledgeable about and willing to address the domain of inquiry and share their life experiences. The key informants were chosen as knowledgeable representatives of the Taiwanese

American population with their willingness to provide in-depth ideas about the domain of inquiry during several interviews and home visits. The key informants provided particularly rich data about their beliefs and practices bearing on the research questions and the domain of inquiry. The informants enjoyed talking about culture and care practices. In contrast, the general informants were not as fully knowledgeable as the key informants about the domain of inquiry, but they had general reflective knowledge to share and were representative of the Taiwanese Americans. Their ideas were important and provided information to reflect on key informant ideas to see if they had relevance or were generally Taiwanese public knowledge.[10] The criteria used to select key informants were as follows:

1. Born and educated in Taiwan and migrated to the United States
2. Twenty-one years old or older
3. Lived or worked in the United States for 5 or more years
4. Knowledgeable about the central cultural institutions related to the domain of inquiry
5. Willing to participate in the study for two or three interviews lasting approximately 3 hours each

The criteria for selecting general informants were as follows:

1. Born and educated in Taiwan and migrated to the United States
2. Twenty-one years old or older
3. Lived or worked in the United States for at least 5 or more years
4. Willing to be interviewed for approximately 2 hours on one occasion

Keeping with the ethnonursing method, six key and twelve general informants were purposefully selected for this study from a large urban city in the midwestern United States. There were eleven females and seven males. The age range of the key and general informants was 28 to 86 years with an average of 53.7 years. Ages of the key informants ranged from 46 to 86 years with an average of 56.16 years. Ages of general informants ranged from 28 to 68 years with an average of 49.25 years. All informants had a length of residence in the United States from 5 to 27 years with an average of 16.1 years, with the majority living in the United

States less than 20 years. The key informants had lived in the United States for a longer period than the general informants. The immigration of Taiwanese people to the United States was a recent development with most arriving in the mid 1970s. Ten informants were parents whose children also immigrated to the United States. Among these parents, 60% came to this country after their children arrived in the United States, and so their United States residence time was shorter than their children's.

Data Collection

Data were obtained through Leininger's ethnonursing enablers namely the Stranger-Friend Enabler and the Observation-Participation-Reflection Enabler.[11] Semi-structured interviews focused on the researcher's domain of inquiry (DOI) and on the informants' emic views, beliefs, and values in their worlds with their care meanings and expressions along with any etic views of professional care. The Sunrise Model[12] was an enabler used to examine the major tenets of the Culture Care Theory dimensions, and was also used for culturological and clinical health care assessments. Leininger's Stranger-Friend Enabler[13] was used to guide the researcher to enter, participate in, and leave the field research. The purpose of this enabler was to ensure accurate, reliable, and credible data as a researcher sought emic (insiders') ideas of their culture while examining the researcher's etic views and influence on the informants. As the researcher became a trusted professional friend, the informants' secrets or in-depth truth statements were shared with the researcher.

All interviews were conducted by the researcher in English, Mandarin, or Taiwanese, depending on the preference of the informant. While many informants could speak English, most preferred to be interviewed in Taiwanese because they felt more comfortable using their mother language. Most interviews were conducted in a home, although a few were conducted at a restaurant for the convenience of the informants. The lunchtime interviews gave the researcher a good opportunity to observe the informant's beliefs about food in relation to health care, as well as activities in the home setting. During the interviews, the researcher continuously reaffirmed or confirmed information by restating the informants' statements to clarify distinctive and accurate meanings and expressions of their responses. With the informant's permission, the author used a tape recorder and made notes of each interview session, which were later destroyed to protect the confidentiality of informants. Translation from Taiwanese into English was completed by the researcher immediately after the interview was completed to provide accurate recall of data. The researcher fluently speaks all three languages (English, Taiwanese, and Mandarin).

Data Analysis and Evaluation Criteria

Leininger's Four Qualitative Phase Analysis Guide was used to examine systematically and rigorously the researcher's domain of inquiry and major theoretical tenets.[14] This method was used for data analysis to identify major themes and provide final synthesis of data findings. Actual data analysis was an on-going process that began at the time of collecting raw data with the first interview and recording all data in the field journal until the last contact or interview with informants. The qualitative ethnonursing Four Phases of Data Analysis includes Phase I, raw data collection and documentation; Phase II, identification of code descriptors and components; Phase III, patterning and component analysis; and phase IV, development of major themes and summary findings.[15]

Since qualitative research is different from quantitative research, specific criteria for evaluating qualitative findings were essential, and so Leininger's six criteria for evaluating qualitative studies were used to evaluate themes and findings of this research study.[16] The six criteria included credibility, confirmability, meaning-in-context, recurrent patterning, saturation, and transferability and were used throughout the collection and final data analysis.

Orientational Definitions

The following definitions as defined by the theorist and adapted by the researcher for this study were used to guide the researcher in discovering and evaluating data from interviews with Taiwanese American informants.[17]

1. *Culture Care*: refers to the subjectively and objectively learned and transmitted values, beliefs, and patterned lifeways that assist, support, facilitate, or enable Taiwanese Americans to maintain their well-being and health; to improve their human condition and lifeways; or to deal with illness, handicaps, or death.

2. *Worldview*: refers to the way the Taiwanese Americans look out on the world or their universe to form a picture of a value stance about their life or world around them.

3. *Cultural and Social Structure Dimensions* refers to the dynamic patterns and features of interrelated structural and organizational factors of the Taiwanese culture (subculture or society). These include religious, kinship (social), political (and legal), economic, educational, technologic, and cultural values, and ethnohistorical factors, as well as how these factors may be interrelated and function to influence human behavior in different environmental contexts.

4. *Environmental Context* refers to the totality of an event, situation, or particular experience that gives meaning to human expressions, interpretations, and social interactions in particular physical, ecological, sociopolitical, and/or cultural settings.

5. *Generic (folk or lay) Care* refers to culturally learned and transmitted, indigenous (or traditional), folk (home-based) knowledge and skills used by Taiwanese Americans to provide assistive, supportive, enabling, or facilitative acts toward or for another individual, group, or institution with evident or anticipated needs to ameliorate or improve a human lifeway or health condition (or well-being) or to deal with handicaps and death situations.

6. *Culturally Congruent (nursing) Care* refers to those cognitively based assistive, supportive, facilitative, or enabling acts or decisions that are tailor-made to fit with individual, group, or institutional Taiwanese cultural values, beliefs, and lifeways to provide or support meaningful, beneficial, and satisfying health care or well-being services.

7. *Taiwanese Americans* refers to individuals who were born and raised in the country of Taiwan, or who identify themselves to be of Taiwanese descent or heritage, and have immigrated to the United States.

8. *Emic* refers to the folk, local, or "insiders'" knowledge of a culture.[18]

9. *Etic* refers to the "outsiders'" knowledge and often professional views of health care.[19]

Ethnohistory of Taiwan

Taiwan is an island in the western Pacific Ocean between the East and South China Seas, being located midway between Japan and Korea to the north and Hong Kong and the Philippines to the south. Taiwan stretches about 245 miles from north to south and 90 miles from east to west.[20] With the land area of 13,900 square miles, it is about the size of Switzerland. About two-thirds of the island is covered with forested mountain. Taipei is the largest city in Taiwan and the capital of Taiwan.

Perhaps the fact that Taiwan is surrounded by the Pacific Ocean, thus being isolated both geographically and socially from its neighbors, accounts for its "separatist tradition." The island was initially inhabited by nine different cultural groups of aborigines considered to be of Malay or Polynesian origin. Until the Ming dynasty (1368–1644) Taiwan was not yet clearly identified in Chinese court records, but about 1430 the admiral-explorer Cheng Ho determined its exact location, after which its present name was used in official sources.[21]

During the 16th century the Portuguese named the island *Formosa*, which means *beautiful isle*. After the Portuguese sighted but bypassed Taiwan, the Dutch and the Spaniards began setting up trading stations, missions, and forts on the island. In 1661 the Dutch were driven out by the pirate Koxianga who later made the island a refuge for supporters of China's deposed Ming dynasty.[22]

In 1895 Taiwan was ceded to Japan as booty in the wake of the Sino-Japanese War and entered another colonial period for 50 years. Japan's colonization of the island was done in the face of strong hostility from both Taiwanese and aborigines. Japan began to *Japanize* the island by making Japanese the official language of government and education. Even today, many older Taiwanese people can speak Japanese. After World War II Taiwan was restored to National Chinese control.[23]

In 1949 as a result of a civil war on Mainland China, the Chinese communists defeated Chiang Kai-Shek's Nationalist forces and took control of China. Chiang moved his government to Taiwan and under the Kuomintang Party kept the idea of reuniting with China an important goal of the group. After Chiang Kai-Shek and his eldest son died, numerous social and political reforms developed. Today, Taiwan is struggling between seeking independence and/or reunification with Mainland China.[24] Presently in the year 2000, President Cheng is holding to independence amid threats from the Chinese for their control and to be part of Mainland China. Currently, Taiwan is considered a free society and whether this will change remains unknown.

Because of numerous invasions by other countries and colonization, Taiwan is a country of mixed cultures, including the native Taiwanese, traditional Chinese, and Japanese. At present, Taiwan has a population of more than 22,000,000 people[25] that is divided into four main ethnic groups.[26] The first group, the aborigines, were originally identified to be similar to Indonesians in language and lifeways. Ethnohistorically, these earliest inhabitants are considered to be of Malay or Polynesian origin. The next two groups of early Chinese immigrants or "Taiwanese" are the Hakka, who came from south China near Hong Kong, and the Fukienese, who came from China's Fukien Province directly across the Taiwan Straits.

By the year 1000 A.D., there were a large number of Hakka settled in western Taiwan. These people spoke the Hakka dialect and regular Taiwanese that is a derivative of the Fukien dialect and Mandarin.[27] The Fukien began migrating across the Taiwan Strait nearly a thousand years ago with many making the journey between the 14th and 17th centuries. Being separated from China for so many years has made the Hakkas and Fukien culturally distinct from other Chinese.

Finally, the fourth group is comprised of Chinese from various parts of China who came to Taiwan after World War II. They are often referred to as *mainlanders*. Although growing western influences have inundated the country, the Taiwanese have preserved their identity and a considerable part of their traditional premodern culture. As more Taiwanese migrate to the United States, it is important for nurses to assess and understand the cultural history of the people and their health care needs and practices that are culturally specific to Taiwanese immigrants with acculturation factors. Nurses can also anticipate a variety of responses in the 21st century related to the current struggle between Taiwan and China.

Chinese immigration to the United States began over 150 years ago. In 1850 there were only a few thousand Chinese inhabitants in the United States. In 1880 the Chinese American population grew to over 100,000 and has continued to increase to over 1.6 million in 1990.[28] In 1990 the Chinese were the largest of more than 20 Asian groups residing in the United States. Most Chinese immigrant statistics combine people from Mainland China, Hong Kong, and Taiwan. Before 1991 limited data were found on the number of Taiwanese immigrating to the United States.[29]

In the late 1950s and early 1960s an estimated 250,000 to 300,000 Taiwanese-Americans immigrated to the United States. In 1981 congressional legislation established a specific quota of 20,000 entrants annually from Taiwan. From 1991 to 1996 approximately 76,000 Taiwanese immigrated to the United States.[30] Thus there are more Taiwanese in the United States today, and their cultural history and lifeways are very important for nurses to understand.

In the past several years the problems and needs of Taiwanese and Chinese Americans have received increasing attention among social scientists. As the Taiwanese population continues to increase in the United States, the distinction between Chinese Americans and Taiwanese Americans needs to be understood. The history of Chinese immigration and the characteristics of Chinese immigrants have changed drastically since the first immigration. Not only has the total number of Chinese immigrants increased, but also the composition of recent Chinese immigration is strikingly different from previous ones. Early Chinese immigrants were laborers who were predominantly uneducated men and women. In contrast, recent Taiwanese and Chinese immigrants are often highly educated and skilled in the professions.[31] Early studies of Chinese immigrants may help to understand the historical context of the Chinese in the United States at various time periods and the cultural differences between Mainland Chinese and Taiwanese.

■ Social Structure Factors
Religion and Philosophy

There are several religions in Taiwan, and most Taiwanese people adhere to more than one set of beliefs. The aborigines have practiced nature and animal worship, while many of the Chinese immigrants have subscribed to Buddhism or Taoism, the two primary religions of Taiwan. The Dutch introduced Protestant Christianity to Taiwan, the Spanish brought Catholicism, and the Japanese brought Shintoism.[32] Today, 93% of the Taiwanese population is a mixture of Buddhism, Confucianism, and Taoism; 4.5% are Christian; and 2.5% represent other religions.[33]

Buddhists and Taoists usually embrace Confucianism, which is more of an ethical system and philosophical moral code of personal behavior relating to human relationships. A Christian minority of less than a million are divided between Roman Catholic and Protestant churches. A Taiwanese person may call himself a Buddhist, a Taoist, or even a Christian, but never ceases to be Confucian. The Confucian philosophy has become an inseparable part of the society and thinking of the Taiwanese people.[34]

Confucianism is important to understanding the Taiwanese. It provides values and an ideology of everyday life for Taiwanese people. Confucianism focuses primarily on the importance of interpersonal relationships based largely on Confucian teachings and philosophy in which individuals must perform their roles in a society based on fixed principles of authority. Five categories of interpersonal relationships based on authority are parent and child, king and minister, husband and wife, elder brother and younger brother, and friend with friend.[35] Filial piety is an important part of the moral philosophy of Confucius.[36] Confucian teaching gives meaning to living, dying, family life, childbearing, maintenance of health, and cause of illness as principles and guides for living.

Kinship and Family Structure

The philosophy and teaching of Confucius is deeply ingrained in the Taiwanese way of life. The family is a unit of a clan, as well as the foundation of society. Social life is based on human relations within the family. As a result, group ties are strong, and it is expected that the individual will work hard to contribute toward the success of the family. The most important aspect of traditional family consciousness is the father-son relationship. Traditionally, the family is strongly patriarchal and hierarchical and with marked role differentiation based on age, gender, and generation among the family members. Authority in the Taiwanese family has been largely based on respect for age (especially elders) as the extended family lived in one house. Respect for elders continues to be important and extends throughout society as the elders often hold nominal positions in businesses or government.[37]

Confucianism teaches that filial piety is the basis of all conduct, and followers are educated along this principle. Because of parental demands, strict obedience is a son's moral obligation to serve his parents with sincerity. Based on this tenet, the rule of seniority applies: a child obeys the parents, a wife obeys her husband, and a younger brother obeys the older brother. Age indicates dominance within families, and older adults expect to be respected and supported by their children.[38] Of course, these traditional Taiwanese values are under pressure as Taiwan continues its economic prosperity as one of the wealthier countries in the Asia region.

Language Uses

Chinese groups in Taiwan speak different dialects; namely, Fukien Taiwanese speak Taiwanese, and the Hakka speak the Hakka dialect. Both Taiwanese groups also speak Mandarin Chinese, which is the official language in both Taiwan and China, but some older Taiwanese do not speak Mandarin Chinese well and may speak Japanese. Aborigines speak a language resembling Malayan, and, in addition, many speak Taiwanese, Mandarin Chinese, and Japanese. Hence, Mainland Taiwan's population is trilingual or multilingual. Many Taiwanese people (except elders) speak English today in the United States, and they have been socialized to speak more than one language or dialect. The nurses should be alert to these language differences.

Economic, Political, and Cultural Value Factors

Several historical studies have been conducted on Taiwanese Americans and the history of Taiwan.[39–43] Ng recently completed a book on Taiwanese Americans with an emphasis on their community organizations, information networks, religious practices, cultural observances, the growing second generation, and the contributions of Taiwanese Americans to American society.[44] Hu examined the relationship between Taiwan's polit-

ical culture and social stratification factors.[45] He documented the transformation of the political structure from the evolution of authoritarianism to the early stages of democratization and to the latest developments in democracy. These recent sources of knowledge are important background social structure information to further nurses' in-depth perspective of Taiwan.

Education

The importance of education is highly valued by both the Taiwanese government and families. During the first half of the 20th century when Japan ruled Taiwan, they extended educational opportunities beyond the elite to average citizens and workers. Next to Japan, Taiwan now has one of the best educated populations in Asia with more than 100 institutions of higher learning.[46]

Ying conducted a social psychological study on Taiwanese college students in the United States.[47] He confirmed that traditional Chinese values play an important part in shaping the behavior of Taiwanese college students and discussed the dominance of collective behavior over individual needs. Taiwanese college students have been taught to obey authority since their childhood. Taiwanese students generally find difficulty in experiencing Western cultures that emphasize the importance of the individual person. In a study by Sodowsky, Maguire, Johnson, Ngumba, and Kohles, worldviews of white Americans, Mainland Chinese, Taiwanese, and African students are compared.[48] They conclude that some international students' worldviews were different from the traditional values of their respective cultures. The studies indicated that students perceptions may be changed by exposure to a pluralistic modern society.

Technology

Over the past 50 years Taiwan has transformed itself from an agricultural island to a high-tech industrial economy. During this time Taiwan has progressed through various stages, including the use of agriculture to support industry during the 1950s when import restrictions were imposed, the export years of the 1960s, the building of infrastructure through the Ten Major

Construction Projects during the 1970s, the liberalization of government and private businesses leading to internationalization of the 1980s, and, finally, the explosive growth of information technology (IT) in the 1990s. Today, Taiwan is the world's third largest IT producer where two out of every five notebook computers in the world are made. It is also the fifth largest computer chip producer globally. Taiwan has transformed itself from the toy producing king to the IT power with its focus on the semiconductor industry, computer component production and assembly, and electronic consumer goods.[49]

Review of Literature

Research on Nursing and Caring

Nursing studies have been conducted on care of Taiwanese Americans. Liang and DeChesnay[50] studied Taiwanese who were temporary residents of the United States and found that, while language was often problematic, of more concern was the lack of understanding about Taiwanese culture that led health care providers to make inappropriate suggestions to their patients. Shyu, Archbold, and Imle[51] studied the caregiving process of Taiwanese families and found a balance point needs to be reached between the health care provider and patient that involves recognizing, weighing, and making judgments about competing needs. Nursing actions and strategies need to be developed that are in balance or congruent with traditional Taiwanese culture. Sun and Roopnarine[52] conducted a study on childcare behavior of Taiwanese families that verified a distinct gender-differentiated pattern of involvement in child care and household activities. They found that the Taiwanese society reflects rigidity in filial piety and gender roles. To date, there were no transcultural care studies of the Taiwanese focused on the use of Leininger's Culture Care Theory with the ethnonursing research method and related transcultural nursing knowledge.[53]

Cultural Themes from This Study

In keeping with a systematic data analysis method,[54] several patterns and themes were abstracted from a large database focused on the domain of inquiry of this study. Only the themes will be reported because of space constraints.

Theme 1: Cultural care was reflected in development of national and cultural identity

Care expressions were derived from the informants' cultural beliefs, political and economic values, and worldview of their national Taiwanese identity. Important issues among Taiwanese American informants was their national identity related to their ethnohistory, worldview, and environmental context that contributed to a strong sense of Taiwanese cultural caring identity. The researcher observed that the issue of reunification was a sensitive matter with all informants. While all key and general informants did not express specific personal preferences regarding Taiwan's quest for independence or reunification with China, it was clear that the relationship between Taiwan and Mainland China was an important factor shaping the lives of Taiwanese and their responses. As Taiwan's quest for democratic changes continues, differences in the political systems between Mainland China and Taiwan grow wider. While all informants were unwilling to discuss preferences toward reunification, all key and general informants did express a desire for democracy and an open political system. They felt this needed to be nurtured (cared for) by those Taiwanese who live and are educated abroad for a long period and then return home to help local people.

The most significant political influence described by older informants has been World War II and the Chinese Civil War in 1949. These war events lead to uprooted families experiencing psychological, emotional, and physical stress. National and cultural themes were revealed in the following informant statements. One key informant stated: "I have been educated in the way where I identify myself as Taiwanese instead of Chinese. Care and politics are different: China is Communist and Taiwan is Democratic." Another key informant stated: "Although I have a green card, and in some social activities I am called a Chinese American, I always think of myself as Taiwanese." Another key informant stated: "China has mainly Chinese culture. Taiwan has a mix of native Taiwanese, Japanese, and American cultures. The lifestyle is so different." The criterion of credibility was confirmed by all key and general informants throughout by their verbatim statements. Hence, caring was frequently referenced with cultural identity.

Theme 2: Cultural care was reflected in the value of harmony and balance in daily life based on Taiwanese ethnohistory, social structure, and worldview to prevent illness and maintain well-being

The findings from all key and general informants revealed that cultural values of Taiwanese people are rooted in the search for harmony and balance as a caring modality. Taiwanese believe keeping unity between man and heaven is an essential part of existence and is integral to how the world is viewed. Harmony, balance, and unity emanate with the individual, but are expressed in a family and collective expression at a societal level. An appreciation of nature is important to achieve harmony as a caring modality in one's life.

The majority of Taiwanese American informants believe that taking care of oneself can be hard work, but results in good health. Taking care of oneself means proper eating, sleeping, rest, and exercise. Trying to do too much at one time is stressful and leads to poor health. Taiwanese believe in the concept of "balancing," which means not trying to do too much at one time. The verbatim informant descriptors are reflected in the following statements about lifeway and proper eating as caring for self and others and were confirmed through the criteria of recurrency and saturation.

One key informant stated: "The most important cultural values to me are having a simple life with simple desires. If you have restraint in your desires in this world, you can live easily and keep peace of mind. Don't show off or have an attitude of self-importance about yourself." Another key informant stated: "Life consists of cause and effect. If you do something bad, it will come back to you. You will be punished." The third key informant stated: "The last time I caught cold, I felt so weak. I had no energy. So, I made a bowl of noodles and added three spoons of red pepper in the soup and ate everything. I thought hot soup and hot pepper can make me sweat. Cold means my body is cold so I need some hot food in my body to expel the cold." A fourth key informant stated: "My father told

me that garlic, ginger, green onion, and hot pepper are not only for seasoning, but are good foods to prevent illness and maintain health. These foods can keep the body in good balance" as a caring practice. All key and general informants established these findings as credible and confirmed this theme.

The informants repeatedly stated that the search for harmony and balance is often divided into matters that are either internal or external in nature and are often referenced in Taiwanese diets and medicine. The forces of Yin and Yang (the dual principles of male and female, or positive and negative) have reinforced the importance of hot and cold in Taiwanese food and medicine. These principles are part of a philosophy that fosters a balance of humans with nature and are reflected in the Taiwanese worldview. These statements were expressed by six key informants with agreement by all general informants. Ten of 12 general informants viewed illness as an imbalance between Yin and Yang. Yin and Yang theory suggests that to maintain caring for good health, one needs to have good eating habits, as well as proper goals in life. Body equilibrium is maintained on a hot day by eating cool foods like fruits and vegetables and avoiding meats, oil, fatty dishes, and alcohol. All key and general informants confirmed that on cool days plenty of stimulating foods should be eaten like meats and high-protein meals along with alcohol. Herbs and other home remedies were widely used by Taiwanese American informants to restore balance that related to culturally congruent eating and lifeways. The qualitative criteria of credibility, confirmability, meaning-in-context, and recurrent patterning of this theme substantiated the observational and verbatim findings with all key and general informants in their daily living.

Theme 3: Culture care means preserving traditional folk health care beliefs and practices along with the use of Western health care practices for healthy outcomes

All key and general Taiwanese American informants held that health was one of the most important aspects of life. Informants related that one must preserve good health through caring for self and others, for without it one could accomplish very little. Taiwanese Americans were willing to spend a great deal of time, effort, and money to obtain Chinese medicine for promotion of health and prevention of illness. Since Taiwan's society is very competitive, one is usually not excused from the usual demands of work and family obligation, even when ill. Consequently, Taiwanese believe it is very important to prevent illness. They will go through much effort to do so.

Over 90% of key and general informants believed that chemical substances in the body could endanger health. Many informants held that Western medicine was chemically based while Oriental medicine was more natural. A few key informants said that Taiwanese Americans believed that Western medicine could actually prevent health but taking Oriental herbal medicine promoted health. In addition, some general informants felt that Western medicine treated local symptoms while Oriental medicine took a more holistic caring approach and attitude by taking care of the entire body—a holistic caring mode.

In Taiwanese culture, traditional healing practices often exist side by side with modern medicine, which was confirmed by 94% of all Taiwanese American informants. Additionally, 94% of all Taiwanese American informants used various Taiwanese home remedies such as acupuncture, cupping, bar-kuan, Salonpas, and plant and animal treatments like deer horn and ginseng. Others spoke of using Oriental and Western medicine together based on availability. Two-thirds of all informants feel that, because of a lack of Oriental medicine resources in the United States, they had no choice but to use Western medicine.

The following verbatim informant descriptors were documented from key and general informants as follows. One key informant said the following:

> Our ancestors used traditional Chinese herb medicine for thousands of years. There is a long history with how this approach benefits the human body. You just cannot ignore this history. Perhaps the folk healers may not have much formal education, but they do have a lot of experience and history as their guides. I feel this approach really helps treat my health problems.

Another female key informant stated the following:

> Every Taiwanese American family must have some folk medicine. I have some folk medicine with me which I brought from my country. There are some

powders for a stomachache, a pain-relieving patch, and some ointments for mosquito bites. Western medicine uses so many chemical substances that may have some quick results. But, Chinese medicine is more natural and has less side effects.

Another key informant stated, "Chinese medicine is easier on the body. Western medicine can be too strong. You can take Chinese medicine everyday but with Western medicine, it can hurt the body over a longer period of time." One general informant said, "During the cold weather, I will drink herb tea. I think taking Chinese herb medicine definitely promotes health and prevents illness." Another general informant stated, "I believe that Chinese medicine consists of more natural elements that will not harm our bodies. Whenever I don't feel well, I will take folk medicine by myself." One key informant stated, "I believe that Western medicine may be professional and scientific with evidence to cure many diseases, but this is still not the natural way. Basically, I don't like to take Western medicine because it's artificial and chemical." Still another general informant stated, "If I have a really serious disease or I need surgery, I may go to see a Western doctor. Afterwards, I will use both traditional and Western ways to take care of myself." From the above verbatim statements, theme 3 was confirmed. These statements showed strong use today of generic (emic) medicine and care modes to recover from illness and remain healthy. Caring was expressed through knowledge about the use of traditional medications.

Theme 4: Caring was expressed as an obligation for family members with different gender role responsibilities

Traditionally and still today, Taiwanese American families have been patriarchal, patrilineal, and patrilocal. The family structure was highly valued by Taiwanese American informants. Within the extended family union religion, lifeways, goodness, and respect for self and others was learned. The value of family and role expectations was confirmed by all key and general informants. The informants stated that still today the head of the Taiwanese American family is the father. Descent of the children is also through the father who represents discipline and firmness. Informants stated that Taiwanese American mothers have traditionally remained at home during the childbearing years and have responsibility for organizing and maintaining the household and ensuring that a positive and nurturing environment is present in the home. Credibility and confirmability, as well as meaning-in-context, were established by key and general informants who verified the importance of the family and gender role responsibilities through verbatim descriptors showing recurrency, meaning-in-context, and saturation.

One key informant stated, "The father and the oldest son have the main responsibility of taking care of the family. My wife has the responsibility of taking care of our home and making sure the children are okay. I have two jobs now because I want my wife and my children to have a better life." Another key informant stated, "Taiwanese are very family centered. You have to put your family in first place and put yourself second." One general informant stated, "My parents worked so hard and tried to save every penny for us. Now I am doing the same thing for my kids." Another general informant stated, "The mother's responsibility is to take good care of the children, prepare healthy foods, and support her husband in his work. After I got married, I felt it important to put more focus on our family and not put all my time and energy into work." Another general informant stated, "In the traditional Taiwanese ways, the male was head of the family, school, and many other institutions. In my family, my father made most of the decisions when he was alive. Now my oldest brother has taken on some of that responsibility." Thus, a caring ethos through the family and with the fathers providing protective care could be substantiated.

Theme 5: Caring was expressed as unconditional emotional and physical support for Taiwanese loved ones

The culture care meanings and expressions of Taiwanese Americans were closely linked to the worldview, ethnohistory, and Confucianism. Frequently, caring was described by informants as loving someone by providing an action, but not necessarily by verbal response. The Confucian philosophy of societal respect and treatment of others as family members manifests itself in unconditional acceptance. The data revealed that caring was characterized as a process of continuous

overt activity and deeds that reflected the inner expressions of love. These care meanings and expressions were described in the following verbatim statements by key and general informants through the criteria of recurrency and saturation.

One key informant stated: "When you love someone, you must love them. You will just do anything that can help the person and try to make them happy." Another key informant stated:

> Taiwanese people express their love in different ways. Some are not very verbal about displaying their love, but you can feel it from their actions. I seldom hear words of love from my parents, but they sacrifice their whole life for me.

The other key informant stated:

> I call my parents once a week. My mother always chatters a lot on the phone with me, but my father prefers to write. They don't tell me by words that they love me, but I can feel they love me so much.

One general informant stated: "In my culture, people often don't say so much about love and care for a person. You can tell they love you by what they have done for you and how they look at you." Another general informant stated:

> In Taiwanese culture, caring can come from inside our bodies and mind or as outward expressions. When we care for someone, we are concerned about their complete mental and physical health. Only caring is more than an outward expression. Caring comes from the soul, which is an inner expression.

The five themes just presented support Leininger's theory that caring is important for the health and well-being of humans. Caring was discovered from different dimensions of the social structure, the worldview, and cultural values and beliefs. Leininger's Theory of Culture Care with the above research (themes) findings led to the use of the three modes for transcultural nursing actions and decisions as discussed next.

 ## Three Nursing Modes of Actions and Decisions

In accordance with Leininger's theory, three modes were predicted to guide nursing actions and decisions. They are 1) culture care preservation and/or maintenance, 2) cultural care accommodation and/or negotiation, and 3) cultural care repatterning and/or restructuring.[55]

First Mode: Culture Care Preservation/Maintenance

Culture care preservation is reflected in the importance of family relationships as filial love for Taiwanese Americans. Culture care means family closeness, and care is family centered. Nurses need to use this family closeness through family presence, support, and help. The family decision about treatment may be more important than the individual's decision. It is necessary to include family members in every aspect of care. Family members need to be involved in all stages of a patient's health situation—from preventing illness to maintaining health. Culture care preservation and maintenance of family love (filial love) by including significant family members in caring and treatment activities are essential.

Second Mode: Culture Care Accommodation/Negotiation

Harmony and balance as culture care must be accommodated or negotiated for the Taiwanese Americans. For example, illness is viewed as an imbalance between Ying (cold) and Yang (hot), and so a nurse needs to provide this balance of hot and cold to be a sensitive caregiver. Nurses need to accommodate this value by allowing and providing clients Taiwanese diets and medicine to keep internal and external equilibrium.

Holism and spiritual life values as caring ways need to be accommodated or negotiated for Taiwanese Americans. Holism as a value manifested itself among older-generation Taiwanese Americans who do not separate illness of the body from illness of the mind and learn about the whole person within a cultural context. This mode includes nursing care that recognizes and promotes the connection between cultural, psychological, and spiritual care, as well as physical care. For those Taiwanese Americans who believe that having a peaceful mind as caring brings health, nurses need to accommodate and facilitate the use of spiritual care with professional nursing care practices for healthy recoveries.

Third Mode: Culture Care Repatterning/Restructuring

Cultural care repatterning or restructuring may be difficult for nurses who do not understand Taiwanese Americans. Taiwanese Americans utilize various treatments, including Western medicine and Oriental medicine. Some treatments are accomplished through self-care, while others are provided by professional caregivers. All Taiwanese Americans in this study expected quick results from Western medicine. It is, therefore, important for nurses to emphasize the importance of taking medicine when there may be no immediate visible effect. Taiwanese Americans often have beliefs about causes of illness and what treatments should be used, which may not be consistent with those of Western health care. This implies that nurses may need to develop an understanding of Taiwanese cultural beliefs about care and health so they can effectively work with the patient to accept or reject Western care practices. However, it would be culturally incongruent for the older-generation Taiwanese Americans to violate their traditional beliefs about health care and practices. Restructuring nursing actions would be needed where traditional Taiwanese folk health care and professional nursing practices are in conflict or if changes are indicated from traditional to professional care.

In addition, repatterning or restructuring nursing actions need to be conducted by helping clients understand the possible consequences and side effects of combining Western medicine prescribed by their physician with Oriental herbal remedies. Careful and sensitive repatterning or restructuring care practices also provides a sense of trust between patient and health care provider that develops from an understanding and acceptance of the client's cultural beliefs.

■ Conclusion

This study was based on Leininger's Culture Care Theory of Diversity and Universality with the domain of inquiry focused on describing, analyzing, and explaining cultural care meanings and expressions of Taiwanese Americans with the ethnonursing method. Contrasts between Taiwanese Americans and traditional Taiwanese in the homeland were briefly discussed to show comparative views. This study examined the lifeways and worldviews of Taiwanese Americans rather than merging all Chinese (Taiwan, mainland, Hong Kong, Singapore, etc.) into one cultural group. An island state such as Taiwan is very different from mainland China in economic, social, and political climates. Taiwan's advanced industrialized economy and democratic political system is vastly different from the third-world, centrally planned climate of mainland China. Therefore, some wide variations in the culture care meanings and beliefs between Taiwanese Americans and Chinese Americans were discovered, but a maxi study could highlight more details.

Five major themes were discovered from the data analysis of this ethnonursing research:

1. Cultural care is reflected in the development of national and cultural identity.
2. Cultural care is reflected in the value of harmony and balance in daily life based on Taiwanese ethnohistory, social structure, and worldview to prevent illness and maintain well-being.
3. Culture care means preserving traditional folk health care beliefs and practices along with the use of Western health care practices for healthy outcomes.
4. Caring is an obligation for the physical provision of family members with different gender role responsibilities.
5. Caring is expressed as unconditional emotional and physical support for loved ones.

The Theory of Culture Care was substantiated showing the great importance to use a holistic theoretical framework with generic and professional care and social structure factors. The ethnonursing method and Leininger's enablers were crucial to discover Taiwanese Americans' care meanings and expressions. Just as vast cultural differences exist among the people of European countries, there is also great diversity in social structure and lifeways among the populations of Asian nations. There were, however, more universal (similarities) than diverse findings from this study. The ethnonursing research method was important to uncover these subtle differences so that nurses can provide culturally congruent care to a diverse Asian and Asian American population and to Taiwanese Americans in particular.

References

1. Leininger, M., *Care: The Essence of Nursing and Health*, Detroit, MI: Wayne State University Press, 1984.
2. Leininger, M., *Transcultural Nursing: Concepts, Theories, Research, and Practice*, Blacklick, OH: McGraw-Hill Book Company, 1995.
3. Leininger, M., "Ethnomethods: The Philosophical and Epistemic Basis to Explicate Transcultural Nursing Knowledge," *Journal of Transcultural Nursing*, 1990, v. 1, no. 2, pp. 40–51.
4. Leininger, M., *Cultural Care Diversity and Universality: A Theory of Nursing*, New York: NLN Press, 1991.
5. Ibid.
6. Ibid.
7. Ibid.
8. Leininger, op. cit., 1990.
9. Ibid.
10. Leininger, op. cit., 1991.
11. Ibid, p. 83.
12. Ibid, p. 43.
13. Ibid, p. 82.
14. Ibid, pp. 105–106.
15. Ibid.
16. Ibid, pp. 112–115.
17. Ibid, pp. 47–49.
18. Ibid, p. 32.
19. Ibid, p. 32.
20. Copper, J.F., *Taiwan: Nation, State, or Province?* San Francisco, CA: Westview Press, 1996.
21. Ibid.
22. Rubenstein, M.A., *Taiwan: A New History*, New York: M.E. Sharpe, 1999.
23. Ibid.
24. Robinson, T.W., "America in Taiwan's Post Cold-War Foreign Relations," *The China Quarterly*, 1996.
25. *The World Almanac and Book of Facts (2000)*, World Almanac Books, A Primedia Company, 2000.
26. Copper, op. cit., 1996.
27. Ibid.
28. *The World Almanac*, op. cit., 2000.
29. *Statistical Abstract of the United States*, US Department of Commerce, Bureau of the Census, 1998.
30. Ibid.
31. Ng, F., *The Taiwanese Americans*, Westport, CT: Greenwood Press, 1998.

32. Copper, op. cit., 1996.
33. *The World Almanac*, op. cit.
34. Copper, op. cit., 1996.
35. Ibid.
36. Chan, W., *A Source Book in Chinese Philosophy*, Princeton, NJ: Princeton University Press, 1973.
37. Copper, op. cit., 1996.
38. Ibid.
39. Ibid.
40. Ng, op. cit., 1998.
41. Rubenstein, op. cit., 1999.
42. Shambaugh, D., *Contemporary Taiwan*, Oxford: Clarendon Press, 1998.
43. Wachman, A.M., *Taiwan: National Identity and Democratization*, New York: M.E. Sharpe, 1994.
44. Ng, op. cit., 1998.
45. Hu, C., "Social Stratification and Changing Political Culture: The Case of Taiwan," *American Sociological Association*, 1999.
46. Rubenstein, op. cit., 1999.
47. Ying, Y.W., "Use of the CPI Structural Scales in Taiwan College Graduates," *The International Journal of Social Psychology*, 1990, v. 36, no. 1, pp. 49–57.
48. Sodowsky, G.R., K. Maguire, P. Johnson, et al., "Worldviews of White American, Mainland Chinese, Taiwanese, and African Students: An Investigation into Between-Group Differences," *Journal of Cross Cultural Psychology*, 1994, v. 25, no. 3, pp. 309–324.
49. *The Taiwan Economic News*, ROC Government Information Office, June 2000.
50. Liang, H. and M. DeChesnay, "Culturally Competent Care for Taiwanese Temporary Residents," *Home Health Care Management and Practice*, 1998, v. 11, no. 1, pp. 33–37.
51. Shyu, Y.L., P.G. Archbold, and M. Imle, "Finding a Balance Point: A Process Central to Understanding Family Caregiving in Taiwanese Families," *Research in Nursing and Health*, 1998, v. 21, no. 3, pp. 261–270.
52. Sun, L.C., and J.L. Roopnarine, "Mother-Infant, Father-Infant Interaction and Involvement in Childcare and Household Labor Among Taiwanese Families," *Infant Behavior and Development*, 1996, v. 19, no. 1, pp. 121–129.
53. Leininger, op. cit., 1995.
54. Leininger, op. cit., 1991.
55. Ibid, pp. 48–49.

CHAPTER

26
Transcultural Nursing and Health Care Among Native American Peoples*

Lillian Tom-Orme

According to Leininger the goal of transcultural nursing (TCN) is to provide culturally congruent and competent nursing care to diverse peoples through the discovery, understanding, and use of transcultural knowledge, practices, and theories.[1,2] In the formative years of TCN, Leininger, the founder of the field of transcultural nursing, held that it was important to blend the worlds of nursing and anthropology to expand and advance the new discipline of transcultural nursing.[3,4] It was important to consider the role of culture and its influences in the nursing profession.[5] She also held that nurses need to discover emic (insider's) and etic (outsider's) viewpoints of nursing and cultures and to compare and contrast the differences for quality health care. Leininger has challenged nurses to study in-depth cultures and the different ways cultures provide care, as well as the commonalities that might lead to universalities in the future.[6] Although her

pioneering work in TCN began in the 1950s, nurses and other health care professionals are just beginning to adopt, accept, and appreciate the important role of culture in the health field. The major challenge continues for nurses to lead the health professions in learning as much as possible about world cultures, universal care patterns, and to build on evolving transcultural nursing knowledge and research findings to provide culturally based and responsible care to clients.

In this chapter the TCN care concepts and practices that the author believes are highly relevant to care for Native American peoples will be discussed. On interacting with Native American peoples, health care professionals will discover that there are tremendous diversities and commonalities among indigenous populations in terms of their language, cultural lifeways, rituals related to health and illness, and care expressions.[7,8] As of September 2000, the United States Census Bureau estimates that there are 2.4 million Native Americans making up 0.9% of the total United States population.[9] According to the National Indian Health Board, there are presently 554 federally recognized tribal nations throughout rural and urban areas in the United States, including those on and off reservations.[10] Many Native Americans are bilingual, speak only their native language, or are learning their native language for the first time. Many tribal nations lost their languages during the forced assimilation period of the 1800s and the early 1900s, but Native Americans are beginning to reintroduce the language through formal efforts from grade school to tribal community colleges. The author is proud that she remains fluent in Diné, which is an Athapaskan language,

---

*The term Native American is used in this paper to refer to American Indians and Alaskan Natives. The American Indians are tribes of the continental United States while Alaskan Native refers to Indians in Alaska, both Aleut and Eskimo. In some literature sources, Native Americans may also include natives from all the United States territories including the Pacific Islands (Hawaii, Samoa, and Fiji). However, for the purposes of this paper Native American only refers to American Indians of the continental United States and Alaska. When "peoples" is used in this chapter such as Native American peoples it is to respect the diversity among all tribes or groups referred to by these terms based on their treaties and sovereignty rights. The US government has drawn up treaties with over 500 tribal nations. The peoples of these tribal nations speak different languages and have different cultural values, beliefs, and practices.

and, as is true for many Southwest Native American peoples of her generation, has English as her second language.

It is important to remember in this chapter that many tribal nations use their own indigenous names rather than names assigned to them during colonial times. For instance, the Spanish term Navajo is used widely in the literature, but Navajo people of the Southwest have always referred to themselves by their indigenous name, *Diné*, or *the people*. Likewise, the Northern Utes of the Uintah-Ouray reservation call themselves *Nuntz*; the Yakima have changed their name to *Yakama*.[11] Accordingly, in this chapter the preferred tribal names for Native Americans will be used as much as possible. Other general ideas about Native American peoples are discussed along with use of specific examples. The Theory of Culture Care will be used as a general theoretical guide to explain their cultural values, beliefs, and practices related to care and health.

Health Status and Health Needs

Native Americans suffer from many preventable illnesses and diseases.[12] In recent times, chronic diseases have become increasingly prevalent such as obesity, diabetes, cardiovascular disease, cancer, and hypertension. In fact, type II diabetes has become an epidemic in the latter half of the 20th century. It is well known that the *O'odham Akimel* (Pima) have the highest prevalence of diabetes in the world; over one-half of those over 35 years of age have type II diabetes. However, relatives of the O'odham, who live in Mexico, have been found to have almost no diabetes.[13] This finding indicates that environmental and lifestyle factors may play major roles in the development of diabetes. Recently, type II diabetes has begun to increase among Native American children, particularly those with a family history of the disease or those with a mother with gestational diabetes and those who are obese or who have hyperinsulinemia.[14,15] Parallel to the increasing risk factors of a sedentary lifestyle and over-consumption of calories, cancer and cardiovascular diseases (CVD) have also increased. Cardiovascular diseases have become the leading cause of mortality, while cancer-related deaths have moved from number three to number two in the past decade.[16,17]

Interestingly, cancer types and rates vary considerably among tribal nations and by region.[18] Cigarette smoking and lung cancer incidence rates are highest among American Indian women of the Northern Plains and Alaska.[19,20] Hodge, Fredricks, and Kipnis noted that among some tribes in California, smoking rates were at least 40%.[21] Cancer is rapidly becoming a serious concern among native populations, particularly among Alaskan Natives. The most current data for 1993 to 1997 show that the most commonly diagnosed invasive cancers among Alaska Natives were lung, colon/rectal, breast, prostate, and stomach.[22] Alaskan cancer incidence rates for lung, nasopharynx, most organs of the digestive system, and kidney now exceed those of the United States as a whole. The rate of breast cancer has increased among Alaskan Native women such that it is now as high as that of all white women living in the United States. Alaskan Native, Navajo, and Northern Plains women have a cervical cancer rate at least twice that of white women.[23,24] The rate of injury caused by motor vehicle accidents remains high; this is attributed to driving while intoxicated and/or nonuse of seatbelts.[25] The Native American rate of alcoholism is 627% greater than the general United States rates.[26] These facts about known illnesses, diseases, and injuries of these people are very important for transcultural nurses to know, assess, and understand.

The Worldview of Native Americans

With the author's transcultural presentations and research consultations, nurses have been encouraged to think of Native Americans in circles or circuitous ways rather than from a linear perspective, as the former is congruent with their values, beliefs, and lifeways. All too frequently health care providers (except for nurses prepared in TCN) tend to use linear thinking and restrictive theoretical models with Native Americans that fail to fit with the peoples' beliefs and lifeways. Native Americans strongly believe that life's experiences occur in concert with the circles of the changing four seasons, the rhythm of the dances and music, the solar system, the homes made by humans and animals, and the pathways of life from birth to death.[27–29] The Sunrise Model with the Theory of Culture Care Diversity and

Universality is a congruent paradigm that fits the circular ways for Native Americans to view and respond to their world.

A general fundamental belief of Native Americans is that all things in life are connected and interconnected; this belief also supports the value of circular thinking.[30] In nursing and transcultural nursing, connection is linked to relationships with clients, with families, with other peers and colleagues, and is likened to nursing care activities such as touching, listening, client-focused nursing, and holism.[31-33] Strickland, Squeoch, and Chrisman show how the concept of holism is exemplified in their research on promoting women's health.[34] They emphasized education for Native American women and health care providers, using a wellness rather than an illness prevention approach, by focusing on the health of all women to show interconnectedness rather than targeting only women in a specified age group. Through the holistic approach the importance of self-care for the good of the community is promoted, thereby integrating health promotion into an environmental and spiritual balance. This collective care of women in the community is a priority over the isolation of individuals outside the circuitous orientation. Likewise, Leininger's Theory of Culture Care emphasizing multiple holistic social structure factors, environmental context, language use, and ethnohistory reflects the qualitative holistic theory prespective. Crow has supported the holistic and circuitous approaches in nursing education as ways to foster Native American students' learning needs and to meet their expectations.[35] These nursing approaches could include focus groups, storytelling, talking circles, and the use of silence.[36-39] These approaches are preferred over didactic or standardized testing approaches.

Language and Communication

Understanding a culture's patterns of communication, as well as being familiar with their language, is important to establish rapport and acceptance.[40,41] Transcultural nurses and other health care providers who are working with Native American peoples need to become familiar with their native languages as this shows a genuine effort to understand health, illness, and human experiences and care needs.[42,43] There are usually many influences or variations in the local native language; however, nurses need to learn a few words to communicate care as respect and interest in helping people.

Use of traditional language is usually reflected in a person's worldview. Knowing a person's preference for language is critical within the health care professions. To have messages understood and prescriptions followed, the nurse or health care provider must ensure that both the provider and the client understand each other. In many cases this is not always planned or given serious consideration. For example, the Diné have a strong preference to speak their indigenous language and some cannot speak or understand English. Yet, many health care professionals, including nurses who come to the reservation, do not speak their language and therefore must attempt to communicate through translators. Often the translators are inadequately trained, and, in addition, many English words cannot be translated into the Diné language or vice versa. Also, if a health condition is described or somehow communicated, the perception of what was translated may be entirely altered and delivered in an unintended manner. Diné understand this and tell many humorous stories. One story shared with me by a Diné health care administrator is a good example of why not to use a young grandchild as a translator. A grandchild accompanied his grandfather to the clinic. The Anglo nurse asked the grandchild to serve as a translator to find out from Grandpa if he was still having diarrhea. After some discussion between the two in the Diné language, the young child remarked, "My Grandpa," he says, "he don't give a s— anymore!" The nurse was quite taken aback by what he considered graphic language by a small child, but the child should not be expected to know the medical term congruent with the nurse's knowledge.

Another reason to avoid burdening young children with this task is that often children become privy to personal information about adult relatives, information heretofore kept from the children and valued by elders as private. Although children participate in many community-based social activities, their innocence is strictly valued and maintained in religious or illegal situations.[44]

Purnell and Paulanka differentiate between translator and interpreter by the level of training and depth of knowledge about a language.[45] A translator may only restate what is said in one language from another, while an interpreter not only decodes words but also provides the meaning of the message. It is always best to use caution when relying on an interpreter as there is much diversity in social classes, relationships, sensitivity to certain issues, and dialects. Also, the context of the interview setting may affect the translated communication.

Other communication patterns relevant to Native Americans include the care practice of allowing for periods of silence. This time allows individuals to reflect and to formulate ideas from their native mind-set to one that might be more appropriate to dominant Anglo cultures.[46] Leininger's research has also found silence as a dominant domain of care.[47] Consistent with silence is the generic or folk caring practice of "being with" or presence. In the Diné care practice of presence one might say, "I sat with her to make us both feel better." This may be most pertinent during times of ill health or grief; however, care as presence is practiced in a variety of settings for physical, emotional, and spiritual comfort.[48,49]

Body language, hand movement, eye movement, lip movement, and head movement are common nonverbal ways to communicate among many Native American peoples. Unfortunately, communication patterns are misunderstood and used stereotypically by Western people who refer to the stoic and passive ways of Indian people. Struthers and Littlejohn found that Native American nurses consider and prefer their communication patterns to be more relaxed, peaceful, reflective, and respectful rather than loud, direct, and prescriptive.[50]

One example of how Native American peoples value nonverbal communication among themselves and with their surroundings comes from Standing Bear's account of the Lakota people's preparation for a buffalo hunt.[51] He illustrated the power of silence among humans and animals, as well as their surroundings. He stated the following:

One word was sufficient to bring quiet to the whole camp. The very presence of quiet was everywhere. Such was the orderliness of a Lakota camp that men, women, and children, and animals seem to have

a common understanding and sympathy. It is no mystery but natural that the Indian and his animals understand each other very well with words and without words. There were words, however, that the Indian uses that are understood by both his horses and dogs. As long as the hunters listen, the animals will listen also.

This example may not directly apply to communication between a health care provider and patient, but the values of shared respect and silence among the community can be found among a support group of family or community members. Thus, a transcultural nurse may provide communicative care by facilitating an environment in the home or health care institution where proper respect and silence are highly regarded by both the health care staff and native peoples for healing to take place. A non-Indian person may have difficulty in understanding the above example. However, during the author's youth, many examples of appropriate and respectful behavior were taught that included examples of animal behavior. Some examples were to run but quietly like the deer, to be strong like the bear, or to have keen awareness and eyesight like the hawk or eagle.

This is not to say that all communication is quiet and respectful. During times of celebrations, Native American tend to be like others, boisterous and joyous; some dances call for shouting; and many other occasions such as sports activities call for uninhibited celebratory behavior. Therefore, transcultural nurses must be nonjudgmental and avoid stereotypes surrounding communication patterns when planning nursing care.[52]

Another transcultural concept that many nurses may not regard as important is cultural care preservation.[53] Through songs and dances, Native Americans relive their traditions and pass them on to younger people. Songs and dances are also performed during times of illness or health. The Diné maintain strong generic care traditions today; they call in a medicine person to recite prayers and sing special songs for healing. Through song and dance, people believe they communicate with the healing spirits. The gift of song is considered a true blessing. Those who know special songs are revered to strengthen others in times of need or for support. This is an example of generic care that needs preservation through recognition and support by transcultural and all other nurses. Many creation stories of Native American peoples include a song for different events and occasions. Songs are sung for rites of passage, for healing, and during times of illness or stress and celebrations of the seasons. Nurses and other health care professionals may witness singing and chanting in hospital rooms or in settings where communication with healing and guiding spirits are sought. These generic folk care practices call for respect and understanding of indigenous cultural communication traditions.

Humor is another manner of communication that remains strong among most Native American peoples. Humor is also thought of as a generic practice/folk care practice to alleviate stress, as well as to temporarily or permanently heal worries or sadness. Health care professionals working with Native Americans will discover the value of humor as care in daily events. In spite of the seriousness of an illness or life's challenges, Native American people will use humor as care to deal with the situation. Nurses must learn to appreciate Native American humor and to integrate this generic care practice into professionals nursing care when it is appropriate. When a client or family uses humor with nurses, it is a good sign that trust has been established.

In her research Strickland has advocated for the use of focus groups to collect and describe group norms; however, a modified version of the traditional focus group may be preferred to accommodate Native American communication patterns, which would be useful in planning nursing care.[54] For instance, small-group prior to larger-group discussions may actively engage participants and still respect the presence of elders by calling on them at the end of the session to show acknowledgement of cultural values, beliefs, and practices.

 Family/Kinship Factors and Dimensions

Although many Native American families do not live in an extended family household anymore, many remain strongly oriented toward being part of an extended family and community network. For example, whenever Diné greet another, they state their matrilineal and patrilineal clans (parents) and add their maternal and paternal grandfathers' clans. Also, any time care decisions are necessitated by family illness or rites of passage (birthdays, graduations, funerals, etc.), the extended family network is called into action to provide care. Therefore, the extended family and clan networks remain strongly involved in care practices among the Diné, as well as other Native American peoples. Traditionally, health care delivered by the Indian Health Service focused on the ill person alone. Increasingly, more attention has been paid to the ill person and his or her family and extended family as health care recipients, and generic nursing care decisions and actions have been designed to extend beyond individuals to include the active participation of the community. This focus extends beyond self-care to family care or even collective care in a community that values this. Thus, culturally congruent care by transcultural nurses must be more macro oriented to include community care activities.

Family is extremely important to Native American peoples. The Diné have a saying that to be poor is to be without family or kin. Family consists of extended members who share commonality through maternal and paternal grandmothers' family, and clan members are expected to provide care by visiting an ill person while at home, in a hospital, or in a long-term care facility. Most native people believe that presence or "being with" encourages that person to regain health and balance. When the Diné family member is institutionalized for a length of time, particularly off the reservation, family members have serious concerns about the person's health and well-being. Care as presence among familiar kin is believed to contribute positively to health. If this is not possible in strange places and among unfamiliar people and sterile environments, transcultural nurses need to be aware of this and to provide care that is culturally congruent to promote health, healing, and well-being. In the absence of family, transcultural nurses may call a local Native American organization to arrange for a guest who speaks the language of the client or some family member who could provide care by being present. If unsuccessful, a nurse could provide the presence or provide familiar taped Indian songs or stories.

Living near an urban environment, I have occasionally provided care by visiting hospitalized Diné to speak with them in our native tongue, to bring them a gift, and to offer my home to their relatives. If I find that a family is related to me by clan, I am obliged to provided generic cultural care by greeting them with appropriate terms and treating them just like my blood relatives. These generic care practices are important to Native American people, as they are part of the recovery or health maintenance process.

Relationship with Environment

Native American people have lived for centuries in a variety of settings across the United States before they were confined to reservations or terminated as tribes. In diverse locations and climates, they adapted to and learned to use plants, wildlife, and materials for food, clothing, utensils, and home building. The use of paint, feathers, beads, or amulets of various materials may be found on clothing or on a client's body. These sacred items are representations of Native American peoples' relationship with their surroundings and are powerful and meaningful forces to them in the universe. Some examples of Diné practices include the use of ash or clay to paint the body, an eagle feather when honoring a person, or juniper beads to prevent bad dreams. Nurses need to provide care by showing respect for these cultural beliefs and practices and to support cultural care preservation, one of Leininger's theoretical modes for nursing actions and decisions for culturally congruent care.[55]

Many Native American indigenous practices are learned during childhood and reinforced throughout adulthood. Typically, Diné children living on the reservation wander throughout the landscape to find various gifts of nature for amusement. The author's children have heard many of her childhood stories about how the environment was explored for play and entertainment. She played in the dirt and mud, climbed rocks, splashed in the water, ran among the bushes and trees, collected plants and insects, rode horses and donkeys, learned to swim in the river, picked berries and nuts, dug for roots, and learned to plant and care for crops. She also participated in ceremonial activities after being told how to listen, act, and respect the rituals. Thus, children are taught at an early age to become resourceful and to respect the environment for its generosity. The Native American world is an interactive one where the person is considered to be only a small part of larger expansive surroundings. Other beings, inanimate and animate, are also considered to be part of

this interactive balance of relationships. Preservation of care practices is pertinent to maintain health and balance, which begin in childhood and remain throughout the life cycle. Transcultural nurses and all nurses need to understand these close ties to the environment and provide and respect assistance to maintain and promote these Native American lifeways and rituals.

As a middle-aged adult today, the author's respect for the environment has deepened, and she has continued to enjoy nature by jogging or walking outside to seek peace of mind, to gain balance, and to enjoy the Creator's or Great Spirit's gifts. Transcultural care providers, including nurses, need to recognize this whenever they are invited by Native American people to give professional care in their community. Rather than teaching "aerobic exercise" as preferred by Western society, a more acceptable Native American approach might be to stress self-care and care to significant others through walking or jogging. Such activities give peace and balance to an individual that is health promoting and culturally congruent with native people's cultural beliefs and lifeways. The author always tells the story of how her grandfather taught her that while she ran she should not only run for exercise but also to celebrate life by shouting, throwing rocks, embracing the new day, and looking forward to what new opportunities the new day would bring.

Spirituality and the Use of Traditional Medicine

Spirituality is an integral part of being a Native American or a natural and integral part of their Native American existence.[56,57] Spirituality is a caring mode among Native American peoples. It is important to promote healing and to create harmony and is complementary to Western healing modes. Spirituality is emphasized with Native Americans as it also promotes self-awareness about one's body or condition and connects with and harmonizes one's lifeways.[58] Spirituality is viewed by Native Americans as essential to their existence; therefore, all gatherings and business meetings are opened and closed with prayers. Native people are always grateful for the camaraderie and presence of fellow Native American people who share similar cultural beliefs and practices. Native Americans encourage their young to offer sacred objects as gifts to the Creator in a variety of settings; these gifts may include traditional tobacco, corn pollen, water, salt, plants, and others. Care as spiritual connectedness is uniquely strong and its presence is felt among the Native American people during gatherings; they are generally very comfortable and peaceful with one another. Some Native Americans may not speak the same language and live miles apart, but through spiritualism they find a sense of equality and family belonging. Thus, transcultural nurses need to preserve spirituality among Native Americans as a dominant feature in care decisions and actions to provide culturally sensitive and appropriate care.

Struthers and Littlejohn have described the spiritual benefits of the annual Native American summits.[59] After returning from these gatherings many Native American nurses have realized they provide a unique forum to discuss Native American nursing issues but also to share and explore cultural and spiritual care experiences in their own ways. These annual gatherings have been times to honor Native American nurses and to reconnect with and strengthen their spirituality, as well as to promote healing. Moreover, these summit caring experiences are important to share knowledge and skills, mentor new nurses and students, and support each other. The nurses share cultural wisdom and help reintegrate nurses as a cooperative group, which honors and strengthens the traditional learning circle. Thus, spirituality is an integral part of Native American nursing care. Crow supported these views in her contrasts of Native American and Western worldviews of nursing education.[60] Crow stated that the Native American educational worldview and culture are not necessarily consistent with that of the Euro-American worldview and culture; therefore, learning and performance of Native American students are sometimes unfairly evaluated. Thus, in a culturally acceptable learning environment, where teachers understand the Native American students and their preferences for learning methods, both teachers and students benefit from the experience.

 ## Traditional Medicine and Health and Healing Modes

To Native American peoples health is a balance of the physical, mental, spiritual, social, and cultural factors within the individual or community. Traditional medicine and healing modes have always treated these dimensions as important to promote harmony and healing and are still thriving in many Native American communities. Today, many use traditional Western allopathic medicine and Native American Church (NAC) care practices by self-treatment using over-the-counter medications and making a visit to the nearest healthcare provider. If a serious condition exists, family members are consulted to assist in making a decision for costly or major procedures or professional health care. Traditional medicine may be used first when the condition is caused by a natural phenomenon or when the Western treatment being considered has been effective based on previous experience. Transcultural nurses need to respect the client's and family's decisions if they choose one or both practices. Today, it is unlikely that Native American people will use traditional practices exclusively. Nurses can provide care by supporting the client's interaction with the traditional practitioner, NAC roadman, priest, or other denominational leaders. In eliciting information about the people's use of health practices outside of modern professional health care, transcultural nurses might ask such questions as, "What other treatments or healing practices do you use? Tell me about the necklace or feather (amulet) that you are wearing and how it may help you. When you were told that you have diabetes, what were your first thoughts? What do you do to feel better?" Asking open-ended questions in a nonhurried manner communicates acceptance, caring, and a willingness to learn about the client's traditional or generic care beliefs and practices.

Today, Native American peoples generally do not understand how life's activities such as eating and preferences for modern conveniences could be blamed for chronic health conditions and physical illnesses.[61,62] However, when exploring further, one will find that these people have their own cultural explanations, which include abandonment of tribal traditions, a loss of spirituality, adopting Anglo ways, increased use of chemicals (fertilizers and pesticides) on plants, and cultural taboo violations.[63] Patience, understanding, and persistence are important values in providing transcultural care practices. They need to be learned and used to provide culturally congruent health education and nursing care with Native American peoples.

■ Food Beliefs and Practices

As in most cultures of the world, food use and preparation are important to Native American peoples. In traditional times, most Native American peoples relied heavily on natural foods gathered from their local environments. Today, many continue to rely on these traditional foods, while some have almost completely abandoned traditional foods. Native Americans from the southwestern United States have valued and used corn and its products in many dishes and rituals as it is a traditional food with many symbolic meanings. For instance, corn pollen is used in Diné and Apache ceremonies. Pueblo people also use corn in food preparations and in dances. Likewise, Hopi people use corn in stews, in *piki* bread, and cornmeals. The Hopi who now live in northern Arizona are known for perfecting dry farming in arid conditions to grow corn for their very important rituals and for food consumption. To these native peoples, corn plays an important role in their food use and sacred knowledge and is considered a healthy food. In addition, Diné have herds of sheep, which provide food and wool for weaving rugs. Sheep and goat meat contain high amounts of fat, and nurses may need to help the Diné to use such meats in moderation or to decrease the fat content in preparing different dishes. Culture care negotiation is indicated as a compromise rather than teaching the complete elimination of meat, which the people desire and have eaten for many years.[64]

Northern Plains people of the United States believe that the buffalo was given to them as a sacred being to provide for their sustenance and rituals. Many of their cultural practices depended on the buffalo such as their dances with clothing that they make from buffalo skin. Traditionally, they organized socially and developed their cultures around the buffalo migration with respect for all that the buffalo brought and represented to them. Today, there are only a few buffalo left and so the plains peoples no longer structure their lives in accordance with the buffalo migrations. However, many continue to hold feasts and other gatherings to honor the old traditions, including reverence to the buffalo. It is important to know the ethnohistory and its relationship to food to provide generic care practices. Native American people feel accepted and respected by any health care providers who accommodate their traditional care practices. The elders, particularly, remain closer to traditional ways with their philosophy of life and very much appreciate health care providers who give culturally congruent care.

As with many cultures of the world, Native Americans have their own food categories and prescriptions. Certain foods are reserved for various stages of the life cycle. Many food prescriptions and taboos are followed during pregnancy, which is a very important phase of life. Pregnancy is believed to be a special time in which "strong" foods are prescribed for the mother and unborn baby. Among the Diné, strong foods consist of traditional foods such as corn, berries, lean meat, and bland food. Fatty, salty, and sweet foods are prohibited during certain rituals, illnesses, or rites of passage. Transcultural nurses need to take a careful nutrition history and to incorporate some of these preferred foods into their care plans and practices. Children usually eat all foods eaten by adults, and they often share foods with adult relatives and eat as much as they want. The Diné believe in feeding small children adult foods such as mutton, stews, or tortillas as they are considered strong foods required for growth. Elders have their own food patterns because of their poorer dentition, gastrointestinal changes, and preferences for smaller portions. Southwest tribes prefer cornmeal and berries prepared in various ways. Transcultural nurses and other care providers need to know the traditional food categories for each stage of the life cycle to provide culturally congruent and acceptable care. Nurses may need to practice cultural care restructuring or repatterning to make food modifications if fatty food intake is contraindicated for health reasons.[65]

When Native Americans are institutionalized, they long for familiar foods and the company of their families during mealtimes. Nurses need to acknowledge this and accommodate and negotiate ways for families to bring in occasional traditional meals. When the author's grandfather was placed in a long-term care facility almost 100 miles away from his home, he longed for many familiar things, but requested food from home every time he was visited by a family member. He described nursing home food as having "no taste and like rubber." He also asked about people from home, his animals, and other news. These are opportunities to provide cultural care preservation and to provide cultural congruent care.

Nurses must learn about people's preferences for foods, food categories, food use during various rituals, food taboos, and foods considered to have favorable health benefits at different times in the life cycle. In the author's research among the Diné people with diabetes, she found that all foods were considered to be gifts from the Creator or Great Spirit; therefore, what Anglos call "junk food" was not a category shared by the Diné.[66] Instead nurses must teach that this food group does not provide proper nutrients for growing children, and foods in this group are detrimental to the health if consumed frequently and in large amounts. Again, nursing actions and decisions for culture care repatterning or restructuring are indicated.

Relevance of Ethnohistory in Nursing and Health Care

Knowledge of native people's history was one of the themes that Native American nurses identified as important to know.[67] This knowledge brings a better understanding about Native American clients, explains some contemporary behaviors, and enhances the establishment of trust between nurse and client. The history of Native Americans is replete with cultural imposition practices in educational settings, in religious realms, in the political-legal process, as well as in the institutions that provide health care. Ortiz, a contemporary Acoma poet noted, " . . . a link to the past that is important for me to hold in my memory because it is the only memory by knowledge that substantiates my present existence."[68] Native American peoples are present and past oriented. Their ethnohistory is important to establish their origin and existence, as well as their cultural lessons learned over time. When Native Americans are asked to introduce themselves, often they take time to acknowledge tribal affiliation, family, and upbringing and how these factors have affected their current lifeways over time. Likewise, Ortiz described his childhood education in a boarding school setting and his realization of the separation from his home and familiar surroundings of places and people. He wrote the following:

> Naturally, I did not perceive this in any analytical or purposeful sense; rather, I felt an unspoken anxiety and resentment against unseen forces that determined our destiny to be an Indian, embarrassed

and uncomfortable with our grandparents' customs and strictly held values. We were to set goals as American working men and women; single-mindedly industrious, patriotic, and unquestioning, building the future that insured that the U.S. was the greatest nation in the world. I felt fearfully uneasy with this, for by then I felt the loneliness, alienation, and isolation imposed upon me by the separation from my family, home, and community.

There is a long history of negative experiences of epidemics, annihilation of entire villages or tribes, forced migrations, and government-sanctioned cultural assimilation practices in Native American history. These historical accounts of survival are shared with children, often through oral history or storytelling so they can pass this intergenerationally on to their children. Historical accounts create and ingrain memories for many generations to come. Ortiz held that the past is brought forward to the present to build a better future.[69] It is for these reasons that elders are valued as they have endured brutal, oppressive practices; experienced the toughest life conditions; and, therefore, have lessons to teach about survival, cultural continuity, perseverance, and dignity. The elders have been trailblazers whose values of strength, persistence, and longevity are emulated. Through acknowledgment of people's ethnohistory, transcultural nurses can provide respect and trust and use generic care practices in the community or with collective groups of Native Americans.

These same lessons exist in health care today, just as Native Americans endured epidemics and hardships of the past. Many believe that the present epidemics of chronic health problems must be faced with strength and persistence. Native Americans remain ever hopeful that life's cruel lessons keep them strong and cohesive and that their traditions will not be lost. Transcultural nurses need to understand the rich and diverse tribal history that provides a context to understand collective peoples and how they define their current lifeways. Understanding the Native Americans' past and present lifeworlds also provides and communicates respect to the people for whom nurses care, and most of all it provides an atmosphere of caring and opens a way for dialog and trusting relations between Native American clients and nurses. Ortiz's summary of cultural preservation depicts this care practice with these words, "We have always had this language, and it is the language, spoken and unspoken, that determines our existence that brought our grandmothers and grandfathers and ourselves into being in order that there be a continuing life."[70]

Summary

In this chapter the author has identified some of the major cultural beliefs, practices, and values as relevant to Native Americans to provide culturally congruent care. Leininger's Theory of Culture Care Diversity and Universality was used to guide the discussion about holistic care with the use of the three modalities of culture care preservation/maintenance, accommodation/negotiation, and repatterning/restructuring. Such knowledge is critical to provide meaningful, sensitive, and knowledgeable care to Native Americans. In using the Culture Care Theory, one can discover multiple factors such as kinship, politics, economics, and high technology that influence the health and well-being of Native Americans. Dominant care constructs for Native Americans include care as *respect, presence among familiar kin, silence, singing special songs, humor,* and *spiritual connectedness*. These care constructs need to be recognized as pertinent and critical by transcultural nurses and other health professionals and need to be included in nursing actions and decisions and other health care planning endeavors.

Tribal communities, whether on reservations or in urban settings, need to be actively involved as partners in their own health care to preserve their emic perspectives. Tribal nations have goals to elevate their health and well-being to the highest possible level. This can be accomplished through the provision of culturally appropriate, competent, and congruent nursing and health care to Native American peoples of this country. In accordance with Leininger's theory, we must acknowledge and respect both the diversity and commonalties that exist among tribes so that stereotyping is avoided. While making cultural assessments, nurses must identify and explore with each tribe their unique beliefs and culturally specific preferences for nursing care. It can be unequivocally stated that, when providing care to Native American clients and communities, one must keep in mind that the holistic approach is preferred to promote the physical, mental, spiritual, and social health of persons, families, and communities. Transcultural nursing is a subfield within the nursing profession, as well as the health care arena, that provides a very important basis for the provision of culturally congruent care to promote the health of Native American peoples.

References

1. Leininger, M., *Transcultural Nursing: Concepts, Theories, Research, and Practices*, New York: John Wiley, 1978.
2. Leininger, M., *Transcultural Nursing: Concepts, Theories, Research, and Practice*, Columbus, OH: McGraw-Hill College Custom Series, 1995.
3. Leininger, M., *Nursing and Anthropology: Two Worlds to Blend*, New York: John Wiley, 1970.
4. Leininger, M., *Culture Care Diversity and Universality: A Theory of Nursing*, New York: National League for Nursing Press, 1991.
5. Leininger, Op. cit., 1970.
6. Leininger, Op. cit., 1995.
7. Tom-Orme, L., "Native Americans Explaining Illness: Storytelling As Illness Experience," in *Explaining Illness: Research, Theory, and Strategies*, B. Whaley, ed., Lawrence Erlbaum Associates, Inc., 2000, pp. 237–256.
8. Weaver, H.N., "Transcultural Nursing with Native Americans: Knowledge, Skills, Attitudes," *Journal of Transcultural Nursing*, 1999, 10(3), pp. 197–202.
9. U.S. Census Bureau, *Resident Estimates of the United States by Sex, Race, and Hispanic Origin: April 1, 1990 to July 1, 1999 with Short-Term Projection to September, 1, 2000*, Population Estimate Program, Population Division, Washington, DC: U.S. Census Bureau, 2000.
10. Indian Health Service, *Regional Differences in Indian Health, 1998–1999*, Washington, DC: U.S. Department of Health and Human Services, 1998–1999.
11. Strickland, C.J., M.D. Squeoch, and N.J. Chrisman, "Health Promotion in Cervical Cancer Prevention Among the Yakama Indian Women of the Wa'Shat Longhouse," *Journal of Transcultural Nursing*, 1999, 19(3), pp. 190–196.
12. Tom-Orme, L., "Native American Women's Health Concerns: Toward Restoration of Harmony," in *Health Issues for Women of Color: A Cultural*

Diversity Perspective, D. Adams, ed., Thousand Oaks, CA: Sage, 1995, pp. 27–41.

13. Valencia, M.E., P.H. Bennett, E. Ravussin, et al. "The Pima Indians in Sonora, Mexico," *Nutrition Review*, 1999, 57(5 pt 2), pp. S55–57.

14. Dean, H., "NIDDM-Y First Nation Children in Canada," *Clinical Pediatrics*, 1998, 37, pp. 89–96.

15. Fagot-Campagna, A., N.R. Burrows, and D.F. Williamson, "The Public Health Epidemiology of Type 2 Diabetes in Children and Adolescents: A Case Study of American Indian Adolescents in the Southwestern United States," *Clinical Chim Acta*, 1999, 286(1–2), pp. 81–95.

16. Indian Health Service, *Trends in Indian Health—1996*, Washington, DC: U.S. Department of Health and Human Services, 1997.

17. Indian Health Service, Op. cit., 1998–1999.

18. Cobb, N. and R. Paisano, *Cancer Mortality among American Indian and Alaska Natives in the United States: Regional Differences in Indian Health, 1989–1993* (IHS Publications No. 97-615-23), Rockville, MD: Department of Health and Humans Services, 1997.

19. Ibid.

20. Glover, C.S. and F.S. Hodge, "The National Cancer Institute's Interventions in Native American Communities: Background and Overview," in *Native Outreach: A Report to American Indian, Alaska Native, and Native Hawaiian Communities* (NIH Publications No. 98-4341), C.S. Glover and F.S. Hodge, eds., Bethesda, MD: National Institutes of Health, 1999, pp. 1–21.

21. Hodge, F.S., L. Fredericks, and P. Kipnis, "It's Your Life—It's Your Future Stop Smoking Project," in *Native Outreach: A report to American Indian, Alaska Native, and Native Hawaiian Communities* (NIH publication No. 98-4341), C.S. Glover and F.S. Hodge, eds., Bethesda, MD: National Institutes of Health, 1999, pp. 67–74.

22. Lanier, A.P., J. Kelly, and J. Berner, "The Alaska Native Women's Health Project to Reduce Cervical Cancer," in *Native Outreach: A Report to American Indian, Alaska Native, and Native Hawaiian Communities* (NIH Publication No. 98-4341), C.S. Glover and F.S. Hodge, eds., Bethesda, MD: National Institutes of Health, 1999, pp. 67–74.

23. Lanier, A.P., J.J. Kelly, P. Holck, et al. *Alaska Native Cancer Update 1985–1997: By Sex, Age, Service Unit and Year.* Anchorage: Alaska Epidemiology Center, May 2000.

24. Indian Health Service, Op. cit., 1998–1999.

25. Denny, C.H. and D. Holtzman, *Health Behaviors of American Indians and Alaska Natives: Findings from the Behavioral Risk Factor Surveillance System, 1993–1996*, Centers for Disease Control, Atlanta, GA, 1999.

26. Indian Health Service, Op. cit., 1998–1999.

27. Bear Heart, *The Wind is My Mother: The Life and Teachings of a Native American Shaman*, New York: Berkley, 1996.

28. Tom-Orme, Op. cit., 2000.

29. Struthers, R. and S. Littlejohn, "The Essence of Native American Nursing," *Journal of Transcultural Nursing*, 1999, 10(2), pp. 131–135.

30. Ibid.

31. Leininger, Op. cit., 1978.

32. Leininger, Op. cit., 1995.

33. Struthers and Littlejohn, Op. cit., 1999.

34. Strickland, C.J., "Conducting Focus Groups Cross-Culturally: Experiences with Pacific Northwest Indian People," *Public Health Nursing*, 1999, 16(3), pp. 190–197.

35. Crow, K., "Multiculturalism and Pluralism Thought in Nursing Education: Native American Worldview and the Nursing Academic Worldview," *Journal of Nursing Education*, 1993, 32(5), pp. 198–204.

36. Tom-Orme, Op. cit., 2000.

37. Strickland, Op. cit., 1999.

38. Hodge, Fredericks, and Kipnis, Op. cit., 1999.

39. Crow, Op. cit., 1993.

40. Tom-Orme, Op. cit., 2000.

41. Weaver, Op. cit., 1999.

42. Tom-Orme, Op. cit., 2000.

43. Tom-Orme, Op. cit., 1994.

44. Aamodt, A.M., "Sociocultural Dimensions of Caring in the World of the Papago Child and Adolescent," in *Transcultural Nursing: Concepts, Theories, and Practices*, M. Leininger, ed., New York: John Wiley & Sons, 1978, pp. 239–249.

45. Purnell, L.D. and B.J. Paulanka, eds., (1998). "Purple's Model for Cultural Competence," in *Transcultural Care: A Culturally Competent Approach*, Philadelphia: F.A. Davis Co., 1998.

46. Tom-Orme, Op. cit., 2000.

47. Leininger, Op. cit., 1991.

48. Plawecki, H.M., T.R. Sanchez, and J.A. Plawecki, "Cultural Aspects of Caring for Navajo Indian Clients," *Journal of Holistic Nursing*, 1994, 12(3), pp. 291–306.

49. Tom-Orme, Op. cit., 2000.

50. Struthers and Littlejohn, Op. cit., 1999.
51. Standing Bear, L., "At Last I Kill a Buffalo," in *Growing Up Native American: Stories of Oppression and Survival, of Heritage Denied and Reclaimed—22 American Writers Recall Childhood in Their Native Land*, P. Riley, ed., New York: Avon Books, 1993, pp. 107–114.
52. Weaver, Op. cit., 1999.
53. Leininger, Op. cit., 1991.
54. Strickland, Op. cit., 1999.
55. Leininger, Op. cit., 1991.
56. Bear Heart, Op. cit., 1996.
57. Struthers and Littlejohn, Op. cit., 1999.
58. Hernandez, C.A., I. Antone, and I. Cornelius. "A Grounded Theory Study of the Experience of Type 2 Diabetes Mellitus in First Nations Adults in Canada," *Journal of Transcultural Nursing*, 1999, 10(3), pp. 220–228.
59. Struthers and Littlejohn, Op. cit., 1999.
60. Crow, Op. cit., 1993.
61. Tom-Orme, L., "Diabetes in a Navajo Community: A Qualitative Study of Health/Illness Beliefs and Practices," unpublished doctoral dissertation, University of Utah, Salt Lake City, UT, 1988.
62. Tom-Orme, Op. cit., 1994.
63. Ibid.
64. Leininger, Op. cit., 1991.
65. Ibid.
66. Tom-Orme, Op. cit., 1988.
67. Weaver, Op. cit., 1999.
68. Ortiz, S., (1993). "The Language We Know," in *Growing Up Native American: Stories of Oppression and Survival, of Heritage Denied and Reclaimed—22 American Writers Recall Childhood in Their Native Land*, P. Riley, ed., New York: Avon Books, 1993, pp. 29–38.
69. Ibid.
70. Ibid.

27
Lithuanian Americans and Culture Care

Rauda Gelazis

Lithuanian Americans in the United States constitute a culturally distinct group of people which has not been extensively studied to date, in nursing or in other fields. The many recent changes in Lithuania, culminating with its dramatic struggle for independence from Soviet domination and oppression, have revitalized interest in Lithuania and the other Baltic countries. Accordingly, nurses are aware of the country, its struggles and needs, but few have substantive knowledge of Lithuanian culture. Transcultural nursing knowledge is essential in order for nurses to understand the people as a basis to learn about their nursing care needs and especially to develop professional nursing care that will provide culturally congruent care to Lithuanian Americans.

During the last four decades Leininger has developed and done research in transcultural nursing to establish a knowledge base for nurse teachers and practitioners for the specialty field. Her Culture Care Theory emphasizes understanding the cultural dimensions of human care. To achieve this goal the worldview, ethnohistory, social structure, language, cultural values, and care systems need to be studied to discover ways to provide care. The major theoretical premise of Leininger's Theory of Culture Care is that knowledge and understanding of a people's culture care beliefs, practices, and values are essential to develop sound professional nursing care that is culturally congruent.[1] The theory predicts that nursing care that fits the client's lifeways will be more satisfying, effective, and lead to well-being.[2] Moreover, a lack of culturally congruent care can lead to cultural conflicts, noncompliance, and additional stress for clients. As nurses become more aware of the importance of transcultural nursing in a world in which many peoples are struggling for cultural

independence and survival, it is important to understand the many diverse cultures who need quality nursing care practices.

In this chapter the author presents some transcultural nursing insights and knowledge about Lithuanian Americans with practical applications for nursing care. This specific, culturally congruent care knowledge is based upon the author's research findings using Leininger's Culture Care Theory with Lithuanian American people, and from the author's lifelong personal experience with the Lithuanian culture.

Theoretical Framework

The theory of Cultural Care Diversity and Universality emphasizes the centrality of cultural perspectives of care to nursing.[3] The theorist postulates that if culture care values, expressions, and forms of care are known, the health or well-being of individuals or groups will be evident.[4] The goal of the theory is to provide culturally congruent nursing care or care that fits with the client's culture and lifeways.[5] In order to achieve this goal, Leininger describes three dominant modes to guide nursing care: culture care maintenance or preservation, culture care accommodation or negotiation, and culture care repatterning or restructuring.[6] These modalities give full consideration to the client's lifeways while at the same time providing professional information to clients to make choices and decisions of what professional ideas and practices will be viewed most helpful to them.

Leininger has identified care as essential to the growth, well-being, and survival of human beings. In order to understand fully the patterns of culture care, the professional nurse needs to closely study the social structure, language uses, symbols, and meanings about care of a given culture, for it is human care that makes a difference in well-being. However, values and beliefs about care are usually covert and embedded in the worldview and social structure of a particular culture. The Sunrise Model, as developed by Leininger, helped the researcher focus on the various aspects of worldview, cultural, social structure, and health system dimensions that influence care and health in the various cultural contexts identified.[7] These diverse social structure factors were investigated by the author with Lithuanian Americans in a Midwestern metropolitan area in the United States.[8] The author used the ethnonursing research method in order to tease out and make known care phenomena for nursing care practices largely from the people's emic perspective using the tenets and premises of the theory of Culture Care Diversity and Universality, looking for similarities and differences among the people.[9] The ethnonursing method is designed to focus specifically upon learning from the people about actual and potential nursing phenomena through eyes, ears, and experiences.[10] The author used the ethnonursing research method to study Lithuanian Americans in order to obtain data and to understand the peoples' views and beliefs about care and ways that these influenced health or well-being. The recommendations for culturally congruent, professional nursing care are based on this research. Since no previous nursing studies of Lithuanian Americans were found in a literature review, this research stands as an important first nursing care study with the culture.

■ Ethnohistory of Lithuanian Americans

A brief ethnohistory of the Lithuanian Americans' homeland on the Baltic Sea will be presented, followed by a focus on Lithuanian Americans in the United States. Ethnohistory helps to set the context to explain and even predict some of the findings about Lithuanian Americans and their care expressions and needs. Lithuanian Americans are a relatively small culture in the United States when compared with other major cultures such as African Americans, Hispanic Americans, and European Americans. This culture has been highly influenced over several generations by the dominant culture of the Anglo-Americans in the United States.

Lithuanian Americans have been able to deal with most conflicting intercultural values in a positive manner.

Lithuania — Baltic Sea Homeland

Lithuania, at present, is 25,200 square miles in area (about the size of West Virginia) with a population of 3,723,000, and a density of 108 persons per square mile.[11,12] The capital of Lithuania is Vilnius. Lithuania has a seaport, Klaipeda, on the Baltic Sea. Lithuania is bounded on the north by Latvia, Belarus on the East, Poland on the South, and the Baltic Sea on the West. In the past the economy was based on agriculture. The people are predominantly of the Roman Catholic religion.

Lithuanians, along with Latvians, are the only remaining remnants of the family of Baltic people who have inhabited the shores of the Baltic Sea for over 4,000 years. The other Baltic tribes of Old Prussians and Yatvingians became extinct during the later part of the Middle Ages through wars with the Teutonic knights and through assimilation into the Germanic tribes. Lithuanian prehistory goes back to 1500 B.C. when Lithuanians were already living in their present homeland. They were called "Aestians" (the Honorables) and were pagan nature worshippers.[13] Their earlier religious beliefs included worship of the sun and other natural phenomena. Artifacts symbolizing the sun god have been recovered, such as amber which came to represent the healing properties of the sun.[14] Evidence of goddess worship has also been found in the artifacts of these peoples.[15] In the Mesolithic and Neolithic eras the Aestians lived as tribes until the fifth century A.D., when a loose federation was formed headed by a pagan high priest. In the thirteenth century (1251) the tribes were united under Mindaugas, who defeated the Mongols. Mindaugas and many Lithuanians were baptized into Christianity and gradually became Roman Catholics. Roman Catholicism has been the dominant religion of the people since the thirteenth century.[16] Lithuania was a powerful nation for several centuries and spread over northeastern Europe. In the sixteenth century Lithuania joined with Poland and later declined in power. During the seventeenth and eighteenth centuries Lithuania was under Polish or Russian rule. Because of its key position on the Baltic Sea, various countries tried to gain power over Lithuania. In the nineteenth century the Russians attempted to eradicate the Lithuanian language and culture by forbidding the teaching of the language and banning printed matter in the language. By the end of the 19th century, Lithuanian serfdom which the Lithuanians experienced under the Russians ended. Lithuanians held tenaciously to their own language, and national leaders emerged to promote Lithuanian identity and language.

Lithuania became an independent state in 1918, but it was forcibly annexed by the Union of Soviet Socialist Republics in 1940. During the time of independence Lithuania, though still largely an agrarian country, had begun to make strides toward modernization and industrialization.[17] When the Communists took over, all private ownership was eliminated and all farming and industry were taken over under the direct rule of the communist government.[18] In 1941, hundreds of thousands of Lithuanians were deported in cattle cars to Soviet prison camps in Siberia.[19] The deportations to Siberia and political oppression continued for almost fifty years.[20]

The Lithuanian language is one of the oldest Indo-European languages.[21] It is part of the ancient European language family called the Indo-European languages.[22] The prehistoric Indo-Europeans left no written records such as did their Egyptian and Mesopotamian contemporaries.[23] The Indo-European language discovery came from clues during the opening of trade with India around 1585. At that time an Italian merchant named Filippo Sassetti discovered that Hindu scholars could speak and write an ancient language as venerable as Latin and Greek and he called this language Sanscruta (Sanskrit).[24] Scholars later studied this language and believed it to have the same roots as Latin and Greek. Sanskrit, or the Indo-Iranian branch of the Indo-European languages, and Lithuanian are both satem-languages, meaning that the primitive Indo-European K' has developed similarly in both languages.[25]

Lithuanians Come to the United States

After World War II Lithuanian emigration to the United States represented the attempts of thousands of Lithuanians to find freedom from political, religious, and economic oppression. Most post-World War II immigra-

tion occurred from 1940 to 1951, but there had been other migrations of Lithuanians to the United States in the latter part of the eighteenth and early nineteenth centuries. The famine of 1867–68 and land reforms in Lithuania had been responsible for earlier emigration to the United States. Those who came in the early nineteenth century came here to better their economic, political, and religious conditions, but many returned to their homeland after saving some money and rejoined families left in Lithuania. The choice of returning to their homeland had not been available to the Lithuanians in the United States until 1991, when Lithuania was recognized as an independent nation after the fall of the Soviet empire.[26]

Throughout the world there are approximately 800,000 Lithuanians in exile in various countries. There are about 650,000 Lithuanians in the United States, living mostly in industrial and metropolitan centers in the Eastern and Midwestern parts of the country. There are also Lithuanians in Brazil, Argentina, Uruguay, Canada, Australia, and Great Britain.[27] Today, over fifty years after the loss of independence and freedom, Lithuanians throughout the world struggle to maintain their language and culture and try to help Lithuanians in their homeland resist the influences of a Soviet communist regime.[28]

In Lithuania there was a pattern of Russification of the Lithuanian language while the country was under Soviet rule.[29,30] In the West, there are influences from the countries where Lithuanians settled after escaping.[31] In the United States, for example, there is now a generation of Lithuanians who have had to be bilingual almost from birth and for whom the Lithuanian language has never been their sole language. Under such conditions, the Lithuanian language becomes difficult to maintain and expression becomes somewhat stylized and awkward due to the fact that speakers use translation in their thought processes.[32]

In recent years Lithuania regained its freedom.[33] Under the Soviet Union's policy of glasnost, or openness (1988–1989), Lithuania began to push for independence. On March 11, 1990 the Act of the Restoration of the Lithuanian State was signed, declaring independence from the Soviet Union.[34,35] In 1991, with the dissolution of the Soviet regime, the United States and many other countries have recognized Lithuania as an independent, sovereign nation. Today Lithuania is striving to become economically stable and is developing economic ties with Europe, the United States and other nations.[36]

Lithuanian Americans living in the United States today consist of Lithuanians and their families who came to America after World War II, in the period of 1949 to 1951, as well as Lithuanians who came to the United States before World War I, and the descendants of the Lithuanian immigrants in the late nineteenth century.[37] They supported the movement for freedom in their homeland in any way they could over the years. Since the declaration of independence by Lithuania, support and assistance for their homeland continues. The most recent wave of immigration to America came in the 1990s and consists of people immigrating to study and to better their economic status.

Review of Literature on Lithuanian Americans

A review of literature on Lithuanian Americans revealed few research studies about this cultural group. The few existing studies of the culture have found that the Lithuanian people value their religion, family, hard work, frugality, hospitality, and possess a strong regard for its culture, traditions, and particularly the Lithuanian language.[38–41] Lithuania has a very old culture and has withstood centuries of invasions and attempts at annihilating its people and identity.[42] Lithuanian scholars and anthropologists such as Gimbutas have studied various aspects of the culture, such as its myths.[43] Its ancient culture was once matriarchal and even to this day women are highly regarded in the culture.[44] To date, no nursing or ethnonursing studies have been published about this culture. This author has conducted research about Lithuanian Americans and the findings are consistent with the few studies mentioned here.[45]

Several more recent ethnographies of Lithuanian Americans focus on the ethnic identity of the people in different parts of the United States. Baskauskas studied an urban enclave of Lithuanian refugees in Los Angeles.[46] She noted that even though Lithuanians participate in American economic, educational, and political systems, they also pursue their other major cultural and social objectives. Lithuanian American refugees viewed their culture as equal to if not better than the surrounding one and had no desire to ex-change it for the other. They have established stable and important social relations with others outside their group. Baskauskas noted that Lithuanians were among those selected to immigrate after World War II due to a seeming behavioral similarity to the population already present in America, but that the expected acculturation/assimilation did not seem to occur. Baskauskas postulated that post World War II Lithuanians who came here were refugees, rather than immigrants who left their homeland by choice. Refugees who had been displaced by the war and could not return to their homeland due to the Soviet Communist occupation may constitute a group differing from immigrant groups. Her study was done in the early 1970s before the interest that African Americans generated in finding their cultural roots. In the 1980s there has been a considerable change in attitudes toward cultural differences and cultural and ethnic pride in one's cultural heritage that has to some extent replaced the attempt of cultural groups to quickly become part of the melting pot.

Gedmintas in 1979 studied the ethnic identity among Lithuanian Americans in the urban industrial setting of Binghamton, New York.[47] Gedmintas concluded that ethnicity and ethnic identification, far from being all or nothing categories, vary according to social conditions. He noted that ethnicity, or ethnic interaction, may fade in importance in comparison to ethnicity at other levels, but the potential for ethnicity is maintained through the retention of ethnic identity as part of the individual's basic social identity. Gedmintas also found that although Lithuanian ethnicity has been declining (among third generation Lithuanian Americans), "Eastern European" ethnicity had gained in comparative importance. In other words, ethnicity as a social phenomenon had not disappeared among the Binghamton Lithuanians, but rather it had shifted in emphasis.

This author also noted that the Lithuanian Americans who were included in her study also held strongly to a Lithuanian identity. The population studied was in another urban center of the United States, and the study was considerably later than the Baskauskas and Gedmintas studies, but some of the findings still hold true. The author found, for example, that Lithuanian identity was very important to Lithuanian Americans of various age groups and generations. Furthermore, during the study, Lithuania regained its independence from the Soviets, and there was an impetus for renewed interest and pride in being Lithuanian. With these changes, the author continues to study Lithuanian Americans and Lithuanians.

 ## Research Findings Related to Worldview, Social Structure, and Other Dimensions

The author conducted research with Lithuanian Americans using Leininger's theory of Culture Care and the Sunrise Model[48] as guides to study the theory. The theory and model helped guide the author's research with both key and general informants who were first and second generation Lithuanian Americans. All social structure dimensions were studied with Lithuanian American informants in their native and in the English languages. Ethnonursing research methods were used to conduct qualitative research with Lithuanian Americans in an urban Midwestern area. The data were analyzed according to Leininger's four-phase analysis, wherein the data are studied for patterns, and eventually themes pertinent to the study emerge. An interview guide based on the social structure features of the theory and the Sunrise Model was used with both key and general informants. Observation and participation in various events in the Lithuanian American community also added important data to the study. The cultural values which were identified from the informant data and observations were the following: 1) family closeness; 2) deep religious beliefs and convictions (Roman Catholic); 3) education; 4) hard work (*darbštumas*) and industriousness; 5) conscientiousness (*saziningumas*); 6) thriftiness and good use of material resources; 7) endurance and perseverance, in spite of hardships; 8) charity to others and hospitality (*vaišingumas*); and 9) pride and emphasis on a continuation of their language and culture despite previous long-term attempts to oppress or annihilate the language and many social structure features. Each of these cultural values will be discussed in relation to culture care.

Kinship Factors

The value of family closeness and kinship was very evident.[49] Lithuanian American informants spoke of the importance of family in their lives. Frequently, family ties were maintained over time and distance. Since many informants had relatives in Lithuania where, until recent years, travel and communication were restricted by the Soviets, the difficulty in maintaining ties were a source of worry and concern. Many informants had for decades sent whatever material help they could to their relatives in Lithuania. This forced separation from loved ones was described as painful by informants. Informants spoke of being close to extended family members such as grandparents, aunts, uncles, and cousins. Informants frequently visit with relatives and described getting support through them. Divorce is not very common and informants placed value on intact family structures. Some informants linked strong family and kinship ties with strong religious beliefs and practices.

Care patterns and meanings related to kinship patterns for Lithuanian Americans were evident in the finding that care is expressed and intertwined with daily lifeways and expressed in interactions with family and friends. Care meant presence, and this was evident in the family interactions. For example, fathers described staying home when children became ill in order to give support through their presence. Persons also described that they showed care to each other in the family "in the everyday small things that you do for each other that you show care for one another." Care is also shown by listening and sharing with one another. Most Lithuanian Americans interviewed, and in participant observations, indicated that care in terms of family was very important to them.

Many said that it was support from relatives and friends that added to their ability to persevere despite difficulties such as illness. Informants who had been ill felt that Lithuanian friends visited frequently and let them know in other small ways that they cared. Being charitable to others was also a value expressed by informants. For example, many had helped their relatives in Lithuania.

Religious Factors

The majority of Lithuanian Americans are Roman Catholic. Informants described their strong faith as the reason they could endure years of hardship, especially informants who lived through World War II and who had to start their lives in America after escaping the Communist regime. Informants with prison experiences under communist or Nazi regimes talked of faith and a hope for the future as important to maintaining themselves in a state of well-being during their imprisonment. This is consistent with the writings of Franklin, in which the author describes survival in deplorable conditions of a concentration camp and emphasizes the key to survival is the meaning one gives to an experience.[50] Other informants pointed with pride at the attempts of Lithuanians to retain their religious beliefs despite mistreatment and punishment under an atheistic government in Lithuania for fifty years. *The Chronicles of the Church in Lithuania* were described as the written account of the peoples' persecution and suffering for their religious beliefs. Participant-observation of the Lithuanian American community revealed that much of the community's activities centered around the two Catholic parishes in the area studied. Many cultural events, for example, took place at the parish auditorium. The Lithuanian elementary and high schools were both held in parish buildings. Religious life is also closely tied to cultural preservation, language, and education as well as other aspects of Lithuanian American life, such as political and welfare organizations.

Religious values and beliefs permeate the daily lives of Lithuanian Americans and are the basis for care expressions. Informants described charity to others and "helping in times of need" as part of the care patterns they experienced. For example, informants described attending a prayer group with a friend with a chronic physical illness. Hospitality, which is a hallmark of caring in Lithuanian Americans, is viewed as an important way to show care to friends and strangers. Even persons of modest means make a great effort to share whatever they possibly can with guests and visitors. Also, the Lithuanian community has several organizations whose purpose is to help those in need. Lithuanians are known for their hospitality (*vaišingumas*) and take pride in this. Lithuanians in America as well as in Lithuania were noted to be very hospitable toward guests. Informants remarked that as students they had traveled to other cities and had been cared for by Lithuanians who hardly knew them. Persons who have visited Lithuania all commented on the warmth and sincerity of the people and how visitors were always received with feasts of food and drink. Friends and relatives

had saved and pooled their resources for weeks in order to receive people hospitably. It is considered poor manners to refuse food and drink and guests are encouraged numerous times to partake of what is offered. Some jokingly told of times when they were new in American and had at first politely declined to eat, waiting to be asked a third or fourth time, only to find out that Americans usually offered only once. This made them think that this was a sign of non-caring until they realized that this was the usual custom in America.

Educational Factors

Education was described as important to informants, both younger and older. Older informants described sacrificing in order to be sure that their children could attend college. Younger informants shared their pride in completing college and working productively in various professions. Many informants pointed out that the sciences and technology were often selected for study because these were viewed as important fields. Material wealth was not emphasized, though informants were pleased that their lives were comfortable. Many of the older informants described coming to America decades ago with very little and becoming successful in a new world through considerable effort and hard work.

Care is evident in the many sacrifices that families make in order for children to be well educated. Parents with young children spoke of supervising children's homework and participating in school activities. Older parents spoke with pride about the educational successes of their children and described many sacrifices they had made to make sure the children received the best education possible. In turn, children expressed considerable respect and gratitude to their parents. Thus the caring was reciprocated, that is, from parents to children and children to parents. For example, most adult children do everything possible to care for elderly parents at home. Nursing homes are seen as a last resort. If nursing home care is required, attempts are made to have placement in Lithuanian-based nursing care facilities.

Economic Factors

The value of hard work (*darbštumas*), industriousness and being conscientious (*sazíningumas*) in any work that is done was noted by the informants. Many informants also noted that this value had changed greatly in Lithuania under the communist regime. Under the communist system it was noted that people no longer had any incentive to work since all of the farms were put into collective farms and all industry was put under the Soviet government. Some of the informants who had visited Lithuania, or who had visitors from Lithuania, had noted the different view toward work. As one informant, who had recently emigrated, noted, "If you work hard here in America, you have something to show for it, but if you work hard there (Lithuania under Soviet rule) you still had nothing." Now that Lithuania has regained its independence, hope was expressed that many of the older values would eventually return to the people.

Lithuanian Americans also described themselves as thrifty and used material resources well. For example, many informants had small vegetable gardens or had fruit trees and canned these products. Some informants sewed or had family members who sewed in order to save money on clothing. Particularly the older informants described being able to endure and persevere through severe hardships.

Care is linked to economic factors in that persons expressed care economically when possible. Relatives in the homeland were sent money, food, and clothing when possible. In Soviet-ruled Lithuania, for example, severe restrictions were placed on what could be sent by mail. Lithuanian Americans circumvented the restrictions by obtaining visas to visit relatives and would come to Lithuania loaded down with clothing, money, and other gifts for relatives. Recently, because Lithuania is independent, travel as well as sending packages have opened up, and Lithuanian Americans continue to demonstrate their care by sending and taking considerable material goods to Lithuania.

Cultural Values and Lifeways

Another value mentioned by all informants was pride in their culture and language. Younger informants described their participation in various dance and folkensembles and expressed the fact that they felt enriched by experiences with these groups. Older informants in particular expressed concern about passing on the language and traditions of the Lithuanian culture. The

informants were also politically aware, particularly regarding the changing situation in Lithuania and the Baltics and other Soviet republics. When Lithuania regained its freedom, Lithuanian Americans rejoiced despite knowing that many future hardships would be faced.

Lithuanian Americans demonstrate care by showing continuing respect and value by their heritage to the point where considerable time and effort is placed on activities and organizations that serve to continue Lithuanian-ness (*lietuvybe*). For example, families described participating in Lithuanian Saturday school, Lithuanian youth religious groups, Lithuanian scouts, parish choir, and Lithuanian sports groups, folk dance and song ensembles. These activities are done during weekend or evening hours after a full work or school schedule. Much appreciation was noted on the part of children, as they grew older, for the opportunities that these activities provided so that not only the Lithuanian heritage-was perpetuated, but participants noticed that their world was widened by these additional activities. Many Lithuanian organizations and gatherings occurred in various cities in America as well as other countries. For example, parish choir members of various ages participated in Rome in the celebration of the anniversary of Lithuania's Christianity. This occasion put them in contact with other European people and cultures. Others spoke of traveling to South America with dance and singing groups or to Australia for Lithuanian scouting jamborees.

Political Factors

Lithuanian Americans of various ages expressed an interest in the political life of their homeland as well as of America. Young people in particular spoke of the importance and need to go outside the political sphere of Lithuanian American communities and enter the politics and influence of America. During the time of the study Lithuania was pressing for its independence from the Soviet Union. Lithuanian Americans throughout the country actively demonstrated, wrote and phoned their representatives in Washington, D.C. in order to get the United States to recognize Lithuania as independent. The author participated in a demonstration in Washington, D.C. as part of her participant observation and noted that considerable unity and organization was evident in the demonstration. For example, bus-loads of people met on the given date in front of the Lincoln Memorial. The feelings expressed by the demonstrators also included elements of political humor in the various placards carried by demonstrators. Examples of such humorous elements were phrases to the President such as "Mr. President, Lithuania doesn't grow broccoli" (the demonstration occurred shortly after the President had taken a firm stand against broccoli, but was seen as not taking a supportive stand toward freeing of the Baltics), or "Read my lips, Soviets, get out of Lithuania!" Lithuanians tended to use subtle humor and humorous approaches to deal with oppressive situations.

Caring was expressed in this sphere by Lithuanian Americans, in so far as many organizations exist in the Lithuanian American community to be sure that the needs of the people are met. Care is seen as both individual and in organized caring community efforts through Lithuanian organizations. An example was the Lithuanian Golden Agers Club, which made sure that information about all available resources for the elderly was given to and understood by members so that the proper agencies would be turned to when needed.

■ Culture Care Meanings

The dominant meanings of care for Lithuanian Americans were the following: 1) care as presence or "being there" for someone else; 2) care as helping in times of need; 3) care as concern for or watching over another (*prieziura*); 4) care as worrying about (*rupestis*) another; 5) care as hospitality toward others; 6) sharing with others (other-care); 7) flexibility to adapt; 8) cooperation with others; 9) praying with others; and 10) using subtle humor. The research showed that care meanings for Lithuanian Americans were embedded or part of daily lifeways and patterns. Care was part of the structure of the Lithuanian American community, for many organizations existing in the Lithuanian American community provided aspects of care to the people. Care was frequently described as being an integral part of everyday life and expressed in daily life patterns between family and friends in the little things that are said and done in family interactions. Care meanings and patterns were closely linked

to Lithuanian American cultural values as highlighted earlier.

Among the important care meanings for Lithuanian Americans was care as presence or being there. For example, informants said that they valued visits from friends when ill and that at times fathers would take time off from work to be at home with ill children. Presence was seen as an important care expression in family celebrations and important family events, from baptism to funerals. Care as presence meant making the extra effort to be with another in times of need.

Care as helping others in time of need was another major finding. Informants described the Lithuanian American community as a caring community. Help in need was provided both by individuals and through organizations. For example, food was brought to the family during acute or long-term illnesses. Spiritual support at such times was evident through visits not only from the parish priest, but from friends and neighbors who visit regularly for prayer and reflection. Organizations, such as the Golden Agers Club, also provide help to members when needed in concrete ways, from providing transportation for medical care to providing information and needed material support.

Frequently care was identified as a watching over or concern for (*prieziura*). This concept connotes care that is broad in scope and includes various aspects of care for a person. It refers to assessing what is needed and providing for the need as possible. For example, an informant described care as "an attitude . . . it's from the soul; an orientation."

Another term frequently used for care was worry about or concern about another (*rupestis*). Along with the concerned attitude is working toward providing the needed element of care. One informant described this as "Care is an on-going thing . . . it's taking care of someone, making it your first priority, also a responsibility."

Care meant sharing with others and was related to the high value placed on hospitality. Informants often described times of sharing with others despite lack of material wealth. Great value was placed on giving of oneself in terms of time or listening to another's problems. Important to this process is doing "little things" for someone else to show care, such as staying with young children so that a young mother can have a few hours to herself. One informant described this kind of caring as "an attitude . . . it's from the soul . . . it's an ongoing thing like when you notice something is needed, you take care of it." Persons are graciously and hospitably received by Lithuanians, even of modest means, because the emphasis is placed on the attitude of caring about others and not on the lavishness of the hospitality offered a guest.

Care as lived in a community of Lithuanian Americans was clearly supported by descriptions of closeness felt by the members of the community. For example, even younger informants frequently stated that they felt understood and accepted and had developed a special closeness for other Lithuanian Americans. Young Lithuanian Americans met frequently and interacted with each other from various parts of America and even other parts of the world, because their involvement in various Lithuanian American organizations made such contacts possible. Informants saw care as cooperation with others with flexibility to meet survival conditions, especially in a new country and culture. Many of the older informants, for example, had to take any job they could find when they first came to America, despite their previous educational preparation or profession. For example, professional musicians, teachers, professors, etc., worked in factories in America. To survive one had to maintain a cooperative and flexible caring posture and attitude. Humor was seen as vital to other survival adaptation processes, especially in situations where direct confrontation was not seen as a productive or desirable end. Humor helped to buffer difficult situations and frequently was subtle in nature. Subtle humor could be used as part of caring forms of communication in difficult situations.

 ## Transcultural Nursing Actions and Decisions Using the Three Modes for Culturally Congruent Care for Lithuanian Americans

Culturally congruent professional nursing care for Lithuanian American clients should reflect the nurse's knowledge of the clients' values and lifeways. Several nursing care actions and decision guides may be drawn from knowledge of culture as well as care meanings and values. Much of nursing care will involve the model of culture care preservation and/or maintenance.

Culture Care Preservation

Since Lithuanian Americans place value on education, and to some extent on science and technology, most Lithuanian Americans were aware of current medical and some nursing practices. The nurse needs to make certain that medications and other instructions are well understood. Because family is highly valued, for example, elderly clients may be living with family members. The nurse needs to include significant family members in caring for the client and in giving home-going instructions. Elderly clients will be likely to follow instructions from professionals very closely. This tendency may relate to the value and respect given to education and educated persons. In teaching Lithuanian Americans it is important to get feedback from them about what they heard and correct any misunderstandings. Informants, in describing how they followed instructions from physicians, have remarked that even the physician was surprised that instructions were followed so closely. Lithuanian Americans take pride in preserving their language and are likely to use Lithuanian when speaking to each other. This preference should be respected. Remembering that the people have been oppressed for years should help the professional nurse understand the reasons for the strong desire to preserve their language and culture. English is spoken by most Lithuanian-Americans and language is not generally a problem unless the client is elderly or recently from Lithuania. Spiritual beliefs are important to the people and should be incorporated into their care.

Because presence means caring for Lithuanian Americans it is important for the nurse to spend time with them. While technical care may be important, presence is highly valued and many informants spoke of listening as an important aspect of care. Therefore professional nurses should make a point of listening to the client and family members. Lithuanian Americans also value flexibility and several informants remarked that they preferred to have nurses who were able to adapt procedures or who were not rigidly holding to the rules of the institution.

Lithuanian Americans use few folk remedies and adhere to prescribed Western medical treatments and medications. Some informants spoke of using herbs and teas at times, such as chamomile tea for colds and linden blossom tea for fever. The nurse does need to assess each client in order to determine what, if any, folk remedies are being used and be sure that no effects are present which may counteract the medications prescribed.

Culture Care Accommodation

Culture care accommodation or negotiation would be used by nurses as well. Primarily this mode may involve accommodating family members and including them in the nursing care when possible. For example, in the case of hospitalized clients, family members may come long distances to be with the client. The nurse needs to accommodate the nursing care to their presence by extending visiting hours and giving family members a role in their care. Lithuanian Americans try to respect rules and regulations and may hesitate to ask for any special treatment, therefore, the nurse will frequently need to be astute enough to anticipate the needs of the client and family.

Culture Care Restructuring

Culture care restructuring and repatterning, referring to changing lifeways by repatterning would not be beneficial with this cultural group. Should any changes need to be made in lifestyle or pattern, the nurse needs to assess how such changes would be received by the client and plan for the changes together with the client and family. For example, if a client needed to change dietary habits because of high cholesterol level, the nurse needs to take a diet history. Since many of the traditional Lithuanian foods may be high in fat and cholesterol, the nurse may need to plan with the client and his/her spouse and family how the modifications in diet would be possible and still include some favorite dishes. Many Lithuanian American informants mentioned that as part of maintaining well-being, physical health and exercise were important. In the case of repatterning some aspects of their lives for the sake of health, most clients could be cooperative with changes,

provided that the nurse is considerate of their preferences and culture care values, needs, and beliefs.

■ Summary Reflections

The theory of culture care was most valuable to study and document lifeways of Lithuanian Americans undergoing many changes in the United States. The theory of Culture Care Diversity and Universality and the Sunrise Model served as the basis for gaining an understanding of this culture and for making culture care guidelines to support the health and well-being of the people.

This chapter focused on Lithuanian Americans and their cultural values, as well as care meanings and values which were shared with the author in doing postmasters and doctoral research with this cultural group. An ethnohistory of Lithuanian Americans helped to explain some of their cultural lifeways and beliefs. Leininger's theory of culture care and the ethnonursing qualitative research method were the basis of explicating the guides for culturally congruent care of the Lithuanian American. Culturally congruent care may include any or all three modes of professional actions. All three, culture care preservation, accommodation, and repatterning were considered, and specific recommendations were made for each mode. The professional nurse can use the above information to provide culturally congruent care for Lithuanian Americans in his/her nursing practice. The author continues her research on this culture. These on-going studies will be published in the future so that professional nurses and others in health care can give culturally congruent care for Lithuanian Americans.

■ References

1. Leininger, M., "Leininger's Theory of Cultural Care Diversity and Universality," *Nursing Science Quarterly*, v. 1, no. 4, 1988, pp. 152–160.
2. Leininger, M., *Culture Care Diversity and Universality: A Theory of Nursing*, New York: National League for Nursing Press, 1991.
3. Leininger, op. cit., 1988, p. 155.
4. Ibid., p. 156.
5. Ibid., p. 155.
6. Leininger, op. cit., 1991, pp. 42–44.

7. Leininger, op. cit., 1988, p. 156.
8. Gelazis, R., "The Effects of Political Oppression on a Culture: A Study of the Lithuanian American," presentation at the fourteenth Transcultural Nursing Society Conference, Edmonton, Alberta, Canada, 1988.
9. Leininger, op. cit., 1991, p. 75.
10. Ibid., p. 79.
11. Urbonas, J., "Lithuanians," in *Ethnic Groups in Michigan*, vol. 2, J.M. Anderson and I.A. Smith, eds., Detroit: Ethnic Heritage Center, Ethnic Press, 1983.
12. LIETUVA: Journal From the Republic of Lithuania, 1991, v. 1, p. 10.
13. Sabaliauskas, A., *Mes Baltai*, Kaunas, Lithuania: Šviesa, 1986.
14. Gimbutas, M., "The Ancient Religion of the Balts," *Lituanus*, 1985, v. 4, pp. 97–109.
15. Gimbutas, M., *The Language of the Goddess*, San Francisco: Harper and Row Publishers, 1989.
16. Gerutis, A., ed., *Lithuania 700 Years*, New York: Manyland Books, 1969.
17. Šapoka, A., *Lietuvos Istorija*, Kaunas, Lithuania: Švietimo Ministerijos Knygu Leidinio Komisija, 1939.
18. Sruogiene, V.D., *Lietuvos Istorija*, Chicago: Terra, 1950.
19. Prunskis, J., *Lietuviai Sibire*, Chicago: Lithuanian Library Press, Inc., 1981.
20. Urbonas, op. cit., 1983.
21. Skardzius, P., "The Lithuanian Language in the Indo-European Family of Languages," 1 and 2, *Lithuanian Bulletin*, 1947, v. 5, nos. 9–10; 11, pp. 3–4.
22. Fraenkel, G., *Languages of the World*, Boston: Gin & Co., 1967.
23. Thieme, P., "The Indo-European Language," *Scientific American*, 1958, v. 199, no. 4, pp. 63–74.
24. Ibid., p. 65.
25. Klimas, A., "Lithuanian and Sanskrit," *Lithuanian Bulletin*, 1947, v. 5, no. 9–10, pp. 78–79.
26. Krickus, R.J., "Hostages in their Homeland," *Commonweal*, 1980, v. 80, February 15, pp. 75–80.
27. Senn, A., *The Lithuanian Language*, Chicago: Publications of the Lithuanian Cultural Institute, 1942.

28. Krickus, op. cit., 1980.
29. Šilbajoris, R., "City and Country in Recent Soviet Lithuanian and Russian Prose," *Journal of Baltic Studies*, 1985, v. 16, no. 2, pp. 118–127.
30. Mickunas, A., "Kad Tik Ne Zmogus: Filosofija Dabarties Lietuvoje," *Metmenys*, 1986, v. 51, pp. 145–162.
31. Bilaišyte, Z., "Ieškant Prasmes: Kalba, Istorinis Palikimas ir Tikrove," *Metmenys*, 1986, pp. 3–20.
32. Ibid., p. 5.
33. Ramonis, V., *Baltic States vs. the Russian Empire: 1000 Years of Struggle for Freedom*, Lemont, IL: Baltech Publishing, 1991.
34. Zumbakis, S.P., ed., *Lithuanian Independence: The Re-Establishment of the Rule of Law*, Chicago: Ethnic Community Services, 1990.
35. Ramonis, op. cit., 1991.
36. Ibid.
37. Urbonas, op. cit., 1983.
38. Alilunas, L.J., *Lithuanian in the United States: Selected Studies*, San Francisco: R. & E. Research Associates, Inc., 1978.
39. Budreckis, A.M., *Eastern Lithuania: A Collection of Historical and Ethnographic Studies*, Chicago: Morkunas Printing Press, 1985.
40. Dunduliene, P., *Lietuviu Etnografija*, Vilnius, Lithuania: Mokslas, 1982.
41. Bindokiene, D.B., *Lietuviu Paprociai ir Tradicijos Išeivijoje*, Chicago: Lithuanian World Community, Inc., 1989.
42. Gerutis, op. cit., 1969.
43. Gimbutiene, M., "Baltu Mitologija," *Mokslas ir Gyvenimas*, January 1989, v. 1, pp. 37–38.
44. Bindokiene, op. cit., 1989.
45. Gelazis, op. cit., 1988.
46. Baskauskas, L., *An Urban Enclave: Lithuanian Refugees in Los Angeles*, New York: AMS Press, Inc., 1985.
47. Gedmintas, A., *Dynamics of Ethnic Identity Among Lithuanian-Americans in an Urban Industrial Setting*, dissertation, Binghamton State University of New York, 1979.
48. Leininger, op. cit., 1991.
49. Ibid.
50. Frankl, V.E., *The Will to Meaning*, New York: New American Library, 1969.

28

Japanese Americans and Culture Care

Madeleine Leininger

Cultures are dynamic and do change over time.   LEININGER, 1989

During the past four decades, Japanese lifeways, values, and business activities have changed in several areas and are of great interest to people worldwide. Some major reasons for heightened global interests in Japan are their active business ventures, their marketing, and their political-economic tourist activities in many countries. Japan has had a very active growth and expansion period, which is one of the most significant in the world. Japan's gross national product has expanded about 10% annually from the mid 1950s, and by the late 1960s, Japan was the third largest economic power in the world and remains so today.[1–3] Japan has become a big business culture with modern cars, railroads, planes, and a host of microtechnologies. It has one of the most rapid and modern transit systems in the world. Japan is a culture that has established many international trade practices and marketed its scientific material products worldwide. Most significantly, it has one of the highest literacy rates in the world and publishes more books annually than most countries. Grossberg states that "Japan is one of the world's most creative and innovative societies, and that is no small collateral with which to face the future."[4]

Amid these highly successful developments, one will find lifestyle variations in rural and urban communities and in different countries where the Japanese live. Their lifestyles vary from their traditional values and beliefs to that of modern Western practices. Today, the Japanese are living and working in many countries in the world, but many still retain some traditional practices because of their coherence, meaning, and relevance to their extended families and country.

Some of these traditional Japanese cultural values are seen in their communal work activities and their strong cultural home living patterns. There is strong cultural pride related to their long, unique, and distinguished cultural history. It has been these strong cultural values and living modes that have sustained them, but also challenged them to a modern period of rapid economic development and growth. These cultural values, rapid developments in technologies, and other changes are of particular interest to health care professionals, but especially to transcultural nurses as they work with Japanese living in many places in the world today. In 1999 the homeland population was 126 million, and 99.4 million are of the Japanese culture—hence, the strong country ties.

In the United States there are over 800,000 Japanese living in the country and approximately 6,000 Japanese who are yearly tourists in the country.[5] Many Japanese Americans live on the West Coast, Pacific Islands, and especially in Hawaii. American nurses are aware of many Japanese living and working in their communities and seeking healthcare services. Nurses are learning traditional and current beliefs and lifeways so they can provide culturally congruent care to Japanese clients and their families.

In this chapter emphasis is given to the Japanese Americans, many of whom were born in Japan and migrated to the United States to live and work. Since the early 1960s the author has spent time in Japan on several occasions. She has studied the Japanese culture and their health care and lifeways in Japan and the United States. The author will briefly highlight Japanese ethnohistory, worldview, social structure, cultural values, environmental aspects, and other factors influencing nursing care practices. The Theory of Culture Care with the Sunrise Model and the importance of understanding cultural variability among Japanese in the United States and elsewhere will be emphasized. Providing culturally competent nursing care is discussed with the three theoretical predicted modes of action or decision. The reader is also encouraged to read other literature about a culture that is changing in many ways.

▦ Brief Ethnohistory of the Japanese

Anthropologically, the ethnohistory of the Japanese in their homeland is exceedingly fascinating with thousands of years of evolutionary development. Japan's history can be briefly divided into four periods as known by the Japanese and social science scholars, namely, the primitive period, ancient period, middle ages, and modern periods.[6] The *primitive* period was the beginning period in which the people were involved largely in rice cultivation and with internal warfare that united many small territories within the country. The *ancient times* covered approximately the 4th to 12th centuries, with the people united into a single nation under an emperor; this was the time of interaction with the Chinese and the rise of the nobility. The *middle ages,* from the 12th to the 19th century, was characterized by warriors who were used by the nobility to regulate or control the people. If the warrior was outstanding in the view of the emperor, he became a *shogun.* The feudal system prevailed in the 17th century with many warring groups, which led to a period of isolation during which the country developed its own educational, industrial, and socioeconomic institutions.

Very little was known about Japan by the West until the middle of the 19th century when the American Commodore Perry went to Japan and influenced Japan's entering the modern period.[7] There were many periods and dynasties that rose and fell over the long history of Japan, and they shaped Japanese lifeways. The Meiji period led to the end of isolation, and trade was established with selected other countries. Japan captured the most desirable features from other countries, especially military influences of Britain and

Germany. Japan was soon at war with China, Korea, Russia, and, finally, during World War II, with the United States. These brief glimpses of the ethnohistory of Japan have great implications for understanding the past and current cultural values and lifeways of the people.

Anthropologically, it is held that the Japanese are mainly of Asian ancestry with a mixture of Malay origin. They apparently came from different areas of the Asian continent and from the South Pacific to inhabit the islands more than 10,000 years ago.[8,9] There is archeological evidence that early paleolithic man inhabited the islands as early as 200,000 years ago. Among the early islanders were the Ainus. Some ancestors still live in Tokkaido today with only 16,000 Ainus remaining, and, according to Hane, the Japanese language appears related to Polynesian and Altaic languages.[10]

Land and Islands

Japan consists of four major islands and nearly 4000 smaller islands with a total size of about California. Most of the 127 million Japanese people live on a small portion of the land, as two-thirds of the land is uninhabitable. Japan is the fifth most densely populated country in the world, with 721 people per square mile compared with 56.6 in the United States.[11] Thus, the Japanese people who immigrated to the United States or to any place in the world have been used to living in small and compact geographic areas. This factor has influenced their goal to live in harmony with their neighbors and to form self-sufficient communities with similar cultural values, as well as to explore other places to live in the world.

Thousands of Japanese male immigrants began coming to the United States beginning in 1885 from Japan and Hawaii, but from 1908 to 1913 it was limited by the Gentleman's Agreement.[12] In 1924 the American immigration curtailed Asian immigration. Many of the first immigrants were young men with a rural agricultural orientation who took on farming, but others worked in gardening, landscaping, and small businesses such as fruit, fish, and vegetable markets. With the Exclusion Law of 1924, the Japanese male immigrants had a difficult time getting an American spouse, which led to many single, elderly men in the United States in the early immigration days.

Intergenerational Groups

It should be noted that the Japanese Americans are one of the few cultures to identify themselves by the generation in which they were born. These generational groups are distinguishable by age, language, experiences, and values. They are the following: *Issei* are the first generation living in the United States, *Nisei* are the second generation, *Sansei* are the third generation, and *Yonsei* are the fourth generation.[13] These different groups help to understand intergenerational family cultural values, beliefs, and patterns of behavior and are often referred to by Japanese in common communication exchanges. The *Issei* upheld strong family traditional values and practices and could endure hardships, whereas the *Sansei* and *Yonsei* have adopted many nontraditional values, particularly American and other Western views. The Anti-Japanese Law of 1913 prohibited *Issei* from owning land in America, which was difficult for them to accept. The *Nisei* generation, who were strong in education and obedience, maintained a hard work ethic, and they were not forced to attend segregated schools as were Indian, Chinese, and other U.S. immigrants from Southeast Asia.

Japanese Americans were evacuated from their homes and placed in government relocation centers during World War II. This caused many serious problems with the tragic disruption of family interdependency and the loss of Japanese businesses, farms, and homes. The relocation camps were declared unconstitutional in 1945. In 1991 President Bush proclaimed forgiveness to the Japanese relocates and offered financial recompense for the harm and related problems caused. World War II and the relocation camps led to much distrust between Americans and Japanese for many years. It has taken nearly 50 years to heal partially the distrust between the two nations, and at times factors arise that reactivate degrees of distrust. *Nokkei* was often used to refer to all Japanese Americans.

During the past two decades, there has been a large influx of Japanese tourists, students, and many businessmen into the United States, but especially into Hawaii and California. The Japanese have actively bought land, hotels, industries, and large homes and established car and high-tech businesses in the country. Initially, some Americans were anxious about these activities and felt threatened by aggressive overseas Japanese interests, buying and marketing power, and trade agreements. Today, many Americans greatly value the Japanese people and are enjoying learning about their traditional and changing cultural lifeways, group entrepreneurship, and successful achievements in transnational marketing. Japanese have also been active to present their exquisite cultural and artistic work as glassware, music, and paintings—all enjoyed by Americans.

Sunrise Enabler with Culture Care Theory

Dominant Cultural Values

Japanese Americans have been coming to America since World War II, with signs of intergenerational variability and degrees of acculturation. My research and observations of the Japanese over the last several decades have revealed signs that Japanese value their traditional lifeways and retain many of these values in their thinking, business, and daily living activities.[14] From my observations and direct participant experiences with the Japanese, there are cultural patterns among the Japanese key informants such as the following dominant *cultural core values*:[15]

1. Duty and obligation to kin and work group
2. Honor and national pride
3. Patriarchal obligations with respect
4. Team group work goals
5. Ambitiousness to achieve
6. Honor and deep respect toward elders
7. Politeness, self-restraint and control, patience, and forbearance (*gaman*)
8. Nonassertiveness in interaction (*entyo*)
9. Group compliance
10. High educational standards and values
11. Futuristic expansion plans worldwide

These cultural core values are important for understanding Japanese Americans as they influence their lifeways and caring expectations. The Sunrise Enabler shows how these values interface with social structure and theory factors.

Worldview

Japanese Americans view the world with harmony and congruence between one's *internal* and *external* environments. This essentially means being attentive to harmony factors within and outside oneself. The Japanese worldview includes collective group harmony by being attentive to kin and work group lifeways rather than becoming preoccupied with individual concerns. While serving as a transcultural nurse consultant in a Midwestern industrial car plant, it was interesting that the employees from Japan were often misunderstood because of their collective group management philosophy and mode of operation. In contrast, Euro-American employees focused on individual needs, achievements, and rights and found that the Japanese collective group work values and group consensus was difficult to accept because of their strong focus on individual behavior. Such differences in cultural values often pose similar problems for Japanese nurses working with Euro-American nurses. In addition, the Japanese American's worldview supports group interdependence, family support and protection, and group performance. As the Japanese continue to travel worldwide as tourists or land seekers, one finds their worldview is being expanded from a small village to a worldwide global perspective.

Technology and Economics

Since technology and economics are closely related in the Japanese culture, they will be discussed together. Technology and economics are of great importance to Japanese in their homeland and overseas. Japan and the United States are two of the strongest cultures in the world, giving high relevance to the development, use, and marketing of technologies for economic growth and education. Since World War II the Japanese have been leaders in developing, refining, and perfecting a wide variety of technologies and then exporting them worldwide. Japanese technological products such as many kinds of electronic equipment, radios, television, cameras, and cellular phones are found in homes, businesses, and in other public places. In addition, automobiles, buses, trains, and a vast array of microcomputer products are manufactured in Japan and sold worldwide. The Japanese have been very successful in marketing their technologies and in stimulating worldwide competition with high technologies, offering reasonable, efficient, and compact products. Lowering costs and maintaining quality products with new innovations have been important Japanese production goals for local and world markets. The Japanese continue today to be active international exporters and are known for small and efficient cars and technologic products such as cameras, audiovisuals, cellular phones, and many electronic products.

Japanese American clients in hospitals or clinics expect the latest, best, and most efficient machines, instruments, and other technologies to be used for surgery and human caring. Most Japanese clients have been able to pay for such modern technologies and modern professional treatments. High technologies and their many computer products have had great economic gains for the Japanese. Their technologies are diverse and creative and are sought after in world markets.

Kinship, Social, and Political Factors

The Japanese traditional extended family structure had remained strong in the past, but today it has been influenced by United States Western values and lifeways. Many Americans and other Western lifeways have been incorporated into the current youth generation. Knowledge of traditional Japanese family and kinship structure patterns and their ways of kin ties and caring modalities need to be assessed with current changes. In the past, the oldest son was important, and the father was the head of the household who arranged marriages and occupations for his children. The oldest son and his wife usually lived in the father's family home. With the birth of a son, the daughter-in-law attained recognition and was expected with the son to care for the elderly parents. Still today, the husband with less patriarchal dominance continues to be the dominant breadwinner of the family, and the wife is expected to care for the children. Today, Japanese marriages and courting practices vary, having been influenced by Western ideas. Only a few marriages are arranged in the traditional way. Intercultural marriages are increasing. However, most brides and grooms are of the same cultural heritage because of desired values, descent benefits, property, and inheritances.

Japanese living in America are seeing many diverse American patterns of parenting and marriage roles and models, and so some changes are occurring, especially with family-parent role responsibilities. However, many newlywed Japanese couples value remaining close together and patterning their lifeways to support traditional parental values and norms. Divorce is not seen as good for the children, but it may occur. In general, Japanese parents highly cherish and desire children, but are flexible to let them try American ways. The parents treat their small children with indulgence, much attention, and leeway for their actions, especially male children. They use limited physical punishment with children. The firstborn male (primogeniture) child is still valued in Japan and in America with special ritual acknowledgements and favoritism to male children and adults.

Japanese women remain the principal caregivers in the home. They are nurturing women who look after, anticipate, and protect the needs of children, their husband, and close kin. The Japanese American mother today usually bears two children. The mother today often works outside the home, but is responsible for the care of the children by either herself or a caretaker. Surveillance, affection, protection, and active attention are manifest caring practices with the children. Mothers are often seen shopping for their sons and daughters and showing concern for their children's needs. The concept of *amaeru*, which means to depend on another's benevolence, is often observed in child-rearing practices between mother and child.[16] Doi holds that this practice of *amaeru*, or *learning to be dependent on another's goodness and kindness*, especially from females, is related to neuroses with Japanese.[17] However, the author interprets these as culturally learned caring modes of Japanese mothers.

Japanese immigrant women coming to America are finding many freedoms. Several Japanese women interviewed told me about their freedom to be employed and to encourage their husbands to help with child care responsibilities like Americans. Hane recently gave a summary of the status of women in Japan. He contends that while the legal rights of women have been strengthened, their political, social, and economic conditions have not improved measurably in Japan.[18]

Male supremacy still prevails in Japanese offices, and women are struggling to get executive male positions. Temporary work status and the responsibilities of raising children in the home seem to keep Japanese women from executive roles, university positions, and other top positions outside the home. While legal social reforms in Japan have been passed to give women equal status, legal ways to eliminate discriminatory practices are slow to become a reality in Japan and in some places in the United States. In 1999 about one-half of the married Japanese American women held jobs,[19] and more Japanese women are employed today. Japanese men still like their wives to be content in the home with the children so that men can retain their executive positions and often work long hours at their offices. It is also important to realize that Japanese men seek and attend some of the best colleges, whereas Japanese women have only recently begun to pursue graduate studies. The husband's commitment to his company and to collective Japanese group work remains important for success. Such work should not be handicapped by his wife's outside work, male informants told me. Japanese men work very hard and long hours and sometimes suffer from mental exhaustion. The wives said that their husbands are often so tired that on Sunday they are not interested in social activities. Male success in their work is of the highest priority in the United States and in Japan.

Education

Traditionally and today, Japanese highly value education and will assist their children to get the best education possible. Japan has a 100% literacy rate today with excellent standards of education.[20] Education is a Japanese lifeway that is highly valued and esteemed throughout one's life. Education of the child begins with preschool and later with college entrance exams for admission. Students study diligently to prepare for rigorous higher education entrance examinations in Japan. If they perform well in the tests, they can enter outstanding colleges. Test-taking is, however, very stressful to most Japanese students because they want to excel, get high grades, and be admitted to good schools.[21] Male students are especially high achievers, hoping to get future positions desired by their family and corporate groups.

The cultural value of *saving face* remains important to Japanese in education, kinship, and testing. Saving face is somewhat comparable with Anglo-Americans trying to maintain their reputation or good image. Americans have difficulty recognizing and understanding the importance of the Japanese concept of saving face. Since Americans emphasize the individual, the idea that the Japanese group and family are more important than the individual seems strange. The Japanese student is concerned about saving their self-esteem with their family, work group, or the company where employed. They tend to be more other-directed than self-focused. Japanese are quite concerned for their group or family members and do not want to cause them embarrassment or shame. Saving face, therefore, becomes an important *caring cultural expression* for Japanese, whether they live in Japan or in the United States. Saving face is not, however, a mental illness or a psychotic or neurotic condition. It is also possible that a Japanese individual may take his life to save face because of great shame brought to one's family and group. Thus, the concept of saving face needs to be kept in mind for transcultural nurse administrators, clinicians, managers, teachers, and others working with Japanese people.

Political and Legal Systems

The current political system in Japan is parliamentary (Diet) with a prime minister and independent supreme court. The party functions as conservative liberal democratic systems in both houses of parliament. The emperor inherited political status since World War II with the allied occupation. The Japanese legal system and politics are kept separate so that fair hearings are maintained. Judges are appointed, not elected, on the basis of their educational preparation and expertise rather than political selected influences. While in America, the Japanese citizens follow the American political process in government affairs, but they often remain influenced in their thinking and actions by their traditional political values and practices. It is evident that in the last decade young Japanese Americans are becoming more relaxed and seem less interested in formal traditional political ritual behavior, but they still cherish the cultural values of honor, politeness, and justice for harmonious living and coherence among Japanese and others. These adults are beginning to study and assess the issues and values of the American democratic process and modes of functioning in the United States and Japan. Young Japanese Americans dislike, however, getting involved in major loud debates or destructive political and legal games as they are counter to harmonious working ways of the Japanese culture.

In Japan, recent political reforms have been directed toward democratization by reducing traditional power and making the executive branch more responsible to the people. Adults have become more responsible for democratic activities using new political strategies. Changes are occurring to support women's political and legal rights and more employment opportunities for women. Most Japanese Americans in the United States and in other countries keep in close contact with their homeland, especially as related to government and organizational changes. Several informants told me they want to keep some of their "homeland political practices" and Japanese interest groups to maintain the strength of their cultural heritage within an evolving democratic system.

Religious and Philosophic Orientations

Shintoism, Buddhism, and Confucianism are the traditional religious and philosophic beliefs in the Japanese culture. Still today the temples and shrines are being used for healing purposes. Each religion or philosophic orientation has contributed in different ways to the thinking, living, and healing of the Japanese. Efforts to live in harmonious relationships with each other and to remain well in their geographic areas or communities have been important. Shintoism is one of the early Japanese religions, which developed from local legends, rituals, and myths and provided guidelines for living many years. Many of the shrines in Japan are Shinto and are where newborn children are registered and presented approximately 1 month after birth. The Shinto shrines are also where the people come for special ceremonies when the child is 3, 5, and 7 years of age and for healing.

In the 6th century, Confucianism came with Buddhism from China. Confucianism emphasizes the promotion of harmony in the social and natural order and to follow daily ethical rules of behavior. Buddhism seeks the truth through two extremes of asceticism and self-indulgence. It teaches how to attain *nirvana* through meditation and relaxing the mind and body to see life as it really is. Nonviolence is important, as well as privacy, quietness, and self-control with Buddhism.[21a]

Buddhism teaches that death is inevitable and a part of all living things because humans inevitably disintegrate and come to an end. People are instructed by Buddha not to make big plans for living without full awareness of death. In Buddhist thinking the person accepts death with confidence and strength and does not fight it. Today, there are only a few Buddhist and Shinto priests in Japan and elsewhere, and those available have taken secular positions to survive.

Roman Catholicism and the Protestant faiths have increased in Japan in recent decades. There are also many new religious sects that draw from Buddhism, Shintoism, and Christianity. Japanese religion's formal ritual seems to be waning because of cultural influences of Western religions. However, today one does find Japanese praying at the Buddhist temple or at a Shinto shrine, especially for healing needs or to deal with trouble. Bus tours with Japanese elderly were noted going to temples and shrines that specialize in healing older people or to bring harmony into their lives. Hence, Buddhist shrines are important in Japan today.

In the United States there are only a few temples or shrines for Japanese Americans. I found that young Japanese in America tend to use Christian churches because of their interest in what they call the "newer" Christian religions, but elderly Japanese continue to rely on their traditional religion. Several older Japanese Americans told me they wanted to return to their native country to die with traditional Buddhist ceremonies, but young adults want to have Christian burials here. In general, traditional religion plays a major role with elderly Japanese, but the youth seek diverse religions in the United States. The philosophic and religious values of practicing nonviolence and maintaining peace and harmony remain important values to Japanese in the United States.

■ Generic and Professional Health Care Systems

In Japan both generic and professional health systems are found. Most of the traditional generic and folk practices came originally from China. They gradually became a part of the Japanese culture until the Meiji Restoration when the country was no longer isolated from other people in the world.[22] After this time Japanese men studied abroad, which led to the introduction of many Western ideas and especially the German model of professional medicine.[23] Many Western medicines and nursing and treatment modes have been brought to Japan and are used in the country. However, several generic home remedies are used when Western practices fail or have limited meanings and therapeutic effectiveness.

The generic folk system includes Chinese *Kampo* medicine, which has been used since the 6th century. Kampo is a holistic approach of all body systems and includes the use of the therapeutic folk practices of acupuncture, herbal medicines, moxibustion, and spiritual exercises.[24] Kampo provides an answer to a familiar traditional way to receive care and treatment, but its strengths also complement the weakness of Western biomedicine.

Generic home care practices are still found in some Japanese hospitals, especially when family members provide client care. Family members often care for clients after they are hospitalized. There are many home remedies that mothers use as primary home care or as prevention modes. Ginger, sake, and egg are used for a cold, and herbal teas are a "cure-all" for many conditions. Headaches are treated with sesame oil and ginger oil rubbed on the head. Finger massage and exercise are valued to prevent illness and maintain wellness. The yin-yang (hot-cold) theory is important in Japanese care, especially during pregnancy and with medical and surgical conditions. Acupuncture is increasingly being used in Japan and is used by Japanese in other countries where available and when professional Western treatments are ineffective.

For the Japanese there is not a split between the body and the mind. When illness occurs, it is often expressed in somatic complaints, depression, or stress.[25] The healing approach is to restore harmony, order, and control through specific caring ways in one's environmental context.[26,27] Harmony is highly valued as a healing mode and to control one's emotions. Appropriate cultural and social behavior are required to regain harmony and alleviate stress. Today, Japanese businessmen in the United States and in their homeland seek places to rest, often in hotels, to restore harmony for health. Several informants said they will stay in a quiet place for several days to relieve themselves from present-day stresses and to regain their coherence with life. They like hotels with no external distractions such as radios or television programs.

Japanese clients who are hospitalized seek physicians who have excellent expertise in surgery and in medical treatments. Clients like to be introduced to physicians and then choose them rather than vice versa to get proper attention and services.[28] Medications are requested mainly to help clients control excessive pain and gain well-being. The goal or form of therapy is usually to facilitate care repatterning of life or to reintegrate oneself into one's social group in meaningful ways. Most importantly, transcultural health professionals and especially psychiatric nurses need to be aware that to verbalize negative feelings about family members in psychotherapy seldom leads to successful outcomes. It is not appropriate to express negative feelings about the family or to dichotomize or manipulate the mind and body. Instead, harmony of mind and body need to be restored through the sociocultural harmonization, care repatterning, and ritual activities that facilitate coherence with Japanese values.[29] Ohnuki-Tierney states that the average length of stay in Japanese hospitals in 1977 was 42.9 days, which contrasted with 8 days in the United States and was the longest in the world.[30]

Japanese have national health insurance, and employers are required to provide insurance for their employees and to pay 10% of the medical costs. Physician's fees are low as they are set by the government. Christopher states:[31]

> The Japanese tend to visit doctors more often than Americans do. And preventive medicine is more widely practiced in Japan. School children get mandatory medical and dental checkups, and as a result of vaccinations and inoculations administered at school or through neighborhood organizations Japanese of every age are better protected against disease than the citizens of most other countries.

The professional health care system in Japan is based on a holistic approach that physicians and nurses use in care to clients. In recent years, Japanese have been prepared in baccalaureate degree nursing

programs, adopting both Western and United States ideas with traditional caring practices. Japanese nurses remain attentive to family needs and practices in the hospital and in the home. Physicians are educated and do major and minor surgeries. According to Lock, an anthropologist who has studied Japan services:[32]

> Patients are socialized, as are their physicians, to think holistically about their bodies, to focus on somatic rather than psychological levels of explanation and to expect the family, place of work, and other social units to participate actively in health care except for the actual diagnosis and specialized treatment of diseases. The Japanese public is also, for the most part, extremely well versed in a scientific approach to the body. Pluralism in the organization of medical care and in medical practice is the norm in Japan, but despite the great diversity apparent in hospitals and clinics, there are nevertheless certain striking and dominant features which can be discerned in a variety of clinical settings and which form the basis for uniquely Japanese approaches to health care.

Culture Care Meanings and Action Modes with Culture Care Theory

From the above ethnohistory worldview, social structure, and health system features, cultural care considerations can be identified with the Theory of Culture Care. The reader has entered the emic world of the Japanese whether in the United States or in other places to consider ways to provide culturally congruent and specific care to clients for their well-being and health. The culture can be identified from the data presented in this chapter, especially from the Japanese worldview, social structure, and dominant cultural values stated previously. Other research data can also be used.

From studies using the Culture Care Theory with 20 key and 35 general Japanese American informants, specific culture care meanings and action modes were identified as dominant common or universal core care features to guide nursing care practices.[33] They are the following:

1. Respect for family, authority, and corporate groups
2. Obligations to kin and work groups

3. Concern for group with protection
4. Prolonged nurturant care for self and others
5. Control of emotions and actions to save face and prevent shame
6. Looking to others for affection (amaeru)
7. Indulgence from caregivers
8. Endurance and forbearance to support pain and stress (keeping restrained in expression)
9. Respect for and attention to complaints
10. Personal cleanliness
11. Use of generic folk therapies (kampo medicine)
12. Quietness and passivity

Many similar patterns with some intergenerational variations were observed with informants while staying in Japan. These dominant care values are considered to help Japanese families or individuals. They are the guides to action or nonaction. In planning or providing care, the nurse would first do a culturalogic assessment and consider the cultural context. After the nurse reflected on general ideas about the Japanese culture, worldview, ethnohistory, social structure, generic and professional care practices, and general culture values as presented in this chapter, the nurse makes care plans and actions with the client and family. The client's identified specific care needs would be given full consideration with the theoretical three modes of action and in a cooperative way with client and family.

The three theoretical modes of action and decision derived from the above ideas presented in this chapter are important in the care of the Japanese American client and will be discussed next.

Culture Care Preservation and Maintenance

Culture care preservation and maintenance would be used with respect for the client in ways to provide peace and harmony. This care mode would be especially important for the Issei or elderly Japanese American client who wanted peace, quietness, and harmony. For example, the nurse would be attentive to the Japanese elderly's needs by showing respect for and honoring their ideas regarding care they believed essential. Respect as care is an essential care construct for all Japanese clients, but especially the client's family and kin. Family members should be included as participants in care

to their elders. For example, the daughter might be expected to bathe her mother or to provide personal hygiene. The nurse would let the daughter fulfill her obligations to her mother by accepting the family member's anticipated need. Honor and respect must also be maintained and preserved to those in authority, as well as those who know home remedies and foods held best for their family. The term *oya-koko* is often used to refer to "caring for parents," which may be used by family members in talking to the nurse.

Another area to provide culture care preservation and maintenance is to be attentive to ways of *saving face* or to prevent unnecessary shame or embarrassment. Reducing the Japanese client's self-esteem or confidence should be avoided, especially in conversations with them or in casual discussions in the hallways. The nurse would especially watch so that one does not confront the Japanese client directly or blame them in front of family members, work groups, or in a public context. Japanese tend to feel like they are always indebted to their family and work group, so saving face is very important.

Culture care preservation would also be considered with foods the client desires to regain health and harmony and to prevent illnesses. The Japanese client's preference for fish, steamed vegetables, fresh fruit, rice, and herbal teas would be given full consideration by nurses and dietary staff. Maintaining Japanese exercises and daily life activities in a quiet environment is also important. Recognizing and preserving *gaman* as efforts by the client to be patient, to persevere, or to show self-control would need to be maintained, as well as the concept of *amaeru*.

Most importantly, the nurse would need to plan for ways to preserve and maintain Japanese health in a peaceful environmental context so that healing can occur. Rest as healing is extremely important for Japanese clients to regain their health and harmony with those in one's environment. Work stresses in America and Japan are clearly apparent today. Thus, many Japanese in executive positions may request a private room if hospitalized. Finding a quiet place in the hospital is quite a challenge as some American hospitals tend to be noisy and busy places. Loudspeakers, many treatment activities, and limited time to rest without interruptions from staff or physicians require creative strategies.

Culture Care Accommodation

Culture care accommodation is essential for the families and for special needs. This means letting family members participate in care practices with the client. Family members may want to give direct care to their kin and make decisions about their care except where professional nursing actions or decisions are very critical to use special knowledge. For example, family members may want to be responsible for feeding and exercising their kin. They may want to use home remedies such as herbal tea, sake, and massage. Some folk therapies *kampo* and spiritual therapies may be requested by healers. Combining professional nursing care with generic care practices is essential for potential therapeutic outcomes. At all times, the nurse remains open to discussing folk (generic) remedies and other care practices with the client to observe their limitations or benefits. If some folk practices seem deleterious to the client, the nurse has an ethical responsibility to share such professional ideas with the client and family.

The nurse will be expected to assess and help with Japanese pain and stress needs. Often, Japanese clients may be restrained and endure considerable pain. Sometimes, they may request medications if under stress to save face or to deal with stressful demands in the work place. Somatic complaints may be anticipated as one expressive pain pattern. Clients' needs would be considered and discussed with them, trying to blend their ideas with professional practices. Japanese clients may avoid a lot of pain medications because of fear of drug addiction. The nurse should give attention to physical complaints, but should avoid talking about physical and mind-body (somatic) expressions as separate entities. Instead, the nurse should maintain a *holistic or total care* viewpoint by respecting the total person who is functioning with a particular lifestyle and environmental context.

In providing culturally congruent care for the Japanese client in the United States or elsewhere, it would be important to use culture care accommodation so that the Japanese client can use traditional (*kampo*) or alternative care services. Supportive care from kin and employment groups may be important, as well as assessing and respecting their group suggestions. Some male corporate work groups like to provide special foods for their sick group member. The concept of *amaeru*, or looking to others for affection and offering help, is very important in regaining and maintaining the client's health because it expresses group and family care, which is more other-care directed than self-care focused. Personal cleanliness is also valued and should be given to the client in quiet and proper ways, or the client's family may wish to provide cleanliness practices.

Culture Care Repatterning/Restructuring

This is difficult to know until the nurse first discusses with the client what they want to repattern or restructure of the daily cares. For example, I recall a Japanese American pregnant woman who wanted to adopt some professional maternal-child care practices. I worked directly with her in a co-participatory way to determine what specific changes in care she desired to alter or repattern. The areas the client wanted me to help her change from her traditional Japanese ways were the following: 1) to avoid using the traditional Japanese abdominal binder after birth (this has been used by her mother and kin for years); 2) to have her "shy husband" and mother-in-law remain in the delivery room with her, but not to have them directly help with the physical delivery of the baby or assist with labor pushes. It was especially taboo for Japanese men to be involved with the actual delivery of the baby, and it was also counter to men's ideas of self-esteem and gender role activities; and 3) be more physically active after delivery rather than staying in bed. (The usual Japanese stay had been 3 weeks). These were major areas that the client wanted to repattern. With the repatterning, the mother-in-law and husband became more involved, but only in certain activities. The extended Japanese family members had to be reeducated about the shorter stay of the mother in the hospital to allay their fears and to reduce the mother's somatic complaints. The mother had to be reassured along with other female kin about not using the abdominal binder after delivery or for long periods. This was a client-family nurse repatterning plan that had very favorable outcomes. The client was extremely pleased with the transcultural care. This was creative transcultural nursing with culture care repatterning, and it led to culturally congruent care that fit with the client's and the family's expectations of "good" nursing care. There were no restructuring areas of care.

Summary

In this chapter the reader has been presented with an overview of important cultural information about the Japanese worldview, ethnohistory, religion, kinship economic, cultural values, and care meanings and actions. Also discussed were educational, technological, and political-legal factors influencing care expressions with Japanese, but primarily those in the United States. Such information needs to be considered with other Japanese clients with the theory and the three modes of action or decision making. The theory of Culture Care with the Sunrise Model can be a highly valuable guide to the nurse to holistically assess, plan, and provide nursing care to fit the Japanese client's needs and satisfactions. Entering the world of the Japanese client requires holding knowledge of the culture and consideration of action modes with the individual, family, or group. The extent of acculturation and intergenerational value changes also must be considered. Variations in culture care will always need to be considered according to the extent of acculturation along with the environmental contextual factors. Such nursing care practices can prevent cultural imposition by the nurse and avoid major cultural clashes and unfavorable consequences between the Japanese client and the nursing staff. Recently, an undergraduate nursing student completed a clinical experience with a Japanese American family. She said the following, which summarizes this chapter.

> This transcultural nursing experience was extremely valuable to me. I had such great difficulty caring for the Japanese patient until I studied transcultural nursing. I had been using Euro-American professional practices, and this did not help the client or family. Through the guided mentorship experience, I learned to "cue-in-to" observations and the meaning of culture-specific and congruent care. I also learned how to use the Theory of Culture Care to guide my work and to provide creative transcultural nursing care. Now I have an entirely new way to practice nursing and with Japanese clients. I can see how important transcultural nursing concepts, principles, and research findings are in patient care.

References

1. Farley, H.P., *Japanese Culture*, Honolulu: University of Hawaii Press, 1984.
2. Hane, M., *Modern Japan. A Historical Survey*, Boulder: Westview Press, 1986, pp. 6–30.
3. Norbeck, E., *Changing Japan*, New York: Holt, Rinehart and Winston, 1965.
4. Grossberg, K., *Japan Today*, Philadelphia: Institute for the Study of Human Issues, 1981, p. 8.
5. U.S. Department of Commerce, Bureau of Census, Tourism, Visitors, 1996.
6. Nakamura, O., *Nippon: The Land and Its People*, Japan: Nippon Steel Corporation, 1984.
7. Ibid.
8. Norbeck, op. cit., 1965.
9. Hane, op. cit., 1986.
10. Ibid., p. 6.
11. U.S. Census Bureau Website, May 2000.
12. Kitano, H., *Japanese Americans: The Evolution of a Subculture*, 2nd ed., Englewood Cliffs, NJ: Prentice-Hall, Inc., 1976.
13. Hashizume, N. and J. Takana, "Nursing Care of the Japanese American Patient," in *Ethnic Nursing Care: A Multicultural Approach*, M.S. Orque, B. Bloch, and L.S.A. Monrroy, eds., St. Louis: C.V. Mosby, 1983, pp. 219–243.
14. Leininger, M., *Culture Care Diversity and Universality: A Theory of Nursing*, New York: National League for Nursing Press, 1991.
15. Leininger, M., "Nursing Care of a Patient from Another Culture: A Japanese American Patient," in *Transcultural Nursing Concepts, Principles, and Practices*, New York: John Wiley & Sons, 1978, pp. 335–350.
16. Doi, L., "Amaeru: A Key Concept for Understanding Japanese Personality Structure," in *Japanese Culture*, R. Smith, ed., Chicago: Aldine Publishing Co., 1961, p. 132.
17. Ibid., p. 86.
18. Hane, op. cit., 1986.
19. *The World Almanac and Book of Facts*, Mahwah, NJ: Premedia Reference, Inc., World Almanac Books, 1999, p. 814.
20. Ibid.
21. Leininger, M., "Nursing Care of a Patient from Another Culture: A Japanese American Patient," *Nursing Clinics of North America*, 1967, v. 2, pp. 747–762.

22. Emiko, Ohnuki-Tierney, *Illness and Culture in Contemporary Japan An Anthropological View*, New York: Cambridge Press, 1984.

23. Long, S., "Health Care Providers: Technology, Policy and Professional Dominance," in *Health, Illness, and Medical Care in Japan: Cultural and Social Dimensions*, E. Norbeck and M. Lock, eds., Honolulu: University of Hawaii Press, 1987, pp. 66–88.

24. Ibid.

25. Lock, M., "Japanese Responses to Social Change—Making the Strange Familiar in Cross-Cultural Medicine," *Western Journal of Medicine*, 1983, v. 6, pp. 829–834.

26. Leininger, M., *Ethnocare of Japanese Americans in an Urban Context*, unpublished study, Detroit: Wayne State University, 1990.

27. Leininger, op. cit., 1991, pp. 337–350.

28. Emiko, op. cit., 1984.

29. Ibid.

30. Ibid.

31. Christopher, R., *The Japanese Mind*, New York: Fawcett Columbine, 1983, p. 237.

32. Lock, M., "The Impact of Chinese Medical Model on Japan," *Social Science and Medicine*, 1985, v. 21, no. 8, p. 945.

33. Leininger, op. cit., 1991, pp. 5–73, 358.

Other Suggested Readings

- Ishida, D., et al., *Japanese Americans in Transcultural Nursing: Assessment and Intervention*, St. Louis, MO: Mosby Yearbook, 1995.

- Sharts-Hopko, "Birth in the Japanese Context . . . The Experiences of 20 American Women Who Gave Birth in Japan," *Journal of Obstetric, Gynecological and Neonatal Nursing*, May 1995, v. 24, no. 4, pp. 343–351.

29

Jewish Americans and Russian Jews Culture Care

Madeleine Leininger

Discover the past within the context of today.

The Jewish people, their religion, and related culture care beliefs, values, and lifeways need to be understood by nurses and other health personnel. The long cultural history of the Jewish people with their migrations into different places in the world for freedom, to practice their religion, and to preserve their family lifeways needs to be understood to facilitate culturally congruent care. In this chapter Jewish American culture will be discussed with the Culture Care Theory and the Sunrise Model to identify culture-specific nursing care practices appropriate to Jewish clients. The major emphasis will be on Jewish Americans living in the United States, but many ideas have relevance to Jews worldwide. Knowledge of Russian Jews is also important, so this chapter has two parts, Part A focuses on Jewish Americans and Part B focuses on Russian Jews.

■ Part A: Jewish Americans

Ethnohistory

Understanding the Jewish culture begins with a brief account of their ethnohistory. The term Jewish primarily refers to people of identifiable religious beliefs and cultural practices that generally characterize the people. Since the 6th century B.C., the term "Jew" was given to members of the tribe of Judah. It refers to the descendants of Abraham, the first of the three Patriarchs and the founder of the Jewish nation.[1,2] The term "Jew" is not identical in meaning to "Israeli," for the latter refers to people of political citizenship of the state of Israel.[3]

Since the beginning of time Jewish people have been singled out and persecuted for their religious rituals, beliefs, and practices. For example, in 210 B.C. the king of Syria was upset by the Jews' strange monotheistic beliefs and their tendency to remain separate from others. Other rulers wanted the Jewish people to stop infant circumcisions and begin eating pork.[4] Although the Jewish people have often been threatened by others, they maintain their religious beliefs, rituals, and prayers to survive spiritually. Most Jews have continued to observe their holy days, maintain social group solidarity, and retain specific cultural beliefs to preserve their health and well-being. Moreover, some Jewish people in Europe and in America have created a degree of autonomy by developing and establishing their own educational institutions, social welfare programs, and support systems. Since the Hebrew language was sacred and reserved for prayer and special interpretation of scripture, the Yiddish language, which combined Hebrew with German, was developed and often while in exile.

Since the mid 1600s Jewish migrations from different places in the world continue to grow, especially to the United States of America. By the 1800s the German Jews migrated in large groups to America, which led to the homogeneity of American Jews.[5] Many of these European Jews began to build elite Jewish retailing businesses in the United States with the people bound by their Jewish cultural ties and interests. For example, in the late 1800s nearly 90% of all wholesale clothing firms in the United States were owned by Jews.[6] Most of these immigrants settled in New York and others in Philadelphia and Chicago, and these cities represented

58% of the Jewish population. The Jewish network of providing supportive culture care among their groups was noteworthy and contributed to maintaining their survival and well-being. Some theorists hold that the Jewish people became more at home in the United States and became more aware of their strong cultural ties than Jewish people living in other places in the world.[7] Indeed, the importance of the United States as a center for Jews and their Jewish cultural life increased markedly with the impact of the Nazi genocide of the Jewish people.[8] Jewish persecution has also been experienced not only with the Nazi persecution, but also by Jews in Communist regimes such as the former Soviet Union, which had the second biggest Jewish settlement in the world. Jewish people have shared these tragic life experiences, especially the Nazi Holocaust, as they established themselves in different places in the world.

During the post World War years the Jewish people maintained their strong convictions and religious practices. Many preserved their dress, beards, and earlocks as they dispersed across the United States. In addition, the Jewish people have retained their reverence for learning and diverse intellectual pursuits. They have taken positions in academic institutions and in many scholarly fields and public endeavors. Jewish people became leaders in religious studies, music, fine arts, and the motion picture and entertainment industries in the United States.

Jewish membership has grown in numbers in the United States and worldwide. Their influences have been often identified with legislation to support the underprivileged, defending their own civil liberties and civil rights, nurturing their Jewish kin ties worldwide, and promoting international trade policies. The ethnohistory of the Jewish people reflects many struggles to survive, grow, and maintain their cultural identity and place in the world. The nursing student will find readings about the past and present Jewish cultural history of much interest and as background to understanding the Jewish culture.

Worldview

Continuing with the use of the Sunrise Model to examine Jewish lifeways and care, the worldview becomes essential. The author holds that every culture has a worldview or a way of "looking out on" the world or the universe. The Jewish worldview is frequently viewed as one of suffering and surviving in different places in the world. The long history of persecution and discrimination and the need to retain Jewish religious values, beliefs, and practices are often expressed when talking with Jewish informants. The strength of their cultural identity and not yielding to a dominant culture has been manifest over time. Most children of Jewish parents try to retain a strong sense of cultural pride and ethnocentrism about their valued lifeways, but younger Jewish adolescents are waning today. Most Jewish people find their worldview keeps them closely united, ethnocentric, and cautious of movements or leaders who may cause them to suffer or lose their cultural identity. Most importantly, their worldview is reflected in their beliefs of four ways to become and remain Jewish. They are 1) being born of a Jewish mother, 2) marrying a Jew and accepting Jewish norms and lifeways, 3) converting to Judaism, and 4) being fully integrated into a primary Jewish group with sustained loyalties and retention of cultural norms. Those who fail to live with these norms are questioned whether they are "true Jews."

Education and Religion

Since Jewish religion and education are closely interwoven, they will be discussed together. Religion, with its complex dimensions, is central to the Jewish people. Judaism is a monotheistic religion based on the interpretation of the laws of God as found in the Torah and explained in the Talmud. Jewish laws prescribe the lifeways of people in their activities, diet, education, and ceremonial activities throughout the life cycle. There are *three* major religious groups within Judaism: *Orthodox, Conservative*, and *Reform*. There is also a fundamentalist sect called *Hasidism*. The history and ethnogeographic aspects of these three groups are generally held to be that Orthodox Jews originated in Israel, Conservative Jews began in Eastern Europe, and Reform Jews started in Germany, Hungary, France, and England around 1830.[9] The Orthodox Jews are the strictest group and firmly uphold religious values and practices. The Reform Jews are more flexible. Conservative Judaism falls between Orthodox and Reform in upholding religious values and life-ways. In the United States, Reform Judaism is more evident with membership approximately 70% of all Jews. Conservative Judaism constitutes 20% and Orthodox Judaism about 10% of Jews in the United States.[10]

In recent years attendance at religious services in the synagogue in the United States has been slightly decreasing, and home rituals have become flexible. There are often five traditional religious rituals with the home services: 1) lighting Sabbath candles Friday evening, 2) having or attending a Seder on Passover, 3) eating kosher meat, 4) using separate dishes for meat and dairy foods, and 5) lighting Chanukah candles. Having the children participate in these home ceremonies and keeping them instructed in the tenets of the religion are important. Jewish boys have always been expected to be educated from an early age in the same tradition as their fathers. Maintaining intellectual pursuits, valuing education, and being charitable are important features of Jewish lifeways, especially for the enculturation of males and females.

Judaism is largely based on observance of the Torah laws as given to Moses by God on Mount Sinai. The purpose of the Torah is to teach the Jewish people to act, think, and feel within the Jewish laws. Klein holds that classical Judaism has no word for "religion"; the closest counterpart in the Jewish vocabulary is "Torah."[11] The Torah supports the belief that all aspects of living, including worship, business affairs, use of leisure time, and maintaining rites of passage such as the *bar mitzvah*, are important. Marriage and death are part of the mandate that Jewish people are to serve God in everything.

Religious beliefs and the education of Jewish people support the sanctity of life and related cultural values as ways of living. Jewish people hold that their bodies are God's; one's body is on loan from God and must be returned to God at death. The Jewish people are, therefore, observant of the Talmud and must keep themselves in a good state of health by caring for themselves and others. They are duty bound to exercise, get sleep, eat well, avoid drugs and alcohol abuse, and not commit suicide. Moreover, they are obligated to help others to prevent illness, injury, disabilities, and death.[12] Another important belief is that the body God

has given them is good and should be a source of holiness and pleasure as long as enjoyment is within God's rules.

The Jewish people observe a number of holy days such as Rosh Hashanah (the Jewish New Year); Yom Kippur (Day of Atonement); Chanukah (the Festival of Lights); Passover; Shavuot (the Festival of the Giving of the Torah); and Purim. These holy days and a few others are important for Jewish clients to observe. For example, surgery and medical treatments should not be performed on holy days or on the Sabbath unless there is an emergency need.

The Jewish Sabbath, which begins at sundown Friday and lasts until dark on Saturday, is the holiest day. It is a day of rest, which signifies that God rested after creating the world, and so Jewish people are expected to rest on the Sabbath day. Orthodox and Conservative Jewish people may avoid using modern technologies in the home. Some Orthodox Jewish people might not travel except on foot or might relinquish using the phone, elevator, or electric bed. They may not want to handle business or money matters on the Sabbath and holy days. These values need to be respected as culture care accommodation in nursing care practices.

The importance of attaining holiness is not only by one's intellect but also to have energy to perform God's expectations. For example, eating has a divine dimension as the traditional Jewish people observe dietary kosher laws and not eating pork or predatory fowl, nor mixing meat and dairy products during the same meal or from the same dish. Moreover, only fish with fins and scales are allowed, and shellfish are prohibited. Preserving the proper dietary laws is important to attain holiness and to maintain their culture lifeways. The term kosher is often misunderstood by non-Jewish people who view it as a type of food. However, it means that all animals must be ritually slaughtered to be kosher, that is, properly handled and preserved. According to Jewish law, there is a prohibition against ingesting blood such as raw meat or bloody substances, but this does not apply to receiving blood transfusions.

The synagogue is the place for prayer, and it is an inte- gral part of the prayer services to study the Torah. The synagogue is the center for religious study and the formal education of children and adults. The rabbi is active in many activities in the synagogue. Judaism is not embodied in the synagogue, but in the Torah. The rabbi and other males often wear a small black cap or *kippa* and sometimes a prayer shawl or *tallith*. Today, most Jewish men and women sit together in prayer services in the synagogue.

In the Jewish culture there are other special religious services that need to be understood by nurses. The *bris* is a traditional birth ritual in which the male child is circumcised by a religious leader or *mohel* shortly after brith. This ritual varies today in how it is observed and who performs the ritual, that is, a rabbi or sometimes a pediatrician is involved in the bris. The bris is actually a religious celebration of brith and the naming of the child. It is common practice to name the child after a recently deceased relative.

When the Jewish young enter adulthood, there are two other religious events. For males, this event is called *bar mitzvah* and for the females *bat mitzvah*.[13] These are both important occasions with big celebrations for young males and females. These ceremonies mark the induction of the individual into full adulthood with their spiritual role expectations. For young males, their spiritual role responsibility includes mastery of scripture reading. Many families and friends help young males and females celebrate these events as the young adults take on their new status and role responsibilities in Jewish culture.

Unquestionably, education is greatly valued and expected for Jewish people throughout the life cycle. Intellectual achievement is highly respected and viewed as important. Education is expected of all Jewish people, for it leads to spiritual growth, as well as to economic, social, and cultural well-being or success. Jewish men are expected to be well educated, and in recent decades Jewish women are likewise expected to pursue advanced education and to move into special employment and community leadership roles. Education is strongly valued because it can transform and protect the individual. It also gives Jewish people a strong appreciation for their cultural heritage. Indeed, a well-educated Jewish person has opportunities and benefits that have served them well in the United States. In general, the Jewish people have always valued education, and this comes largely from their religious beliefs and cultural expectations. Jewish parents continue to set high educational standards for themselves and their children.

From the above religious and educational dimensions, the nurse recognizes important considerations to understand and to use in providing culturally congruent care. Unquestionably, the nurse needs to practice culture care preservation with Jewish clients in preserving their holy days, the Sabbath, and ritual life-cycle activities. Culture care accommodations may also be needed to provide their expected foods and for other nursing care needs of Jewish clients. Culture care repatterning and restructuring tend to be less needed, except for "fallen away" Jewish youth.

Major Cultural Values

Based on the author's use of the Culture Care Theory and research findings of Jewish Americans and from research from other sources over several decades, several dominant cultural core values have been identified.[14] These findings are based on the ethnonursing qualitative research method with many key and general informants over time. Some intergenerational variations are evident among the three different Jewish groups. However, these cultural core values have remained evident with Reform and Conservative Jewish informants. The *dominant core Jewish cultural values* to guide nursing practices are the following:

1. Maintaining respect for Jewish religious beliefs and practices
2. Maintaining the spiritual centrality of family with patriarchal respect and the importance of the mother for generic caring values in sickness and well-being
3. Supporting education and intellectual achievements
4. Maintaining intergenerational continuity of the Jewish heritage
5. Being generous and charitable with contributions to the arts, music, and many community services
6. Achieving financial and educational success
7. Being persistent and persuasive in religious values and cultural norms
8. Enjoying art, music, and religious rites

These core values can be viewed as important "holding care values" as the nurse works with Jewish clients to plan and provide culturally congruent care. Individual and family variations may exist among the different Jewish people, especially in relation to their geographic and environmental contexts. The above cultural core values remained with the informants and were confirmed as important to providing quality nursing care practices.

Kinship and the Generic (Folk) and Professional Health Care

The family is the core of the Jewish lifeways buttressed by religious beliefs and cultural values. The Jewish family is viewed as closely united showing closeness, unity, and the stability influenced by Jewish religious laws and intergenerational values. For example, one is expected to honor one's father and mother and to care for one another in the family. The family values and the relationship between a husband and wife are based on the importance of mutual aid, harmony, peace, and good will. However, if dissension and conflict occur between a husband and wife with fighting and anger, the marriage can be dissolved, but it must be done according to the Jewish religious laws to be valid.[15,16]

The cultural anthropologist, Harland, discusses in Haviland's book that the original Jewish descent groups who immigrated to New York from Eastern Europe were known as "family circles."[17] These family circles included all the living descendants with their spouses of an ancestral pair. They were linked by males and females to establish ambilineal descent (or different group) membership to avoid problems of divided loyalties and interests.[18] Each family circle had a name, usually the surname of a male ancestor, and they met regularly throughout the year. This was an innovative way to be organized to maintain family solidarity and mutual aid to one another. The Jewish family traditionally recognizes patrilineal descent and is pleased and excited for the first male child as this establishes *primogeniture* or acknowledgement of intergenerational Jewish male descent.[19,20]

A Jewish marriage is an elaborate festivity that unites two families. In traditional wedding ceremonies, a glass is broken (*kheysa*) to symbolize the fragility of marriage. Many gifts are given to the couple, and there is much interaction between the Jewish families and friends at the wedding ceremony. The married couple is expected to keep the marriage together forever, and divorce is not encouraged.

The Jewish woman remains very important in the Jewish family, especially as the key caring or nurturant person to the nuclear family.[21] She is the cornerstone of the family's spirituality and maintains optimal family health or well-being by her generic caring activities and rituals. Any person born of a Jewish mother or converted to Judaism is revered as a Jew. It is the Jewish mother who remains close to the children. She will offer chicken soup to a Jewish sick person and is an active listener and advisor to family members. The father and mother are usually active to bring the family together on the Sabbath and on all special holy days, as well as on other special family occasions to increase family unity and well-being. It should be noted that Jewish women teach their generic caring ways to other women. Many women maintain key leadership roles in Jewish organizations and in community activities doing charitable deeds and helping in contemporary local, national, and international activities.

In the Torah it is said that Jews should be fruitful and multiply, and so most parents have at least two children. In the past, contraception and abortion were seldom permitted unless the woman's health was threatened. Traditionally, Judaism did not endorse abortion on demand, but today some liberal Jews permit abortion. With a rabbi's permission artificial insemination may be done. Judaism holds that the fetus is a human being and has full sanctity of life. Efforts are, therefore, made to preserve infant life as a high priority at birth and throughout the life cycle. The parents and grandparents are usually very thrilled to have a child, and much attention is given to the newborn. While the family uses wine as part of their religious and family rituals, it must be used in moderation. Good Jewish persons do not abuse use of alcohol. Jewish people have had a low incidence of alcoholism, which some hold is related to strong family caring modes and religious beliefs to control and regulate alcohol use and general behavior.[22]

Technology

The use of technology as a part of the American way of living is more acceptable to Jews today than in earlier days. Today, Jewish families are seeking and using some of the latest technologies for their homes, but especially to support their health or well-being. Some

Orthodox Jews are reluctant to use modern technologies. The nurse needs to do a cultural assessment to determine the use of technologies in client care, especially on the Sabbath and holy days and with Orthodox Jews.

Providing Congruent and Acceptable Nursing Care

In this last section, some major nursing care considerations are presented for the nurse to provide culturally congruent care. Both generic (folk) and modern professional services need to be considered with Leininger's three modes of action and decision. They will be discussed next.

Jewish people tend to rely on both generic (their home remedies) and professional health knowledge. This is in keeping with Jewish intellectual, scientific, and humanistic interests. In the past, generic home remedies were relied on considerably while living in unfavorable places and with discrimination practices. Today, generic care exists as mother's care is still viewed by many Jews as highly desired and comforting. In the author's research many of the folk care practices are evident. Jewish informants recalled "old" folk conditions and healing rituals with practices such as the "evil eye," cupping for chest colds, and the use of amulets as objects to protect the person; however, some are not used nor endorsed today. The charm or amulet symbolizing the "hand of God" is still frequently worn by a Jewish person for good luck and protection. In addition, many mothers relied on their "good home remedies" for colds such as chicken soup and other home practices as primary care practices for their children and adult friends. Combining professional medicines and folk care needs careful thought to prevent adverse reactions.

The Orthodox Jewish dietary religious laws prohibit eating milk and meat at the same meal, which can be viewed as part of generic religious and traditional practices. Eating unleavened bread (*matzah*), vegetables, herbs, and fruits is also a generic health promoting mode, as is drinking small amounts of wine. How foods are prepared and consumed are of symbolic religious significance, which the nurse needs to note to preserve and maintain well-being and acceptance. The dietary practices with the Jewish mother's generic caring patterns and techniques are very important for transcultural nursing practices, which should be respected for their care meanings. Food symbols such as eating of *matzah* at Passover symbolizes the time the Jews were forbidden to eat leavened bread, and the wine is a symbol of joy and gladness when they fled Egypt in the olden days.

From my research with the Jewish people the following *care meanings and action modes* were identified with 24 key and 36 general informants and are discussed in relation to the three theoretical modes of care.[23] The *culture care meanings and action modes* to be incorporated into nursing care are as follows:

1. Expressing one' feelings and views openly
2. Getting direct and the best help possible
3. Accepting shared sufferings
4. Supporting maternal nurturance, i.e., overfeeding, permissiveness, overprotection, advice, and special foods
5. Giving and helping others in need as social justice (*tsdokeh*)
6. Performing life-cycle (birth, marriage, and death) rituals
7. Being attentive to others
8. Caring for one's own people (Jews)
9. Teaching Jewish values to family and others

These care meanings and action modes are derived from cultural findings related to the worldview, ethnohistory, social structure factors, and other ideas already discussed about the Jewish cultural values. The culture care meanings and action modes can provide for culture-specific and competent care for Jewish clients, recognizing variabilities among individuals and groups. Creative care to members of the three different Jewish groups is important among and between Orthodox, Conservative, or Reformed Jewish clients. The care needs to be tailor-made to fit the three care modes of the Culture Care Theory with the clients.

With respect to the three major care modes, it was evident that culture care preservation and accommodation would be emphasized unless the clients have greatly modified their lifeways or changed their religious beliefs. Religious and family life values would be especially important to preserve to help Jewish clients recover from an illness and to help them regain and maintain their health or well-being. If these care values are maintained, one can reasonably predict client care satisfactions and beneficial nursing outcomes.

The nurse needs to be attentive to the Torah laws that guide Jewish health and well-being for culture care accommodations for the following:

1. Dietary practices in the methods of food preparation by not mixing meat and dairy dishes
2. Respecting the Sabbath and major holy days
3. Maintaining, respecting, and accommodating modesty and the dignity of the body
4. Respecting the sancity of the life of the newborn and those of all ages
5. Using generic or folk home remedies that are believed to be beneficial with professional health care with assessed beneficial outcomes

The sensitive and knowledgeable transcultural nurse would be aware of the importance of letting Jewish clients openly talk and express feelings and would listen to their concerns. At times, some Jewish clients can be very demanding, assertive, and persuasive in regard to "their needs." The latter has been especially annoying to some nurses in the hospital. Jewish clients tend to complain about the pain and are assertive and demanding for relief of pain by the nurse's services. If some Jewish clients are shunned or avoided, they may feel discriminated and resent noncaring responses. It is well to deal directly with clients' requests and views and to set limits with repeated requests if unable to meet multiple expectations. The nurse will also observe that female family members tend to be overattentive to their sick family member with their affection, nurturant attitudes, feeding the client, and performing home care rituals, which may be viewed as intruding into the nurse's professional role in the hospital setting. The Jewish mother can assist with or participate in the nursing care rather than be excluded, shunned, or avoided.

In general, the culture care values of *being attentive to, providing frequent nurse presence, offering nurturant expressions, and providing care directly* are important care values to guide nurses in care activities. The Jewish client will expect good care and will usually complain if it is not acceptable. Recurrent nursing problems frequently expressed by nurses in caring for Jewish clients are their demands for attention, their limited tolerance for pain, and their need to be sure

nurses follow medical regimes. While it would be well to practice culture care accommodation acts, it is also important to consider culture care negotiations or repatterning of the client's ways to improve health such as repatterning for overuse of drugs, medications, or injections. With different care modes, the Jewish client may learn other ways to handle perceived and actual pain for improved health. For example, the author recalls that a family member demanded that pain medication be given every 1 to 2 hours after surgery. The nurse helped the Jewish client by negotiating a plan to increase the time interval gradually unless intense pain is evident. Sometimes, the nurse can redirect or repattern demands for pain relief by reexamining past shared Jewish sufferings and ways the Jewish people have handled sufferings in the past through their religious beliefs. Other creative strategies can be used when one understands the cultural and religious beliefs and values and psychophysical needs or expectations. Sometimes, ritualized decisions and timed actions are beneficial in repatterning nursing care. The nurse must also be aware that not all clients in the postsurgery recovery room should be treated alike because of cultural variability, and the Jewish client may have intense pain that needs to be relieved.

Another area of nursing care for Jewish clients that requires knowledge of *emic* Jewish understandings and development of creative strategies is providing competent care to the dying client. Care to the dying Jewish client is of major importance and will briefly be highlighted because it is significant to providing culturally congruent nursing practices for client and family satisfactions. A number of literature sources and research studies such as Lamm, Sohier, Leininger, and Boyle and Andrews point to this important need.[24–27] Cultural variabilities with Jewish individuals and families of the three Jewish groups need full consideration with dying clients. An important point to remember is that the family is expected to remain with the dying client as a sign of caring, showing respect for the family member. There is also a spiritual obligation to watch over the person as he passes from this world into another. Prayers are recited by Jewish family members seeking the blessing of God, the "True Judge" at the time of death. Many Jewish clients prefer to die in their homes. The nurse should respect this request if possible as it facilitates family rituals and obligations to the dying member in their familiar environmental context. More-over, in the hospital the family is often concerned about proper care while the client is dying in a strange set-ting. Nurses and physicians need to understand Jewish generic care to the dying family member, and if they are so busy with professional activities and treatments, they can miss the opportunity to give culturally based care. Since death is inevitable, medical and nursing practices should be congruent with the family expecta-tions. Medicine and treatments that artificially and ex-tensively prolong life are usually not desired by Jewish families. Euthanasia is prohibited and viewed as mur-der. Comfort care and alleviation of pain are essential to the dying Jewish client.

After death, an autopsy and donation of body or-gans may be permitted, but only for particularly good reasons. The decision is usually made in consulta-tion with the family, physician, and rabbi. Only es-sential organs remain, and these organs or body tis-sues must be returned for burial as the whole body must be buried. Cremation is generally not accep-table for it is not in keeping with Jewish laws. The body is to be washed and buried in a simple coffin within 24 hours. For the next 7 days there is intense mourning (*sitting shiva*), followed by an 11-month mourning pe-riod with daily prayer (*kaddish*). *Kaddish* is also said on the anniversary of the death.[28]

Some transcultural care points after the death of the Jewish client are the following: 1) the body is ritually washed (*taharah*) by the family or members or some-times the nurse in the hospital. If the person is in the funeral home, the *chevra kadisha* and Ritual Burial Society may do the ritual washing; 2) the eyes and mouth are usually closed by family members or friends, and a sheet is placed over the face; and 3) a candle is often placed near the head and sometimes around the deceased person. If the Jewish client is Orthodox, there is often the custom of placing the body on the floor and positioning it so that the feet face the doorway. Non-Orthodox Jewish families will not usually expect the body to be placed on the floor. The family, relatives, and friends may ask forgiveness of the deceased for any harm or discomfort they may have caused during the client's lifetime. At that time many psalms are re-cited by family and relatives. The family will need to have a quiet place to pray, and the nurse should be sen-sitive to and accommodate this anticipated need. The rabbi is usually called, and he will usually notify the

chevra kadisha (burial society). The latter will typically take care of the body with the funeral director.

From the time of death until burial, the deceased is with a watcher (*shomer*) who is generally a family member or personal friend. This person recites from the Book of Psalms. All deceased are buried in the same type of garment whether wealthy or poor. The shrouds are of muslin, cotton, or linen and symbolize simplic-ity, dignity, and purity. The deceased are wrapped in a prayer shawl (*tallith*) with one of the fringes cut. Gifts and flowers are generally discouraged, but money do-nations can be sent to charity or Jewish organizations and are appreciated. The Jews value charity because it can protect them from spiritual death and it is in keeping with social justice goals. In accordance with Torah laws, the burial of the Jewish person always takes place soon after death. A mourning period exists for several months. One will find the relatives, especially immediate family who espouse traditional Jewish values, often wearing black or dark clothing.

From the above cultural values of the Jewish peo-ple, the nurse realizes the importance of transcul-tural nursing knowledge to guide the nurse in provid-ing culture-specific care or congruent care to fit the client's cultural values and religious care meanings. It is through these culturally based practices that the nurse becomes truly professional to Jewish people. This kind of nursing care helps clients recover from illnesses or die with dignity according to the Jewish beliefs. Since Jewish clients are especially cognizant of their religious and cultural values, they expect nurses and other health care providers to respect their needs.

Professional nursing practices can be transformed to meaningful culture care practices. Such transcultural nursing knowledge and skills are beginning to be used in nursing in culture-specific ways with beneficial and satisfying outcomes. Most importantly, the nurse who understands the Jewish client will find nursing care to be less difficult and more effective when one knows the *why* of cultural care with Jewish values and lifeways.

 ## Part B: Russian Jewish Culture Features

In the late 1980s and after *perestroika* large numbers of Russian Jews applied to leave the Soviet Union for the United States and Israel, before which only a small number were allowed to emigrate. This short cultural summary will be focused on Russian Jews who came to the United States and on glimpses of their traditional historical lifeways, beliefs, and values back in Russia to reflect on differences between the two cultures.

Ethnohistory and Language

The majority of the Soviet or Russian Jews that came to several United States cities were from Belarus and Central Russia and were Ashkenic in cultural orientation. It is important to clarify here that the Jews from the former Soviet Union comprised two cultural groups, the *Ashenasima* and the *Sephardin*. The former are European Jews whose ancestors were from Germany and lived in the Ukraine, Russia, and Belarus. The Sephardic Jews came from Spain and lived in the central Asian area. Prior to the 1917 Communist Revolution, the Russian Jews lived in rural poor areas known as the Pale or Jewish Settlement.[29] However, after the Revolution they moved to larger cities and sought higher education in professional fields. One should be aware that most Russian Jews left the former Soviet Union because of increasing fears of anti-Semitism, threats to life, and for economic reasons. Jews from the former Soviet Union speak the Russian language, but they also speak the language of the republic they lived in such as the Ukraine. Some elders speak Yiddish, the language of most European Jews.[30]

Russian Jewish refugees highly value their families, children, and the elderly. They have very strong family relationships, usually having only one to two children because of limited money and poor housing. Many families lived in three-generation households with the grandparent watching the children while the parents worked. When they came to the United States, they often brought their elderly family members. The general Russian Jewish values of family, high achievement, education, love of conversation, hospitality, friendship, and belonging to a community with obligations were important in their lives.[31]

Health and Caring Modes

With respect to health and caring in the Soviet Union and in Russia, pregnant women have regular prenatal (mandatory) testing and check-ups. They can have an 8-week leave of absence from work before delivery of their child and extended leave with partial pay for 3 years. Child immunizations are mandatory—hence, pregnant mothers and children get fairly good health attention in which culture care maintenance of check-ups should be highly supported.[32]

The diet consumed by former Russian Jewish people from the Soviet Union had saturated fats with the use of butter, sour cream, and fatty meat, which was eaten frequently and in large amounts. Because of this high-fat diet, gallbladder disease and high bad cholesterol were evident along with heart diseases and diabetes. Alcohol and smoking occurs in the Russian Jewish culture and with many young people. *Culture care repatterning* is much needed with respect to foods, alcohol consumption, and smoking—all these need to be repatterned for better health.

Soviet Russian Jews entering the United States expected free health care as they had had in their assigned polyclinics in the Soviet Union. Many were disappointed to find no free health care and that they had to learn how to enter, pay, get health insurance, and receive health services in a seemingly complicated United States health system. They also discovered that United States physicians and nurses had higher social status than in the Soviet Union. This also contrasted with their homeland polyclinic health care providers of whom the majority were women. The social structure features in the homeland were quite different as they had district clinics and hospitals. They also separated children and adults in each region for health care. They could seek another physician if they were not satisfied at one place. In the Soviet Union, people often stayed in the hospital on an average of 3 weeks; while in the United States only a few days in the hospital was permitted with managed care practices.

In the Soviet Union, Russian Jews knew how to do *bribing* as a means to get care or medical services and to be assured of safe and on-going good care. Nonverbal hand gestures were often used for bribing nurses and physicians to get good care. Still another important difference faced by Russian Jews was that in the Soviet Union patients were not told they had a fatal disease such as cancer, as this meant a death sentence. However, in the United States they soon learned that patients were told immediately about a disease with a poor prognosis or death outcome by physicians, nurses, or others.[33]

Russian Jews were very familiar with the use of generic folk home remedies, herbal treatments, and traditional medications. They also used mud baths and mineral waters to remove body impurities and promote healing. In the United States physicians and most health personnel were skeptical of relying on generic folk practices. This was another big adjustment, but as transcultural nurses and others are prepared to know and use selected generic, available herbs, and healing modes, the Russian Jewish client is more happy as they know what has worked in the past. Culture care accommodations for new practices and culture care preservation and maintenance are being encouraged by transcultural nurses with generic medicines and care practices, blending generic care with compatible and appropriate professional care modalities. Nurses also were told how Russian Jewish families got medications in the past from "black markets" for ill family members with great costs and some dangers from the black market procurements. Today, health care in the Soviet Union is somewhat better, but the costs are very high for medicines and health care, and there are few professional nurses.

Historically and still in many places, Russian Jews do not accept the concept of mental illness.[34] Mental illness is shameful and a cultural taboo topic within and outside the family. It was also dangerous to admit that someone in the family had mental problems as early mental institutions in the Soviet Union were believed to be unofficially under the KGB auspices and used for punishment for civil disobedience from the government.

Currently, Russian Jews who have been refugees or immigrants are adapting quite favorably to the American culture. They are very grateful for being in a free, open, and protected society. However, transcultural nurses and other health providers need to use transcultural concepts, principles, and the theoretical three modes to provide culturally congruent care to help Russian Jews in health care services for improved and favorable health outcomes.[35]

A few summary points can be stated to provide culturally congruent and beneficial care to Russian Jews:

1. Use appropriate traditional generic care, medicines, and treatment modes with appropriate professional services and with ways to prevent and maintain health care.
2. Learn ways to do bribing cultural care gestures and with culture care negotiation strategies.
3. Use culture care repatterning with education to change old diet practices to improve health along with exercise.
4. Culture care preservation of family closeness and relationships are essential.
5. Remember the stigma of mental health programs, and find new ways to provide culture care to the mentally ill or the distressed and be alert to post-refugee depression and anxieties.
6. Use and focus on holistic transcultural nursing with a friendly caring approach with all assessments and communications. (They favor holistic care to the partial and fragmented body-mind emphasis in the United States hospitals.)
7. Provide culture care accommodation strategies to link new Russian Jewish immigrants lifeways with those that have already been established within beneficial USA health care practices.

Summary

In this chapter important transcultural nursing and related discipline knowledge has been presented on the Jewish Americans (Part A) and Russian Jews in Russia and after immigrating to the United States (Part B). The focus has been on using the Culture Care Theory with the holistic perspective and the three modes of culture care decisions or actions. Respecting specific and differential cultural variations within and between these cultural groups is important to tailor-make care for health, dying, and other client congruent outcomes.

References

1. Green, J., "Death with Dignity: Judaism," *Nursing Times,* 1989, v. 85, no. 3, pp. 64–65.
2. Samuel, R., *A History of Israel: The Birth and Development of Today's Jewish State,* London: Steinmatzky, 1989, pp. 1–30.
3. Tweddell, C. and L. Kimball, *Introduction to the Peoples and Cultures of Asia,* Englewood Cliffs, NJ: Prentice-Hall, Inc., 1985, pp. 88–89.
4. Samuel, op. cit., 1989.
5. Goren, A., *The American Jews: Dimensions of Ethnicity,* Cambridge: The Belknap Press of Harvard University Press, 1982.
6. Ibid.
7. Ibid., p. 89

8. Sklare, M., *America's Jews*, New York: Random House, Inc., 1971.

9. Ibid.

10. Dorff, E., "Judaism and Health," *Health Values*, 1988, v. 12, no. 3., pp. 32–36.

11. Klein, I., *A Guide to Jewish Religious Practice*, New York: KTAV Publishing House, Inc., 1979.

12. Dorff, op. cit., 1988.

13. Ibid.

14. Leininger, M., "Selected Culture Care Findings of Diverse Cultures Using Culture Care Theory and Ethnomethods," in *Culture Care Diversity and Universality: A Theory of Nursing*, New York: National League for Nursing, 1991, pp. 345–366.

15. Donin, H.H., *To Be a Jew*, New York: Basic Books, 1972.

16. Greenberg, S., *A Jewish Philosophy and Pattern of Life*, New York: Jewish Theological Seminary of America, 1981.

17. Haviland, W., *Cultural Anthropology*, San Diego: Harcourt Brace Jovanovich College Publishers, 1992, p. 271.

18. Ibid.

19. Finkelstein, L., *The Jews: Their Religion and Culture*, New York: Schocken Books, 1971.

20. Goldsmith, E.S., and M. Scult, eds., *Dynamic Judaism: The Essential Writings of Mordeau M. Kaplan*, New York: Schocken Books, 1985.

21. Schlesinger, B., *The Jewish Family: A Survey and Annotated Bibliography*, Toronto: University of Toronto Press, 1971.

22. Leininger, op. cit., 1991, p. 366.

23. Ibid., p. 366.

24. Lamm, M., *The Jewish Way in Death and Mourning*, New York: Jonathan David Publishers, 1969.

25. Sohier, R., "Gaining Awareness of Cultural Differences: A Case Example," in *Transcultural Nursing: Concepts, Theories, and Practices*, M. Leininger, ed., New York: John Wiley & Sons, 1978, pp. 433–450.

26. Leininger, op. cit., 1991, p. 366.

27. Boyle, I. and M. Andrews, *Transcultural Concepts in Nursing Care*, Boston: Scott, Foresman, Little, Brown, College Division, 1989, pp. 405–409.

28. Ibid.

29. Ivanov, M., "Russia, Take Heart," *Russian Life*, May 1997.

30. Richmond, U., *From Nyet to Da: Understanding the Russians*, Yarmouth, MA: Intercultural Press, 1992.

31. Markowitz, F., *A Community in Spite of Itself: Soviet Jewish Émigrés in New York*, Washington, Smithsonian Institute, 1993.

32. Gold, S., *Refugee Communities: A Comparative Field Study*, Newbury Park, CA: Sage Publishing Co., 1992.

33. Brod, M. and S. Heurtin-Roberts, "Older Russian Émigrés and Medical Care," *Western Journal of Medicine*, 1992, V. 157, no. 3, pp. 333–337.

34. Bodsky, B., "Mental Health Attitudes and Practices of Soviet Jewish Immigrants," *Health and Social Work*, Spring 1988, pp. 130–136.

35. Leininger, M., *Culture Care Diversity and Universality: A Theory of Nursing*, New York: NLN Press, 1991, pp. 1–118.

Additional Suggested Readings

Zborowski, M., *People in Pain*: San Francisco: Jossey-Bass, 1969.

Abraham, A., "Organ Transplantation and Jewish Law," in *Science in the Light of Torah*, H. Branover and I. Attia, eds., Northvale, NJ: Jason Aronson, 1994.

Benson, E., "Jewish Nurses: A Multicultural Perspective," *Journal of the New York State Nurses Association*, 1994, v. 25, no. 2, pp. 8–10.

Rabinowicz, T., *A Guide to Life: Jewish Laws and Customs of Mourning*, Northvale, NJ: Jason Aronson, 1994.

Fischel, J. and S. Pinkser, *Jewish-American History and Culture: An Encyclopedia*, New York: Garland Publishing, 1992.

30

India: Transcultural Nursing and Health Care

Joanna Basuray

Health care in India is interwoven into the complex Indian cultural fabric. In this chapter there will be a broad presentation of the numerous cultural groups of India. India's health care is pluralistic despite the strong bent toward allopathic medicine and a Eurocentric health care model. From a nursing perspective it is important to understand that modern care and curing in India have been significantly influenced by the older Ayurvedic, Unani, and homeopathic health systems, framing a complex issue in nursing education and practice.

An overview of India's cultural and social structural dimensions is studied with Leininger's Culture Care Diversity and Universality Theory, which includes ethnohistorical, geographic, religious, and cultural belief systems, as well as social structure factors such as family/kinship, education, economy, technology, and politics. Nursing care is discussed through decision making and action modes within the Culture Care Theory, namely, 1) culture care preservation and/or maintenance, 2) culture care accommodation and/or negotiation, and 3) culture care restructuring and/or repatterning.[1] The Culture Care Theory provides a naturalistic and comprehensive means to study in-depth and holistically transcultural nursing care. The theory is directed toward discovery of existing beliefs, values, and lifeways of cultures.[2] An understanding of India's complexities and variability is essential for transcultural nursing. This chapter will therefore present an overview of the diverse nature of India to understand and discover ways to provide culturally congruent health care practices. The reader is asked to study health care in India not from one group's cultural worldview but from cultural factors of the health care context throughout the country. Since professional nurses and other health care providers in the United States and other countries are expected to provide meaningful and often first-care practices to Indian clients within or outside their country, the holistic content in this chapter is important to understand the Indian culture to advance transcultural health care in India. The author was born in the Indian subcontinent, but has lived her adult life in the United States and has deep research interest in both cultures.

Geography and Ethnohistory

India is shaped like a large, inverted, triangular land in Asia and is bordered by the Himalayan range in the north, Pakistan and Kashmir on the northwest, and Bangladesh, China, and Tibet on the east and northeast (Fig. 30.1). The Bay of Bengal on the east, the Indian Ocean in the south, and the Arabian Sea on the west surround the remaining peninsula.[3] Both the climate and the seasons are variable with regions such as with the northern plains, Himalayan mountain ranges, the central highlands, the desert of Rajastan, the Deccan plateau of the peninsula, the river valley in Assam, and the two large east and west coasts. Seasons vary from dry, hot, and cold in the northern plains to humid and temperate on the east coast and tropical in the south. Monsoons and hurricanes annually bring chaos through flooding and breakouts of infections while cooling the hot, dry temperatures and providing water for crops. Monsoons are preceded by hot and dry spells from April to May.[4] The ecologically diverse country offers the health care provider the adapted lifestyle of people in urban and rural settings. For example, nurses observe great variations in diet and clothing from region to region with fish as the protein source near the Bay of

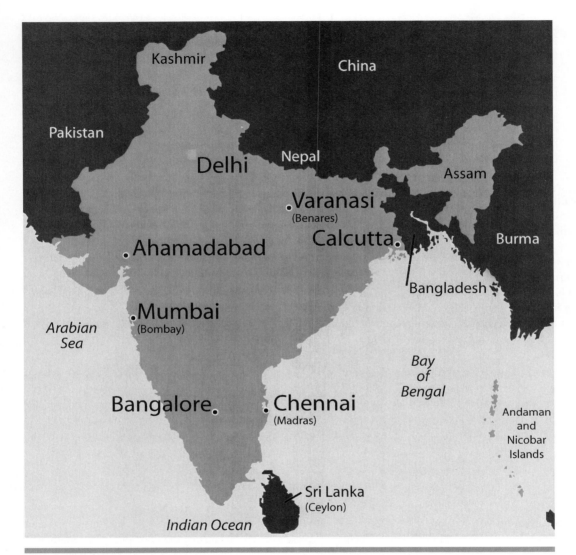

Figure 30.1
Map of India.

Bengal. However, in the northern and cooler climate, the nurses will find the use of meat as primary source of protein and heavier clothing (including animal skin and fur) for protection. Likewise, nurses are challenged to provide culture care to people encountering diseases and poor nutrition from ecological imbalances such as soil erosion and severe droughts.

 People of India

The population in India reached one billion in 1999 with approximately 50 million births per year (Indian Census Bureau). Nurses need to acknowledge the universal concern of increased population growth in relation to resources for health care and nutrition. Most large cities such as Mumbai, Calcutta, and Delhi are overcrowded, but 74% of the population resides in rural areas.[5] The mixed groups across India consist of Indo-Aryans comprising 72% and Dravidians 25%.[6] Although outlawed by the government, the caste system still prevails, especially in Hinduism both in India and elsewhere that Indians migrated. Presently, 16% of people within the caste system are listed as members of Scheduled Castes and 8% as members of Scheduled Tribes. The term *Scheduled* under Indian law refers to those who are designated as economically and socially disadvantaged and therefore protected and entitled to benefits from the government.[7]

The caste system was developed by Aryans more than 3000 years ago and traditionally was related to the occupation of people. Four major categories of castes were assigned: the highest rankings were the *Brahmins* or priests; *Kshatriyas* were warriors and rulers; *Vaishyas* were landowners and merchants; and *Shudras* were artisans and servants. A fifth category, the "untouchables," were later called the Scheduled Castes, and were assigned menial tasks related to body wastes and dirt.[8–10] Knowledge of the caste systems is essential for nurses in addressing the complex roles the different caste systems have in health beliefs and healing practices.

India has been settled over time by diverse groups of people.[11] The Aryan migration took place in the second millennium. The subcontinent was ruled by different kingdoms until the 17th century when for the first time the entire country was unified under the Mughals who were nomadic or seminomadic groups mostly from Mongol, Turkish, Persian, and Arabic backgrounds. These people continued to develop the agricultural economy of the land and introduced the Islamic religion along with Persian, Urdu, and Hindi languages. The Europeans succeeded in getting a strong hold on India in the 17th century.[12] The British colonized India in the 18th century and moved India toward industrialization. Colonization in India, as with most countries, primarily served the colonizers' interests in power and economy.[13] Today, India's official language is English. Among a series of significant changes brought by the British was the creation of infrastructure for research, education, technology, transportation, and government, which propelled modernization of the country. India

practices democracy with increased education and improved economy. Since the 1980s the middle-class population has markedly increased.[14]

 ## Cultural Values, Language, and Lifeways

Language

The Indian government recognizes 18 languages out of 180 languages and more than 500 dialects. The official languages are Hindi and English.[15] Political regions may teach their own language in schools in addition to Hindi. English is taught in most urban schools, so most educated Indians can converse in English. In the home the language or dialect depends on family/clan social structure and preference.

Children are schooled for 10 to 12 years. Public education is free and mandatory until the age of 14 years.[16] Government-run primary education was opened for all Indians during the British rule in the 1800s and English became the standard language. The nurse is expected to preserve the indigenous languages through use of translations and through choice repatterning of language uses for women. In rural communities official documents and forms require some modifications, but face-to face interviews are important for meeting the nursing care needs of specific cultures.

The Indian educational system is directed by the central government and is administered through state and local governments.[17] Private schooling is largely based on the specific cultural group's religions. Private nursery schools are increasing in numbers today with the growing middle class. Post-secondary education in India is based in technical/professional schools, colleges (government, religious, and private), or universities.

Nursing and Medical Education

In 1947 nursing education became standardized under the supervision of the Indian Council on Nursing.[18] In the past, nurses, midwives, and public health nurses were called "health visitors," and Christian missionary hospitals or other schools managed nursing education.[19,20] The Indian Council on Nursing is a formal organization that sets the standards for the education and practices of nursing programs. Presently, continuing under the western health care framework, Indian nursing curriculum consists of two levels, the professional and the paraprofessional programs: a 3-year diploma in general nursing and a 4-year Bachelors of Science in Nursing degree. Most of the nursing education is hospital based. The second level of nursing education is called the Auxiliary Nurse Midwives and multipurpose technicians. Graduate programs in nursing are very few in number. The council officially oversees educational programs, serving as an advisory body and conducting periodical inspections of nursing programs.[21–23] Indian nursing is primarily a female profession within a health care system dominated by the medical profession. Rao reported that the Indian nursing profession, despite its isolated grassroots initiatives for improving health care, continues to struggle in its development of the professional image in that the nursing care of patients/strangers by women is often "looked down upon" and nurses are not often represented by the upper class or caste.[24] Additionally, there is a lack of professional autonomy and a poor infrastructure in education and practice.

In the large cities nurses with high academic degrees are valued with status comparable to the British or American nursing education graduate model. For nurses who practice or care for clients in rural India, knowledge of generic health care practices is essential to provide culturally congruent care. It is a challenge for nurses from the United States to use generic care with professional care.

The regulatory body for physician education and the practice of medicine is the Medical Council of India with the curriculum of four and a half years to follow the British medical school model.[25] Like nursing during the British colonial rule, physicians were initially trained to serve the British expatriates rather than the general colonized population. However, in medical education the scope of practice moved away from curative to preventative practices and encouraged a trend of higher physician to patient ratio in the 1970s. However, as the employment market was reduced both in India and abroad, it led to competitive private practices and misuse of the medical practices through inappropriately trained medical graduates who established businesses in urban areas. According to Krishnan, the preventative model in medical practice has not been

fully realized within the infrastructure of education and practice. Furthermore, social factors that influence health and health care practices of the general population group are presently ignored in the assessment of health conditions, which leads to minimal positive effects on the actual and prevailing health needs of the people.[26]

Social, Political, Economic, and Technological Factors

In 1996 India was known as the *World's Largest Democracy*, with 354 million voters and more than 500 political parties, including its own army, navy, air force, marines, and reserved forces.[27] In economic growth India has been in constant transition since its independence. It has shifted from being a largely agriculture-based society to a modern, technologic, and industrial manufacturing economy. India, however, remains largely rural.[28]

Knowledge of the people's modes of transportation and technologies are critical to understanding and accessing health care facilities to accommodate and receive appropriate care and treatment. Health care facilities that are closest to clients' communities increase the access to care, especially during trauma and emergencies and for nurse availability. The Indian government railways have been modernized since 1991 for large cities. There is also available waterway transportation along the coast and inland, as well as modern airline travel. Transportation by road is the most common type of transportation with different motor vehicles such as two- and three-wheeled automobiles, minibuses, buses, and trucks. Bullocks, camels, elephants, and other animals, as well as human rickshaws are also transportation modes. Telephones exist but only for few households.[29] Recently, cellular phones have become popular.

To facilitate trade and commerce, India depends on international aid, which is largely supplied from the World Bank. Japan is India's largest donor in international aid. Since the 1970s nongovernmental organizations (NGOs) have become well known for assistance of the poor by serving those areas that are neglected by government services. Nurses play an important collaborative role in many NGOs through their volunteer work within communities. NGOs provide services to the poor, helping them to meet their needs and those demands of their political leaders. Pachauri observed that NGOs are mostly involved as grassroots experiments, developing "self-reliance" without changing national policies.[30]

Kinship and Social Factors

In this section social structures will be discussed using Leininger's Sunrise Model to identify major influences on health care beliefs, values, and lifeways. To provide holistic care the social and cultural factors need to be explored and understood with other dimensions. This is especially important for India as the cultural and social structures are complex and diverse. Class, castes, and similar groups (including Hinduism) have existed for a long time and are an integral part of the culture. Influences of caste and class have varied social, psychological, and financial effects on the cultural groups of India. India has a stratified social structure. This means that there are different hierarchical status factors at different levels to understand in this society. Wealth determines the class status of men in a group. India's families are patriarchal with recognized hierarchical relationships. This hierarchy pattern is usually transferred into workplace and bureaucratic institutions. Kinship structure is complex and kinship relations are noted by calling an older colleague *uncle* or *auntie* as a classification term. In the majority of communities extended kinship family groups exist with preferred joint family systems. The family, community, clan, or caste lifeways are interwoven into the daily life of the individual and into the workplace and academic settings. In health care similar patterns exist, and so nurses can expect clients and colleagues from India to be related to others through their similar kinship and stratified social interactions and norms.

In childrearing practices families teach hierarchy or stratified relationships to their children. Collaborative and shared cooperative responsibilities are taught to them, especially with respect for kin and older-aged family members. Although birth is always celebrated, males remain largely preferred today. Sons are expected to conduct funeral rites. National and international concern for female children has been evident because many Indian girls have been found underfed or have become victims of neglect and even murder.

Some selective abortions and female infanticide continue to be practiced,[31,32] which leads to ethical and moral conflicts among the Indians and among clients, health care providers, and religious pro-life agencies. Nurses may have to face ethical personal dilemmas about male preferences and abortion issues. It is often difficult to respect the family's values when it is against the nurse's own religious and cultural beliefs, and so cultural conflicts exist with nurses in care practices.

Making cultural nursing assessments in India is complex and holistic. Traditional cultural values are often closely adhered to, but some cultural variation may be identified. For example, with the practice of veiling (purdah), Hindu and Muslim women follow complex and traditional rules of body veiling and the avoidance of public appearances, especially before relatives and strange men. Almost all women dress modestly, and unmarried Muslim women refrain from appearing in public without a chaperone.[33]

Marriage is an important event in Indian society. For many the gesture of negotiating and conducting a marriage is a critical and major event. Arrangement for marriage can be complex among different cultural groups, classes, and clans in different regions of the country. Negotiations for a future, prearranged marriage sometimes begin with the birth of a child. Marriage celebrations often may continue for a week. Each cultural or religious group conducts their own variation in marriage rituals. For Muslims, and with Hindus in some parts of the south, marriage to cousins is allowed. Preference is given to similar-caste and upper-caste alliances through Hindu marriage. For the past several years, the age of brides has increased to late teenage years or older. Bride dowries are part of the marriage contract that includes jewelry, household goods, and money for the woman's wealth that are given by the bride's family to the groom's family and are important in the marriage arrangements. At present, crimes of mistreatment and bride burning are mostly dowry-related issues.[34] Divorce as a mutually consented process is traditionally not recognized in India, and both Hindus and Muslims vary in the application of the divorce law. Nurses need to be knowledgeable about brides' dowries and divorce values and how to promote culture caring preservation and accommodation with respect to a woman's dignity and status. Respect for women and mens' beliefs and values regarding modesty, marriage, and divorce with their cultural interpretations of wealth and status are also important to understand.

Purity is an intriguing and important cultural concept and value among diverse religions of India. For example, with Hinduism purity in daily life is believed and acted out in various prescribed caste hierarchies and sociocultural statuses. The "what" and "who" are pure if associated with high status, whereas "what" and "who" are polluted if associated with low status. Gold is valued as purer than copper. The lowest ranking caste member in Hinduism is given the occupation of sweeper (janitor), whereas a high-status Hindu is expected to wear properly laundered clothes, take daily baths in flowing water, and eat foods with one's own appropriate caste group. Contacts with impure objects and handling body wastes, including products of death, are left for those of the lowest caste(s). Furthermore, the menstrual period for Hindu and Muslim women is seen as unclean. So, during the menstrual time women are not allowed to cook, worship, or touch holy books. These laws of purity are not always followed properly by many Hindus and Muslims since it is generally considered as oppressive for modern, educated Indians and non-Indians. Maintaining purity-related behaviors by individuals and families, however, remains and is traditionally related to the social structure and transcultural spiritual and physical connections for healing.

Nurses knowledgeable about Indian cultural values, beliefs, and care phenomena of stratified and marginalized groups can provide meaningful care that fits the culture and transcultural nursing concepts, principles, and research findings. Since ancient times, particular groups of people such as holy men or *eunuchs/transvestites* (Hijras) have been recognized as having different lifestyles and statuses. Traditionally, Hijras are often employed for fulfilling particular roles in a household or in public. Historically, Hijras have varied servant roles in households where seclusion of gender (women) is observed. In public roles many become entertainers. Hijras are commonly excluded as a social group and live in their own communities or colonies and in Hinduism are treated as a lower caste and as a social and religious taboo.[35] It is of interest that Indian literature lacks records of homosexuality or the exploration of homosexual lifestyles in India. Currently, it is rare to find literature or films on social

reform or published studies on homosexuality. There are marginalized groups everywhere, and nurses need to be sensitive to the related issues to attain and maintain culturally congruent care for Indian clients. Overall, nurses must be astute to the individual and group differences and variabilities that exist with prescribed cultural values and health needs of clients from Indian heritage, especially those seeking health care in the United States or other countries.

Village unity is a governmental policy that is emphasized where common facilities are shared, for example, the water ponds and grazing grounds. The headman is seen as leader and advisor on such governance and social matters. The local residing Hindu priest or a Muslim holy man has the same honor. Nursing care is often positively affected by the inclusion of village and tribal heads in decision making and achieving desired health care goals.

 ## Religious, Spiritual, and Philosophical Factors

One of the strongest areas of the social structure in the life of people is their religious and spiritual beliefs and health practices. In 1991 82% of India's population was Hindu.[36] India has the fourth largest Muslim population in the world (12.1%). The remaining Indian population is 11% and includes Christians, Sikhs, Buddhists, and Jains. Judaism and Zoroastrianism are followed by very small numbers of people.[37] Religious beliefs in India are very diverse and would require an in-depth presentation, which is beyond space limitations. Nurses are encouraged to study all religions and to be knowledgeable of differences and similarities.[38] With Hinduism, Buddhism, and Jainism the concept of the enlightened master exists in the monasteries. Enlightened masters commonly practice seclusion, engage in rigid austerities, ascetic disciplines, teach, meditate, or travel in pilgrimage to holy places. Devotees, likewise, seek learning, offer food and worship, and travel to retreats to participate in group activities with the master.[39,40]

Belief in fatalism, animism, and astrological signs are followed by many people of different religions. Khare describes care and curing practices in India as moral, personal, goal-oriented activities along with Hindus, Muslims, Christians, and Sikhs. These groups use traditional care and cure practices and seek holy persons and sacred places, but they will also use selected modern professional health care practices.[41] Some of these principal religious groups will be briefly highlighted next.

Hinduism

For most Hindus, an important practice is to choose a personal God or Goddess for devotion. In West Bengalis it is Durga and Kali (manifestations of goddess Parvati), whereas for Gujratis it is Ganesh, son of lord Shiva and Parvati.[42] Most devotees are polytheistic, which means they worship all or part of the vast pantheon of deities, some of whom have existed since ancient Vedic times. In daily practice, a devotee concentrates prayers to one deity or to a small group of deities with whom one has a close personal relationship.

There are worship behaviors that involve the blessings from deities for health promotion and healing. Acts of worship or *puja* consist of a range of rituals offering prayers before an image of the deity or a symbol of a sacred presence. *Puja* begins with the personal purification and invocation of a god/goddess, which is followed by offerings of flowers, food, or prayers. At home women usually perform daily *pujas*. Through *puja*, gifts become sacred. Sacred ash, saffron, or red vermilion would often be smeared on the foreheads of the devotees. In the absence of using these objects, people can stop for a moment to pray or stop at a roadside shrine and fold their hands offering invocations to their gods. Worship includes stylized dancing, hymns, and poetry.

Local deities are usually past or present admired human beings who are believed to protect people from evil and harm. These deities are enshrined in various places in rural areas such as under trees or in entryways of homes. Religious rituals are usually directed toward purity (water) and toward pollution (avoidance of dead flesh or body fluids). Those who avoid the impure are accorded increased respect. Worship is neither mandatory nor congregational. The temple and its maintenance are sustained through devotees and followers' donations. Brahmin priests perform life-cycle rituals such as transitions in life, pregnancy, birth, marriage, and death. Pilgrimage is a religious activity valued by followers and priests. In India there are numerous sites for pilgrimages, and each year thousands of people take pilgrimages. The most popular site is Varanasi, the north bank of Ganges River. Throughout the year schools and offices close for festivals that occurs for several days, and each region has its own holidays or celebrations. For example, in Bengal a major celebration for goddess Durga takes place in October.

Becoming knowledgeable and respectful of the clients' religion, beliefs, rituals, and practices is essential to provide culturally congruent care. Meeting the daily care needs will require culture care accommodation to allow time for prayer and purity rituals. It will also be an important care mode to provide accommodation with the use of amulets, rituals, and symbols. Restructuring or changing religious beliefs and rituals that have been firmly maintained in India over time would not be appropriate except perhaps to some related religious activities requested by the group or community. Outside of India, professionals who are Brahmins may be called to assist with rites and rituals in homes or for individuals. It is important for nurses to anticipate and know about their values, beliefs, and rituals for purity or blessings and to facilitate uses to provide desired culturally based human care.

Islam

Islam is India's largest minority religion. It is historically patriarchal with selected roots in some aspects of the Judaic and Christian religions. Muslims arrived in India in 712 AD.[43] Muslims follow a religious calendar and their festivals are derived from the lunar calendar of 354 days. Sunism (Sunni) and Shiaism (Shia) are the two major denominations of Islam in India. A few Sayeeds reside in India (direct descendants of Mohammed). Another related path is that of Sufism, mystical followers of God, who seek direct vision of oneness with God and display characteristics different behaviors in meditation and worship than the mainstream Muslims.[44]

Local Islamic saints have shrines and living saints are called *pirs*. *Pirs* are sought for spiritual assistance, infertility, stress in marriage, and illness and death. They offer prayers, provide amulets, and give advice to people. Traditionally, face engravings or pictures of saints are not favored for shrines, mosques (place of worship), or homes. Muslims celebrate two main holy days a year: *Eid-ul-fitr* (feast of breaking of the fast or *Ramadan*) and *Eid-ul-Zuha* (feast of sacrifice, based on the account of prophet Ibrahim's willingness to sacrifice his son Ishmael). Celebrations take place for several days. An animal sacrifice, especially the sacrifice of a goat and sheep, is a significant part of religious celebrations. Charity to the poor is an esteemed and expected activity for the Muslim. At birth, a newborn in a Muslim home receives prayer in his or her ear by a paternal uncle. After birth, a mother is kept in seclusion for 40 days, massaged and fed foods considered rich in nutrients such as milk based. An infant's hair is shaved and weighed (the value of which in silver is donated to charity), and this is followed by application of saffron water on the shaved head. This is also the time for naming the baby. All Muslims practice circumcision of the male infant. Another Indian tradition is the use of *henna* (herbal dye), by applying it to the palms of the hands and soles of the feet, as a good omen when used in marriage and other ceremonies by women. For children and adults, *henna* is also known for its cooling effect on the head, palms of the hands, and soles of the feet during hot summers.

Religious instructions for Muslim women include seclusion, which is practiced in traditional homes where homes are constructed to partition male and female quarters. The veil or *hijab* worn by Muslim women symbolizes modesty. To adhere to female seclusion, women prefer female nurses and female physicians as health care providers. Clothing, an essential symbol of modesty in Muslim India, often comes with unique differences according to geographic region and in aggregates of ethnic groups. Women prefer culturally relevant modifications of the dress code, which varies according to the individual's or family's conservative and nonconservative practice and beliefs. Seclusion is also observed during the menstrual cycle, and women are not allowed to pray or visit the mosque to observe purity. Culture care restructuring should be instituted to prevent physical problems or complicated matters for women, for example, in performing breast self-exam or in seeking a female physician and nurse for women's health concerns. Other care-accommodation goals for religious worship are providing space and material items such as prayer beads or a prayer mat. Culture care accommodations by nurses for gender differences are important to show respect and dignity, especially

through the nurses' ability in articulating their understanding of the beliefs and values of Muslim clients to the clients' family members. Overall, it is important to know that Islamic studies (formal or nonformal) serve as an integral component of Muslim life in health and well-being or to prevent illness, consistent with the goals of Leininger's Culture Care Theory.

Sikhism

Sikhism started in the early 16th century by Guru Nanak through a concept of reform derived from Hinduism. About 79% of Sikhs reside in Punjab province, but many Sikhs live abroad.[45] The philosophical message of Sikhism is universal love, devotion to God, and equality to all men and women. Sikhs worship and receive teaching in *gurdwaras* or temples. Baptismal ceremonies are conducted to include a vow in Sikhism in defending the faith at all times. To show faith and devotion, the hair is not cut, and symbolic material items such as a long knife, a comb, a steel bangle, and short breeches are worn by men. After marriage couples abstain from tobacco and alcohol. Religious ceremonies are rich with songs, music, and poetry. There is no official priesthood within Sikhism; instead, communities of believers rely on the holy book and make decisions accordingly.[46] Sikhism offers several paths for followers. Culture care maintenance and preservation should be sensitively observed by nurses in caring for them and respecting the Sikhs moral codes. Nurses need to allow for devotional time, preserve religious symbols, and maintain their desired religious practices. Daily rituals would be accommodated by nurses promoting the daily ritual practice for the followers' health and healing.

Christians

Christianity is largely practiced in much of southern India primarily by Roman Catholics from Europe. Other than influences by Portuguese traders and missionaries from various countries, the British ruled India for 300 years during which the Protestant beliefs dominated the country. Most of the converts to Christianity have been from the lower castes and classes of the Hindus and Muslims. During colonialism the British had converted some entire villages to Christianity.[47] Christians' places of worship such as churches and chapels remain and are still maintained by Indian Christians across India.[48] Some Christian groups adhere to all Western practices through their clothing, language, and material symbols, while others have combined indigenous (largely, Eastern) and Western Christian cultural beliefs and practices into their daily living. Christians' beliefs are similar to the British and European religion even though some worship times are divided with religious practices in English or the local Indian provincial language.

Christian missionaries were primarily responsible for initiating health care facilities for the common public and for education of girls.[49,50] Several British parochial schools and colleges still exist. In nursing, the pluralistic health care services pose interesting challenges for nursing practice, which nurses in India and abroad need to observe as pluralistic health care practices. Christian beliefs and practices are found in nursing education. Culture care accommodation is expected. Cultural clashes can occur if the nurse's educational preparation and personal values are in conflict such as with European/British allopathic education and ethical issues. The author has noted that British colonial nursing education has had a major impact on the nursing profession in India with residual effects of oppression, colonialism, and cultural imposition practices.[51] Nurses would be expected to use culture care repatterning and restructuring to incorporate generic Indian care practices with British practices as discussed below. In addition, culture care preservation and maintenance in religious practices would be imperative to present meaningful culturally congruent care practices.

■ Professional and Generic Health Care Practices and Issues

Generic Indian care practices incorporated with selective professional practices are a major area for nurses to consider. Indian health traditions within a holistic framework date back to the 3rd millennium BC and remain important. Modern health practices in India are based on ancient Vedic scriptures to Buddhist curative practices and Islamic medical science.[52] Some of these practices can be found in the 18th and early 19th century practice of Western medicine with their trained physicians who addressed the needs of the expatriates and colonizers. However, during the colonization eras

limited services such as immunizations and curative treatment centers were opened to the indigenous Indian public.[53,54] Western health care systems gained status with colonization, but the indigenous health care systems and generic folk care was looked down on with arrogance.[55-57] Since India's independence in 1947 from Britain, diseases and related mortality rates remain high with health care services being glaringly inadequate despite some improvements in India's infrastructure in health care and personnel.[58,59]

Three types of India's allopathic health services exists today, namely, 1) government, 2) private, and 3) voluntary. Increasingly, privatization of health care now comprises 78% of physicians' services. In the urban setting, the middle and upper-middle class receive adequate health care from the government and private sectors. Today, some commonly identified health problems in urban settings are tuberculosis (largely the result of overcrowding and poor ventilation), malaria, and urban filariasis (from stagnant pools of water). Primary health centers are public and are largely used in rural settings, staffed by Indian physicians, nurses, and allied health workers. In addition, the public health care service is supplemented by 7000 government and private voluntary organizations.[60,61]

Economically, most Indians cannot afford health insurance to cover hospitalization costs. Most Indians are unaware of the insurance plans unless supported financially by friends or relatives except for a few who receive reimbursements through limited insurance plans.[62,63] Nurses will find a competitive market in the health care services. The poor people still continue to get care under government health care services, while the wealthier use private professional health services. In light of these facts, nurses have an important role to practice culture care preservation and maintenance and also cultural care accommodation for keeping a desired balance between modern Western and generic indigenous Indian health care services, specifically in rural settings. Culture care restructuring is needed in educational preparation of nurses and physicians; this should include generic and professional health care, which is needed for the Indian clients and with acculturation considerations. Establishing trust between clients and nurses through collaborative work with generic and modern professional Western health practitioners is important to provide culturally congruent care.

Throughout India, the two most dominant systems in generic health are Ayurvedic (meaning science of life) and Unani (Galenic medicine) herbal medical practice. Nearly 80% of India's population live in rural regions and have increased access to both systems. A variety of institutions offer education about indigenous medical practice.[64]

The Indian government acknowledges generic health care practices such as Ayurveda and Unani\ Siddha under the title Indigenous Health Systems. Educational, research, and practice methods have been established for these and others (such as homeopathic medicine). Indigenous pharmacology involves the study of the whole plant or its parts: the leaves, stem, seeds, root, bark, fruit, and/or flowers. Plants are studied for their tastes, the composition, and properties, as well as substance potency and postdigestion state formulating the unique pharmacological activity of the substance. Lad, Mukhopadhyay, and Noble and Dutt described that traditional health systems in India function through two social streams, *lok swasthya paramparas* and *shastriya*. In *lok swasthya*, or "peoples" health culture, villagers use the readily available local resources of flora, fauna, and minerals. Housewives use these substances for preparing nutritional food and home remedies; birth attendants, bonesetters, and acupressure practitioners also use these resources, as well as traditional herbalists. The *Shastriya* is the professional knowledge of Ayurveda, Siddha, Unani, and a Tibetan theory and practice.[65,66] Generic health care has lasted for years, but support from the World Health Organization (WHO) is important. Transcultural nurses should seize the opportunity to support an integrated or complementary approach of modern professional allopathic systems of health with the generic indigenous systems to provide culturally congruent and beneficial care.

The Ayurvedic professional discipline contains seven main branches today: general medicine, pediatrics, psychiatry, ear, nose, and throat (ENT), toxicology, geriatrics, and reproduction. Siddha was developed within the Dravidians culture of the pre-Vedic period.[67–69] Siddha means "achievement," and siddhars were saintly figures that achieved results in medicine through the practice of yoga. It is important for nurses to understand how nature and healing are connected through generic health practices in India. For example, the human body is composed of universal elements such as fire, earth, space, air, and water. Likewise, assessment, diagnosis, and treatment methods depend on the data obtained from the food consumed by the clients, as well as their environment, meterological considerations (astrological signs), age, sex, race, habits, mental status, habitat, diet, appetite, and physical condition.

Arabs and Persians introduced the Unani medicine around the 11th century AD. Today, India has the largest, educational and research institutions for the study of Ayurvedic, Unani, and homeopathy health systems, which are essentially generic or traditionally derived systems. Greece was the original home to the Unani health system. Arabs developed the knowledge and practice through extensive use of physics, chemistry, botany, anatomy, physiology, pathology, therapeutics, and surgery. Mukhopadhyay reported there are several thousand trained midwives, bonesetters, and herbalists practicing in India.[70] The reader needs to be aware of the important task of transcultural nurses to balance nursing practice between the Western professional health systems and generic health, for clients from India or in India, despite the present-day dominance of the Western health professionals and systems in India. Therefore, nurses educated in the professional Western health systems have the big task of learning the generic care practices to interface them with professional practices to be congruent, accessible, and promising in the 21st century. Leininger's three modalities are essential in this endeavor.[71]

With the present nationwide and international focus on the health of women and children and with high infant and child mortality rates, nurses and others need to address general cultural, social, and economic factors that impact on the health of women and children such as the following: 1) mother's literacy level, 2) household's access to a sanitary human waste system, 3) religion or tribe membership, and 4) economic status. Sex preference for males and discrimination against women are prevalent in most states.[72] The neonatal death rate in India is high despite the fact that immunization of pregnant women is becoming an effective intervention.[73] Still another consideration is that violence against women is often times accepted, unrecognized, and unreported.[74] Both the government programs and NGOs have contributed to international health services organizations like WHO and the United Nations to bring this issue to the foreground with deep concerns especially regarding women's dependency on sons and being unpaid for work.[75,76] Nurses are advised to be increasingly vigilant in advocating women's just and moral rights to health in nursing practice through professional educational programs and protective activities. Thus, the religious, cultural, social, and educational status of the mother play a major role in the Indian women's health conditions, all of which need active consideration to provide therapeutic, transculturally congruent nursing care.

The European colonists brought homeopathy to India, which is based on the concept of the law similarly described by Hindu sages in the 10th century BC and Hippocrates in 400 BC. The homeopathic system of health care became organized through Samuel Christian Friedrich Hahnemann, a German physician in the early 1800s, who discovered homeopathic remedies tailored to the individual and not the symptoms with a detailed set of assessment protocols. In homeopathy, physical, mental, and emotional assessments are critical in the diagnosis of health conditions. The discipline is practiced through three principles: 1) health is a natural state of human beings, 2) specific remedy applications increase the healing power of medicine and reduce its toxicity while simultaneously potentiating it through various levels of dilution and titration methods, and 3) the patient rather than the illness is the focus of diagnosis. With clients the concept is mostly applied for health promotion and prevention of illness. Presently, India has 121 homeopathic medical schools, and students usually earn a medical degree (MD). It is primarily practiced by physicians, and the clients maintain health by following instructions provided by physicians and pharmacists.[77,78] General health care literature lacks descriptions of the nurse's role and activities in homeopathy, but nursing education and practice is subsumed under the Indian health system of medical programs. In the United States and in several European countries homeopathy is gaining popularity. It is therefore important for nurses to understand the general use of homeopathic remedies in homes and clinics usually as naturalistic caring.

Spiritual health and healing in India are largely viewed as a complex ritual in which the patient and family participate. Given the different religious practices, each provides a unique framework for the individual's spirituality that is linked to the beliefs of the particular system practiced. Throughout India it is common for both the educated and the illiterate groups of cultures to use generic amulets, poultices, and astrologers and to seek supernatural causes for illness along with the professional practices. Some may reject either health care system. With India's pluralistic health care systems, professional Western medicine permeates the larger culture and with advances in technology that most nurses follow today.

In a classic study Gould identified that, because of Indians' relationship to their past with changing rulers, the continuous introduction of different cultures over time occurred. Villagers who wanted modern medical treatment avoided the treatment, dreading a visit to an outpatient clinic or being "hospitalized." There was an aversion to hospitals or institutionalized health care and physical structures in which Gould holds that Western medical practice brings with it impersonal behavior with the professional role.[79] Today, professional health care and personalized care patterns with generic care need to be integrated into medical and nursing practice. Transcultural nurses who value providing culturally congruent care need to consider generic health care practices that are therapeutic, safe, and desired. This means including remedies, herbal cures, and meditation that are safe and congruent with modern and changing professional practices. Leininger's Culture Care Theory and modes of care are a valuable therapeutic guide toward health and well-being.

Nutritional and Environmental Factors

Cultural and environmental factors are important and are related to overpopulation and the production and distribution of food in India. Nutritional disorders exist such as protein deficiency and pathological conditions exist such as kwashiorkor and marasmus. Indians have nutritional deficiencies caused by the lack of iron (anemia), vitamin A (keratomalacia or nutritional blindness), vitamin B (leading to angular stomatis, glossitis, and goiter conditions). Infants and children are the most vulnerable to nutritional deficiencies of iron and vitamin A.[80] Staple diets that consists of rice, wheat, maize (jawar), or bajra lead to an unbalanced diet for many Indians and serious nutritional disorders such as pellagra from deficiency of nicotinic acid in the diet when maize (jawar) is consumed in large amounts.[81]

Cultural and environmental factors affecting nutrition include breast-feeding practices, weaning practices (timing, duration, quantity, and type of weaning foods); and intrafamilial food distribution. Males usually get more food than females in India. Women suffer largely in their general health from cultural practices in which they are the last to get family food.[82] Several studies show that low-calorie diets and the lack of vitamin and mineral intake continue into pregnancy, leading to anemia, nutritional disorders, and low birth weights of their offspring.[83] Evidence shows that females achieve poor growth largely because of discriminatory feeding practices in several states.[84] The occupational status of the mother and the nature of the mother's occupation (including the distance from home), the family structure (nuclear or extended family), the decision-making process within the family, and food taboos all influence the malnutrition of people. Today and in the future, nurses need to assess these dimensions and use the three modes in the Culture Care Theory for restructuring or repatterning to provide culturally congruent care. Educating women and men on the importance of adequate nutrition through educational programs within the communities is essential. Education should be provided by both male and female health care professionals for effective results. Education about adequate nutritional intake and the selection of nutritional foods, especially for women and children, is needed. This would require careful restructuring and repatterning by nurses and collaborating with supportive organizations such as the NGOs. The use of culture care maintenance or patterning actions could be used to promote and maintain community projects related to oral traditions and useful generic care practices. Having clients tell their stories and sharing experiences that are held meaningful are important to maintain the best practices that are safe, nutritional, and culturally acceptable. The culture care accommodation or negotiation, for example, would be used in establishing

community-wide nutritional food service that is free to the poor. Offering cooking demonstrations for preserving nutrients through cooking along with basic education with the illiterate population, and emphasizing knowledge about market products and discriminate use of nutritious food could lead to congruent care. This will require the nurse to negotiate and participate with the heads of families, elders, and males as their traditional consent norms are essential to consider unless deferred to the sons.

Poverty is a major factor for malnutrition in India, and most vulnerable are the infants, preschool children, and expectant nursing mothers. Recent reports confirm reduced incidences of kwashiorkor, marasmus, and blinding vitamin A deficiency,[85] as well as a reduction of malnutrition, in some parts of south India because of the higher literacy rate of women and families. Other factors influencing poor health are drinking unclean water, poor sanitation facilities, illiteracy, and ignorance about safe health practices. Good health practices with food distributions are essential considerations for culture-based repatterning and restructuring in the country. Chronic gastrointestinal conditions from infections exacerbate the nutritional problem in a vicious cycle.[86] Most recently, AIDS is being increasingly found in 10% of the 10 million infected with the HIV virus, which is likely to increase the illness-death patterns in the future.[87]

Other environmental and cultural health concerns are important, such as alcohol addiction, which is leading to poor health and poverty of many people. Occupational health hazards are seriously affecting agricultural laborers (both men and women) who are exposed to pesticides, fertilizers, and infections such as hookworms through skin breakdown in the feet. Industrially based environmental hazards often lead to chronic and acute injuries, respiratory conditions, and disabilities from working in mines, quarries, pits, riverbeds, and forests.[88] In large urban areas, slums foster poor health and are cultural stressors that often lead to mental illness, addiction to alcohol and tobacco, and social diseases.[89]

■ Summary

In this chapter an overview of India has been presented with the general use of Leininger's Culture Care

Theory to provide a holistic perspective for culturally congruent care practices. The reader is urged to continue study on this complex but interesting culture. In the process, nurses need to be mindful that lifeways of Indians are different from region to region with similarities and differences as predicted in Leininger's theory. Despite the diversity, some larger commonalties show the strong relationship of religious/spiritual facets in influencing health and the value of kinship ties and interactions. Class and caste play a major role in the socially upward mobility of individuals and family; thus both patterns of similarities and differences prevail. Leininger's three theoretical modes of culture care actions and decisions can provide a sound basis to improve and facilitate culturally congruent care by reflecting on social structure factors, public education, individual literacy, economic support, nutrition, poverty, and generic and professional care practices. These modes are a valuable paradigm for new perspectives for transcultural nursing practice and for nursing education in India.

Transcultural nursing knowledge remains imperative to attain and maintain culturally congruent care for the health and well-being of Indian clients. This is the goal of Leininger's Culture Care Theory, which served well for this researcher to discover these dimensions with the Indian culture. An exciting challenge awaits nurses in the future as more nurses become prepared in transcultural nursing to serve diverse cultures such as India. Such knowledge will greatly expand the nurses' worldview and knowledge of ways to provide culture-specific and therapeutic care within the modern Western nursing education frameworks to promote generic and professional transcultural nursing knowledge and skills. Leininger's Culture Care Theory[90–92] can serve as a systematic, rigorous, and comprehensive theoretical and practical framework for discovery and for improving care in India and other countries. Understanding the worldview, ethnohistory, social structures factors, and generic and professional care in India and other cultures is imperative to arrive at credible, accurate, and meaningful culture care decisions and actions. Such transcultural nursing knowledge and skills are imperative in our changing pluralistic and multicultural world to become a competent transcultural nurse practitioner, teacher, colleague, researcher, and/or consultant.

References

1. Leininger, M., *Culture Care Diversity and Universality: A Theory of Nursing*, New York: National League for Nursing Press, 1991.
2. Leininger, M., *Transcultural Nursing: Concepts, Theories, Research and Practice*, 2nd ed., New York: McGraw-Hill, Inc., 1995.
3. Chapman, G.P., "Change in the South Asian Core: Patterns of Growth and Stagnation in India," in *The Changing Geography of Asia*, G.P. Chapman and K.M. Kaker, eds., London: Routledge, 1992, pp. 10–43.
4. Katiyar, V.S., *The Indian Monsoon and Its Frontiers*, New Delhi: Inter India, 1990.
5. Premi, M.K., *India's Population: Heading Towards a Billion*, Delhi: B.R. Publishing Co., 1991.
6. Chapman, op. cit., 1992.
7. Heitzman, J. and Worden, R.L., eds., *India: A Country Study*, 5th ed, Washington, DC: Federal Research Division, Library of Congress, 1996.
8. Klass, M., *Caste: The Emergence of South Asia Social System*, Philadelphia: Institute of the Study of Human Issues, 1880.
9. Kolenda, P.M., *Caste in Contemporary India: Beyond Organic Solidarity*, Menlo Park, CA: Cummings, 1978.
10. Latif, S.A., *An Outline of the Cultural History of India*, Hyderabad: The Institute of Indo-Middle East Cultural Studies, 1958.
11. Ibid.
12. Wolpert, S., *India*, Berkeley, CA: The University of California Press, 1991.
13. Reynolds, R., *The White Sahibs in India*, Westport, CT: Greenwood Press, 1970.
14. Singh, S.N., *Rocky Road to Indian Democracy: Nehru to Narasimha Rao*, New Delhi: Sterling, 1993.
15. Heitzman and Worden, op. cit., 1996a.
16. Yadeva, S.S., and Chandney, J.G., "Female Education, Modernity, and Fertility in India," *Journal of Asian and African Studies*, 1994, v. 29, no. 1, 2, pp. 110–119.
17. Ghosh, S.C., *Education Policy in India Since Warren Hastings*, Calcutta: Naya Prakash, 1989.
18. Bhattacharya, B., "Nursing and Midwifery Regulation in India," *The Indian Journal of Nursing and Midwifery*, 1998, v. 1, no. 1, pp. 9–14.
19. Basuray, J., "Nurse Miss Sahib: Colonial Culture-Bound Education in India and Transcultural

Nursing," *Journal of Transcultural Nursing*, 1997, v. 9, no. 1, pp. 14–19.

20. Paul, J.J., "Religion and Medicine in South India," *The Sudder Medical Missionaries and the Christian Medical College and Hospital Vellore: Fides et Historia*, 1990, v. 22, no. 3, pp. 16–29.
21. Bhattacharya, op. cit., 1998.
22. Indian Nursing Council, "A Status on the Proposed Expansion Plan of Indian Nursing Council," New Delhi: 1997.
23. Trained Nurses Association of India, *Nursing Year Book*, New Delhi: 1994.
24. Rao, A.R., "Nursing Education," in *State of India's Health*, A. Mukopadhayay, ed., New Delhi: Voluntary Health Association of India, 1992, pp. 319–324.
25. Krishnan, P., "Medical Education," in *State of India's Health*, A. Mukopadhay, ed., New Delhi: Voluntary Health Association of India, 1992, pp. 303–316.
26. Ibid.
27. Echeverri-Gent, J., "Government and Politics," in *India: A Country Study*, 5th ed., J. Heitzman and R.L. Worden, eds., Washington, DC: Federal Research Division, Library of Congress, 1996, pp. 429–506.
28. Sinha, R.K., *Planning and Development in India*, New Delhi: Har-Anand, 1994.
29. Heitzman and Worden, op. cit., 1996a.
30. Pachauri, S., ed., *Reaching India's Poor: Non-governmental Approaches to Community Health*, New Delhi: Sage Publications, 1994.
31. Jeffery, P., *Labour Pains and Labour Power: Women and Childbearing in India*, Manohor: Zed Books, 1989.
32. World Health Organization, "Executive Summary on Pre-Congress Workshop on Elimination of Violence Against Women," On line, WHO, 1999, pp. 1–25.
33. Jacobson, D., "Family and Kinship," in *India: A Country Study*, 5th ed., J. Heitzman and R.L. Worden, eds., Washington, DC: Federal Research Division, Library of Congress, 1996, pp. 240–266.
34. Diwan, P., *Dowry and Protection to Married Women*, New Delhi: Deep & Deep Publishers, 1987.
35. Jacobson, D., "Caste and Class," in *India: A Country Study*, 5th ed., J. Heitzman and R.L. Worden, eds., Washington, DC: Federal Research Division, Library of Congress, 1996, pp. 297–183.
36. Heitzman, J., "Religious Life," in *India: A Country Study*, 5th ed., J. Heitzman and R.L. Worden, eds.,

Washington, DC: Federal Research Division, Library of Congress, 1996, pp. 121–174.
37. Ibid.
38. Leininger, op. cit., 1991.
39. Heitzman, op. cit., 1996.
40. Schumacher, S. and Woerner, G., *The Encyclopedia of Eastern Philosophy and Religion*, Boston: Shambhala, 1993.
41. Khare, R.S., "Dava, Daktar, and Dua: Anthropology of Practiced Medicine in India," *Social Science Medicine*, v. 43, no. 5, 1996, pp. 837–848.
42. Latif, op. cit., 1958.
43. Ibid.
44. Heitzman, op. cit., 1996.
45. Ibid.
46. McLeod, W.H., *The Sikhs: History, Religion and Society*, New York: Columbia University Press, 1989.
47. Basuray, op. cit., 1997.
48. Reynolds, op. cit., 1970.
49. Basuray, op. cit., 1997.
50. Flemming, L.A., "Between Two Worlds: Self Construction and Self Identity in the Writings of Three Nineteenth-Century Indian Christian Women," in *Women As Subjects: South Asian Histories*, N. Kumar, ed., Charlottesville, VA: University Press of Virginia, 1994, pp. 81–107.
51. Basuray, op. cit., 1997.
52. Khare, op. cit., 1996.
53. Arnold, D., ed., *Imperial Medicine and Indigenous Societies*, Oxford: Oxford University Press, 1989.
54. Basuray, op. cit., 1997.
55. Arnold, op. cit., 1989.
56. Basuray, op. cit., 1997.
57. Watson, K., *Education in the Third World*. London: Croom Helm, 1982.
58. Mukhopadhyay, A., ed., *State of India's Health*, New Delhi: Voluntary Health Association of India, 1992.
59. Arnold, op. cit., 1989.
60. Mukhopadhyay, op. cit., 1992.
61. Baru, R.V., *Private Health Care in India: Social Characteristics and Trends*, New Delhi: Sage, 1998.
62. Sanyal, S.K., "Household Financing of Health Care," *Economics and Political Weekly*, 1996, v. 31, no. 20, pp. 12–16.
63. Berman, P., "Rethinking Health Care Systems: Private Health Care Provisions in India," *World Development*, 1998, v. 26, no. 8, pp. 1463–1479.

64. Heitzman and Worden, op. cit., 1996a.

65. Lad, V., *Ayurveda: The Science of Healing*, Santa Fe, NM: Lotus Press, 1994.

66. Noble, A.G., and Dutt, A.K., *India: Cultural Patterns and Processes*, Boulder, CO: Westview Press, 1982.

67. Larson-Presswalla, J., "Insights into Eastern Health Care: Some Transcultural Nursing Perspectives," *Journal of Transcultural Nursing*, 1994, v. 5, no. 1, pp. 21–24.

68. Mukhopadhyay, op. cit., 1992.

69. Noble and Dutt, op. cit., 1982.

70. Mukhopadhyay, op. cit., 1992.

71. Leininger, op. cit., 1991.

72. Pandey, A., M.K. Choe, N.Y. Luther, et al., "Infant and Child Mortality in India," National Family Health Survey Subject Reports, 1998, v. 11, pp. 96–99.

73. Gupta, S.D. and Keyl, P.M., "Effectiveness of Prenatal Tetanus Toxoid Immunization Against Neonatal Tetanus in a Rural Area in India," *Journal of Pediatric Infectious Diseases.* 1998, v. 17, no. 3, pp. 316–321.

74. Lata, P.M., "Violence Within Family: Experiences of a Feminist Support Group," in *Violence Against Women*, S. Sood, ed., Jaipur: Arihant Publishers, 1990, pp. 223–235.

75. Lingam, L., ed., *Understanding Women's Health Issues: A Reader*, New Delhi: Kali for Women Publisher, 1998.

76. WHO, op. cit., 1999.

77. Mukhopadhyay, op. cit., 1992.

78. Tyler, M.L., *Homeopathic Drug Pictures*, Sussex, England: Health Science Press, 1942.

79. Gould, H.A., "Modern Medicine and Folk Recognition in Rural India," in *Culture, Disease and Healing: Studies in Medical Anthropology.* D. Landy, ed., New York: Macmillan Publishing Co., 1997, pp. 495–503.

80. Ali, M., "Nutrition," in *State of India's Health*, New Delhi: Voluntary Health Association of India, 1992, pp. 1–50.

81. Edmundson, W.C., P.V. Skhatme, and S.A. Edmundson, *Diet, Disease and Development*, New Delhi: Macmillan India, Ltd., 1992.

82. Pachauri, op. cit., 1994.

83. Ali, op. cit., 1992.

84. Ibid.

85. John, T.J., "Health Care and Medical Research in India—A Thumb Nail Sketch in the Lancet," *Current Science*, August 1998, v. 75, no. 3, pp. 181–183.

86. Mitra, A., "Towards a National Nutritional Policy," Proceedings of Nutritional Society of India, 1980.

87. John, op. cit., 1998.

88. Mukhopadhyay, op. cit., 1992.

89. Ibid.

90. Leininger, op. cit., 1991.

91. Leininger, op. cit., 1995

92. Leininger, M., *Transcultural Nursing: Concepts, Theories, and Practices*, New York: John Wiley & Sons, Inc., 1978.

31

Canadian Transcultural Nursing: Trends and Issues

Rani H. Srivastava and Madeleine Leininger

Transcultural nursing remains the most holistic and comprehensive and yet particularistic means to help cultures. LEININGER, 1984

The purpose of this chapter is to provide an overview of past and current statuses of transcultural nursing in Canada. The intent is to give a current picture of trends and some issues that merit theoretical, research, and clinical consideration today and for the near future. This chapter is not intended to cover fully, nor in detail, all issues or contributing literature related to the development of transcultural nursing in Canada. Most importantly, the chapter reveals the authors' direct experiences and knowledge along with input from several Canadian nurses who have published, contributed to, or shared their ideas on the topic over several decades.

Transcultural Nursing within a Multicultural Legislative Context

Transcultural nursing has had a slow and episodic development in Canada over the past several decades.[1] It has been caught within the dominant and firmly embedded linguistic and sociolegislative ethos of multiculturalism, which will be discussed in this first section. Multiculturalism has been used by Canadians in linguistic and cultural diversity terms to deal with diverse issues and as a referent for immigrants and cultural minorities. Not always have the meanings and uses been clear, but the term is widely used in Canada.

According to 1996 data, 11.2% of Canadians are viewed as minorities. (The term minorities is used here and often in the literature to refer to people who are visibly non-Caucasion and are "underrepresented" in the population.) An additional 4% percent are indigenous.[2]

In 1992 statistical data showed that only 2% of Canadians who were over the age of 65 cited their cultural origin as Canadian; while others identified a variety of other cultures as their heritage.[3] While the immigration rate has not changed drastically over the last two decades in Canada, the immigration patterns have shifted considerably. In the cultural history of Canada, initially most immigrants came to Canada from Europe, but by the late 1980s, nearly 70% of the immigrants came from Southeast Asia, Central and South America, Africa, and China.[4] This was a major shift in the Canadian population from previous decades. Immigration is clearly evident in large urban cities such as Toronto and Vancouver, but is found across all of Canada. Toronto has been recognized as one of the most culturally diverse cities in the world. Moreover, it is expected that within a few years minorities (or underrepresented groups) will represent 51% of the Toronto population.[5] Multiculturalism has been identified as a significant factor in Canada in understanding, working with, and accommodating cultures to live together in relative harmony. Multiculturalism has been a major issue for all Canadians, and particularly for nurses and other health professionals who are expected to work closely with all cultures. Although transcultural nursing was greatly needed to guide nurses in their thinking, decisions, and work, the general multicultural ethos of dealing with day-to-day diversity issues related to immigration seemed to dominate their thinking and action modes.

Multicultural concerns and policies began with a focus on the English and French languages and preserving cultural lifeways of established Canadians who had lived in the country for a long time. Soon, general concerns quickly spread to the many different immigrant cultures in Canada. According to Elliott,[6] the multiculturalism theme and trends have gone through four phases. In Phase One (early 1970s), there was a period of *cultural preservation of cultures' values and lifeways*. Communities with diverse cultures received government support for programs to preserve their language and lifeways.[7] The result was an emphasis on cultural celebrations, and the majority of Canadians came to view multiculturalism as "the 3Ds," namely, *diet, dance* and *dialect*.[8]

By end of the 1970s, the second phase was evident with a shift in emphasis from preserving traditional multicultural values to *cultural sensitivity and recognition*. Previously, multiculturalism seemed to belong to the individual ethnoracial communities, but now more attention was paid to promoting awareness and understanding various cultural groups. Group relations were largely addressed through information about different cultures. For example, the City of Toronto Public Health Department developed community profiles, and the Canadian Council of Multicultural Health (CCMH) was created as an organization to address issues across cultures. While there was a desire to learn about different cultures, little thought was given to how to use the information with different cultures.

In the 1980s Phase Three was evident with the primary focus as *antiracism*. In 1982 the Canadian Charter of Rights and Freedom recognized multiculturalism as a constitutional right, and so racial and cultural equality was protected by law. However, during this period considerable debate occurred between the interpretation and understanding of multicultural and antiracist policies. The former focused on equity, understanding, and opening doors, whereas the latter demanded "leveling the playing field" by affirmative action and positive hiring.[9] In health care the emphasis was on reducing treatment and related inequities due to ethnicity.[10] Thus the language of "equity" became the dominant discourse. The construct of culture and transcultural approaches were viewed as "soft" because they were seen as focused only on understanding cultures and using a "cookbook approach" to care or treatment. In contrast, antiracism was "hard," addressing inequities and demanding action or, as some critics argued, "creating

defensiveness." Much energy was spent on differentiating between multicultural and antiracist approaches to groups.

Unfortunately, the construct of culture and its full meaning and uses got lost in the language of power, inequity, and differences. This was particularly evident in talks about sexual orientation, gender, and disability where the issues were viewed in the debate as inequities. Although the multicultural approach was held to be broad and comprehensive,[11] there was limited in-depth knowledge of the cultures and no theoretical foundation to understand and use ideas in practice. In the meantime, the field of transcultural nursing care was continuing to develop and will be discussed later in the chapter. Still another factor that limited full advancement of multiculturalism and uses of transcultural nursing knowledge was the narrow interpretation of culture, often seen as being limited to rituals, language, and food. These limited views of cultures led to stereotyping, generalizations, and narrow perspectives. So after 25 years of policy development and previous phases of focus, Canada is said to have entered *Phase Four*, viewed as integration and establishing "multicultural citizenship."[12] However, multicultural, antiracist, and transcultural nursing approaches in health care continue to be periodically debated in Canada for understanding and linguistic uses. The reality is that there is an urgent need to find ways to understand and help cultural strangers and to integrate the many cultures of Canada into a harmonious, functioning society using sound cultural care research-based data in practice.[13,14]

◼ Transcultural Nursing in Canada

In the mid 1960s Leininger, the founder and pioneer leader of transcultural nursing, came into Canada and began to initiate ideas, definitions, and functional concepts.[15–17] One of the early definitions described transcultural nursing as "the comparative study and analysis of different cultures and subcultures with respect to nursing and health-illness caring practices, beliefs, and values, with the goal of generating scientific and humanistic knowledge and to use this knowledge to provide culture-specific and culture-universal nursing care practices."[18]

While some Canadian nurses were aware of different cultures, they had limited knowledge about specific cultures and care phenomena to transform ideas into transcultural nursing. Conceptualizing transcultural nursing as a formal area of study and practice was difficult to envision but was needed for direct care to diverse cultures.[19-21] Leininger worked with multicultural leaders such as Ralph Masi, a physician, who was taking an active leadership role to promote multicultural knowledge and practices. On different visits over three decades, she shared transcultural nursing concepts, principles, theory, and ways to practice transcultural health care with nurses, physicians, and other providers. Most of all she helped Canadian health care providers to realize the urgent and growing need for establishing a body of research-based knowledge and skills to provide culturally congruent care to native Canadians and many immigrants. She visited schools and institutions and gave lectures and workshops across most provinces from 1967 to 1989.

In those early days Canadian nurses and physicians saw diversity among the immigrants and native Canadians who needed health care. The concept of "mosaic" was used to refer to groups of immigrants and natives living in a geographic area, with the cultures retaining their visible traditional heritage. This idea was also supported by multicultural legislative viewpoints and led to the idea of tolerance, curiosity, and celebrating the traditions of indigenous people and some immigrants. Canadian nurses supported this view, and the mosaic image with different cultures trying to live together was promoted along with a few transcultural nursing ideas. The crux of the problem was the lack of graduate-prepared transcultural nurses to understand fully the constructs and application of follow-up with Leininger's theory and future needs and challenges. Hence, a slow and uneven development of transcultural nursing in Canada has occurred over the past several decades.

With the development of transcultural nursing in United States, there were a few committed Canadian nurses eager to use the Theory of Culture Care and Leininger's concepts, principles, and practices. Two Canadian transcultural nursing models were published.[22,23] These were largely focused on immigrant clients and reflected the traditional worldviews of the countries from which the people came (such as Portugal and Africa). Leininger served as a consultant to Yoshida's research project with children in the mid 1970s, which became the first major transcultural nursing study in Canada.[24] These Canadian studies and models had a cultural focus, but needed in-depth culture and care knowledge to provide culturally congruent care with theoretical and research findings. Discovering and integrating cultural and caring knowledge into transcultural nursing practices from traditional nursing was a difficult challenge for most nurses. Both care and culture needed to be fully studied, understood, and then synthesized into meaningful transcultural nursing knowledge and practices.[25-27]

Grasping the full meaning and understanding of transcultural nursing with clients of many different cultures required teachers and mentors to be prepared in transcultural nursing. There were very few graduate-prepared nurses in transcultural nursing in Canada. Gradually, Canadian nurses saw the need for transcultural nursing knowledge and practice, but it was still difficult to realize this goal because of the lack of prepared transcultural nursing faculty, programs, and mentors.[28] Thus, the most serious problem was the lack of courses and programs in transcultural nursing in Canada. There were also some nurses who saw transcultural nursing as "unnecessary" or "irrelevant" to nursing, even though they were trying to care for many cultural strangers in Canada.

Today, the Canadian nursing profession recognizes cultural diversity, but has not established substantive formal courses and programs in transcultural nursing. Some Canadian nurses are not fully embracing and understanding the nature and scope of transcultural nursing to provide culturally congruent care. Canadian nurses are further developing their roles, but many are still focused on diseases, symptoms, and medical management of diseases. Unquestionably, these practitioners, especially family practitioners, need transcultural nursing concepts, principles, and competencies to provide holistic and meaningful care to families of different cultures. There are, however, more Canadian nurses interested in and wanting transcultural nursing, but they have limited support and programs to help them.

Interestingly and paradoxically, there have been several distinguished Canadian nurse leaders vitally interested in international nursing organizations, and they have given outstanding leadership in organizations such as the International Council of Nurses. Some of these nurses were active in developing and maintaining the Canadian International Development Aid in foreign projects.[29] Indeed, Canada was one of the early countries in the world to take leadership to help other countries with their nursing needs, standards, and practices. It, therefore, seemed ironic that these leaders did not recognize and support the field of transcultural nursing, especially to help prepare Canadian nurse leaders to be effective in unfamiliar cultures in many international and overseas endeavors. Most of these nurse leaders relied on their Canadian practical and extensive professional home experiences. Thus, transcultural nursing was a large and missing area for Canadian nurses in international work until almost the 1990s, when a few Canadian nurses enrolled in transcultural graduate programs in the United States.

Initiatives such as the development of community profiles and events were undertaken with efforts to know native and immigrant communities through social and other policy information exchange sessions. There was also an explicit focus for many government and local health care organizational initiatives to help the indigenous native Canadians (Indian cultures). However, without theoretical perspectives and research findings, and understanding of the diversity and universality of cultures in relation to health care as the central focus of nursing, the knowledge and discipline thrust was missing.[30–32] The use of the Theory of Culture Care Diversity and Universality was much needed to advance nursing and health care services. Nursing and other health care professionals and health organizational administrators struggled for years to discover ways of knowing and providing culturally based care to meet consumer needs and demands.

As noted by Leininger[33,34] and Masi,[35] this struggle led to misunderstandings and misconceptions about culture and the ways to develop culturally congruent care practices. A recurrent misconception was the belief that a few linguistic phrases and a few culture ideas would be sufficient to care for clients of strange cultures. Others believed that experiences and direct encounters were all that was needed to become competent. Still others held that international exposures (experiences) to very different cultures would be sufficient to learn about cultures and provide appropriate care. Some nurses held that culture was the same as ethnicity and needed only sociological insights. Others questioned understanding of cultural variations within

and between cultures as unnecessary. There were also those who believed that all individuals were very unique and that any attempt at describing and knowing them as of a large or small culture was stereotyping and nonbeneficial. Also, there were those nurses who did not value theories and research in nursing because "only direct nursing experiences were important."[36]

Thus, until recently the idea of gaining in-depth and specific, theoretical research–based knowledge of cultures, with care as the essence of nursing practice, was limitedly evident to Canadian nurses. How to gain transcultural nursing competencies, as well as to change myths and misconceptions about cultures and nursing, seemed overwhelming to many nurses. Integrating transcultural knowledge into all practice areas for specific cultures and health organizations such as hospitals seemed too great a task. However, the greatest need was first to study systematically cultures and their specific care beliefs, values, and lifeways to become confident and competent transcultural nurse practitioners. Most assuredly, a theoretical approach was much needed to identify and study culture and care of Canadian immigrants and native indigenous people who had long lived in Canada. Rosenbaum's transcultural nursing research study of Canadian Greeks in the early 1990s was a first major step and an excellent example to show the value of the Culture Care Theory to discover new knowledge and practices.[37] A few other studies followed and will be highlighted later. The study of language and culture care expressions and their meanings in relation to caring/care context was also much needed for the new transcultural paradigm of Canadian nursing knowledge and practices.

Recently, in the Canadian society several mainstream organizations have developed specific multicultural initiatives or outreach activities to encourage the community to use their services. Even when community representatives have been involved in the development of these initiatives, there is often a lack of knowledge and understanding of specific cultures and their care needs within particular environmental contexts. For example, the staff of a multicultural diabetes program hired representatives from Korean, Chinese, Portugese, and a number of other cultures to develop and deliver a diabetes program, all speaking different languages. The assumption was that language was the only barrier and all would accept the approach offered.

While the cultural representatives did not object to a group format that was advised by the Western psychologist, there was deep concern about discussing cultural and personal concerns in the group and with strangers. The cultures found the experience uncomfortable and felt restrained to share.[38] While this example is presented in simplistic terms and may not reflect a comprehensive picture of all that happened, the example is used to highlight issues and approaches to care that are frequently heard in the community. This example illustrates cultural imposition of practices and Western ways to approaching health teaching to immigrants. It also assumes that the culture care needs of cultures can be met simply by involving one individual from a culture to represent and speak for the cultural needs of the community and that Western group process methods can be effectively used for mixed cultural groups. Such assumptions and practices need to be reexamined and guided by transcultural nursing experts.

Currently, in urban centers such as Toronto and Vancouver, there are many "ethnospecific" agencies to serve the needs of specific communities, but there is often limited collaboration between these specific agencies and mainstream health organizations. In some ways the responsibility for providing culturally congruent care seems to have shifted to these ethnospecific organizations with the majority of health professionals continuing to practice in traditional ways with limited or no transcultural research or general knowledge to provide culturally congruent care.

 ## Specific Issues in Transcultural Nursing

In looking more specifically at transcultural nursing issues in Canada, transcultural nursing as a formal area of study and practice for nursing is a major issue to be addressed. Despite the cultural demography of the large Canadian society with many diverse cultures and subcultures, there are far too few books and articles addressing Canadian cultures and culturally based care. Current books on Canadian nursing issues such as Kerr and McPhail[39] and others do not identify transcultural nursing or culture care as a distinct, major, and essential domain for Canadian nurses to address and study. Even if culture care is identified as a relevant and essential topic in a continuing education conference or

workshop, a 1- or 2-hour lecture is insufficient to guide nurses to provide transculturally based care.

Canadian nurses as a profession have been rather slow to recognize the importance of systematic and rigorous study, teaching, and research in transcultural nursing. Yet, there are great opportunities to provide culturally based health care within and outside the country. Until recently, there has been no policy or position paper on transcultural nursing or culture care at the Canadian national level. Recently, there was acknowledgement by the Canadian Nurses Association (C.N.A) in the newsletter *Nursing Now*[40] with a general challenge about cultural diversity, but there were no references to many available transcultural nursing articles, theory, or research and educational programs to guide Canadian nurses toward cultural knowledge and competencies.

At the provincial level, the Registered Nurses Association of Nova Scotia (which is the regulatory and the professional body for nurses in Nova Scotia) has recently published a document entitled: "Multicultural Health Education for Nurses: A Community Perspective."[41] This document presents the community participants' and the nurses' perceptions about their needs in relation to culturally sensitive care; however, it offers no substantive knowledge and limited guidance on how to meet those needs. Another example is the College of Nurses of Ontario (the regulatory body for nurses in Ontario that is responsible for setting the standards of practice), which has recently published a document entitled: "Guide to Providing Culturally Sensitive Care."[42] This document is more encouraging as it reflects Leininger's[43–45] transcultural nursing framework, but provides limited information on transcultural care principles and concepts and the use of available transcultural research knowledge that has been published over the past four decades in transcultural nursing. The focus of these provincial documents is largely on "cultural sensitivity," which is limited and only a beginning awareness of transcultural nursing knowledge.[46–48] While the terms such as cultural diversity, cultural competence, and cultural effectiveness are used,[49] the documents are very general with limited use of specific transcultural nursing knowledge. The complexities of diverse Canadian cultures and the specific use of transcultural nursing knowledge as a specialized and generalized area of professional practice have yet to be developed and systematically used in people care.

In general, much work lies ahead in Canada to meet the repeated challenge of the past five decades that *all* nurses need to be prepared in transcultural nursing today and in the future to be relevant, safe, competent, and effective to serve cultures.[50–54] Leininger contends this challenge needs to be met by 2015 because of the increase in global migration, consumer demands, and expectations and thus the potential for cultural health care violence in health care practices.[55] Boyle holds that transcultural nurses are needed to provide leadership in areas such as managing lifestyle changes and reaching out to cultures.[56] With Canadian immigration and refugee policies and patterns, along with the diverse communities that constitute Canada, these challenges become imperative and offer great opportunities for Canadian nurses to become transcultural nurse generalist or specialized practitioners in this global and essential field.

 ## Nursing Education and Transcultural Nursing

As one reviews available information about transcultural nursing education in Canada in the year 2000, one finds that there are no specific graduate transcultural nursing programs and only a few undergraduate and graduate courses on culture and health. The concept of culture is generally assumed to be "integrated" into the curriculum and nursing practices. However, transcultural nursing concepts, principles, research findings, and practices need to be made explicit and reinforced throughout the nursing curriculum. Moreover, specific transcultural learning experiences that are meaningful and draw on available transcultural nursing research knowledge and practices are needed. An encouraging start has been Toumishey's[57] work, but it is only an introduction to the general area of multicultural health care. Far more emphasis is needed to teach and follow through on transcultural nursing care in the classroom and clinical field areas. The emphasis on differences, equity, power, and racism are too limited to understand holistic transcultural nursing care. Calls and letters from nursing students show an eagerness to learn about transcultural nursing and become certified as a transcultural nurse specialist and how to use theories and

concepts such as those from the Culture Care Theory in their programs.[58]

To determine further the prevalence of transcultural nursing courses in Canadian universities, one of the authors, Srivastava, did a search on the Internet and found in the year 2000 only four courses were specifically titled transcultural nursing.[59] As a Canadian faculty member, Srivastava realized that without the support of formal courses in transcultural nursing, students will struggle to learn about transcultural nursing and how to use the ideas. They currently struggle to find reference sources through the literature in the Canadian nursing libraries (only a few carry transcultural nursing literature and the discipline's journal) and Internet websites. Fortunately, Transcultural Nursing Society's website, *www.tcns.org*, has been a great help to some nurses since 1999. The Internet search also revealed that twelve Canadian schools of nursing offered an undergraduate course with the word "culture" in the title. Of these twelve, five courses were labeled "transcultural health" and three courses referred to international, multicultural or cross-cultural health. Only four Canadian schools of nursing identified a transcultural nursing course within their course listings, with limited information about these courses. There were a few courses focused on caring and curing, but only one incorporated the idea of cultural similarities and differences in practice to make caring or curing a reality in practice or education. With respect to Canadian graduate programs specifically in transcultural nursing, there were none found in the Internet survey and from other written inquiry surveys. There were five universities that offered graduate courses, but only one had a course entitled "transcultural nursing," and the other four used the terms multicultural or "cross-cultural health" largely from an anthropological perspective. Granted this was not an in-depth, inclusive or extensive study, but it provided a general picture of undergraduate and graduate Canadian nursing education with respect to transcultural nursing in the year 2000, shows a limited number of offerings and emphasis on transcultural nursing. Of concern was that the few courses identified were electives, and none were a required nor an integral (or explicit) part of the curriculum and clinical practices.

A major factor curtailing the development of transcultural nursing education in Canada has been the lack of sufficient numbers of faculty prepared through graduate (master's, doctoral, or post-doctoral) preparation in transcultural nursing. This is a critical problem and urgent need to make transcultural nursing a reality in Canada. A cadre of prepared faculty are needed to teach many nursing students who are eagerly awaiting such preparation to provide culturally based nursing care practices in Canada. Granted there are Canadian nurses who engage in international experiences, but very few have been prepared through graduate studies in transcultural nursing to be fully recognized as transcultural nurse leaders, teachers, researchers, or consultants.

Recently, a few community nursing texts such as that of Stewart speak of the importance of "understanding culture,"[60] but the discussion is largely focused on cultural assessment, and there is no substantive knowledge or way to show how to provide culturally congruent care. There is limited reference to the extensive body of transcultural nursing research-based and theory-based knowledge that has been available and used for several decades in the United States and elsewhere in the work. MacDonald has stated "culture is often presented to nursing students almost as an afterthought" and is not consistently taught and brought into nursing education and practice.[61] Sometimes, culture has only an anthropological focus with no linkage or conceptualization to transcultural nursing.

The Canadian literature reveals limited major writings on transcultural nursing with limited use of constructs or principles to guide nursing students, educators, administrators, or consultants. Transcultural nursing literature in Canada, written in reference to specific cultures and in the diverse Canadian context, by Canadian nurse authors is virtually absent. A key reference for Canadian nurses has been Waxler-Morrison, Anderson, and Richardson,[62] which offers insights into cultures in western Canada. Recently Davidhizar and Giger published a text entitled *Canadian Transcultural Nursing: Assessment and Intervention.*[63] While this book title looks encouraging, the authors (who are not transculturally prepared) fail to address the major cultures in Canada (only minor ones), and there is no theoretical base or specific use of transcultural nursing principles to guide nurses. The major emphasis in the book is on cultures and assessment of cultures, but not transcultural nursing per se. Canadian nurses need to study the wealth of transcultural nursing literature to gain basic and advanced research-based knowledge from transcultural nursing scholars prepared in the discipline and to use the knowledge for quality cultural care.

Preparation of Transcultural Leaders

One of the most encouraging realities is that there have been a few Canadian nurses prepared specifically through doctoral education in transcultural nursing (under Leininger and others), and these nurses have contributed some excellent transcultural nursing research knowledge to the field. These Canadian leaders have studied cultures in Canada and overseas and are very helpful to nurses and especially to Canadian nurses. Rosenbaum studied culture caring patters related to grief and loss of older Greek Canadian widows with the Culture Care Theory and the ethnonursing method.[64] She discovered new concepts and knowledge about grieving and death with this study. Cameron studied the influence of extended caregiving on the health of elderly Anglo-Canadian wives caring for physically disabled husbands and discovered new insights about caregiving.[65] MacNeil undertook a major and unique transcultural nursing study of Baganda (African) women as AIDS caregivers using the Culture Care Theory and ethnonursing research method.[66] Her findings were the first in-depth AIDS research on caregiving in Africa. These pioneering studies serve as scholarship models to guide Canadian and other nurses in transcultural nursing. They also point to the beginning research base of knowledge for Canadian transcultural nursing. Canadian nurses are urged to read these studies and other transcultural nursing research to grasp the importance of comparative transcultural nursing knowledge using theory and research. One must also note the work of Dr. Joan Anderson who is an active anthropologist and who continues to apply anthropological concepts and research to guide nursing and general health services in Canada. Dr. Pam Brink is a nurse anthropologist who wrote a book on transcultural nursing that has anthropology articles useful to nurses.[67] While there are other Canadian nurses with graduate preparation, very few have focused on transcultural nursing theory and research. In general, far more Canadian nurses need to be prepared in the near future in transcultural nursing (master's and doctoral preparation) and to become certified to ensure cultural competencies based on transcultural nursing literature and research in Canada and elsewhere.

In sum, Canadian nursing has been interested in but rather slow to respond to the longstanding need of its multicultural population. The critical need remains for transcultural nursing education, research, and practice to care for the many native cultures who have long lived in Canada and an increasing number of immigrants and refugees from many new countries. Transcultural nursing concepts, theories, and research findings need to be incorporated into professional work with clients and in administrative practices. Transcultural nursing courses and programs could greatly assist nurses in all provinces to guide nursing actions and decisions in providing culturally based nursing curricula, research, education, and other practices. For without a substantive knowledge base one cannot ensure safe, effective and quality transcultural nursing care outcomes. As more Canadian nurses become prepared in graduate courses and programs in transcultural nursing, their teaching, research, and advanced practice will be strengthened. It can also lead to some new or different kinds of leadership in schools of nursing, health institutions, and in public arenas with transcultural nursing philosophy, theory, research findings, and practices. Hence, there could be a new approach to some past endeavors for the new millennium.

Future Challenges for Canadian Nursing

While there are many urgent challenges and boundless opportunities for the future for transcultural nursing in Canada, the greatest challenge is to first become prepared and committed to further transcultural nursing in Canada and then influence other multidisciplinary colleagues for better health care. Explicit philosophical statements, policies, curricula, and education practices need to be developed. There is no question that transcultural health care and providing culturally congruent care is needed and long overdue in Canada with theory-based and research-based outcomes. For indeed, culturally based care is a basic human right and ethical obligation for consumers of all cultures. This mandate will become more demanded in the 21st century. As the direct front line and often most continuous care provider, nursing has a responsibility to provide cul-

turally based care to Canadians and others with the rapid globalization of health care worldwide.[68] Educators, practitioners, and administrators are challenged to identify their accountability and responsibility toward this goal. Educational institutions, research centers, and policy developers need to address specific ways to provide and maintain culturally based care to Canadians. One can also predict that as consumers increase their demands for meaningful care, nurses will be expected to be well prepared and responsive to their transcultural needs. Canada needs more research-based transcultural knowledge to understand and guide national policies and practices with their many immigrants, refugees, elderly, the youth, and young children across the diverse communities. The Theory of Culture Care Diversity and Universality may be one helpful theory to identify holistic and multifaceted aspects of transcultural health care.[69–71]

Still another future direction to tap is the study of differences among and between nurses from diverse cultural backgrounds and from different nursing cultures with their impact on practice, education, and research in Canada. Currently, such differences have received limited study, and yet one can predict that they could greatly influence communication, education, and quality of care to clients. Unquestionably, cultural diversity and some similarities exist among all nurses in Canadian health care agencies. Such cultural differences and commonalities in patterns and meanings of nurses' cultural behaviors in different contexts and with different clients need to be identified to prevent clashes, cultural conflicts, cultural care imposition, and unintentional destructive healthcare outcomes. Racism exists in Canadian nursing, as well as elsewhere, but needs to be studied systematically. With the basic transcultural nursing principle "to know thy self," another imperative challenge faces Canadian nurses. This principle is extremely important today in nursing education and practice exchanges in foreign cultures.[72] Fortunately, Canadian nurses can draw on existing transcultural nursing research, concepts, principles, and other knowledge to deal with many of these issues and challenges. While other traditional and current nursing knowledge from nurse theorists and different schools of thought may be helpful, for example, J. Watson's transpersonal caring,[73] most nursing theories fail to address culturally constituted knowledge and research methods to fit culture care needs. Caring ideologies and practices exist, but caring can only be fully known, understood, and practiced when culturally based research knowledge is known and used for holistic care of human beings.[74] Thus, the future of Canadian transcultural nursing is challenging, but awaits its full development with great potential to a new era of education and practice in this 21st century.

References

1. Leininger, M., *Care: The Essence of Nursing and Health*, Detroit: Wayne State University Press, 1984a.
2. Elliott, G., *Cross Cultural Awareness in an Aging Society*, Hamilton: McMaster University, 1999.
3. Statistics Canada, *Ethnic Origin: The Nation*, Ottawa 1992 Census of Canada, Cat No. 91-315, pp. 128–135, 1991.
4. Statistics Canada, *Immigration and Citizenship: The Nation*, Ottawa 1992 Census of Canada, Cat No. 93-316, pp. 38–71, 1991.
5. Masi, R., personal communication, Toronto: March 2000.
6. Elliott, op. cit., 1999.
7. Ibid.
8. Kulig, J.C., "Culturally Diverse Communities: The Impact on the Role of Community Health Nurses," in *Community Nursing: Promoting Canadians' Health*, M.J. Stewart, ed., Toronto: W.B. Saunders, 1995.
9. Elliott, op. cit., 1999.
10. Dobson, S., *Transcultural Nursing*, London: Scutari Press, 1991.
11. Mensah, L., "Transcultural, Crosscultural, and Multicultural Health Perspectives in Focus," in *Health and Cultures: Exploring the Relationship Policies, Professional Practice, and Education*, vol 1, R. Masi, L. Mensah, and A.K. McLeod, eds., Oakville: Mosaic Press, 1993, pp. 33–44.
12. Elliott, op. cit., 1999.
13. Leininger, M., "Transcultural Nursing: An Essential Knowledge Field for Today," *The Canadian Nurse*, 1984b, v. 30, no. 11, pp. 41–45.
14. Leininger, M., "Transcultural Nursing: Research to Transform Nursing Education and Practice: 40 years," *Image: Journal of Nursing Scholarship*, 1997, v. 29, no. 4, pp. 341–347.
15. Leininger, M., "Transcultural Nursing Workshop," unpublished paper, Manitoba, Canada, 1967.
16. Leininger, M., *Nursing and Anthropology: Two Worlds to Blend*, New York: John Wiley & Sons, 1970.
17. Leininger, M., *Transcultural Nursing: Concepts, Theories, and Practices*, New York: John Wiley & Sons, 1978.
18. Ibid, p. 493.
19. Ibid.
20. Leininger, M., "Transcultural Nursing: Quo Vadis (Where Goeth the Field)," *Journal of Transcultural Nursing*, Summer 1989, v. 1, no. 1, pp. 39–45.
21. Leininger, M., *Transcultural Nursing: Concepts, Theories, Research and Practice*, 2nd ed., New York: McGraw Hill, 1995.
22. Carpio, B., "The Adolescent Immigrant," *Canadian Nurse*, 1981, v. 77, no. 3, pp. 27, 30–31.
23. Davies, M. and M. Yoshida, "A Model for Cultural Assessment of the New Immigrant," *Canadian Nurse*, 1981, v. 77, no. 3, pp. 22–23.
24. Yoshida, M. and M. Davies, "An Innovative Project—Childbearing and Childrearing: Recent Immigrant Families in the Urban Toronto Setting," in *Community Health Nursing in Canada*, M. Stewart, J. Innes, S. Searl, and C. Smilie, eds., Toronto: Gage, 1985.
25. Leininger, op. cit., 1984a.
26. Leininger, M., *Culture Care Diversity and Universality: A Theory of Nursing*, New York: NLN Press, 1991.
27. Leininger, op. cit., 1995.
28. Leininger, M., "Nursing Education Exchanges: Concerns and Benefits," *Journal of Transcultural Nursing*, Jan–June 1998, pp. 57–63.
29. Kerr, J.R. and J. MacPhail, *Canadian Nursing: Issues and Perspectives*, St. Louis: Mosby, 1996.
30. Leininger, op. cit., 1981.
31. Leininger, op. cit., 1989.
32. Leininger, op. cit., 1991.
33. Leininger, op. cit., 1978.
34. Leininger, op. cit., 1995.
35. Masi, R., "Multiculturalism in Health Care: Understanding and Implementation," in *Health and Cultures: Exploring the Relationship—Policies, Professional Practice, and Education*, vol 1, R. Masi, L. Mensah, and A.K. McLeod, eds., Oakville: Mosaic Press, 1993, pp. 11–32.
36. Leininger, op. cit., 1997.
37. Rosenbaum, J., "Culture Care of Older Greek Canadian Widows Within Leininger's Theory of

Culture Care," *Journal of Transcultural Nursing*, 1989, v., no. 1, pp. 37–47.

38. Srivastava, R., personal communication, 1999.
39. Kerr and McPhail, op. cit., 1996.
40. Canadian Nurses Association, "Cultural Diversity—Changes & Challenges," *Nursing Now: Issues and Trends in Canadian Nursing*. v. 7, 2000. (Available from the Canadian Nurses Association, 50 Driveway, Ottawa, Ontario, K2P 1E2.)
41. Registered Nurses Association of Nova Scotia, *Multicultural Health Education for Nurses: A Community Perspective*, 1995. (Available from RNANS, Suite 104, 120 Elleen Stubbs Ave, Dartmouth, NS, Canada.)
42. College of Nurses of Ontario, *Guidelines for Providing Culturally Sensitive Care*, 1999. (Available from College of Nurses, 101 Davenport Rd., Toronto, ON, Canada, M5R 3P1)
43. Leininger, op. cit., 1984b.
44. Leininger, op. cit., 1991.
45. Leininger, op. cit., 1995.
46. Leininger, op. cit., 1978.
47. Leininger, M., "Strange Myths and Inaccurate Facts in Transcultural Nursing," *Journal of Transcultural Nursing*, 1992, v. 4, no. 2, pp. 39–40.
48. Leininger, op. cit., 1995.
49. Canadian Nurses Association, op. cit., 2000.
50. Leininger, op. cit., 1978.
51. Leininger, op. cit., 1981.
52. Leininger, op. cit., 1985.
53. Leininger, op. cit., 1991.
54. Leininger, op. cit., 1995.
55. Leininger, op. cit., 1997.
56. Boyle, J.S., "Transcultural Nursing: Where Do We Go from Here?" *Journal of Transcultural Nursing*, 2000, v. 11, no. 1, pp. 10–11.
57. Toumishey, H., "Multicultural Health Care: An Introductory Course for Health Professionals," in *Health and Cultures: Exploring the Relationship—Policies, Professional Practice, and Education*, vol 1, R. Masi, L. Mensah, and A.K. McLeod, eds., Oakville: Mosaic Press, 1993, pp. 139–158.
58. Leininger, M., personal and telephone communication, 1995–2000.
59. Srivastava, R., Transcultural Nursing Internet Survey, unpublished document, Toronto, Ontario, Canada, February 2000.
60. Stewart, M.J., *Community Nursing: Promoting Canadians' Health*, Toronto: W.B. Saunders, 1995.
61. MacDonald, J., Preparing To Work in a Multicultural Society, *Canadian Nurse*, 1987, v. 83, no. 8, pp. 31–32.
62. Waxler-Morrison, N., J. Anderson, and E. Richardson, *Cross-Cultural Caring: A Handbook for Health Professionals in Western Canada*, Vancouver: University of British Columbia Press, 1990.
63. Davidhizar, R. and J. Giger, *Candian Transcultural Nursing: Assessment and Intervention*, St. Louis: Mosby, 1998.
64. Rosenbaum, op. cit., 1989.
65. Cameron, C., An Ethno-Nursing Study of Influence of Extended Caregiving on Health of Elderly Anglo Canadian Wives Caring for Physically Disabled Husbands, unpublished dissertation, Wayne State University, 1990.
66. MacNeil J., "Use of Culture Care Theory with Baganda Women As AIDS Caregivers," *Journal of Transcultural Nursing*, 1996, v. 7, no. 2, pp. 14–20.
67. Brink, P., *Transcultural Nursing: A Book of Readings*, Englewood Cliffs, NJ: Prentice Hall, 1985.
68. Leininger, op. cit., 1997.
69. Leininger, op. cit., 1991.
70. Leininger, op. cit., 1995.
71. Leininger, op. cit., 1997.
72. Leininger, op. cit., 1998.
73. Watson, J., *Nursing: Human Science and Human Care*, Norwalk, CT: Appleton-Century-Crofts, 1985.
74. Leininger, op. cit., 1991.

32 Culture Care of the Homeless in the Western United States

Nancy White, Diane Peters, Faye Hummel, and Jan Hoot Martin

Homelessness is a growing problem in the United States. The homeless are people whose dominant feature is the absence of permanent housing. The homeless may have primary residence during the night in a supervised public or private facility that provides temporary living accommodations.[1] However, many homeless have no such facility and live on the street or in any place they can find shelter.

The homeless present a special challenge to nurses, health care providers, and others in health promotion, as well as illness management. They often lack access to primary health care, routine screening, and health promotion services.[2] They tend to delay seeking care or ways to maintain health. One study found that 28% of the homeless admitted not taking medications that have been prescribed for them.[3,4] Physical and mental disabilities are often aggravated by the living conditions of the homeless. They are more likely to be in fair or poor health than those who are not homeless.[5] The homeless have a cultural lifestyle that varies, yet there are often common themes that challenge transcultural nurses to study, understand, and help them in caring ways.

In the United States 75% of the population reports using self-administered or generic care; this includes both activities that substitute for professional intervention, as well as those that supplement professional care.[6] The greatest potential for improving health for the homeless involves finding ways to build on what individuals do to care for themselves and others. In Leininger's theory this is generic care.[7] While the self-management of care movement continues to gain popularity in the United States with the growth of wellness centers, health clubs, and self-help groups, it is criticized as appealing primarily to the culture care values of the Anglo-American middle class. In contrast, the homeless as a culture tend to fend for daily food and clothing in diverse places such as garbage containers, street refuse materials, handouts, and basic material for living and survival. Their use of adaptive resourcefulness is used for self-care, for survival, and for other homeless people. The homeless, as a subculture, reveal generic care features that are important for survival; however, other cultural patterns need to be studied and understood as their lifeways. In fact, little is known about cultural patterns and care needs of the homeless. In this chapter Leininger's Theory of Culture Care is used to identify, analyze, and discuss the dominant cultural care patterns of the homeless.

Purpose and Domain of Inquiry

Since little is known about the care practices of the homeless, their patterns of living, caring modes and concerns, this study is directed toward this goal. Harris and Williams identify that the homeless have not been thoroughly studied with regard to what they are capable of or willing to perform.[8] Neither the substantive nature of how and what they do to care for self or others nor the process of caring are well known. The need to gain an in-depth understanding of practices and especially emic or the local, home, or folk generic ways need to be studied. Studying the group is also essential to identify the strengths, limitations, and often interdependence of the homeless to develop culturally congruent health care programs for them. Both emic (homeless self-care) and etic (the professional help) research-based knowledge is essential with respect to culturally congruent practices of care and care needs for the homeless as a culture or subculture. *The domain of inquiry for this study is focused on the care meanings, patterns, and expressions of the homeless living in a designated homeless shelter.* The following questions were used to explore this domain of inquiry, but are not limited to these in the discovery process:

1. What are the cultural meanings of caring for self and others among sheltered homeless persons?
2. What are the self-care strengths among the sheltered homeless persons that reflect caring for one's own health?
3. What are the care differences and similarities among the homeless?
4. How are the strengths and limitations to taking care of one's own health expressed among the sheltered homeless?
5. Is care offered by designated professional caregivers or by other homeless persons?
6. Are there dominant features of a subculture of the homeless?

Assumptive Premises of the Research

Several assumptive premises, which guided this investigation, were taken from the Culture Care Theory.[9] The following assumptive premises were developed for study of the homeless.

1. Self and other caring is essential for well-being, health, healing, growth, and survival and to face handicaps or death.
2. The homeless are a subculture that has evidence of generic (lay, folk, or indigenous) care knowledge and does not always use professional care knowledge and practices.
3. The homeless develop generic care that serves them for survival.
4. The homeless have dominant care patterns and commonalities, but differences exist.
5. Culturally congruent nursing care of the homeless can only occur when the culture care values,

expressions, and patterns are known and used in meaningful ways by the nurse.

Theoretical Conceptualizations

The Theory of Culture Care Diversity and Universality using primarily the Sunrise Model as a guide to discovery was used in this study.[10] The major tenets of discovering culture care differences and similarities and examining variability within cultural groups are discovered through the use of social structure, worldview, and environmental factors. The Sunrise Model depicts the components of several dimensions of the worldview and of the cultural and social structure of a culture (e.g., kinship and social factors and cultural values and lifeways) as guides to discover how or if these factors influence expressions of care and health. With research-based knowledge of these dimensions with the homeless, nurses should be able to provide necessary and meaningful culturally congruent care using the three theoretical modes of nursing care decisions and actions, namely, culture care preservation, accommodation, and repatterning.[11]

In this study the Culture Care Theory guides the discovery to arrive at meanings and practices of care with the homeless and to determine if a homeless subculture exists. Leininger posits that the folk (indigenous) care system may be quite different from the professional care system, creating an underlying source of conflict between two cultures with regard to health promotion.[12] The researchers' hunches are that generic care may dominate, and there may be limited professional care. The researchers will look for both generic and professional care of self and others. This is critical to improve care to the growing numbers of homeless in the United States. It is also predicted that a homeless subculture exists with distinctive patterns of living such as identifiable cultural norms, special care values, and care practices that differentiate them from dominant cultures.[13]

Review of Literature

Ethnohistory and Demographic Characteristics of Homeless Individuals

In the rural community of this study there are two shelters and a Salvation Army noon meal site to serve the needs of the homeless. The authors' health care experiences with the homeless were limited to observations of occasional visits to the community health care center and local emergency room. The nature of the visits was often acute and crisis oriented. To improve health care services and to include health promotion and illness prevention, understanding of the care practices of the homeless seemed essential. The study was focused on discovering cultural similarities and differences in patterns, values, and beliefs that would contribute to professional nursing care of the homeless. Identifying any shared, learned, and transmitted patterns, beliefs, and lifeways would contribute to understanding the dominant features of the homeless as a subculture.

The review of the literature highlights research and writings. Estimates of the numbers of homeless individuals in the United States range anywhere from 250,000 to 5 million.[14] Because of a combination of social and economic factors, the demography of homelessness has changed in recent years. Reimer, Cleve, and Galbraith found that Anglo-American homeless are of young age, are women and minorities, and more than 30% are families with dependent children.[15] Women and children are the fastest growing subgroup of the homeless population with increased numbers of teenage mothers.[16,17] African Americans, Mexican Americans, and Native Americans are overrepresented among the homeless.[18] Twenty percent of the nation's homeless now live in rural areas, and there is little research describing the care experiences of the rural homeless persons.[19]

Davis holds that the typical homeless man is in his mid-thirties and holds a high school diploma or higher, while the homeless woman is younger, comes from extreme poverty, and lacks education and job skills.[20] Whether the homeless is a subculture or whether it is a culture of extreme poverty is largely not established in the literature. Studies have demonstrated both similarities and differences between homeless individuals and welfare/low-income individuals with homes.[21,22] The increasing number of women living in poverty (two of every three poor are women) may be a contributing factor to the increasing numbers of homeless women in the United States.[23]

Studies addressing the economic factors that contribute to homelessness include reduction in government aid programs, loss of welfare benefits, rapidly escalating rent, the continual erosion of low-income

housing, and the loss of a job.[24,25] Several kinship and social factors have been identified as contributing to homelessness. These involve family conflict, loss of social support networks plus reduced aid programs, and living-place eviction because of behavioral problems.[26,27] For women alone or with children, being homeless was often preceded by violence and/or sexual abuse.[28]

Many distinctions exist regarding what constitutes being homeless. Homelessness may include living on the street or in shelters or living with another family, friends, or relatives.[29] The literature tends to differentiate between episodic homelessness and situational homelessness. In the case of the former, individuals often describe living intermittently in their own home or that of a friend or relative. Usually, conflict, lack of room to accommodate all, or behavioral problems lead to eviction. Situational homelessness is generally the result of temporary economic strain such as the loss of a job leading to failure to pay the rent and ultimately ending in eviction.[30,31] Many homeless persons find it difficult and time consuming to locate low-income housing and are often unable to afford the security deposit and first month's rent on minimal wage earnings.[32,33] Cultural factors leading to homelessness are limitedly identified in the literature and transcultural nursing studies.

Social Structure and Worldview of the Homeless Subculture

Using Leininger's theory and realizing the importance of worldview and social structure factors, the authors explored kinship and social factors, cultural values and lifeways, and economic and educational factors.[34] Clark et al. described two common phenomena among the homeless population.[35] First, they have experienced significant psychological trauma resulting in the breakdown of interpersonal trust and loss of a sense of personal control. Second, they tend to experience life as a "downward spiral" from which stabilization or recovery is difficult. Absence of social support and social networks and isolation characterize the homeless population and differentiate them from low-income welfare recipients.[36] Being homeless fosters dependency on others for food, shelter, and clothing.[37]

Culture care patterns of the homeless are influenced by the culture care values of the dominant culture, for example, the emphasis on materialism means that the absence of a permanent shelter may define one aspect of the culture or subculture. Homelessness may be discovered to be different or may even be nonexistent in other countries and other cultures such as the Philippines and Saudi Arabia. For persons living in poverty, orientation to present time is often an important value. Delayed gratification requires a belief that the future is within one's own control—an unlikely belief for those in poverty and seeking basic necessities.[38,39] Persons lacking economic resources may be more oriented toward "being" (passive) in their activities than "doing" (active). Those living in chronic poverty value lineal group relationships as a result of sharing resources with extended family members or neighbors.[40] For some homeless, the shelter provides a survival place and often a milieu in which social relationships are established that ultimately limit the possible trajectories out of the shelter.[41]

The everyday existence of the homeless in the United States is characterized by several survival concerns, which include acquisition of basic necessities as food and shelter, sleep and protection from the elements, and a search for needed services. Davis contends that many seek to be "invisible" for their own self-protection from those who might cause them physical, psychological, or cultural harm and that they experience a variety of serious health problems that are caused by or exacerbated by their homeless state and that affect their quality of life.[42] The average life expectancy for a homeless person in the United States is 51 years.[43]

Understanding the culture of the homeless and considering their strategies for survival when planning human services should help the homeless to obtain culturally congruent care. The researchers believe that programs that address the needs of the homeless to get culturally congruent care are important along with learning new life skills and health maintenance lifeways. Making shelters "one-stop shopping" centers providing immediate access to a variety of services is one means of making programs culturally accessible to this subculture. While these suggestions appear to be sensitive to the needs of the homeless, further exploration and discovery of culture care meanings is essential to validate this approach.

Reimer, Van Cleve, and Galbraith demonstrated that waiting for appointments, waiting during appoint-

ments, and the high cost of transportation were barriers to homeless families obtaining preventive health care for their children.[44] A large number of homeless report excessive use of alcohol, drugs, and tobacco.[45,46] Some homeless report spending most of their time searching for food and a place to sleep, seeking medical care only in the case of an emergency, and failing to attend to their own health.[47,48]

Service providers involved in the care of the homeless (nurses, social workers, and hospital administrators) suggested that the following were barriers to health care for homeless people.[49] The respondents cited cost of services and inadequate or no health insurance. They also identified characteristics of homeless persons, lack of motivation for taking care of self, and inability to follow through with treatment recommendations as significant barriers to adequate health care. Ugarriza and Fallon indicate that nurses' victim-blaming attitude (e.g., belief that poor women become pregnant to collect welfare benefits) may deter the health-seeking behavior of the homeless individual.[50] The literature sources provided evidence of several patterns of a subculture of the homeless and support of some of the researchers' hunches.

 Method

The mini-ethnonursing approach as developed by Leininger was used for this qualitative research study based on the emic (insiders') views, as well as some etic (outsiders') views.[51] The setting for the study was a 27-bed homeless shelter located 5 miles from the center of town (population approximately 50,000) and 20 miles from a major interstate highway in the western United States. The shelter is situated in a rural agricultural region located in an area where migrant farm workers travel for employment. Residents of the shelter include families and single adults with residency limited to a 30-day stay. After this, residents have to seek other alternatives, which means relocating to another city since this is the only shelter in the city.

During a typical month at the shelter there are 100 homeless with the majority being males. Nearly 10% are families who comprise approximately one-fourth of the total number of clients. Forty to fifty percent of the homeless are unemployed, and a significant number hold low paying jobs and are awaiting low-income housing. In 1995 nearly as many homeless persons were turned away from as used the shelter because of lack of space. Shelter records available to the authors indicated significant success in finding employment for the unemployed residents (91% of those unemployed were able to gain employment while a resident of the shelter). However, the duration of their employment is unknown.

The authors' contact with the homeless was initiated during a transcultural nursing service-learning experience designed for first-semester nursing students. Each clinical group prepared an evening meal for the shelter and practiced communication skills learned in class. During these encounters faculty and students noticed a variety of poorly managed chronic illnesses and common health care problems. As transcultural nurses, the authors wanted to learn more about the homeless and their health care services and needs. The need for a research study was clearly apparent.

Key and General Informants

Permission to conduct the study was obtained from the shelter's administration. The study was approved by the university's Institutional Review Board with careful attention to having consent forms prepared at the sixth-grade reading level and prepared in both English and Spanish. Informants were offered a small fee at the completion of the interviews that acknowledged the value of their time.

Informants were selected for the study based on who might meet criteria for key and general informants. The criteria for selection as a *key* informant included being 1) homeless, 2) a shelter resident, 3) recommended by the shelter director as being knowledgeable about the domain of inquiry, and 4) willing to talk and available for several interviews. The researchers did not include migrant farm workers who used the shelter temporarily and had a permanent residence elsewhere. A total of six key informants from 23 to 45 years of age were purposefully selected. Four women and two men participated in the study. One of the male and female informants were living together in the shelter along with her two children who did not participate in the interviews (ages 6 and 2 1/2 years). Key informants were Anglo-American (three), Mexican-American (one), African-American (one), and Native American (one). Educational preparation ranged from ninth grade to 1 year of vocational training. (See Table 32.1 for key and general informants with age, gender, and cultural heritage.) Each of the informants was interviewed several times by the same researcher.

Four of the key informants participated in the initial interviews and two of them participated in a series of individual and group interviews, which were used as in-depth confirmatory interviews. This plan was necessary because of the unique transitory nature of residency in the shelter. None of the original four key informants were available for final confirmatory interviews.

There were twelve *general* informants in the study. Eight were homeless residents who were interviewed once and provided a reflective emic view of the data from key informants (five men and three women). Six of them were Anglo-Americans ranging in age from 25 to 43 years, and two were Mexican-Americans in the same age group. The other four general informants were two shelter directors, the regional coordinator from this shelter, and a director from another shelter in the region. These individuals were considered to be intimate outsiders knowledgeable about the shelter population, and they were used to provide an etic view and contextual information about life in the homeless shelter. Two of the general informants were Anglo-American and two were Mexican-American.

Data Collection

Using Leininger's Stranger-Friend Guide and the Observation-Participation-Reflection Enabler helped to gain entry into the subculture.[52] Initially, the researchers spent several weeks meeting with the shelter personnel and administrators discussing the project, the research plans, and observing homeless people coming to the shelter. Several times, the researchers prepared evening meals with some participants (each evening a different volunteer group was responsible for preparing and serving the evening meal) and spent time observing the activities and communication patterns of the residents and staff (usually the shelter director and case manager). Clearly, there were cultural patterns and normative rules that both residents and staff understood and followed. For example, children were typically the first to be fed, and the men were responsible for

Table 32.1   Key and General Informants with Age, Gender, and Culture

Age	Gender	Cultural Group	Status
40	F	Anglo-American	Key
34	M	African-American	Key
31	F	Native-American	Key
29	F	Mexican-American	Key
45	M	Anglo-American	Key
23	F	Anglo-American	Key
38	F	Anglo-American	General
43	F	Anglo-American	General
27	M	Anglo-American	General
37	M	Mexican-American	General
31	M	Anglo-American	General
25	F	Anglo-American	General
33	M	Anglo-American	General
27	M	Mexican-American	General
Shelter director	M	Mexican-American	General
Regional director	F	Anglo-American	General
Shelter director	M	Mexican-American	General
Shelter director	M	Anglo-American	General

removing the dining tables and sweeping up after the meal was served. The meal and evening hours provided opportunity for the researchers to sit and talk to residents and to participate in some of the evening activities; for example, basketball was a favorite recreational activity for adolescent-aged girls and boys. Many adult residents took the opportunity to watch sports events on television, wash clothes, and prepare small children for bed. The researchers took many opportunities to reflect on and confirm their observations during meetings and discussions following these events.

Interviews were generally conducted with informants during the hour before dinner was served. The residents would begin to gather outside the shelter from about 5:00 in the afternoon, but were not admitted to the shelter until 6:30 PM. However, the shelter personnel allowed the volunteer informants and the researchers to use the shelter dormitories to conduct the interviews in private during this time. An enabler guide that focused on the domain of inquiry was developed by the researchers, but was revised following pilot testing with informants who found it difficult to understand the meaning of "taking care of self or others to stay healthy." Rather, the use of personal vignettes was helpful to begin discussions. The researcher would ask the informant to describe what they would do if they developed a sore on their foot that was so bad that they could not put on their shoe and were unable to walk. From this point, informants were able to answer questions about things they do to stay healthy, keep from getting sick, get well, feel better, take care of themselves, and so forth. The enabler guide for the group interview was developed based on the initial analysis of the data, but documented individual responses.

In addition to approved use of taped interviews, the informants were also given disposable cameras and requested to take pictures for the next 24 hours that they felt would represent their daily lives as a homeless person. When they returned the cameras, the researchers had the pictures developed. The homeless were asked to explain each photograph, and informants received copies of the photographs.[53] This technique proved to be very effective as pictures with the interviews helped to confirm their patterned, and special lifeways and the photographs contributed to the final themes identified earlier in the preliminary analysis of the initial interviews. The pictures facilitated telling their story as they experienced daily life.

Data Analysis

Leininger's Phases of Analysis for Qualitative Data using the hand/eye paper-sorting method was used to analyze the data.[54] Taped interviews and field notes were transcribed into hard-copy narratives. The researchers individually identified descriptions and components of the narratives, which were followed by pattern and contextual analysis. The researchers met together to compare findings, discuss discrepancies, identify patterns, and formulate major themes. The process continued for several weeks as more interviews were conducted and more transcriptions were available for comparisons. Patterns were shared with key informants during subsequent interviews, and ultimately patterns and major themes were shared with informants during the final group interview to meet the qualitative criteria of credibility, confirmability, meaning-in-context, recurrent patterning, and saturation.[55]

◼ Findings

Findings revealed there were many similarities in shared values, beliefs, and lifeways of the homeless. This gave evidence that the homeless were a subculture. The dominant subculture commonalties were as follows: 1) all of the homeless shared a worldview of daily survival goals, 2) a view that care meant meeting their most basic survival needs, 3) an orientation toward present-day survival, and 4) resourcefulness care for their needs and others in their group. One of the informants describes not getting enough sleep at the shelter because of noise and an early wake-up (5:00 AM). He said, "So, I go to the park and I will sleep for a while there, but when it is real cold I go to the library." All of the homeless knew where they could find water, restrooms, food, and temporary shelter from the elements. The similarities in lifeways were much more prominent than the differences to affirm the subculture of the homeless. Moreover, socioeconomic status (inability to support themselves financially) and their ethnohistory revealed patterns that provided safety for survival. In addition to demonstrating care for themselves, these homeless informants demonstrated care for other homeless in the context of helping them learn the rules of the shelter and how to obtain meals, services, and a place where they could sleep and be safe. The homeless as a subculture closely identified with their own homeless group and saw themselves as different from the dominant culture.[56] The dominant subculture caring characteristics were care as *safety, survival, present-time orientation*, and *helping self and others*.

Five themes regarding these care practices were identified from the data with recurrent supporting patterns of living. For the most part, these themes were universal among the homeless residents in this particular shelter. The first theme: *Taking care of self for the sheltered homeless person meant health promotion and illness management activities and the use of available resources.* The second theme: *Barriers or obstacles to caring for one's own health and the health of other homeless were perceived and real.* The third theme: *Becoming or remaining homeless necessitated establishing a caring lifeway for daily survival.* The fourth theme: *The homeless shelter provided a structured milieu and a patterned lifeway that had to be learned by shelter residents to provide safety, stability, and survival for others and self.* The fifth theme: *Caring for each other was essential for the survival of the homeless.*

The above themes were confirmed by the group interviews and photographs taken by the second set of informants who discussed both the text of the interviews and the photographs with the researchers. These themes, substantiated by Leininger's five criteria, namely, creditability, confirmability, confirmability, meaning-in-context, recurrent patterning, and saturation,[57] were commonalties of the subculture of the homeless and differentiated them from the general culture. Credibility of the themes was substantiated through the researchers' observations and direct experiences with the homeless as their "truths" of living over time. Meaning-in-context was substantiated by repeated observations and experiences and from the interviews. The Observation-Participation-Reflection Enabler was valuable to identify recurrent patterning and saturation of data with the six key and twelve general informant interviews.

The First Theme

The first theme, *taking care of self*, for the sheltered homeless person meant health promotion and illness management activities and the use of available resources. All key informants demonstrated sound knowledge regarding appropriate health promotion activities. There were three care patterns that were identified that substantiated this theme.

The first pattern, *care as health promotion activities*, revealed a significant knowledge base describing a wide range of appropriate care practices such as eating right, getting plenty of rest, and staying clean and well hydrated. Female informants made comments such as "I try to buy milk . . . an important part of staying well and making babies" and "It's just like you need to keep your body with a lot of fluids and stuff so you don't end up sick." One family proudly demonstrated their routine of taking a two-liter plastic bottle filled with water with them each morning and remembering to wash it out each evening. There was some diversity in this pattern in that some informants described in both words and photographs higher levels of self-care practices such as reading books to "exercise their mind" or visiting museums to appreciate the art displays. While some used the library to find relief from the weather, others sought cultural and intellectual stimulation using library resources. Their photographs of statues and paintings confirmed their verbal comments.

The second care pattern, *care as staying healthy*, meant doing as much as possible for themselves before seeking outside help. One informant stated, "When I get really sick, I take a hot bath so I can sweat it out a little." Most informants indicated that if the health problem was beyond their expertise or did not improve with initial self-help, they could as a last resort go to the emergency department for help. They were also more likely to use the emergency department than a free clinic or urgent care center because of the 24-hour availability. In response to an inquiry about what one informant would do if her foot hurt so bad she could not put her shoe on, she responded, "Drive to the emergency. That's awful to say, but . . . my husband says 'you go for the slightest little things.' " These are examples of seeking outside or professional (etic) care if needed. An exception to this was noted by informants who needed regular treatment and/or medications for a chronic condition in that they would often have a designated physician. One informant with epilepsy described regular visits to her primary care physician and maintenance on her seizure medication. These patterns showed some seeking of professional care when their generic resources were not available.

The third care pattern, *care as resource use*, involved discovering what resources were readily available near them and for what resources they were eligible, as well as when to use the resources and how to obtain and access major resources needed. Homeless informants were resourceful and discovered the availability of the various social services such as food stamps, Women-Infants-Children (WIC) benefits, low-income housing office, employment services, location of homeless shelters, parks for resting, and location of museums/libraries to get out of the inclement weather. Photographs from several informants showed the Salvation Army Soup Kitchen in downtown where most of the homeless without work went for daily lunch. Interestingly, the location of this Salvation Army was at least 5 miles from the location of the shelter. To the researchers it was clear that being homeless was like a full-time job. All of the homeless informants left the shelter (according to shelter rules) by 7:00 AM each morning, walked to the park or some social service appointment, and then walked to lunch at the Salvation Army, followed by another appointment to get WIC benefits. Finally, the informants would check with the responsible persons at the job training center or low-income housing authority for available services. They were due back to the shelter for dinner and evening laundry or bathing by 6:30 PM. Public transportation in this rural community was not well developed so walking to all these areas was the only option. These cultural patterns were daily rituals and patterned expressions with all key and general informants.

The Second Theme

The second theme is *barriers or obstacles to caring for one's own health and the health of other homeless were perceived and real*. While knowledge and intentions for caring for self were noted, all informants described situations that were obstacles to getting and receiving care. The first pattern was *having limited material possessions*. Self and other care was difficult as they had limited material items they could carry while on the streets. Learning where to get water and find public restrooms was critical to caring for oneself and others on the streets. One informant included a photograph that indicated public restrooms while another photograph included a sign that said "No Loitering." The latter meant unwanted to the homeless.

The second pattern, *care is expensive and hard to get*, made daily health care difficult to obtain for the homeless. Located on the outskirts of town, the shelter was several miles from any health care services. The lack of money for the homeless was often mentioned and a major reason that professional health care was not obtainable for the homeless. One female key informant recalled an earlier experience while living on a Native American reservation as a homeless person and with no money. Because she did not have financial resources to pay for transportation to the emergency room for care of her son's ear infection, she called an ambulance to take her son into the hospital. The ambulance driver obligingly returned her home after the examination in the emergency department. Without this assistance, access to care would have been impossible.

The third care pattern, *feeling unwanted and undesirable*, made it uncomfortable for most key informants to seek professional care even when it was accessible. Four key and two general informants talked about situations in which they had been treated most disrespectfully or felt that the professional health providers viewed them as undesirable, inferior, and unwanted persons who used too many welfare services. One general informant said, "If I didn't have to walk one and a half hours to get into town, that would be nice. But that's just people not wanting the homeless in their

own city . . . because they don't want us in the town. We are undesirable." One of the shelter directors interviewed said, "They are able-bodied, but they are not able to keep a job because they are chronically irritating, and employers and family won't have much to do with them." Most homeless informants discussed expressions of the homeless not being wanted in professional health services settings.

The Third Theme

The third theme is *becoming or remaining homeless necessitated establishing a caring lifeway for daily survival*. Three key and four general informants described in detail the circumstances in which they or others became homeless and that it was not a caring and desired lifeway. Several offered patterned lifeway explanations. The first pattern was that of *ineffective problem solving to get and maintain care*. This pattern involved a type of explanatory reasoning that was often evident among the informants. For example, one informant described seeking employment as a cook (for which he was trained), but the only position he could find was too far away to justify the time and effort it took to get there. Another described the need to quit his current job in a meat-packing plant to find something that was less boring, stating he could not look for work while still employed. This form of reasoning was self-defeating with respect to what they said they wanted—work, money, and a place to live.

The next pattern was *being controlled by outside forces as a noncaring mode*. All key informants described situations they felt were beyond their control as contributing causes of their homeless state. One female general informant had been sharing an apartment with her son when he was arrested for parole violation, and she was unable to afford the rent without his assistance. This was viewed as noncaring. Several were unaware of anything they might have done to contribute to their eviction, but mentioned the landlord's desire to "remodel" the apartment necessitated their eviction. Others were evicted for failure to pay the rent, and some recounted situations in which alcohol and behavioral problems on their part contributed to their eviction by the person with whom they had been living. One respondent stated, "(we) can't control what's happening to us," and another stated, "You have to do what you have to do—you can't count on anything." The meanings to the informants were noncaring and showed lack of empathy toward the homeless.

The fourth pattern was *being economically deprived as noncaring*. Four key informants identified a 2-year waiting list for low-income housing and even more inaccessible was housing for larger families (more than one bedroom). One respondent told about her need to "marry for housing." Economic deprivation meant absolute lack of income and of working for minimum or part-time wages without benefit packages. Several related this fact as noncaring by outsiders who failed to be caring people. Many held jobs, but could not afford the security deposit and first month's rent (some landlords also required the last month's rent) needed to get of an apartment or house. One female respondent stated, "This time I have a car. Last time when I was homeless, which was 3 years ago, I didn't have a car and I was on foot, had to carry bags around. I had my little dog and no place to go. I couldn't come here because they didn't want dogs in here." This homeless woman still had her little dog and chose to sleep in her car with the dog rather than give up the dog. She perceived having to choose (sleeping in her car versus a bed in the shelter) as evidence of noncaring attitude by the shelter staff. Thus, the lack of money and any substantial employment placed the homeless in precarious daily survival situations.

The final pattern within this theme was *setting unattainable goals that limited being healthy and caring for self over time*. Three key and four general informants made decisions or set goals for themselves that were difficult to realize. One female general informant made a purposeful decision to become pregnant and planned to have a baby. The father of the baby was also a homeless person who had recently been seriously injured in a train accident. Later, the woman found another man willing to be a father to the baby. She expressed no concern that care for herself or her unborn child might be compromised by her homeless state. In response to a question about what brought him to this area, one key respondent replied "Jobs. Well, we heard that uh, the pay is better than it is in South Dakota. See the only jobs in South Dakota is like minimum wage jobs, and it's not enough to make it even pay rent there,

so we decided to come here." He remained unemployed and dependent on the shelter and other resources and was considering "moving on to Utah" when his time at the shelter expired. While most of the informants were constantly striving to get housing and making plans to support themselves and their families, there were major barriers and obstacles at every turn. There were two general informants who preferred being homeless and described being homeless as a worry-free lifestyle and the ability to live without responsibility. These were notable diversity responses from the above more common patterns of key and general informants who wanted and preferred more stable lifeways.

The Fourth Theme

The fourth theme is *the homeless shelter provided a structured milieu and a patterned lifeway that had to be learned by shelter residents to provide safety, stability, and survival for others and self*. This theme was characterized by two patterns of which the first was knowing and following the rules. The rules were explained by both the shelter director and the other residents of the shelter. Etic or local shelter rules required everyone to vacate the shelter at 7:00 AM, and they were not permitted to return to the shelter until 6:30 PM. They were encouraged to shower each night, expected to watch their children and keep them under some degree of control, and the men were expected to sweep and clean off the dining tables after dinner. Women were expected to do laundry. The shelter director and staff assisted the single men to do their own laundry. Drinking, drug use, and disruptive behavior were not tolerated, and persons engaging in these activities were immediately evicted. Mothers were told not to let their children wander off or be out of their sight for the protection of the child. None reported incidents of abuse. Thus, patterned cultural rules and norms existed for the homeless in the shelter and gave them security.

The second pattern was that of feeling safe and protected. All informants described their ability to temporarily relax at the shelter, while feeling safe from harm and assured that their basic needs would be met through the night. One woman said, "It is a weird feeling because of the fact that you don't know where you are going to go or where you are going to sleep. I feel safe here (shelter parking lot) sleeping in my car. I feel very safe here. But if I would have to sleep like down the side of the road somewhere in a different place, I would probably kind of freak because there has been a lot of people getting hurt because of that." Another informant said, "It is hard. It takes a long time for a place to become safe. Like here. I have been here three weeks maybe. I didn't say maybe three words the first two weeks I was here, and now I interact with the people and everything because it has finally become a safe zone for me." They engaged in basketball games and watched television. Many just sat quietly or talked among themselves or read. One woman wrote postcards the entire evening. They described and demonstrated a sense of relief and respite from the daily need to survive to get their basic needs met. If they followed the rules, they could stay until the morning when in the outside world the need for survival would take over again. Mothers expressed a concern for and a desire to have a safe environment for children during and after school hours, especially during the winter.

The Fifth Theme

The final theme, *caring for each other was essential for the survival of the homeless*, was characterized by the pattern of *sharing information and resources among the homeless group*. Key informants willingly shared resource information with each other such as where and when lunch could be obtained at the soup kitchen, the location of public restrooms, and how to get a bus pass. Making certain that the new residents were oriented by more experienced residents of the shelter was another example of caring for others. Respondents spoke about their willingness to share money and goods with those they considered less fortunate. One respondent said how her husband contracted with local farmers to "clean the beets." "He looks for people to work under him. They don't divide the money by how many acres you're doing. They do it, when the fields' done, you split the money equally. This way nobody fights, 'I did more than you.' Everybody just does it and it gets done. You get your money no matter how many rows you did." Sharing limited resources with each other was the rule rather than the exception and demonstrated how the homeless helped each other to survive.

 Modes of Decision Making

As an integral part of the Culture Care Theory, the three modes of decision making and action were studied.[58] They are culture care preservation or maintenance, culture care accommodation or negotiation, and culture care repatterning or restructuring.

Culture Care Preservation or Maintenance

The six key and twelve general homeless informants of this study demonstrated several appropriate and creative care practices to be preserved and maintained, especially those related to these generic/folk care activities for their health outcomes. Nurses should refrain from their desire to "take care of" and "do for" homeless persons and instead preserve their decision-making strategies and cultural lifeways to use their own resources for survival. Generic care and effective illness management strategies are to be preserved, especially to care for self and others, as protective care was important for survival.

Culture Care Accommodation or Negotiation

Several suggestions were made to the shelter administrators regarding modification of their regulations to better accommodate the care needs of the homeless residents. Currently, meals are provided by volunteer groups who prepare low-cost meals such as pasta. Special food needs could be accommodated by providing the residents healthy food selections for conditions such as pregnancy, hypertension, and diabetes. Nursing personnel could give volunteer groups suggestions or guidelines for healthy meal preparation. Shelter rules could be negotiated to accommodate individual needs such as allowing a resident to sleep later when they are ill. These are examples of culture care accommodation by etic shelter staff to provide culturally congruent care. Another area of decision making was to negotiate with individuals for different care practices in the hope of obtaining more favorable outcomes. For example, shelter residents often complained of problems with athlete's foot, but seldom changed their socks. They should be given several pairs of socks and encouraged to change two or three times a day for a more favorable healthy outcome. Members of one fair-skinned family demonstrated facial skin breakdown from prolonged exposure to the sun. Offering them high-index sunscreen and instructions about application before they leave the shelter in the morning would be health promoting. These are examples of cultural care accommodation by blending of emic with etic findings. Nurses can negotiate health prescriptions framed within the context of the homeless individual's values.

Culture Care Repatterning or Restructuring

The informants cited several examples of using emergency department services inappropriately that should be repatterned by using other more suitable resources such as the local, nearby Community Health Center. Establishing a weekly transcultural-nursing clinic at the shelter could provide culturally congruent health care and an alternative to the emergency services department. This nursing clinic could provide care services such as health education and screening that repatterned generic and professional care to benefit the health of the homeless. Asking residents how they are "feeling" or what they are "doing" about their health, to show concern for and about them, and listening carefully to their responses without interruption were important for attaining culturally congruent care. Rather than prescribing professional care, the homeless need to be asked what they are willing and able to do for their own health and incorporate their generic care as a repatterning modality. Providing incremental, repatterned health behavior recommendations was more acceptable than major lifeway changes.

A suggested restructured recommendation for the community was to provide a "downtown" day shelter for individuals and families for homeless services and to provide an opportunity for the homeless to contact various social service representatives. The shelter hours of operation should be repatterned to address the needs of families with children. For example, children ought to be able to go to the shelter after school hours and be safe. Increased funding is needed to provide culturally congruent care for the homeless, and this needs to be considered in repatterning of financial support for the

homeless, as well as in promoting job placements and affordable housing.

Conclusions

The themes and patterns from this ethnonursing study of self and other care among the sheltered homeless were based on data obtained from six key and twelve general informants. The shared worldview of the informants and similar lifeways gave evidence that the homeless were a subculture. The themes demonstrated both similarities and differences within the subculture of the homeless. All key and general informants described examples of care for themselves and others, but differences in their abilities were evident. The findings showed patterns and meanings of caring, but also many noncaring acts in the larger society. The shelter consistently provided a safe and protected environment for survival of the homeless if they were oriented to the rules of the institution. The majority of the informants were situationally homeless and described their goals to find safety, work, and shelter. Two informants identified the worry-free lifestyle of being homeless. There were barriers in taking care of one's own health because of limited resources, geographic and economic isolation, and feelings of being unwanted and undesirable. Care for others was demonstrated by sharing information and resources essential for survival. Culturally congruent care meant acceptance, cleanliness, eating the right foods, respecting lifeways, sharing with others, protecting others/self, and valuing another's ways. Discovering the meanings of the homeless supports the Culture Care Theory and ethnonursing research and method.[59] The cultural meaning of care for the homeless included both health promotion/illness management and feeling safe within the shelter milieu. The informants had health knowledge, and they used and shared resources with each other to achieve their health under precarious circumstances. Care offered by the professional caregivers was very limited and mainly use at the 24-hour emergency department by the homeless. This study substantiates Leininger's Theory of Culture Care tenets showing care diversities and similarities among the homeless as a subculture.

This study illustrated the resourcefulness of the sheltered homeless as they cared for themselves and others under difficult conditions. Professional care needs to be built on the homeless generic/folk care knowledge and ways maximize the health and well-being of the homeless as a subculture to attain and maintain culturally congruent nursing care. Further and ongoing research is recommended to discover changes over time as part of transcultural nursing care goals, knowledge development, and practices for the homeless.

References

1. Stephens, D., E. Dennis, M. Toomer, and J. Holloway, "The Diversity of Case Management Needs for the Care of Homeless Persons," *Public Health Reports*, 1991, *106*(1), pp. 15–19.
2. Norton, D. and N. Ridenour, "Homeless Women and Children: The Challenge of Health Promotion," *Nurse Practitioner Forum*, 1995, *6*(1), pp. 29–33.
3. Clark, P.N., C.A. Williams, M.A. Percy, and Y.S. Kim, "Health and Life Problems of Homeless Men and Women in the Southeast," *Journal of Community Health Nursing*, 1995, *12*(2), pp. 101–110.
4. Hatton, D.C., "Managing Health Problems Among Homeless Women with Children in a Transitional Shelter," *Image: Journal of Nursing Scholarship*, 1997, *29*(1), pp. 33–36.
5. Vredevoe, D.L., P. Shuler, and M. Woo, "The Homeless Population," *Western Journal of Nursing Research*, 1992, *14*(6), pp. 731–740.
6. Lipson, J.G. and N.J. Steiger, *Self-Care Nursing in a Multicultural Context*, Thousand Oaks, CA: Sage, 1996.
7. Leininger, M., *Cultural Care Diversity and Universality: A Theory of Nursing*, New York: National League for Nursing Press, 1991.
8. Harris, J.L. and L.K. Williams, "Self-Care Requisites As Identified by Homeless Elderly Men," *Journal of Gerontological Nursing*, 1991, *17*(6), pp. 39–43.
9. Leininger, op. cit., 1991.
10. Ibid.
11. Leininger, M., *Transcultural Nursing: Concepts, Principles, Theory, Research and Practice*, New York: McGraw-Hill, 1995.
12. Leininger, op. cit., 1991.
13. Leininger, op. cit., 1995.
14. Wagner, J.D., E.M. Menke, and J.K. Ciccone, "The Health of Rural Homeless Women with Young Children," *The Journal of Rural Health*, 1994, *10*(1), pp. 49–57.
15. Reimer, J.G., L. VanCleve, and M. Galbraith, "Barriers to Well Child Care for Homeless Children Under Age 13," *Public Health Nursing*, 1995, *12*(1), pp. 61–66.
16. Davis, R.E., "Tapping into the Culture of Homelessness," *Journal of Professional Nursing*, 1996, *12*, pp. 176–183.
17. Norton and Ridenour, op. cit., 1995.
18. Davis, op. cit., 1996.
19. Wager et al., op. cit., 1994.
20. Davis, op. cit., 1996.
21. Takahashi, L.M. and J.R. Wolch, "Differences in Health and Welfare Between Homeless and Homed Welfare Applicants in Los Angeles Country," *Social Science Medicine*, 1994, *38*(10), pp. 1401–1413.
22. Ziesmer, C., L. Marcoux, and B.E. Marwell, "Homeless Children: Are They Different from Other Low-Income Children?" *Social Work*, 1994, *39*(6), pp. 658–668.
23. Davis, op. cit., 1996.
24. Clark et al., op. cit., 1995.
25. Norton and Ridenour, op. cit., 1995.
26. Kinzel, D., "Self-Identified Health Concerns of Two Homeless Groups," *Western Journal of Nursing Research*, 1991, *13*(2), pp. 181–194.
27. Bassak, E.L., "Homelessness in Female-Headed Families: Childhood and Adult Risk and Protective Factors," *American Journal of Public Health*, 1997, 87, pp. 241–248.
28. Hatton, op. cit., 1997.
29. Wagner et al., op. cit., 1994.
30. Kinzel, op. cit., 1991.
31. Thrasher, S.P. and C.T. Mowbray, "A Strengths Perspective: An Ethnographic Study of Homeless Women with Children," *Health and Social Work*, 1995, *20*(2), pp. 93–101.
32. Berne, A.S., C. Dato, D.J. Mason, and M. Rafferty, "A Nursing Model for Addressing the Health Needs of Homeless Families," *Image: Journal of Nursing Scholarship*, 1990, *22*(1), pp. 8–13.
33. Dehavenon, A.L., ed., *There's No Place Like Home: Anthropological Perspectives on Housing and Homelessness in the United States*, Westport: Bergin and Garvey, 1999.
34. Leininger, op. cit., 1991.
35. Clark et al., op. cit., 1995.
36. Takahashi and Wolch, op. cit., 1994.

37. Park, P.B., "Health Care for the Homeless: A Self-Care Approach," *Clinical Nurse Specialist*, 1989, *3*(4), pp. 171–175.

38. Davis, op. cit., 1996.

39. Humphrey, R., "Families Who Live in Chronic Poverty: Meeting the Challenge of Family-Centered Services," *The American Journal of Occupational Therapy*, 1995, *49*(7), pp. 687–693.

40. Ibid.

41. Dordick, G.A., "More Than Refuge: The Social Worlds of a Homeless Shelter," *Journal of Contemporary Ethnography*, 1996, *24*(4), pp. 313–404.

42. Davis, op. cit., 1996.

43. Ibid.

44. Reimer, VanCleve, and Galbraith, op. cit., 1995.

45. Mason, D.J., M. Jensen, and D.L. Boland, "Health Behaviors and Health Risks Among Homeless Males in Utah," *Western Journal of Nursing Research*, 1992, *14*(6), pp. 775–790.

46. Wagner et al., op. cit., 1994.

47. Burg, M.A., "Health Problems of Sheltered Homeless Women and Their Dependent Children," *Health and Social Work*, 1994, *19*(2), pp. 125–131.

48. Kinzel, op. cit., 1991.

49. Hunter, J.K., C.G. Getty, M. Kemsley, and A.H. Skelly, "Barriers to Providing Health Care to Homeless Persons: A Survey of Providers' Perceptions," *Health Values*, 1991, *15*(5), pp. 3–11.

50. Ugarriza, D.N. and T. Fallon, "Nurses' Attitudes Toward Homeless Women: A Barrier to Change," *Nursing Outlook*, 1994, 42, pp. 26–29.

51. Leininger, op. cit., 1991.

52. Ibid.

53. Leininger, M., *Qualitative Research Method in Nursing*, Orlando, FL: Grune and Stratton, 1985.

54. Leininger, op. cit., 1991.

55. Ibid.

56. Leininger, op. cit., 1995.

57. Leininger, op. cit., 1991.

58. Ibid.

59. Ibid.

33

Reflections on Australia and Transcultural Nursing in the New Millennium*

Akram Omeri

As an Iranian immigrant, I have reflected on my Iranian immigration experience and my identity and feelings of being "the other." I am one of the 23.3% of Australian immigrants, and one of the nearly 17% of Australia's 1996 population from a non–English-speaking country.[1] I was born in Iran, which is a land of diverse topography and climate and of many different cultures with different religions and lifeways. My exposure to multiculturalism began in my birth country with many diverse cultural groups with different languages and religious practices. Iran is a land of very ancient migrations such as Medes, Persians, Parthians, and others.[2] Australia is a land with indigenous Aborigines and many recent immigrants.

Reflections on these facts led me to further explore the experience of immigration in relation to my historical roots. The purpose of this chapter is to explore some current immigration issues and policies related to transcultural nurses providing culturally congruent care with a focus on Derrida's views of the constructs of *otherness and hospitality*.[3-6]

◼ Reflections on Australia

Australia is a culturally diverse society with immigrants and native-born people. The Aborigines and Torres Strait Islanders are the first nation peoples who are rich in culture, languages, and lifeways. The inner cultural strength of these people has been preserved through the years despite colonialism. Australia has grown in population in the past 50 years with immigration. In 1996 23.3% of the Australian population was born overseas, which is a 3% increase since 1971. This was mainly because of the large numbers of immigrants who have come into the country since the late 1980s. In the 1996 census, this percentage had increased to nearly 17% when the total population of Australia was just under 18 million.[7]

One of the most significant changes in Australia over the past 50 years has been the development of public policy from a highly discriminatory *White Australia* policy to a nondiscriminatory immigration policy showing transitions from assimilation to integration and then to multiculturalism. Multiculturalism continues to have a strong emphasis on previous policies of social harmony, but the government recognizes and positively accepts that Australia is, and will remain, a culturally diverse country.[8-10] Australia's diversity is reflected with over 89 languages, 80 religions, and 200 cultures with different lifeways and health care practices.[11] In addition there is diversity in the land, climate, and settings where health care is provided from the remote rural areas to urban settings.

In 1999 the National Multicultural Advisory Council of the Australian government, in a draft policy document, stated ". . . that Australian multiculturalism should be enhanced and refocused to make cultural diversity a unifying force, by placing greater emphasis on *transparency, efficiency, and accountability*." The Council advocates *inclusiveness* as a core policy direction. The report stressed that multiculturalism

* This chapter is based on a modified version of a paper presented at the 26th Transcultural Nursing Annual Research Conference, Legends Hotel, Gold Coast, Australia. 4–6th October, 2000. The author acknowledges Dr Penny Deutsher, Senior Lecturer, Department of Philosophy, Australian National University (ANU) for references and translations of Derrida's work.

should embrace all sectors of the Australian community, including our original inhabitants, namely, the Aboriginal and Torres Strait Islander peoples, as well as all other Australians, whether born in Australia or overseas and of English- or non–English-speaking origins.[12] In addressing the meaning of multiculturalism, the Council recommended the addition of the prefix *Australian* to recognize that the implementation of multiculturalism is uniquely Australian. To achieve the objective set out in its terms of reference, of *ensuring that cultural diversity is a unifying force for Australia*, the Council recommended the following definition of multiculturalism:

> Australian multiculturalism is a term which recognizes and celebrates Australia's cultural diversity. It accepts and respects the right of all Australians to express and share their individual cultural heritage within an overriding commitment to Australia and the basic structures and values of Australian democracy. It refers to the strategies, policies and programs that are designed to 1) Make our administrative, social and economic infrastructure more responsive to the rights, obligations and needs of our culturally diverse population; 2) Promote social harmony among the different cultural groups in our society; and 3) Optimize the benefits of our cultural diversity for all Australians.[13]

The Council endorsed the concept of *Australian Citizenship* as underpinning multiculturalism. It claimed that multiculturalism and Australian citizenship embrace the same values, namely, respect for difference, tolerance, and a commitment to freedom and equal opportunity. *Inclusiveness, Australian multiculturalism, Australian citizenship, social harmony, and productive diversity* have been given as the directions for policy.[14]

Reflections on Nursing in Australia

To interpret multiculturalism and incorporate policy recommendations into Australian nursing necessitates examining what nursing does and professes to do (or not to do) to link it to multicultural nursing practices. The concept of caring has gradually become important in Australian nursing. Leininger in the early 1950s stated that caring is *the essence and heart of nursing*.[15–19] She further challenged nurses worldwide with the statement that: "Care is essential to curing and healing, for there can be no curing without caring." She further held that "... care is culturally constituted and that all human cultures have some forms, patterns, expressions, and structures of care, influenced by cultural values and beliefs."[20] In her theoretical and research work since the early 1950s, she held that care and culture are two major and closely interrelated concepts that needed to be systematically studied as transcultural nursing knowledge and practices. The Culture Care Theory was developed and synthesized and is being used as a new and unique theory to be systematically studied and explicated with the meanings, essences, expressions, and significance of culture care phenomena.[21,22]

This theory with culture and care has relevance to advance Australian transcultural nursing. For if there is anything that can distinguish nursing from all other disciplines, it is the nurse's ability, willingness, and commitment to care more, that is, to care enough to serve people of diverse cultures. Care as the essence of nursing and the unifying core of the nursing profession is being explored as a universal phenomenon in nursing.[23,24] Transcultural nursing is largely based on cultural care phenomena and should be welcomed to advance nursing and especially in a context of culturally diverse Australia. However, nursing has only partially embraced culture care, and therefore many clients from other cultures experience alienation and a feeling of being "other" in the care systems. I also have experienced this construct of *otherness* that so many immigrants experience, and it has become apparent to me as noncaring. Why do our nursing policies not work in practice? Are there directions that nursing could take to become more *hospitable* and more caring to clients and more caring to nurses from other cultures?

To explore the meaning of the phenomena of otherness and hospitality for the discipline and practice of transcultural nursing is important. I found Derrida's views of these constructs of interest.[25] I believe the concept of *hospitality* can be used to discover the reasons for *otherness/noncaring* relating to clients and nurses from non–English-speaking backgrounds. Derrida's most recent work in 1996 included published conversations in which questions were raised related to political asylum, deprivation of citizenship, refugee status, and other issues touching on immigration, xenophobia, and cultural and national identity. Within these contexts Derrida has asked if *hospitality* is possible? In highlighting the relationship between hospitality and coloniality, Derrida argued that all hospitality is conditional, particularly in the context of immigration, political asylum, and colonization. The most obvious response one might want to make to Derrida's views about the concept of hospitality is to note *how culturally specific it is.*[25] The word *hospitality* for Caputo means to invite and welcome the *stranger*. So, personally the question is, *How do I welcome the other into my home?* At the level of the State, however, socio-political questions arise with refugees, immigrants, "foreign" languages, etc. Actually, the word *hospitality* is derived from the Latin word *hospes*, which is from *hostis* and originally meant a "stranger." The term came to mean the enemy or *hostile* stranger who has power. A *host* is someone who receives strangers and who gives to the stranger, but remains in control. *Hospitality* is the welcome that is extended to the guest and is a function of the power of the *host* to remain master of the premises.[26] Thus, a certain stress is built into the idea of a host, who must be a proprietor or the owner of the property from where hospitality is to be given, as the one who offers hospitality to the *other*.

Derrida discusses *hospitality* as being *culturally specific* and not a universal concept. He states that hospitality has an ancient Greek origin related to a tradition of a formal right to hospitality. It was extended in ancient Athens to someone from an unknown city who was accustomed to another set of laws and someone understood as culturally different, *the stranger*. Yet, the Athenians extended hospitality to a *stranger* recognized as not radically *other*. Hospitality was extended only to those identifiable by family name, by the lineage of the family group, or by descendents with the same family name. Hospitality was offered where it was assumed that the stranger had a family and was responsible, rational, and lived by recognized laws, rights, and duties as the Athenians did. In these and other ways, hospitality was "conditional hospitality" because, in this context, hospitality was not offered to someone

"anonymous, someone with no name, no family, no social status, and who is not treated as the stranger, but as the barbaric other."[27]

Based on historical and traditional practices of hospitality two assumptions become evident: first, that *hospitality* makes no sense except in the context both of a pregiven concept of one's proper place, one's home, one's country, one's house, or one's land; and second, that of proper ownership and authority over the dwelling. Hospitality makes sense where someone has the proper right to say to someone else that they may or may not occupy one's own land, country, or place of dwelling. Hospitality assumes a certain relationship to property, authority, law, and legitimacy and to the granting of permission and to occupying the role of the gatekeeper who says, ". . . you may pass." Thus, one might conclude that *hospitality is inherently inhospitable* if it can never be unconditional. The conditions, therefore, for hospitality are property, ownership, authority, gatekeeping, control, order, and regulation. Derrida also suggests that hospitality has often been seen as a patriarchal value, a value system between men, which has been one of its traditional conditions. Other traditions of conditional hospitality, include the ancient Islamic tradition of nomadic communities offering unconditional hospitality to lost travelers, but only for 3 days, after which departure from the community was enforced.[28] Kant, in his 18th century philosophical treatise, *Conditions of Perpetual Peace*, also refers to a concept of universal hospitality. He states that every nation should offer hospitality to every visitor. This seemingly universal concept of hospitality was also conditional as visitors were obliged to conduct themselves peacefully and appropriately and could only be regarded as visitors to the nation, not residents.[29]

In Derrida's work he questions whether hospitality is possible and suggests that *conditional hospitality would be inherently inhospitable*. In the context of immigration, Derrida suggests that only *unconditional hospitality would be truly hospitable*. Derrida asks whether an *unconditional hospitality* could ever be possible in the context of immigration. The focus of Derrida's work with the concept of hospitality is not to emphasise its cultural specificity, nor its Eurocentrism, nor the centrism of a thinking preoccupied with property rights, but instead to emphasize the impossibility of hospitality as in his following passage:

> In unconditional hospitality, the host should, in principle, receive even before knowing anything about the guest . . . (the host) should avoid every question about the other's identity, desire, rules, capacity to work, integration, adaptation . . . From the moment that I pose all these questions and . . . conditions . . . the ideal situation of non-knowledge is broken.[30]

One helpful way to get to Derrida's views on community and identity is to follow his analysis of "hospitality." Derrida's recent work is not so much a call for an impossible pure hospitality, but as a call for the kind of hospitality that might lead to taking on the *responsibility of acknowledgement* that pure hospitality and proper identity are impossible. In rethinking hospitality as impossible, Derrida points to the concepts that seem to presuppose hospitality such as one's own residence, one's proper identity, and one's proper cultural identity. He argues not for the end of all efforts at hospitality, but for the *reconceptualization* of these terms, as in "responding for and to what will never be mine." Actually, Derrida's argument is directed at the white Anglo-European perspective, which has a fundamental investment in designating the *other* as disappropriated; to understanding itself as noncolonized; and as possessing a proper language, culture, identity, and nation as fundamental rights of human beings. What Derrida advocates, in a nutshell, is "democracy," which is supposed to be a very generous "respectable" for every difference imaginable. Therefore, Derrida's argument that hospitality is impossible can be conceptualized not into an articulation of the *other*, defined as that which always resists any presumption that we know, understand, sympathize, or empathize, because the discussion is related to contexts in which Derrida speaks to issues of immigration and coloniality. The question of *the other* is linked to the question of encounters between *different cultures* and *races*, the question of the *raced other* or the *immigrant other*, or the *colonized* peoples. Derrida's politics seem to work in these contexts in opposition to a politics of sympathy or understanding, which collapses into presumptuousness. Derrida offers *negotiations* in the context of our relationship to *the other*, in debates over immigration, legal and illegal residency, and colonialism.[31]

It is the author's contention that Derrida's notion of *hospitality* can be applied to the context of transcultural nursing in Australia and worldwide. The *host*, the nurse or *caregiver* from a dominant culture, is believed to be in possession of property, language, law, authority, and lifeway practices that are based on different ideologies from that of the client or receiver of care, *the stranger* or *the other* in Derrida's term. In this context the nurse from a dominant culture can offer care to "others" or to "strangers" from a transcultural perspective . . . that is both from an *etic* (that of the professional nurse from a dominant culture) and an *emic* perspective (from the client's perspective who may be from a nondominant culture or a culture different from the nurse). Through the use of Leininger's Stranger-Friend Enabler, the nurse can discover the human care of "others" or "strangers." Leininger's Stranger-Friend Enabler encompasses the philosophical belief that the nurse should always assess his or her relationships with the people or clients to get close to them to build trusting relationships with those for whom the nurse is studying or providing care. Leininger anticipated the nurse would need to move from a stranger or distrusted person to a trusted and friendly person during caregiving or in the context of the ethnonursing research process to obtain accurate, culturally sensitive, meaningful, and credible data from clients or informants.[32]

Care as hospitality for others has been discovered in transcultural nursing research studies in several cultures. Leininger has identified hospitality as a care construct in several cultures with the use of Culture Care Theory research. Hospitality as care was found to be important to Greek Americans, Middle Eastern cultures, and some Native Americans.[33,34] Gelazis discovered the culture care meaning of "hospitality to others" in her transcultural nursing studies of Lithuanians living in the United States, as well as among those living in Lithuania.[35]

Leininger initially introduced the Stranger-Friend Enabler for ethnonursing research studies, but it has been widely used for culturalogical health care assessments. Several nurses and others have used the Stranger-Friend Enabler with the Culture Care Theory to obtain information from people of different cultures as one moves from being a stranger to a trusted friend. Use of the Culture Care Theory is important with the Sunrise Model to systematically document actions and decisions to provide culturally congruent care that would be beneficial to clients. The three modes in the theory (culture care preservation and/or maintenance, culture care accommodation and/or negotiation, and culture care restructuring and/or repatterning) have also been extremely useful to provide culture-specific transcultural nursing practices. Identifying which of the three care modalities are beneficial for culturally congruent care involves active participation of clients or the group to identify, plan, and implement appropriate specific caring modes.[36,37]

There is a possibility that *hospitality as care* with Australian nursing may be relevant as the nurse from a dominant culture serves as host for immigrants or to care for cultural strangers. Nurses can learn to identify and provide hospitable care, but it would require that nurses become educated to search for hospitality and know best how to provide it with cultural strangers. These ideas have led to several questions that seem important for nurses in Australia and elsewhere to consider as one moves from strangers to nonstrangers and use the hospitality care construct.

1. What might be the meaning of hospitality and otherness as noncare to nurses with cultural strangers?
2. What might be the reasons for *otherness* or noncare relating to recruitment and retention of indigenous nurses into the nursing profession worldwide?
3. What might be reasons for feelings of *otherness* or noncaring in clients receiving nursing care, particularly those from non–English-speaking backgrounds?
4. What might be the reasons for feelings of *otherness* or noncare among overseas nurse graduates working in Australia?
5. In the culture of nursing what makes nursing *conditional, noncaring, inhospitable, or hospitable* to nurses who practice nursing in countries other than their own?
6. How is hospitality linked to caring and to noncaring as a transcultural nursing phenomenon?
7. How can Leininger's Culture Care Theory with the Sunrise Model and the Stranger-Friend Enabler be used to *reconceptualize*, in Derrida's terms, the "impossibility" of unconditional hospitality as care in Australian nursing and elsewhere?

8. What new directions can nursing in Australia and in the world adopt in this new millennium to promote culturally congruent nursing care?

These questions merit study by transcultural nurses and others to facilitate changes in nursing. There is evidence to suggest that nursing in Australia has moved toward providing care that is inclusive and respectful of multicultural differences to attempt to ensure that caring practices are appropriate and culturally meaningful. However, through further study and practice nurses can become even more respectful, sensitive, and responsible as this already has been demonstrated with several cultures. As responsible professionals in distinguishing themselves as those who care, nurses need to be rightfully and properly challenged to provide hospitable care.

Where are Australian nurses going with plans and directions in this new millennium? More specifically, where is Australian nursing going to further study and advance transcultural nursing knowledge and practices? Given Australia's cultural diversity, there is a need to promote social harmony in health care services and to assure equity of access and appropriateness of care. It is clear that nursing in the future will be shaped by transcultural imperatives. Australia will remain a society of diverse cultures, and it is unlikely that it will return to the discriminatory and closed-door policies of the past. Australian nursing needs to move forward in transcultural nursing with its own development to remain relevant and useful to all people in Australia.

As for my vision of the future, I will paraphrase the immortal words of Martin Luther King: "I have a dream. I say to you today, my friends even though we face the difficulties of today and tomorrow, I still have a dream."[38] I see an era in which transcultural nursing will take the lead in all areas of nursing study, research, practice, and administration in Australia. With growing cultural diversity, there will be no *host* or *stranger* or *other* when immigrants are the norm in populations. Hopefully, it will be a world that acknowledges the injustices inflicted on indigenous people, refugees, and immigrants. It must become a world committed to the principles of human rights and provision of culturally congruent and informed humanistic care. In such a world ethnocentrism, imposition of cultural practices, or racism will have little chance of developing. In the future Australia will see a new generation of nurses with many using a cultural caring ethos and knowledge. The Council for Aboriginal and Torres Strait Islander Nurses (CATSIN) will carry the torch of primary health care for a new and emerging generation of indigenous nurses.[39] This transculturally informed group of indigenous nurses will bring primary health care in culturally meaningful ways to first nation peoples in rural and remote areas of Australia. This new generation will be knowledgeable about the cultural caring modes of traditional cultures and will inform their nursing practices through transcultural nursing studies and research. Prepared transcultural nurse experts will become foundation chairs in Area Health Services in all States of Australia with a new generation of Certified Transcultural Nurse Consultants. This new generation of nurses can guide clinicians in transculturally informed nursing practices in equitable and accessible ways, based on sound transcultural care research and practice to arrive at culturally congruent care that is beneficial to all Australians.

In the new millennium transcultural nursing courses will become imperative for nursing practices in Australia. Faculties of Nursing will need to establish and maintain courses that incorporate philosophy, history, anthropology, arts, languages, and comparative religious practices. Such an expansion of interdisciplinary transcultural knowledge is essential for the understanding of the diverse cultures nurses meet every day in their practices. Members of professional nursing organizations and administrators of health settings and area health services will develop transcultural policies and guidelines. Nurses will need to transform, restructure, and repattern their policies toward competency-based outcomes and care practices that are culturally meaningful as a basis for quality care and to add to or reaffirm existing transcultural nursing research-based knowledge using largely the holistic Culture Care Theory.[40] Monolinguism will no longer be the norm in the new millennium in Australia and the world.[41] A new generation of nurses will speak more than one language and will be well versed in the diversity of cultural caring practices in Australia.

The new Australian generation of nurses will be knowledgeable about uniculturalism, ethnocentrism, and imposition care practices through transcultural nursing studies and practices. These transcultural nurses will lead the way to help other nurses develop culturally congruent, sensitive, and humanistic care practices. They will discover meaningful and culturally specific care as Leininger has advocated for nearly four decades. In this new millennium we shall see and recognize the true worth and gift of transcultural nursing knowledge and leadership. The numbers of nurses from culturally and linguistically diverse backgrounds practicing worldwide will increase proportionate to the diversity of the clients. Many of my dreams are highly congruent with those of my mentor and teacher, Professor Leininger. Leininger has led transcultural nursing and human care cultural movement since the mid 1950s, strongly promoting meaningful and relevant culture care for immigrants and for all cultural strangers and non-strangers to ensure, as her motto states, "...*that cultural care needs of people will be met with nurses prepared in transcultural nursing.*"[42]

References

1. Australian Bureau of Statistics (ABS), *1996 Census of Population & Housing Australia.* 1999 (online). Available: *http://www.abs.gov*.au/websitebs/_415515B4AE63DcbA64A25650600139f9c/.
2. Omeri, A., "Transcultural Nursing Care Values, Beliefs and Practices of Iranian Immigrants in NSW, Australia," unpublished doctoral thesis, NSW, Australia: Faculty of Nursing, The University of Sydney, 1996.
3. Derrida, J., *Cosmopolites de Tous les Pays, Encore un Effort,* Paris: Galilee, 1997a.
4. Derrida, J., "Questions d'Etranger: Venue de l'Etranger"; "Pas d'Hospitalite," in *De L 'Hospitalite,* J. Derrida avec Anne Dufourmantelle, eds., Paris: Calmann-Levy, 1997b.
5. Derrida, J., "Fidelite á plus d'un," and surrounding debate, in *Idioms Nationalites, Deconstructions,* Rencontre de Rabat avec Jacques Derrida, eds., Cahiers Intersignes no 13, 1998, pp. 221–265.
6. Derrida, J., "Une Hospitalite a l'infini"; "Responsibilite et Hospitalite," 1998 (pp. 121–125); avec Michel Wieviorla, "Acueil, Ethique, Droit et Politique" (pp. 143–155) and surrounding debate, in *Manifeste Pour l'Hospitalite,* Autour de Jacques Derrida, ed., Paris: Paroles de l'aube, 1999.
7. ABS, op. cit., 1999.
8. National Multicultural Advisory Council (NMAC), *Australian Multiculturalism for a New Century:*

Towards Inclusiveness, Commonwealth of Australia, Canberra, and Australia: AusInfo, 1999.

9. Castle, S., "Globalization, Multicultural Citizenship and Transnational Democracy," in *The Future of Australian Multiculturalism. Reflections on the Twentieth Anniversary of Jean Martin's The Migrant Presence*, Hage, G. and R. Couch, eds., Sydney, Australia: Research Institute of Humanities & Social Studies, The University of Sydney, 1999, pp. 31–41.

10. Castle, S., W. Foster, R. Iredale, and G. Withers, *Immigration and Australia: Myths and Realities*, St. Leonards, NSW: Allen & Unwin, 1998.

11. NMAC, op. cit., 1999, p. 11.

12. Ibid., pp. 11–12.

13. Ibid.

14. Ibid., pp. 9–15.

15. Leininger, M., *Nursing and Anthropology: Two Worlds to Blend*, New York: John Wiley & Sons, 1970.

16. Leininger, M., *Transcultural Nursing Concepts, Theories and Practices*, New York: Wiley & Sons, 1978.

17. Leininger, M., *Culture Care Diversity and Universality: A Theory of Nursing*, New York: National League for Nursing Press, 1991.

18. Leininger, M., *Transcultural Nursing: Concepts, Theories, Research, and Practices*, 2nd ed., New York: McGraw-Hill, 1995.

19. Leininger, M., "Overview and Reflection of the Theory of Culture Care and the Ethnonursing Research Method," *Journal of Transcultural Nursing*, 1997, 8(2), pp. 32–52.

20. Leininger, op. cit., 1991, p. 35.

21. Leininger, op. cit., 1978.

22. Leininger, op. cit., 1995.

23. Leininger M., *Care: The Essence of Nursing and Health Care*, Detroit: Wayne State University Press, 1984. (Reprinted in 1988)

24. Leininger, op. cit., 1991.

25. Deutscher, P., "Already Mourning the Other's Absence: Deconstruction, Immigration, Colonialism," paper presented at The Future of Australian Multiculturalism, 7–9 December 1998, Sydney, Australia: Research Institute for Humanities & Social Sciences, The University of Sydney, 1999.

26. Caputo, J.D., ed., "Deconstruction in a Nutshell: A Conversation with Jacques Derrida," New York: Fordham University Press, 1997, pp. 107–113.

27. Deutscher, op. cit., 1999.

28. Ibid.

29. Ibid.

30. Ibid.

31. Ibid.

32. Leininger, op. cit., 1991.

33. Ibid.

34. Leininger, op. cit., 1995.

35. Gelazis, R., "Lithuanian Americans and Culture Care," in *Transcultural Nursing: Concepts, Theories, Research, and Practices*, 2nd ed., M. Leininger, ed., New York: McGraw-Hill, 1995.

36. Leininger, op. cit., 1995.

37. Leininger, op. cit., 1991.

38. King, Martin Luther, Jr., *Martin Luther King Jr. Had a Dream* (online), 1999, Available: http://home/diversity/DIVERSITY.htm·

39. National Congress of Aboriginal and Torres Strait Islander Nurses (CATSIN), *Recommendations from the 1998 National Congress. New South Wales Department of Health, NSW, Australia* (online), 1998, Available: http://www.health.nsw.gov.au

40. Leininger, op.cit., 1995.

41. Derrida, J., (1996). *Monolingulism of the Other: Or the Prosthesis of Origin*, translated by Patrick Mensah, Stanford, CA: Stanford University Press, 1998.

42. Leininger, op. cit., 1991.

Transcultural Nursing Teaching, Administration, and Consultation

34

Transcultural Nursing: Curricular Concepts, Principles, and Teaching and Learning Activities for the 21st Century

Marilyn R. McFarland
Madeleine Leininger

During the past four decades transcultural nursing education has transformed many nurses to think and act in culturally safe, sensitive, and effective ways. It is the critical means to transform health care worldwide into meaningful and therapeutic culturally based care outcomes in this 21st century.[1]

Transcultural nursing is changing the ways nurses are discovering and learning about people of diverse and similar cultures with their caring, health, and well-being needs. Learning, teaching, and applying transcultural nursing theoretical and research-based knowledge is one of the most significant developments in the past century and will be even greater in this 21st century. Discovering, understanding, and using transcultural nursing knowledge to care for people has led to new ways of practicing nursing. Comparative cultural knowledge of differences and similarities among individuals, groups, and institutions has challenged nurses to expand their worldviews and to think and act in different ways. Transcultural nursing knowledge and practice have become global and essential imperatives, which are transforming the profession and related health practices into transculturalism. It is therefore imperative that transcultural nursing education be explicitly taught in undergraduate and graduate programs.

In this chapter some major teaching and learning concepts, philosophical views, principles, research, and experiential teaching strategies with suggested content domains will be presented. Most of the ideas have come from the authors and especially from Leininger who has been establishing teaching-learning principles and practices for the new discipline of transcultural nursing since the early 1960s. Leininger's diverse and creative work about the dynamic nature of transcultural nursing has led to some major breakthroughs in transcultural nursing education and practice. The dynamic process and content domains continue to unfold with the richness of cultures unfolding as they move, live, and exist in diverse contexts worldwide. It is this dynamic process that challenges nursing students to think anew and to change practices into a truly transcultural perspective with sensitive culture care action modalities for effective and successful outcomes. For it is through this dynamic teaching and learning process that a new era in nursing is occurring that has the potential to markedly transform nursing education and practice in this 21st century.

Transforming Nursing through Teaching Transcultural Nursing

Since the advent of transcultural nursing in the mid 1950s, nurses have gradually expanded their worldview with a much broader perspective of nursing as they incorporate knowledge about different cultures in the world with transcultural care viewpoints.[2,3] This broader and richer perspective has largely occurred through educational processes and with curricular changes in the undergraduate and graduate nursing programs. As a consequence, a new generation of nurses is learning and practicing transcultural nursing, which is transforming nursing and health care.[4,5] It has been most encouraging to witness this major achievement in some schools of nursing. There are, however, some schools of nursing that have only recently begun to incorporate transcultural nursing knowledge into their teaching curriculum and guided clinical practices. Indeed, much work remains worldwide to integrate and make transcultural nursing a meaningful part of all undergraduate and graduate nursing education. The central goal remains a challenge and imperative to establish transcultural nursing as the major and arching framework of nursing education and practice to serve all cultures worldwide. This has been Leininger's dream goal since initiating the field in the mid 1950s as she saw the world rapidly becoming transcultural. Culturally based care knowledge and health practices were needed for therapeutic outcomes. Since then there has been a transformation of nursing through a dynamic and comparative educational process and philosophy of cultural care and health care. Nurses gradually incorporated this philosophical idea when they realized they were living and functioning in a diverse transcultural world that required new knowledge and practices. Nurses will need to remain sensitive and knowledgeable about many cultures with their different caring ways to practice transcultural nursing. Today, transcultural nurse leaders have promoted active and open teaching-learning about many different cultures in the world and have reexamined past and current teaching content and strategies that may be incongruent and inappropriate for many cultures. Shifting nurse educators and students from a unicultural to a multicultural perspective has been a major challenge because of many past factors that have been so deeply rooted in nursing and because so few faculty have been formally prepared in transcultural nursing. Nonetheless, some significant strides have been made by a core of dedicated and persistent transcultural nurse educators and clinicians who value and realize the critical im-

portance of transcultural nursing worldwide. However, much work remains to educate faculty, students, and clinical staff to expand their worldviews through transcultural nursing education to provide culturally based practices.[6,7] Both general and advanced clinical graduate transcultural nursing education and practices are important to continue the transformation process. A cadre of transcultural nurse generalists and specialist leaders are essential to move nurses forward in this cultural movement of global transcultural nursing education and practices.[8]

A major question for nursing educators worldwide is how best to prepare nursing students and registered nurses so that they are able to provide culturally congruent care practices. This question is of critical importance for new and established nurses trying to function in an intensely multicultural world. For some nurses, this idea may be viewed as impossible. However, efforts must be made to make transcultural nursing an integral part of all nursing education and practice because of the multicultural world nurses serve. Some nurse leaders are committed to learning transcultural nursing, but some nurses believe that they can function without such knowledge by holding onto their personal values and views and manage without learning anew.

■ Some Reasons Why Transcultural Nursing with New Curricular Perspectives Is Imperative

There are several reasons why nursing education and practice needs to shift very soon to teaching and learning transcultural nursing with curricular changes. This shift necessitates some major rethinking, planning, and *establishing plans of action* for transcultural nursing education if nursing is to be relevant to serve clients and students in this multicultural world of the 21st century. Several global reasons have been identified earlier in this book; however, major ideas focused on teaching and curricular changes are needed to be presented here so that faculty will realize why nursing education must become transculturally grounded and taught in all schools of nursing worldwide.

One of the first and most important reasons for transcultural nursing education and concomitant practices is that our world has become intensely multicultural and will be more so in the future, which necessitates that nurses must become transculturally knowledgeable, sensitive, and competent.[9-12] This fact has become increasingly apparent in nursing practice as well as in nursing education, as newly prepared nurses are expected to understand and respond appropriately to people of diverse cultures. They are expected to know and respect cultural differences and similarities of clients to provide culturally effective and safe care. For without culture care knowledge and competencies, one cannot achieve therapeutic outcomes with most clients. Nurse educators must take leadership to teach transcultural nursing care as a moral imperative for health care services today. Transcultural nursing education and curricular changes are a critical mandate to fulfill nursing's role as a meaningful and global service profession. Nurses are expected to respond to clients' health care needs by functioning to serve clients of diverse and similar cultures. Nursing educators are morally expected to meet this global imperative through transcultural nursing education and practice.

A second reason to shift nursing education to a transcultural nursing focus is that most communities and human service institutions are recognizing that they need to make changes to meet population groups of immigrants and refugees and those of other cultures and subcultures who are at their doorsteps seeking to be understood and served. Some older immigrants have often lived and worked in their familiar and folk-supported communities for extended periods. However, today there are many more new immigrants moving into communities, and the diversity of cultures makes communities truly transcultural as described by Leininger.[13] As a consequence, health personnel encounter clients of many different cultures, and they are expected to know their client's cultural backgrounds and care needs to provide culturally congruent health care services. Likewise, nursing students today are caring for clients from many different cultures. Nursing students' cultural values, beliefs, and practices need to be understood in present-day educational settings. Accordingly, curricular and teaching changes are imperative to function in transcultural communities. This is a "new age" of transculturalism, and this "new age" of functioning calls for nursing faculty and administrators to learn about diverse cultures and their care and health needs. For without a shift to transcultural nursing education and service, one can predict many conflicts

and unfavorable or destructive client outcomes. It can also lead to many nursing students being frustrated and dissatisfied with their educational preparation.

Transcultural nurses were the first to carve a new pathway to value, study, and practice transcultural nursing five decades ago along with some faculty, administrators, and curriculum specialists such as Leininger.[14-17] Today, as faculty move forward to prepare a new generation of transculturally educated nurses, they need to first educate themselves to be effective teachers, mentors, curricular facilitators, and role models. Faculty need to be educated about the nature, scope, goals, theories, practices, and desired outcomes of transcultural nursing. Such knowledge is essential to ensure credible teaching and competencies for undergraduate and graduate nursing students. It is also important so that faculty can effectively mentor students in clinical settings and oversee exchanges as they study and care for clients of diverse cultures. The demand for transcultural nursing courses in universities, colleges, and institutes continues with students and nurse clinicians wanting such knowledge and skills in transcultural nursing. If faculty are not prepared in transcultural nursing, students will not learn about ways to care for clients of diverse cultures. This concern is often expressed by nursing students who may get limited teaching about cultures and their care needs. As faculty learn about different cultures in their local and regional communities, it stimulates their thinking to value transcultural nursing curricula and concomitant learning practices for nursing students. Helping faculty become immersed in cultures and to use this knowledge and experience often brings dramatic changes in curricular content and in guiding nursing students or clinical nurses in practice. Learning about "the other" cultures from a skilled transcultural mentor can lead faculty to some entirely new ways to care for clients and new ways for students to function with multidisciplinary staff.

Currently, some faculty say one needs to "be culturally sensitive and competent" with students and clients, but this statement is only a popular cliché unless faculty first learn about diverse cultures and specific care needs and expressions. Transcultural learning can be a most rewarding experience for faculty and can actually change their teaching and guidance modes. Faculty need to learn transcultural nursing principles, values, and practices, as well as how to present this content, to be competent faculty. If faculty and clinical nursing supervisors are not prepared, one can expect imposition practices, ethnocentrism, and serious cultural conflicts and clashes with clients and nursing students. Thus, they need to learn to first educate themselves to be effective and knowledgeable teachers of transcultural nursing.

Currently, fewer than approximately 20% of faculty have been formally educated in transcultural nursing in the United States and even fewer in other countries.[18] However, some faculty have declared themselves educated by their contacts and experiences with cultures but with no linkage to transcultural nursing disciplinary knowledge. There are only 2% of doctoral nursing students in the United States prepared in transcultural nursing.[19] This poses serious problems in teaching and research when these graduates begin to care for clients and are not knowledgeable and competent in transcultural nursing. There are approximately 48% of baccalaureate nursing students and about 9% of master's degree nurses who have had at least a formal course in transcultural nursing or explicit units focused on transcultural nursing phenomena in the United States. There are many associate-degree nursing students genuinely interested in transcultural nursing, and many faculty have been active to incorporate selected concepts and principles for these students in the United States. So, while faculty may proclaim they are "teaching transcultural nursing," many have had no graduate preparation in transcultural nursing and teach what "they feel is important or is common sense" about cultures learned from their home or personal experiences. As a consequence, some nursing students may not have had guided mentors to learn about transcultural nursing and may have been exposed to inaccurate or questionable content that lacks substantive knowledge. Deans and administrators of schools of nursing in the United States are often so busy with financial and other issues that they themselves have not been prepared in transcultural nursing to be culturally competent and, hence, do not recruit faculty with transcultural nursing skills.

Lately, nursing students often demand faculty who are knowledgeable and competent to teach and mentor students in transcultural nursing. Students are keenly aware of culturally diverse communities in which they live and that they must develop competency skills with clients, families, and diverse groups. These nursing students value and want nursing faculty who can help them understand different cultures and demonstrate ways to interact and be therapeutic with clients from diverse cultures. They also want nursing faculty who can adapt their teaching to different cultural strategies, models, and culturally based care phenomena as they realize that traditional unicultural curricular and teaching content are outdated for nurses to function in a multicultural world. Moreover, the teaching strategies and methods of faculty need to change to enter into and learn about diverse cultures and their care and health needs.

Today, nursing faculty can access the body of transcultural nursing literature and have access to transcultural nursing specialists to help them learn about and perfect their knowledge in transcultural nursing. Faculty have opportunities to become immersed in different cultures in their home communities, health centers, and many other places where they can teach and mentor students in transcultural nursing. There are many wonderful opportunities for nursing faculty to become knowledgeable about transcultural nursing and to develop competencies to teach and practice in the field.

It is encouraging to see faculty and students *learn together* about people from diverse cultures with a focus on human caring and health. Much excitement often occurs as faculty gain new knowledge and competencies in transcultural nursing. Nursing faculty and students need to draw on knowledge from the humanities, liberal arts, and social sciences as they grasp a holistic perspective of different cultures and environments with uses of material and nonmaterial aspects of cultures or symbolic referents. For example, knowledge from anthropology is especially critical and so valuable as this discipline has studied and taught about cultures and subcultures for over 100 years. Anthropologists offer valuable insights about material and nonmaterial features of diverse cultures that challenge nursing faculty and students to discover together the meaning and importance of culture care beliefs and practices. Some sociology courses are also helpful, as well as comparative religion, gender, ecology, and ethnohistorical knowledge as background to transcultural nursing. It is, however, the discovery of caring, health, illness, and well-being that is critical in transcultural nursing as discussed earlier in Chapters 1 and 2.

Transcultural nursing faculty have a moral responsibility to learn transcultural nursing with a transcultural care, health, and illness perspective to be helpful to students. Nursing faculty also need to deal with their resistance and prejudices and to extend their knowledge base beyond the biophysical and mental health dimensions of human beings. Discovering cultural influences on care, health, and illness with a holistic perspective is essential. For without a transcultural comparative and holistic view, nursing is too narrow and can lead to an inaccurate understanding of cultures. Learning from transcultural nursing experts can dramatically change faculty, curricula, and teaching content.

A current urgent need in nursing is the *recruitment of graduate-prepared transcultural nursing faculty in schools of nursing worldwide.* Currently, there are far too few faculty to meet the learning needs of culturally diverse students and the health care needs of clients. Rigorous and persistent recruitment efforts for transculturally prepared faculty are needed in schools of nursing for teaching, research, consultation, mentoring, and establishing transculturally based curricula. In addition, guiding students in clinical and community agencies to care for clients from diverse and similar cultures is urgently needed. Transcultural nursing faculty will continue to be in high demand worldwide as teaching and curricular changes shift to multiculturalism. Far more funds and human resources are needed for transcultural nursing faculty and nurse clinicians to meet the current and future needs in transcultural nursing education and practice. Without well-prepared faculty in transcultural nursing, students will be greatly deprived of what they need most to care for people of diverse cultures today and in the future. There is a need for reconstructing nursing curricula and designing and carrying out educational research studies that are transculturally based to facilitate new directions in nursing and health care.

Teaching and Learning Expectations and Methods for Preparing Competent Transcultural Nurses

Since the first class in transcultural nursing was developed and taught by Leininger in 1966 at the University of Colorado, there has been a slow development of transcultural nursing education within and outside the United States. The idea of teaching transcultural nursing "at a distance" began with Leininger, using a transcultural nursing telelecture satellite series within the United States and in Oceania, Pacific Islands, in 1967. This first transcultural nursing "distance" series was an intriguing early mode of teaching to reach nurses worldwide. Today teaching "at a distance" has become a major method within the United States. There are, however, some limitations without the presence of a mentor. There is also the concern of assessing cultural attitudes and biases within total or holistic cultural contexts. However, it is important to teach nurses worldwide. Indeed, "The Internet is the biggest technological change in teaching and learning since the printed book was introduced five centuries ago . . . online learning will constitute 50% of all learning in the 21st Century."[20] This is an exciting and challenging time for transcultural nursing and other areas of nursing to have direct contact with remote or nearby cultures. Nursing programs need to update their courses to meet the needs of growing numbers of students from diverse cultures who cannot complete their degrees in the traditional modes. Nursing students are also eager to use the new technologies of distance learning. Online learning is also an important means to increase the numbers of diverse students and faculty of different cultures in the learning process. Duquesne University School of Nursing has been a pioneer in online courses by using the "information superhighway" to offer new ways of teaching transcultural nursing in RN to BSN / MSN, postBSN certificate, MSN, and post-master's certificate programs, as well as serving students pursuing PhD education. As noted above, only about one-half of all learning will occur online in the 21st century, which leaves room for other teaching modes to ensure quality-based transcultural nursing instruction. For example, if a student wants to learn how to design and implement a culturally congruent nursing care plan for a client, the student could benefit from working with a graduate-prepared transcultural nurse expert in a clinical context. While cultural facts, concepts, and principles can be taught and learned online, learning formats with face-to-face mentorship in institutions and community contexts are essential. Learning by observing transcultural nursing experts care for clients, families, and community groups is highly valued and important.

One must also remember that students in economically poor and culturally different places may not have access to electronic equipment for online education and that it may take some years for this to happen.

Student-faculty learning of transcultural nursing with individuals, families, and community cultures or subcultures with well-planned lectures remains an important teaching and learning method. Students need to learn about complex culture and care phenomena, which are often best taught by transcultural nursing experts. These faculty value working closely with clients and families in hospital or community contexts over several weeks to learn about transcultural nursing in diverse clinical fields with guidance from transcultural nursing faculty. Students can discuss directly with faculty their concerns and biases while working with cultural strangers and using enablers such as Leininger's Stranger-Friend Enabler. Community nursing faculty have been especially eager to learn about transcultural nursing to be effective with Native American, Mexican American, Vietnamese American, and African American clients in the United States. Until recent years, faculty and students in community health nursing in the United States were more aware of cultural differences as they functioned with families and maternal-child problems. They were more sensitive to cultural care factors and more willing to study transcultural nursing than faculty in medical-surgical and psychiatric nursing.

Today, some transcultural nursing specialists are available in hospitals and community agencies to serve as mentors, role models, and consultants to other nurses about transcultural nursing phenomena and cultural variabilities. Both transcultural nurse specialists (prepared through graduate studies) and generalists (prepared in undergraduate programs) can help to make transcultural nursing meaningful in health care settings. Unquestionably, transcultural nurse specialists are in much demand as health agencies are expected to provide culturally competent care for diverse clients. The Joint Commission on Accreditation of Healthcare Organizations (JCAHO) and other accreditation agencies in the United States are now taking hold of the transcultural nursing concept of culturally congruent care, and this is necessitating transcultural nursing experts to help staff meet accreditation requirements. However, one is fortunate to have one or two transcultural nurses in a general hospital or in a university teaching center where they are expected to cover all clinical units, work with noncompliant clients, and help health personnel deal with the myriad of challenges related to serving the culturally different. Hence, there is a critical need for many more transcultural nurses in clinical settings.

To meet the urgent demand for graduate-prepared transcultural nurses in education and service settings, many innovative plans and action strategies are needed. Transcultural nursing workshops, conferences, and special courses have been offered, but more are needed to prepare faculty, clinical staff, and other health personnel for caring for diverse clients in a variety of health care situations.[21-24] Some nurses travel great distances and spend time and money to take intensive short-term undergraduate and graduate transcultural nursing courses to learn transcultural nursing concepts from experts. For example, since 1978 nurses have come from many different countries and states to pursue programs and courses in transcultural nursing from Leininger, the founder of the discipline. Nurses have found these to be extremely valuable as nurses learn holistic transcultural nursing using specific concepts, principles, and research-based findings from theoretical perspectives. Using theoretical care perspectives and learning how to provide culturally specific and congruent care often requires new ways of thinking, learning, and practice. Nurses from Australia, South Africa, the Pacific Islands, Asia, Finland, the United States, the Netherlands, Canada, Europe, and other places have come together to learn from transcultural nursing experts. Nurses who have enrolled in such graduate courses in transcultural nursing have been expected to be leaders and experts in the field, especially in their own countries. They are encouraged to transfer transcultural nursing concepts, principles, and relevant theory and research to their own Western and non-Western culture in meaningful and relevant ways. Transcultural nursing experts know how to teach Western and non-western cultures so that cultural biases or narrow ethnocentric learning and teaching modes can be avoided. Thus, the need and demand for transcultural nursing comparative knowledge and skills is great in most places in the world as nurses recognize that they must provide effective and competent nursing care to clients who are increasingly multicultural. Far more educational programs are needed to meet the critical shortage of transcultural nurses worldwide.

Another teaching and learning approach is to have an exchange program with nurses from different countries reciprocally participating and learning from each other. With this approach prior preparation of students and transcultural faculty is critical so they can use holding knowledge of general concepts, principles, theoretical perspectives, and some research findings about the host cultures. To provide safe, positive, and beneficial learning outcomes, students must be prepared in advance and must know how to use basic transcultural nursing concepts, principles, theories, and practices before being sent abroad or to provinces or districts within a country with culturally different groups. Student and faculty have reported unfavorable outcomes when they are not prepared in transcultural nursing, when they do not have qualified faculty to guide their experiences in overseas exchanges, or when they care for clients from different cultures.[25-27]

Another means to stimulate students and nurses to learn transcultural nursing has been to become certified in the field and to maintain recertification (see Appendix A). Certification was held important by the mid 1980s to help clients of diverse cultures to receive safe and effective care. Certification and recertification was established in 1989 and continues today through the Transcultural Nursing Society Certification and Recertification Committee. Oral and written examinations and a portfolio of experiences with basic and advanced transcultural educational classes and workshops are prerequisites for nurses to be certified to practice transcultural nursing in safe and competent ways. To date, approximately 100 nurses have been certified and recertified to practice transcultural nursing. Transcultural nurse specialists' and leaders' interest in certification has been most encouraging. Graduate preparation in transcultural nursing and direct experiences with clients have been essential to ensure success with the examinations and for nurses to establish their competencies as transcultural specialists, generalists, and consultants. Currently, many of these certified nurses are functioning in diverse clinical nursing practice settings and in schools of nursing. These nurses are skilled at demonstrating ways to prevent culture care imposition practices, as well as cultural clashes, cultural pain, overt prejudices, and other unfavorable

transcultural nursing problems or issues. Well-prepared certified transcultural nurses are making major differences in the quality of nursing care and are providing some entirely new and different ways to practice, teach, and care for people of diverse and similar cultures.

Transcultural nurse practitioners will be expected to function in many different clinical and educational contexts and in teaching and guiding transcultural consultation roles to provide culturally competent and responsible health care. Transcultural nurses are also expected to assess and be effective in diverse cultures of nursing and with the dominant values of the cultures of medicine, social work, and other disciplines that can influence health care outcomes. In addition, they are called to help transform health care systems or to establish new kinds of transcultural nursing institutes, centers, and programs in universities or other academic settings. Transcultural specialists are more and more in demand as the health care professions awaken to the need for culturally competent health care services and educational programs.

Transcultural nursing specialists have initiated transcultural research projects in health settings, schools of nursing, and in private and public community interdisciplinary organizations. Some of their work has been reported in the *Journal of Transcultural Nursing* since 1989 and in other publications. For example, a transcultural nurse specialist is functioning with a private American agency to study women's health care in the United States and overseas. Another specialist is working in a community with new immigrants and refugees. Several are working in community agencies and acute care units in the United States and abroad. Some transcultural clinical nurse specialists are working in urban and rural community agencies to assist teenage mothers with prenatal and neonatal care. There is a demand for transcultural nurse practitioners in primary and tertiary clinical settings. Opportunities in the field for leadership and practice roles for transcultural generalists and specialists are unlimited and largely unfilled. Transcultural nurses however, are expected to identify and carve out their leadership roles in teaching, clinical practices, and research as new agencies discover the relevance and need for transcultural nursing and health care. Establishing new roles, salary expectations, professional expectations, and ways to function in different cultures and institutions are challenges that require active leadership and persistent efforts.

 ## Incorporating Transcultural Nursing into Nursing Education: Approaches and Issues

Incorporating transcultural nursing into undergraduate and graduate programs remains a major challenge in most schools of nursing because of overloaded curricula and the reluctance or resistance of faculty to change curricula into a transcultural nursing one. Transcultural nurses have had to be astute strategists, diplomats, organizers, and politicians to get transcultural concepts, principles, themes, and research-based knowledge into nursing curricula in the United States and in other countries. Accommodating or facilitating the inclusion of transcultural nursing ideas is usually difficult as some faculty tend to tenaciously hold to their traditional areas of content and modes of teaching. Some fear that including what is unknown or vaguely known to them could make them uncomfortable or appear incompetent.

During the past three decades, the authors have found that nursing faculty who are reluctant to incorporate transcultural nursing into the curricula are generally fearful that new courses or content will replace what they usually teach and practice. Some faculty admit that they have limited knowledge about transcultural nursing as they have never been prepared in the discipline. Some hold that they do not need to change as they soon will be retiring. Also, there are some faculty who say, "I've been teaching it [transcultural nursing] for years. I incorporate culture in all the courses I teach." However, the reality is often they are teaching what they believe is culture from personal and home experiences and with no awareness of transcultural nursing theory, principles, and other substantive research-based transcultural nursing knowledge. With virtually no theory and content being taught, transcultural nursing practices leave much to be desired. Some instructors today talk about "cultural diversity" but often with no substantive content about cultural similarities or transcultural nursing care/caring or health. There are also faculty who are not interested in incorporating anything new into nursing curricula such as transcultural nursing as they may believe it is not necessary

or that they do not want to deal with cultural biases or racial issues. Also, there are nurses who may have had a course (or two) in anthropology or sociology and believe this qualifies them to be a transcultural nursing expert. Such faculty problems and concerns have been some major barriers to making transcultural nursing a reality for nursing curricula and clinical practices. However, with state and national board examinations, JCAHO, other accreditation expectations, and certification for practice competencies, faculty are beginning to scurry to incorporate transcultural nursing ideas into nursing curricula and practice. Transcultural nurses remain open and willing to help these faculty in curricular efforts and with new related teaching approaches. In addition, one has to master other hurdles to be effective in curricular and teaching endeavors. It is important to remember that one cannot "integrate" content unless one is knowledgeable in what is to be integrated.

An effective and successful transcultural nurse educator has to assess the political and organizational climate of the school, the faculty, and often the larger educational institution in which a nursing education program exists. Political alignments of faculty along clinical lines such as pediatrics, medical-surgical nursing, community health, and a host of other traditional clinical areas (sometimes more than 50 areas that follow the clinical medical model) impede changing faculty to holistic transcultural nursing. The culture and philosophy of the school and faculty, as well as administrators' attitudes, can make a great difference in incorporating transcultural content into nursing curricula and practice.[28] Sometimes the lone transcultural expert "at home" may not be valued nor used in curricular work or discussions. Lately, outside "experts" with "cultural diversity" expertise have been hired as consultants. Hence, transcultural nurses within institutions may be shunned as they are "too close to home to be considered authorities on the subject." Hence, both nontranscultural and transcultural experts may experience major challenges in schools of nursing.

Four approaches to integrating transcultural nursing content into curriculum are 1) *integrating transcultural nursing concepts and principles into an existing curriculum*, 2) *introducing modules or specified culture care units into a curriculum*, 3) *offering a series of organized and substantive transcultural nursing courses*, and 4) *offering a major program or* substantive track in transcultural nursing. These four approaches will be presented and examples given to assist in fully understanding each approach.

The first approach—to incorporate transcultural nursing content in the curriculum—is to consider existing courses within different clinical areas and to show how transcultural nursing concepts and principles can be integrated into the content and be used in client or family care.[29] Undergraduate and graduate faculty often find this incorporation approach acceptable. One identifies specific transcultural nursing concepts and principles to be integrated into parent-child, medical-surgical, and oncology nursing. This helps to use faculty knowledge, but also transforms traditional ideas and practices into specific transcultural nursing modalities. This approach allows faculty to link their familiar knowledge to new knowledge and assists faculty to gradually learn to use and teach transcultural nursing. It also assists the faculty until they become knowledgeable about cultures and transcultural care and health perspectives woven into a holistic view of clients. Students are the first to voice their views when faculty fail to know the subject matter, especially in clinical areas. Building the transcultural concepts or constructs into several courses in-depth is problematic with the integration approach unless the faculty are knowledgeable and active in facilitating the process. When a transcultural nursing facility expert can teach transcultural nursing concepts across different clinical areas and subjects such as ethics and morals, faculty members begin to realize the depth and scope of the field, as well as the competencies needed to be effective and successful. Most students are happy to see transcultural nursing concepts, principles, and theories taught in their clinical areas with new perspectives of nursing. They are quick to identify the inadequacy of teaching based on unicultural and personal experiences alone or using short cultural encounters or tours.

The second approach to curricular work is to teach transcultural nursing by the use of modules or specified culture care units. With this approach, transcultural nursing faculty are usually responsible for teaching whole units or modules of instruction in undergraduate or graduate programs on transcultural nursing. For example, a unit of instruction might be "Transcultural Nursing Care of Mexican Americans with Hy-

pertension." Such a module is usually part of another course such as physiological nursing. The modular teaching approach requires that transcultural nursing faculty have some stated objectives or goals with specific unit learning activities. They should have plans for ways they believe will be effective to teach and evaluate the content within the culture of the institution. They may also work with other faculty to reinforce transcultural nursing content in their teaching and clinical supervision of students. This approach is often a step before moving to a full course, tract, or program in transcultural nursing. The module or unit approach lends itself to mini-field observations and studies focused on transcultural nursing constructs, theory, and ways to provide culturally congruent care. Some faculty and students view this as a compromise to a full transcultural nursing course and view the units as fragmented and an incomplete way for bright nursing students with anthropological backgrounds to learn about transcultural nursing, especially about specific cultures and their holistic care needs. Students want to know and use transcultural nursing care and health in meaningful ways. Nonetheless, this approach generally stimulates student learning about transcultural nursing and is being used in both undergraduate and graduate schools of nursing in the United States and in a few other countries.

The third teaching and curricular approach is to offer organized and substantive courses, often three to five semester credits, on transcultural nursing in undergraduate and graduate programs. This approach has been the most successful and has prepared nurses to know, understand, and provide culturally congruent and safe care. It has been invaluable to know the close relationship between cultures and caring, which have holistic and meaningful connections. The courses also offer a philosophical, theoretical, and realistic basis to understand why transcultural nursing is imperative and how nurses are in a unique position to care for clients of diverse or similar cultures. These courses on transcultural nursing should be comprehensive and taught by qualified transcultural nurses. A great variety of approaches can be used with one or two course offerings. Most faculty begin with definitions of concepts, principles, and the rationale of the need for transcultural nursing. Students focus on specific cultures and subcultures, identifying the culture care needs of clients within a theoretical perspective. Specific concepts, principles, and theory can be closely linked to the study of specific cultures and related health care needs. Transcultural nursing faculty and students like this approach because they get in-depth knowledge about diverse cultures with field or clinical mentored experiences. It gives students time to assimilate and value transcultural caring as a new and important field of study and practice. When two courses are offered, one course should be taught early in the program and one later by faculty prepared in transcultural nursing.

A basic transcultural nursing course should be required for all undergraduates early in the program so ideas can be used in all experiences. As least one advanced course for graduate students is essential to obtain knowledge to provide culturally competent and responsible care in the field as an advanced transcultural nurse generalist or specialist. Both courses should have field or clinical experiences under prepared transcultural faculty to provide clinical guidance and competency skills. Two courses of two or three credits each are desired in graduate programs that build in-depth from a comparative perspective for the transcultural nurse specialist. The undergraduate course often becomes a foundation for graduate preparation in transcultural nursing. Students are exceedingly pleased with a full course as they are given time to relate the theory, concepts, and principles to practice along with achieving competence in a new area of practice. Many positive comments can be heard such as, "It is exactly what I needed to care for African Americans and others in my clinical practice as I am working in an urban area with 87% African Americans"; "This course has transformed my entire view of professional nursing as I see a whole new and different world in which to practice"; "As a graduate student, I actually had to relearn what I learned earlier as it did not fit the care for these clients"; and "This is the only course that is holistic and puts the clients' total human caring needs together." Most students contend they had to learn nursing anew when they learned about transcultural nursing, but the new ideas seemed "natural" and essential to nursing. Faculty often comment that the courses expand the students' thinking and views of their practice to comparative holistic views of cultural care. They especially found that Leininger's Culture Care Theory and the three modes of care are an exciting and a different way to prac-

tice nursing. Most importantly, transcultural nursing faculty responsible for the courses are usually happy and excited to teach the course and to watch students grow from learning a different and broader view of traditional nursing. Appendices B and C provide some sample course outlines for faculty to consider in teaching transcultural nursing to undergraduate and graduate students.

The fourth teaching and curricular approach is to offer a major program or substantive track in transcultural nursing at the graduate level with a series of courses and related learning experiences. The goal is to prepare clinical specialists in transcultural nursing or broadly oriented generalists for teaching, research, and practice in transcultural nursing. In the early 1970s Leininger launched the first programs and tracks in transcultural nursing for master's (M.S.N.) and doctoral (Ph.D.) preparation. The program was based on sequential courses, including both classroom and clinical field experiences, as part of a graduate program or track preparation in transcultural nursing. This model continues to be used as a guide for transcultural nursing graduate education in this specialty. Such specialized preparation in transcultural nursing remains available in graduate programs in the United States for clinical specialization, advanced practitioner roles, beginning teachers, and new leadership roles in transcultural nursing.[30] (See list of transcultural nursing courses and programs in Appendix D.)

Graduate transcultural nursing specialization is characterized as being comprehensive, complex, and analytical with comparative in-depth knowledge of culturally based phenomena. Students have opportunities to learn about several cultures using theoretical and practical focuses with an emphasis on holistic culture care in diverse environmental contexts. Critical analysis of existing nursing knowledge is studied from Western and non-Western emic and etic perspectives. Graduate field experiences are an expected requirement to discover transcultural knowledge and care needs of specific cultures with well, sick, or dying clients. Field or clinical experiences are with individuals, families, and specific subcultures in different communities and hospitals or in evolving new transcultural centers or institutions.

Nursing students find graduate programs in transcultural nursing highly stimulating and essential to discover new knowledge and to develop cultural competencies through seminars and field-mentored studies and practices. Graduate students specializing in transcultural nursing are eager to be prepared to work effectively with clients of several cultures and to continue studying changes in health care over time related largely to etic and emic discoveries. Many of them have actively worked to advance and change nursing from a unicultural to a transcultural nursing perspective and to introduce or help transform health care systems and organizations based on their research and knowledge. Most encouraging is the trend of these students to pursue doctoral study to increase their care knowledge and research about cultures in different places in the world. Master's degree students are generally certified transcultural nurses who have had 1 or 2 years in the specified programs with a focus in transcultural theory, research, and practice. Some students complete a certificate graduate program in transcultural nursing and become transcultural nurse specialists. Undoubtedly, both master's and doctorally prepared transcultural nurses will be in high demand in this 21st century as transculturalism increases in health care services.

Since faculty often wonder what could be offered in graduate programs, a sample of a transcultural nursing program will be highlighted next. The purpose of the Master of Science in Nursing degree in transcultural nursing provides students with in-depth culture care knowledge and skills to work with individuals, families, and groups from diverse cultural backgrounds. Cultures are studied with similar and diverse care values, beliefs, and lifeways. A variety of creative teaching approaches and methods are used during approximately a one- to two-year program. The seminars are rich learning experiences as students share their cultural-heritage learning discoveries with clients and use of theories to guide their actions and decisions. Graduates of the program are expected to become competent culture care practitioners, clinical specialists, consultants, and teachers in transcultural nursing. As specialists they generally know three or four cultures in-depth from a comparative and explanatory or theoretical stance. They learn how to do ethnonursing studies and different ways to teach and become beginning consultants. Doctoral and postdoctoral courses and experiences are usually tailored to meet students' special research interests and goals.

Some sample graduate seminar titles are as follows:

Nursing and Health Care Environments

Transcultural Health Throughout the Life Cycle

Transcultural Nursing: Theory, Research, and Practice

Field Practices in Transcultural Nursing

Culture Care Theory and Research

Transcultural Advanced Nursing Knowledge and Practices

Research Methods to Discover Transcultural Nursing Phenomena

Comparative Transcultural Nursing Ethics, Morals, and Lifeways

Anthropological and other social science and humanities courses are strongly recommended to expand student learning and to contrast transcultural nursing with these disciplines in theory and practice. Such courses from anthropology, which are often most helpful, are as follows:

Urban Anthropology

Cross Cultural Gender Research

Anthropological Theory

Language and Culture

Magic, Illness, and Health Conditions

Comparative Health and Anthropology

Ethnography of Urban and Rural Cultures

Specific Area Ethnographies

Physical and Genetic Anthropology

Western and non-Western Legal Cultural Practices

Students in both master's and doctoral programs in transcultural nursing gain in-depth knowledge of several cultures and conduct independent field studies or theses using specific theories and research methods. Doctoral students not only are expected to do an original study of a transcultural domain of inquiry but often an overseas study to compare or contrast findings of a very diverse culture with one close to home. Creative and original dissertations in transcultural nursing are expected (see list of doctoral dissertations in transcultural nursing and their focus as shown in Appendix 3-B in Chapter 3, Part II). Graduate seminars build on, reinforce, expand, and deepen student learning, research, and field experiences. Field experiences may be in a community, agency, or health institution or overseas in specific contexts, or some may be done at a distance, using the Internet. Graduate students not only examine in-depth their own cultural biases and tendencies, but learn to value the importance of field mentorship with transcultural nursing experts.

A fifth teaching and curricular approach to advance transcultural nursing is to arrange experiences functioning as researchers, teachers, and consultants within transcultural institutions, centers, or multidisciplinary institutions. With the rapidly growing demand for transcultural nursing education and practitioners worldwide, transcultural institutes and centers are being developed or already established with mini- or multi-disciplinary health focuses. Leininger encouraged and has helped to establish theory- and research-based institutes to prepare highly competent and true scholars in transcultural nursing and health care. Many transcultural nursing scholars in theory, research, and clinical expertise are needed today for institutes to be strong and credible. Some interdisciplinary colleagues such as anthropologists, sociologists, ethicists, and others also participate in these institutes with advanced seminars, research projects, and scholarly debates from a multidisciplinary stance. Regional centers or institutes need to be funded, as well as private or public ones, with scholarships and financial aid to meet the critical shortage of transcultural nurses and other transcultural professionals for rapidly growing health care needs worldwide. Highly motivated graduate transcultural nursing students are recruited to participate in these institutes or centers and to explicate and defend transcultural nursing as a legitimate discipline to serve human cultures. In the near future, many transcultural nursing institutes will be established, but they must have highly qualified and outstanding transcultural nursing scholars to be effective and successful.

Suggested Topic Domains for Undergraduate and Graduate Courses

Since many faculty and students often inquire about general topic domains related to undergraduate and graduate transcultural nursing education, the authors offer some suggestions in Appendix E. These content domains will vary with the institutional philosophy and with cultural areas and interests of faculty and students. Moreover, the scope, depth, and special focuses will vary in undergraduate and graduate curricula with respect to cultures in different geographic regions. Knowledge of common health and care needs of cultures in light of their ethnohistorical backgrounds, environments, and cultural values are important considerations in the development of global, national, regional, or local curricula. For example, in the United States there may be large populations of Vietnamese, Cubans, Native Americans, Hutterites, or others in regional areas that would need to be considered by the faculty such as in Miami, Florida, where there are many Haitians, Puerto Ricans, Cubans, and other Caribbean cultures that speak Spanish or related dialects. The focuses of study in this regional areas could be on transcultural nursing education, practice, and consultation related to Hispanic clients. While schools of nursing will vary with their goals and with cultures living in their geographic area, faculty experts in transcultural nursing will be needed as transcultural nursing becomes a mandate for all nurses by the year 2020 or earlier. Transcultural regional centers could make the most of faculty resources and minimize teaching and research costs.

Transcultural Nursing: A Creative Teaching and Learning Process

One of the exciting features of transcultural nursing is that teaching and learning about culture care and health in relation to nursing is a highly creative and stimulating experience. Transcultural nursing faculty are expected to be open-minded, curious, flexible, and creative in teaching and working with students and cultures. Helping students and faculty learn together from cultural informants and from diverse life experiences about transcultural phenomena is a rich and unique experience. It fits with the principle and philosophy that transcultural nursing is largely based on shared, open emic and etic comparative discoveries that are largely derived from learning about different cultures locally and worldwide. Transcultural nurses generally use an inductive process as they learn from people (emic perspective) of different or similar cultures but also from professionals (etic perspective) for comparative discoveries. Gaining comparative and in-depth insights about cultures with respect to care, health (or well-being), and environmental context are central to transcultural nursing. Establishing and maintaining a cultural ethos of *learning from and about others* in an active listening manner is important. Helping students grasp the totality of cultures rather than "bits and pieces" of physical and emotional aspects of illnesses or symptoms offers a different caring focus. Students are stimulated by and grow in professional abilities with the holistic and comprehensive lifeways of diverse and similar cultures. The Leininger Culture Care Theory with the use of the Sunrise Model and the ethnonursing enablers help students to discover the whole picture of individuals, families, or groups under study. Transcultural nursing faculty are central to help students maintain a strong caring and learning ethos of cultures with sensitivity but with grounded emic and etic knowledge. There is great latitude to be innovative in the teaching and learning processes in transcultural nursing. There are many opportunities to use research-based knowledge now available

with over 100 cultures and their specific care meanings and needs. Such knowledge is used to establish and maintain clinical competencies. Transcultural nursing remains one of the most challenging and creative ways to develop relevant curricula for teaching and learning in the 21st century.

Leininger's Teacher-Learner Conceptual Models and Principles

Over the past several decades Leininger developed the Transcultural Nursing Teacher-Learner Conceptual Process Model (Fig. 34.1) to envision and guide faculty and students in learning together. This model is used with the Transcultural Nursing Learning and Teaching Discovery Modes to learn about diverse cultures (Table 34.1), which can be extremely helpful to guide transcultural nursing and other faculty in their teaching endeavors. In addition, her philosophical premises and principles related to teaching transcultural nursing in undergraduate and graduate programs have been a most helpful guide to faculty and students. These premises and principles are as follows:

1. Faculty and students are *coparticipants in the learning and teaching process* to discover transcultural nursing phenomena. While faculty members assume the major responsibility of facilitating transcultural learning and guiding students using specific observations and

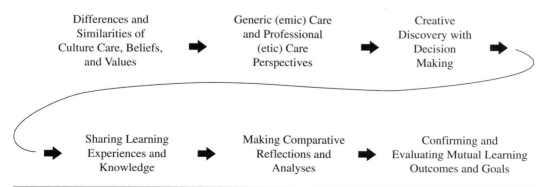

Figure 34.1
Leininger's transcultural nursing teacher-learner conceptual process model.

Table 34.1   Some Transcultural Nursing Learning and Teaching Discovery Modes

1. Direct observations, interviews, participation, and reflection experiences
2. Immersion experiences in the cultural life-care world
3. Reflective learning and critique with mentor(s)
4. Philosophical questions and reasoning
5. Role-modeling with exemplars or experts in action
6. Doing oral and written life histories and stories of cultures
7. Use of symbols and metaphors to learn culture care
8. Learning from simple to complex culture care phenomena
9. Learning ways to integrate and synthesize qualitative culture care data
10. Use of culture care and nurses care stories
11. Learning ways to capture differences and similarities
12. Observing simple, diverse, and complex cultural systems
13. Critical assessment of beneficial and less-beneficial caring with diverse cultures
14. Use of creative modes with the Internet, films, videos, photos, TV programs, new audio-visual and experiential media, and the study of books on the cultures of nursing and peoples worldwide

reflections, the students remain active learners in the process.

2. Students and faculty bring *their cultural or personal heritage and experiences to the teaching-learning context and process,* including their values, beliefs, and lifeways. Cultural heritage factors have special meanings, symbols, and insights that faculty and students need to discover and understand.

3. Nursing students study enculturation and socialization aspects of clients, as well as the culture of nursing and other health professions, to understand cultures and health professions in relation to care and treatments.

4. Student learning is most effective when students become active participants who are willing to become immersed in cultures and open to reflective mentor guidance.

5. Transcultural nursing theories are essential to guide a student's thinking in discovering what one sees, hears, and is told along with other experiences

with clients. It is essential to arrive at culture-specific care validated knowledge. The Theory of Culture Care with the use of the Sunrise Model continues to be a valuable theoretical guide to discover and substantiate knowledge.

6. The use of holding knowledge to study a culture is essential to prevent cultural ignorance and to pick up clues from cultural informants. Building on past similar or diverse experiences helps the learner gain confidence.

7. Transcultural nursing faculty mentors are expected to help students decipher unfavorable biases, marked ethnocentrism, cultural imposition practices, and many other cultural expressions that limit students' effectiveness and success in transcultural nursing.

8. Teaching transcultural nursing should be viewed as a mode of being with students in a caring relationship that is directed toward discovering experiences together and being respectful or helpful to each other.

9. Discovering culture care differences and similarities among clients, students, faculty, and others is an ongoing discovery process for growth in transcultural nursing.

10. Facilitating diverse immersion experiences with cultures under qualified faculty membership becomes an invaluable and powerful means to learn about cultures, self, and others.

11. Discovering, knowing, and analyzing the student's cultural and caring values, beliefs, and patterned lifeways is essential to transcultural nursing to provide meaningful and beneficial client care practices.

12. Teaching transcultural nursing is a creative and humbling special experience that includes learning from others and self in a caring context.

In teaching and learning in transcultural nursing, a great variety of different methods and approaches can be used today such as these found in Table 34.1. Audiovisual and electronic modes along with narratives, epics, and storytelling are used a great deal in transcultural nursing education and in research. All of these teaching modes have been stimulating to students and faculty and lead to rich learning.

The authors have found that if students engage in guided mentorships with transcultural nursing faculty and focus on two or three cultures, they become confident and competent in working with most cultures. We have also found that students without educational preparation in transcultural nursing often have considerable problems when they work with different cultures and experience cultural shock, cultural backlash, cultural stresses, and other problems. Sometimes, students without transcultural nursing preparation who are sent to strange cultures become negative and very biased about cultures largely because they do not understand them. Currently, there is an erroneous and dangerous myth held by some faculty that students do not need to be prepared in advance before going overseas or to work with different cultures. Instead, they believe they can rely on "common sense," "reflections," and direct experiences along with nursing knowledge. Some faculty believe that whatever is communicated and experienced between clients and the students (verbally and nonverbally) can be accurately understood and interpreted without transcultural holding knowledge and insights. Such myths and beliefs need to be reexamined. Indeed, placing students in foreign lands or strange cultures without adequate preparation in transcultural nursing continues to pose problems, including legal difficulties and survival. Several nursing students have returned home in culture shock, disappointed and disillusioned about working with diverse cultures because they lacked transcultural nursing knowledge. This is often evident with students who experience shocking differences between their own culture and that of a community of a very different culture. Hence, students today must be adequately prepared to enter and remain in diverse cultures, to care for clients of these cultures, and to have a positive experience.

There is also another myth—that nursing students prepared in anthropology and sociology can function as transcultural nurses. Anthropology or sociology are different disciplines than transcultural nursing or nursing. Transcultural nursing is both a professional practice and a discipline focused on humanistic care, health, illness, death, the life cycle, and environmental context. In contrast, anthropology is an academic discipline. This fact has been evident when nonnurse anthropologists have taught and guided nursing students in the classroom and in clinical and field areas, but failed to teach or respond to transcultural nursing perspectives. There is also a related myth that "transcultural nursing" and "cross-cultural" nursing are the same.[31]

This myth also needs to be reexamined. Transcultural nursing was deliberately identified and developed by Leininger and others in the early 1960s, and since then the discipline and profession has grown into a highly relevant study and practice field focused on caring. In contrast, cross-cultural nursing has primarily and appropriately focused on advancing anthropological knowledge through different research goals. However, anthropological knowledge, especially from an ethnohistorical perspective, is a rich and valuable knowledge base for transcultural nursing.

■ Current and Critical Issues and Problems Facing Transcultural Nursing Education

In this last section some current critical issues and problems facing transcultural nursing education and curriculum specialists will be summarized. They can be used for debate, for raising faculty awareness and discussion, and for setting goals to help alleviate or resolve these issues. They are as follows:

1. The slow and hesitant shift of educational programs to global transcultural nursing versus the great imperative for transcultural nursing today and in the future.
2. The critical need for many undergraduate and graduate nurses to care for clients of diverse cultures and the need for courses and faculty in transcultural nursing schools.
3. The lack of teaching and research monies to establish transcultural nursing educational and research programs with qualified faculty prepared to do research in transcultural nursing.
4. The lack of knowledge and appreciation by faculty and students for human care as the central domain of transcultural nursing and of all aspects of nursing education and practice.
5. The overemphasis on cultural diversity and the failure to emphasize cultural care and health similarities in transcultural nursing is a major issue. Cultural diversity is only one aspect of transcultural nursing and not the major or only focus of transcultural nursing.
6. The employment of faculty who are unprepared to teach transcultural nursing and mentor students in

transcultural nursing remains of great concern because of the false assumptions that a) anyone can teach transcultural nursing; b) if a nurse is of a culture, then he or she is very knowledgeable about and qualified to teach about that culture; and c) the use of the "common sense" approach is the best teacher of transcultural nursing.

7. Working with nursing faculty and administrators who have strong cultural biases and racist attitudes and who are afraid to work or teach about cultures.

8. The conceptual problems in shifting nursing students and faculty from teaching fragmented, medical, mind-body, symptom-treatment perspectives or using a narrow holistic (mind-body-spirit) focus greatly limits the comprehensive focus of transcultural caring knowledge and practice.

9. The lack of knowledge of the importance and therapeutic benefits of generic (folk) care practices of clients and their relationship to professional nursing or medical knowledge.

10. The tendency to support mainly quantitative paradigmatic research studies in schools of nursing rather than supporting qualitative research methods that have been invaluable to discover complex transcultural nursing knowledge.

11. The use of culture-bound, biased, and inappropriate instruments, scales, and surveys for nursing research and teaching purposes that limits the discovery of culturally based knowledge for many cultures and care phenomena that need to be measured accurately to be known and understood.

12. Inadequate public media coverage to show the importance of transcultural nursing as a significant breakthrough in the 20th century and a major thrust for transcultural nursing care in the 21st century.

13. The lack of focus on transcultural ethical and moral issues with Western and non-Western cultures.

14. Failure to use available transcultural nursing theory-based research knowledge and publications to improve care to diverse cultures worldwide.

15. The mass increase in conducting overseas programs with nursing faculty and students who have had no advanced preparation in transcultural nursing for safe and meaningful health care.

16. The lack of local and national research funds to study transcultural nursing, to change nursing curricula from a unicultural to multicultural focus, and to develop transcultural nursing institutes and centers worldwide.

17. Working with nursing faculty and students whose values and beliefs about Western or non-Western cultures are countercultural, negative, and often inaccurate.

18. The lack of available recognition for transcultural nursing leaders and followers to bring about a new way of educating and providing culturally knowledgeable and competent nurses.

19. Overuse and dependency on tape recordings with cultural informants or clients for teaching and research purposes rather than using direct-talk experiences, field journal data, naturalistic modes of inquiry, and appropriate qualitative discovery methods.

20. Using ethnonursing data, client family stories, field journal notes, and other cultural information for classroom teaching when permission was not granted by the informants.

21. The lack of administrative support from nursing deans and other faculty for transcultural nursing programs and changes in curricula to multicultural content and experiences.

22. The use of nursing diagnoses and misdiagnoses of cultural and health expressions with North American Nursing Diagnosis Association (NANDA) and other classification schemes because of cultural ignorance of faculty.

23. Publishing books and articles under the title of transcultural nursing with inaccurate knowledge of transcultural care practices.

24. Worldwide membership in Transcultural Nursing Society (established in the early 1970s) to shift all of nursing education, research, and practice into transcultural nursing by the year 2015 or earlier for client health protection and benefits.

25. Establishing and maintaining certification and recertification standards and practices on a global basis to protect clients and nurses of diverse cultures and vulnerable populations (the poor and oppressed).

The above are a few current critical issues and needs challenging all nurses, nursing organizations, and the public to take action to function, survive, and grow in transcultural nursing.

In this chapter trends and reasons for the importance of transcultural nursing education have been presented. The imperative mandate is to prepare nurses worldwide in transcultural nursing to meet present and future critical worldwide needs to care for clients of diverse or similar cultures. The ultimate goal of transcultural nursing education is to prepare nurses to become culturally compassionate, competent, responsible, and effective to serve people worldwide. Critical issues were identified so that efforts will be made to maintain transcultural nursing programs grounded in theory-based research, knowledge, and practices. The authors contend that *all nurses need to be prepared in transcultural nursing to serve culturally vulnerable populations and to develop professional competencies in transcultural nursing by the year 2015.*

Time is limited to achieve this global goal, and steps need to be taken soon to prevent destructive or unfavorable cultural care and other problems. Far more nurses need preparation in transcultural nursing because of worldwide multicultural needs and conditions impacting on quality health care services. Several suggested content domains for undergraduate and graduate nursing education and curricula have been offered along with teaching models, methods, and approaches. In the last section some current pressing issues were identified for faculty discussion and global action to advocate transcultural nursing education worldwide. The authors leave the reader to reflect on the belief that the most significant breakthrough in nursing in the 20th century was establishing the new discipline and practice of transcultural nursing, but that the greatest challenge in the 21st century is to prepare nearly five million nurses worldwide to become culturally competent, effective, and satisfied with their endeavors. We hope that this challenge will be realized and valued.

References

1. Leininger, M., "Overview and Reflection of the Theory of Culture Care and the Ethnonursing Research Method," *Journal of Transcultural Nursing*, 1997, v. 8, no. 2, pp. 32–51.
2. Leininger, M., *Transcultural Nursing: Concepts, Theories, and Practices*, New York: John Wiley & Sons, 1978.
3. Leininger, M., *Nursing and Anthropology: Two Worlds to Blend*, New York: John Wiley & Sons, 1970. (First book to link nursing and anthropology). (Reprinted in 1994 by Greyden Press, Columbus, OH).
4. Leininger, M., "A New Generation of Nurses Discover Transcultural Nursing," *Nursing and Health Care*, May 1987, v. 8, no. 5, p. 3.
5. Leininger, M., "Transcultural Nursing: An Essential Knowledge Field for Today," *The Canadian Nurse*, December 1984, v. 30, no. 11, pp. 41–45.
6. Leininger, M., "Cultural Dimensions in the Baccalaureate Nursing Curriculum," in *Cultural Dimensions in the Baccalaureate Nursing Curriculum*, New York: National League for Nursing Press, 1977, pp. 85–107.
7. Leininger, op. cit., 1978.
8. Leininger, M., "Transcultural Nurse Specialists and Generalists: New Practitioners in Nursing," *Journal of Transcultural Nursing*, 1989, vol. 1, no. 1, pp. 4–16.
9. Leininger, M., "Teaching Transcultural Care Theory, Principles, and Concepts in Schools of Nursing," unpublished manuscript, 1992.
10. Andrews, M., "Educational Preparation for International Nursing," *Journal of Professional Nursing*, 1988, v. 4, no. 6, pp. 430–433.
11. Leininger, M., "Report and Recommendations for the First National Conference on Teaching Transcultural Nursing," *Journal of Transcultural Nursing*, Summer 1993, v. 4, no. 11, pp. 41–42.
12. Leininger, op. cit., 1978.
13. Leininger, M., "Transcultural Nursing Care in the Community," in *Community Health Nursing: Caring for the Public Health*, Lundy, K. and S. Janes, eds., Sudbury, MA: Jones and Bartlett, 2001, pp. 218–234.
14. Leininger, op. cit., 1970.
15. Leininger, op. cit., 1978.
16. Leininger, M., "Transcultural Nursing Education: A Worldwide Imperative," *Nursing and Health Care*, May 1994, v. 15, no. 5, pp. 254–257.
17. Leininger, M., "Transcultural Nursing: A Promising Subfield of Study for Nurse Educators and Practitioners," *Current Practice in Family Centered Community Nursing*, St. Louis, MO: C.V. Mosby Co., 1976.
18. Leininger, M., "Survey of Nursing Programs with Transcultural Faculty, Courses and Programs," unpublished survey, Omaha, NE, 2000.
19. Ibid.
20. Draves, W.A., *Teaching Online*, River Falls, WI: LERN Books, Learning Resources Network, 2000.
21. Carpio, B. and B. Majumdar, "Experiential Learning: An Approach to Transcultural Education for Nursing," *Journal of Transcultural Nursing*, 1993, v. 4, no. 2, pp. 32–33.

22. DeSantis, L., "Developing Faculty Expertise in Culturally Focused Care and Research," *Journal of Professional Nursing*, 1991, v. 7, no. 5, pp. 300–309.
23. Smith, S.E., "Increasing Transcultural Awareness: The McMaster-Aga Khan-CIDA Project Workshop Model," *Journal of Transcultural Nursing*, 1997, v. 8, no. 2, pp. 23–31.
24. Baker, S.S. and N.C. Burkhalter, "Teaching Transcultural Nursing in a Transcultural Setting," *Journal of Transcultural Nursing*, 1996, v. 7, no. 2, pp. 10–13.
25. Leininger, M., "Founder's Focus: Nursing Education Exchanges: Concerns and Benefits," *Journal of Transcultural Nursing*, 1998, v. 9, no. 2, pp. 57–63.
26. Leininger, M., "Transcultural Nursing: Quo Vadis (Where Goeth the Field)?" *Journal of Transcultural Nursing*, 1989, v. 1, no. 1, pp. 33–45.
27. Leininger, M., "Transcultural Nursing: Importance, History, Concepts, Theory, and Research," in *Transcultural Nursing: Concepts, Theories, Research, and Practice*, Leininger, M., ed., Columbus, OH: McGraw-Hill College Custom Series, 1995.
28. Andrews, M., "Transcultural Nursing: Transforming the Curriculum," *Journal of Transcultural Nursing*, 1997, v. 6, no. 2, pp. 4–9.
29. Leininger, M., "The Significance of Transcultural Nursing Concepts in Nursing," *Journal of Transcultural Nursing*, 1990, v. 2, no. 1, pp. 52–59.
30. Leininger, M., *Transcultural Nursing: Concepts, Theories, Research, and Practice*, Columbus, OH: McGraw-Hill College Custom Series, 1995.
31. Leininger, M., "Strange Myths and Inaccurate Facts in Transcultural Nursing," *Journal of Transcultural Nursing*, Winter 1992, v. 4, no. 2, pp. 39–40.

Appendix 34–A
Certification and Recertification*

After transcultural nursing was launched in the mid-1950s, the need for transcultural nursing certification was apparent by the mid-1970s. Nurses with limited cultural knowledge and skills were attempting to care for immigrants, refugees, and people of diverse and unknown cultures. There was evidence of some harmful, offensive, and inappropriate care practices with some cultures. Formal courses and programs in transcultural nursing had been introduced to educate nurses, but certification through examinations to verify knowledge and competencies was clearly needed, as well as recertification to maintain competencies.

Accordingly, a Certification Committee was established in 1988 within the Transcultural Nursing Society. The purposes, expectations, and benefits for certification of nurses in transcultural nursing were explicitly stated. Applications with appropriate portfolio documentation were required for transcultural nursing certification. After review of the applications, nurses were notified to sit for written and oral examinations conducted by the Certification Committee. These oral and written examinations helped to assess the nurse's knowledge and abilities to use transcultural nursing principles, concepts, theories, and research-based culture care knowledge with practices to provide culturally congruent care.

A major purpose of certification is to protect clients of diverse cultures from negligent, offensive, harmful, unethical, nontherapeutic, or inappropriate care practices. Other purposes and potential benefits of certification and recertification of transcultural nurses are as follows:

1. To provide quality-based and research-based cultural care knowledge for competent care practices
2. To recognize the expertise of transcultural nurses prepared to care for clients of diverse and similar cultures
3. To protect the public from unfavorable transcultural nursing practices
4. To maintain quality-based standards and policies for transcultural nursing practices
5. To provide and inform the public of the competencies of nurses
6. To serve as transcultural role models

Today, certified transcultural nurses are demonstrating the importance of knowledge and competencies along with confidence, professional pride, and satisfaction to provide culturally congruent quality care to people of diverse or similar cultures. These nurses are prepared to function locally, nationally, and globally through certification and recertification. They are

---

* Revised in June 2001 by the Committee on Certification and Recertification of the Transcultural Nursing Society.

important to protect vulnerable cultures from unsafe practices. Their preparation in transcultural nursing helps them to be effective, competent, and safe with cultures. Recertification is the means to ensure continued competencies in transcultural nursing by maintaining the nurses' knowledge and skills in the field and, especially, to keep abreast of new developments in the field.

During the past two decades many nurses have been certified and recertified. These nurses have gained respect, status, public recognition, and often advancement in their employment because of their unique and valuable service to diverse cultures. Indeed, certified transcultural nurses are meeting a critical need to prevent racial biases, cultural clashes, cultural impositions, and ethnocentric and other unfavorable practices.

The Certification Committee was reorganized in 2000 with a focus on the refinement and updating of standards, policies, examinations, and the general processes for certification and recertification of nurses. This change was essential to meet a rapidly growing multicultural need for worldwide protective and therapeutic care practices. Unquestionably, certification and recertification of transcultural nurses will remain a significant, unique, and imperative global need to provide culturally competent, safe, and responsible quality-based care practices.

Dr. Jeanne Hoffer is serving as the chairperson of the committee along with several members of highly competent certified transcultural nurses. Nurses are encouraged to become certified for consumer and nurse protection in caring for cultures. It is also a valuable means to increase and maintain professional competencies to gain many rewarding satisfactions.

Appendix 34–B
Sample Undergraduate Transcultural Nursing Course

Title: Transcultural Nursing: Concepts, Principles, Theories, Research, and Practices

Credits: 2–3 semester credits

Placement: Early in Undergraduate Program with opportunities to use in diverse clinical settings

Faculty: Graduate (master's and doctoral) Preparation in Transcultural Nursing

Course Description

This basic undergraduate transcultural nursing course is focused on care, health, healing, well-being, and culturally based illnesses. Culture care is the central phenomenon to guide students to learn and use cultural care beliefs, values, and practices of specific cultures and subcultures throughout the life cycle. Students learn how to assess culture care differences and similarities among and between cultures to provide culturally congruent, safe, and competent nursing care. Students learn how to use a nursing theory to discover and guide nursing care practices in living contexts. Specific transcultural nursing concepts, principles, and strategies are learned to facilitate nursing decisions and actions. Contemporary transcultural nursing conditions, gender problems, and diverse issues are identified to assist students in conceptualizing and working through problem areas related to culture care nursing practices in diverse environmental contexts.

Course Goals

Students will be expected to do the following:

1. Identify reasons for the trends, development, and importance of transcultural nursing to establish and improve care to diverse cultures worldwide.
2. Discuss the major historical developments, achievements, and leaders that have shaped the field of transcultural nursing.
3. Apply major transcultural nursing constructs and principles to assess client and family needs and guide transcultural nursing practices.
4. Use the Theory of Culture Care Diversity and Universality with the Sunrise Model and other enablers to provide culturally congruent, sensitive, and responsible care throughout the life cycle and in critical and recurrent culture care incidents.
5. Be knowledgeable about folk (emic) and professional (etic) care and the use of complementary health care.
6. Examine tendencies for cultural and gender biases, ethnocentrism, cultural blindness, and imposition practices.
7. Demonstrate ways to provide culturally congruent, safe, competent, and effective transcultural nursing care with individuals and their families who are

well, who have chronic or acute illnesses, or who are dying.

8. Discuss the use of specific culture care research findings, especially using Leininger's three modes of actions and decisions.

Teaching-Learning Methods or Experiences

A great variety of teaching-learning methods can be used for this course. These methods need to be integrated into all clinical and community experiences after having this foundational course to guide students' observations and practices. Some of these methods are as follows:

1. Direct observations
2. Participation and interaction journals
3. Reflective analysis and discussion of daily cultural life events
4. Use of client-student encounters or situations
5. Use of cultural and transcultural nursing films, videos, and CDs
6. Open discussion on cultural heritage and life experiences
7. Transcultural games, skits, and simulations
8. Use of student experiential accounts
9. Storytelling and narratives related to particular cultures
10. Lecture-discussion exchanges between faculty and students
11. Panel presentations on specific cultures or subcultures from the local community
12. Use of poems, paintings, and drawings related to culture care and health
13. Use of biographies of cultural representatives
14. Use of ethnonursing field journal data

All students are expected to know how to do culturalogical holistic care and health assessments. In addition, students prepare a 15- to 16-page (double-spaced) term paper on a specific culture. This paper should reflect a focused emphasis on transcultural nursing care theory, principles, and concepts, as well as ways to provide culturally congruent care using Leininger's three modes of nursing actions and decisions.

Content Domains with Diverse Teaching Methods and Strategies

I. Introduction to transcultural nursing: cultural diversities and similarities

   A. Student's understanding of purposes and goals of transcultural nursing (historical and current)
   B. Orientational definition of transcultural nursing concepts and constructs
   C. World forces influencing the need for transcultural nursing

II. Discovering the historical factors that led to establishing transcultural nursing (focus on Leininger's Three Eras of transcultural nursing—see references)

   A. Early and later developments in transcultural nursing
   B. Leaders and their specific contributions
   C. Barriers and facilitators in developing the field

III. Discussion of major concepts, definitions, and expressions of transcultural nursing using many examples and life events from different cultures (see transcultural nursing textbooks)

IV. Understanding the importance of language, culture context, ethnohistory, and lifeways of specific cultures in community context with a transcultural nursing focus

V. Identifying cultural life-cycle processes and their meanings (use examples). Examine: 1) assimilation, 2) enculturalism, 3) socialization, 4) acculturation, and 5) gender role and age expectations

VI. Discovering the culture of nursing, the culture of the hospitals, the culture of medicine, and other cultures in health systems

VII. Identifying American cultural values, beliefs, and lifeways and contrasts with other world cultures (comparative analysis)

VIII. Study of Leininger's Theory of Culture Care Diversity and Universality with the Sunrise Model and other enablers to assess and study transcultural nursing phenomena and use of the three modes of Transcultural Nursing Action and Decision

IX. Use of social structure factors, including economic, kinship, religion, legal, education, and spirituality, philosophy and worldview, specific cultural values and beliefs, technologies, and environmental context with the Theory of Culture Care to achieve holistic knowledge

  A. Meaning of environmental context(s)
  B. Importance of language and communication needs
  C. Importance of ethnohistorical factors
  D. Relevance of generic and professional care practices
  E. Use of Leininger's three modes of nursing actions and decisions to provide culturally congruent nursing care, namely: 1) culture care preservation and maintenance, 2) culture care accommodation and negotiations, 3) culture care repatterning and restructuring, and 4) indicators of culturally competent and congruent nursing care

X. Learning how to do culturalogical health care assessments using the Culture Care Theory and Sunrise Model (students gain considerable knowledge and skills in this area by taking different roles in a culture as a client, a family member, or as a nurse)

XI. Discussion of the use of research findings from the literature on specific cultures

XII. Exploring and discovery of comparative life-cycle beliefs, values, and lifeways with gender and age considerations in at least two cultures with focus on human caring and health

  A. Prenatal through early infancy
  B. Early childhood era
  C. Adolescent period
  D. Middlescence
  E. The young-old, old, and advanced years

XIII. Study of special transcultural conditions, meanings, and problems with diverse cultures

such as African, Mexican, Arabs, Polish, Native Americans, Asian-Japanese-Chinese, and others

  A. Expressions of cultural pain in diverse cultures
  B. Expressions of grief and dying in different cultures
  C. Chronic and acute illness and disabilities in diverse cultures
  D. Ethical, moral, and spiritual dilemmas in transcultural nursing
  E. Healing, caring, and curing practices

XIV. Discovering the meaning and realities of transcultural mental health and care needs

  A. Cultural interpretations of normal and deviant behaviors
  B. Culture-bound conditions and healing modes
  C. Misdiagnoses and misconceptions of mental health and illness
  D. Role of mental health healers, carers, and curers

XV. Discovering transcultural nursing as a meaningful and important career

  A. Career opportunities in transcultural nursing in different countries
  B. Transcultural care and specialist functions and roles
  C. Economic, political, and interprofessional issues

XVI. Demonstrate ways to eventually make congruent and effective transcultural nursing decisions, actions, and judgments. Students with faculty mentors need to demonstrate transcultural nursing skills and knowledge.

References

See extensive references cited in the Appendix 34-F of this chapter.

Appendix 34–C
Sample Graduate Transcultural Nursing Seminar

Title:	Advanced Transcultural Nursing Seminar
Credits:	3–5 semester graduate credits
Placement:	Master's and Doctoral Degree Nursing Programs
Faculty:	With Graduate (MSN or PhD) Preparation in Transcultural Nursing and Certification in the field also desired

Course Description

This is an advanced (graduate) transcultural nursing course focused on trends, issues, historical leaders, theories, research methods, and findings related to transcultural nursing as an essential field of study and practice. The Seminar addresses past and current developments of transcultural nursing as a specialty but with general knowledge and practices to provide culturally competent, safe, and meaningful care to people of diverse and similar cultures or subcultures. Theoretical perspectives, concepts, and diverse research methods are discussed with the goal of improving the quality of care to people of diverse cultures. Leininger's Theory of Culture Care is examined, as well as other relevant theories and research findings generated from the theories. Ethnonursing, ethnography, and other qualitative and quantitative research methods are considered to generate and analyze transcultural care phenomena. Cultural differences and similarities in care health beliefs, values, and practices of Western and non-Western cultures are emphasized with an emic and etic perspective to reaffirm, establish, and add to transcultural nursing knowledge. Future directions and issues in transcultural nursing are explored with worldwide perspectives of different cultures and subcultures. Cultures of nursing and medicine are discussed, as well as the students' domains of inquiry as mini- or maxi-studies with theories, methods, and research plans, which are implemented and evaluated.

Seminar Goals

Students will be expected to do the following:

1. Analyze philosophical, historical, cultural, and epistemic factors influencing the development of the field of transcultural nursing with its impact on leaders and cultural conditions

2. Analyze different emic and etic cultural beliefs, values, and practices of Western and non-Western cultures using transcultural nursing constructs, theories, and research findings on different and similar cultures

3. Discuss the use of major transcultural nursing concepts, principles, theories, and research findings as substantive and advanced transcultural nursing knowledge to establish, advance, and improve health care throughout the life cycle during wellness, chronic and acute illnesses, and the dying process

4. Analyze comparative meanings and expressions of diverse and similar cultures of nursing

5. Demonstrate the use of Leininger's Theory of Culture Care Diversity and Universality and other transcultural nursing theories and research methods that contribute to the body of knowledge in the discipline

6. Use selected qualitative or quantitative research methods to study transcultural nursing phenomena of Western and non-Western cultures

7. Analyze in-depth generic (folk) and professional care practices of selected cultures with the goal to provide culturally effective, congruent, and safe care to designated cultures

8. Discuss the importance and method of doing clinical and community services

9. Critique selected theoretical and research findings

10. Have knowledge of ways to do a mini or maxi transcultural nursing study with theory, research methods, and data analysis

11. Analyze critical issues, trends, and problems related to transcultural nursing and describe ways to resolve these issues or problems

12. Have state-of-the-art transcultural nursing knowledge in education, research, consultation, and practice contexts

13. Analyze selected transcultural nursing ethical and moral issues in-depth focused on different cultures or subcultures

14. Use and apply transcultural nursing findings in health care systems, homes, or centers

15. Demonstrate reflective use of transcultural nursing literature related to teaching, curricula,

exchange programs, and consultation, as well as clinical and multi-disciplinary issues

Suggested Seminar Domains

1. Historical, philosophical, epistemological, and cultural factors influencing the development of the field of transcultural nursing as a discipline with specialized and generalized health care services

2. Critical analysis of issues, trends, and problems that have facilitated or impeded the development of transcultural nursing locally, nationally, and globally

3. Pioneering leaders and their contributions to transcultural nursing over the past five decades

4. Relationships of transcultural nursing to anthropology and other related fields as transcultural nursing becomes globalized

5. The cultures of nursing and medicine with cultural conflict and facilitation areas

6. Conceptual models and theories with domains of inquiry to rigorously study transcultural nursing phenomena locally and worldwide

7. Leininger's Theory of Culture Care Diversity and Universality and contributions to the discipline and practice of transcultural nursing

8. Generic (emic) folk and professional (etic) knowledge and integrative or complementary health services

9. Culturalogical care assessments and enablers for individuals, families, and communities to procure data to provide culturally congruent, competent, beneficial, and accessible care practices

10. Roles and issues of transcultural nurse specialists and generalists functioning in nursing education, consultation, administration, and multidisciplinary endeavors

11. Use of qualitative and quantitative comparative research methods to study transcultural nursing phenomena in relation to care, health, illness, well-being, illnesses, and diverse environmental contexts

12. Current ethical, moral, legal, and therapeutic issues related to transcultural nursing research, practice, education, and related problems using NANDA and other classification and diagnostic tools with cultures

13. Current globalization issues in nursing education, administration, finances, and human resources

14. Trends, issues, and problems in nursing education and exchanges and the lack of transcultural preparation on the part of many nurses to be effective teachers, researchers, and consultants in Western and non-Western cultures

15. Intra- and interprofessional cultural clashes, racism, cultural imposition, and ethnocentrism in providing care to clients of different cultures and in transforming health practices to transculturalism

16. Current and future issues, challenges, and concerns in establishing transcultural nursing programs, institutes, centers, and multidisciplinary programs

17. Evaluation of current transcultural nursing contributions and achievements in the 20th century as the significant breakthrough era and strategic plans for the current 21st century of global transculturalism

18. Development of a theoretical research proposal (mini or maxi) with a specific domain of inquiry that demonstrates scholarly and critical thinking, with review of literature, a theory, and research plans.

References for Course (see Appendix 34-F)

Appendix 34–D
Current Graduate Courses or Programs in Transcultural Nursing 2001–2002*

United States

University of Nebraska Medical Center, College of Nursing (Omaha, Nebraska)

- Offers 2 short-term intensive graduate courses (2 credits each) at master's and post-master's level on transcultural nursing and human caring

---

* **NOTE:** Several schools of nursing offer some cultural or transcultural nursing and research, but no full courses or programs over academic terms focused in-depth on transcultural nursing.

M. Leininger (2001)

- Courses may be taken for college credit or for continuing education
- Dr. Madeleine Leininger, Founder of Transcultural Nursing

University of Northern Colorado, School of Nursing (Greeley, Colorado)

- Offers graduate certificate program with transcultural nursing with field studies
- Diane Peters and others

Kean University (Union City, New Jersey)

- Offers graduate courses in transcultural nursing through Transcultural Nursing Institute
- Dr. Dula Pacquiao

Duquesne University, School of Nursing (Pittsburgh, Pennsylvania)

- Offers graduate courses in transcultural nursing, a postmaster's program with focus on transcultural nursing, and a PhD in Nursing with a focus on transcultural nursing (arranged on an individual basis)
- Dr. Rick Zoucha

Augsberg College, College of Nursing (St. Paul, Minnesota)

- Offers graduate courses in transcultural nursing
- Dr. Cheryl Leuning

University of Southern Mississippi, School of Nursing (Hattiesburg, Mississippi)

- Offers graduate courses in transcultural nursing
- Dr. S. Jones and Dr. Hartman

Nazareth University, Department of Nursing (Rochester, New York)

- Offers a graduate course in transcultural nursing
- Margaret Andrews

Australia

University of Sydney, Nursing Faculty, Graduate Nursing Faculty (Sydney, Australia)

- Graduate seminars in transcultural nursing
- Dr. Akram Omeri

Finland

University of Kuopio, Nursing Faculty (Kuopio, Finland)

- Offers study in transcultural nursing
- Faculty Instructors

Appendix 34–E
Suggested Undergraduate and Graduate Transcultural Nursing Knowledge Domains

The content domains below are suggested for teaching transcultural nursing in undergraduate and graduate programs. The scope and depth of content will vary with the philosophy and curricula of the programs, the students' needs, faculty expertise, and the cultures in the area or region. These content domains can be considerably expanded and used in creative ways for teaching transcultural nursing and to plan for specific learning experiences.

1. Discussion of the definition, nature, scope and meaning of transcultural nursing; culture care; and culturally sensitive, competent, and responsible care
2. Examination of the rationale, goals, and importance of transcultural nursing locally, nationally, and worldwide
3. Discussion of the evolutionary phases of transcultural nursing as developed and implemented by transcultural nurse leaders
4. Discussion of dimensions of transcultural nursing to improve people care, advance knowledge, and transform nursing education and practice, including content related to anthropology, nurse specialty areas, and other areas relevant to transcultural nursing and health care
5. Analysis of the progress, challenges, and major barriers to establishing transcultural nursing as a global area of study and practice
6. Discussion of the conceptual ideas and meanings of care, caring, and culture care as central to the transcultural nursing field based on research studies bearing on transcultural nursing
7. Reflections on the conceptualizations of health, well-being, illness, diseases, oncology, and

environmental context in relation to transcultural nursing

8. Discussion of the meaning and clinical/community uses of care concepts, constructs, and principles developed for study in transcultural nursing, e.g., worldview, culture care, health, well-being, bioculturalism, ethnocentrism, cultural imposition, cultural clashes, cultural conflict and shock, cultural context, cultural blindness, cultural pain, cultural taboos, health variations, cultural change, cultural diversities and similarities, culture care values and norms, cultural authenticity, care patterns and expressions, health and well-being patterns and expressions, enculturation, assimilation, rights of passage, culture-bound conditions, prejudice, discrimination, and racism

9. Discussion of the meanings and importance of generic (folk) and professional care, as well as *emic* and *etic* perspectives, to establish and advance transcultural nursing knowledge and practices

10. Discussion of the cultures of nursing, hospitals, and other health disciplines and their impact on nursing care practice decisions, the discipline and the development of transcultural nursing, and health practices

11. Examination of the theories pertinent to advance transcultural nursing, especially Leininger's Theory of Culture Care Diversity and Universality with the use of the Sunrise Model as a central and specific transcultural nursing theory; discussion of other relevant theories useful to advance the study of transcultural nursing and human care

12. Discussion of the principles and guidelines for a culturalogical holistic care assessment providing examples and real experiences of students, researchers, and transcultural nurse practitioners

13. Discussion of the biocultural, biogenetic, social, and ecological dimensions of transcultural health care in diverse environmental contexts

14. Examples of the meaning of providing culturally sensitive, responsible, and competent care; popular meanings and misuses by nurses; and uses of concepts to improve people care

15. Discussion of comparative birth-to-death life-cycle phenomena in relation to transcultural

practices and use with Leininger's three modes: 1) culture care preservation and maintenance; 2) culture care accommodation and negotiation; and 3) culture care repatterning and restructuring

16. Critical examination of past and current transcultural research studies and uses to improve people care, including diverse research methods such as ethnonursing and other qualitative methods, quantitative methods, and other diverse strategies in research

17. Discussion of the ethical and moral dimensions of transcultural nursing in client care, research, and educational processes, drawing on research studies and philosophic stances

18. Discussion of transcultural nursing and international consultation, exchanges, and collaborative practices with issues and trends

19. Discussion of future directions and issues in transcultural nursing, including the globalization and particularization of transcultural nursing in different places in the world with projected benefits

20. Critique of transcultural nursing progress and research literature related to diverse cultures as means to improve the well-being and health of people or to help people face death or disabilities

21. Discussion of the meanings and experiences of transcultural nursing to the student in educational and clinical contexts.

APPENDIX 34–F
References to Support Transcultural Nursing Education and Research

BOOKS

Agar, M.H., *The professional stranger: An informal introduction to ethnography.* New York: Academic Press (1980).

Airhihenbuwa, C.O., *Health and culture: Beyond the Western paradigm.* Thousand Oaks, CA: Sage Publications (1995).

Amoss, P.T. & Harrell, S., *Other ways of growing old: An anthropological perspective.* Stanford, CA: Stanford University Press (1981).

Andrews, M. & Boyle, J., *Transcultural concepts in nursing care* (3rd edition). Philadelphia: Lippincott (1999).

Archer, D. & Gartner, R., *Violence and crime in cross-cultural perspective*. New Haven: Yale University Press (1984).

Becerra, R.M. & Shaw, D., *The elderly Hispanic: A research and reference guide*. Lanham, MD: University Press of America (1984).

Brink, P., *Transcultural nursing: A book of readings*. Englewood Cliffs, NJ: Prentice Hall (1984).

Bryant, C.A., *The cultural feast: An introduction to food and society*. St Paul, MN: West (1985).

Caddy, D., *Culture, disease, and healing: Studies in medical anthropology*. New York: Macmillan (1972).

Carnegie, M.E., *The path we tread: Blacks in nursing 1954–1984*. Philadelphia: Lippincott (1987).

Carson, V.B., *Spiritual dimensions of nursing practice*. Philadelphia: W.B. Saunders (1989).

Comas-Diaz, L. & Griffith, E.E.H., *Clinical guidelines in cross-cultural mental health*. New York: John Wiley & Sons (1988).

Davidhizar, R. & Giger, J., *Canadian transcultural nursing: Assessment and intervention*. St. Louis: Mosby (1998).

Dobson, S., *Transcultural nursing*. London: Acutari Press (1991).

Fadiman, A., *The spirit catches you and you fall down*. New York: Farrar, Strauss, and Giroux (1997).

Giger J. & Davidhizar, R., *Transcultural nursing* (2nd edition) St.Louis: Mosby, 1995.

Glittenberg, J.E. *To the mountain and back: The mysteries of Guatemalan Highland family life*. Prospect Heights, IL: Waveland Press, 1994.

Hayano, D.M., *Road through the rain forest*. Prospect Heights, IL: Waveland Press (1990).

Henderson, G., *Cultural diversity in the workplace*. Westport, CT: Praeger (1994).

Hohn, R., *Anthropology in public health: Bridging differences in culture and society*. New York: Oxford University Press (1999).

Honigmann, J., (1954). *Culture and personality*. New York: Harper & Row (1954).

Kerns, V. & Brown, J., *In her prime: New views of middle-aged women* (2nd edition). Chicago: University of Illinois Press (1992).

Kolenda, P., *Cultural constructions of women*. New York: Sheffield Publishing (1988).

Langness, L.L. & Frank G., *Lives: An anthropological approach to biography*. Novato, CA: Chandler and Sharp (1987).

Lawless, E.J., *God's peculiar people*. Lexington: University of Kentucky Press (1988).

Lefcowitz, E., *The United States immigration history timeline*. New York: Terra Firma Press (1990).

Leininger, M., *Nursing and anthropology: Two worlds to blend*. Columbus, Ohio: Greyden Press (1994). Originally published in 1970 by John Wiley & Sons, New York.

Leininger, M., *Transcultural nursing: Concepts, theories, and practices*. Columbus, OH: Greyden Press (1994). Originally published in 1970 by John Wiley & Sons, New York.

Leininger, M., *Transcultural nursing-1979*. New York: Masson Publishing (1979). This book contains the following proceedings of three National Transcultural Nursing Conferences: 1) Transcultural nursing care of infants and children, 2) Transcultural nursing care of adolescent and middle years, and 3) Transcultural nursing care of the elderly.

Leininger, M., *Qualitative research methods in nursing*. Orlando, FL: Grune & Stratton (1985). First book by nurse researchers.

Leininger, M., *Care: An essential human need*. Detroit: Wayne State University Press (1988). First published in 1981 by Slack, Inc.

Leininger, M., *Care: Discovery and uses in clinical community nursing*. Detroit: Wayne State University Press (1988).

Leininger, M., *Care: The essence of nursing and health*. Detroit: Wayne State University Press (1988). First published in 1984 by Slack, Inc.

Leininger, M., *Ethical and moral dimensions of care*. Detroit: Wayne State University Press (1990).

Leininger, M., *Culture care diversity and universality: A theory of nursing*. New York: National League for Nursing Press (1991).

Leininger, M., *Transcultural nursing: Concepts, theories, research, and practices*. New York: McGraw-Hill and Columbus, OH: Greyden Press (1995).

Leininger, M., *Transcultural nursing: Concepts, theories, and practices* (2nd edition) New York: National League for Nursing Press (1995).

Lincoln, Y. & Guba, E., *Naturalistic inquiry.* Newbury Park, CA: Sage Publications (1985).

MacElroy, A. & Townsend, P., *Medical anthropology* (2nd edition). Boulder, CO: Westview Press (1988).

Meyer, C.E., *American folk medicine.* Glenwood, IL: Meyerbooks (1985).

Micozzi, M.S., *Fundamentals of complementary and alternative medicine.* New York: Churchill Livingstone (1996).

Moore, et. al., *The biocultural basis of health* (2nd edition). St. Louis: Mosby (1990).

Morse, Janice (ed.), *Critical issues in qualitative research methods.* Beverly Hills, CA: Sage Publications (1994).

Norbeck, E. and Lock, M., *Health, illness, and medical care in Japan.* Honolulu: University of Hawaii Press (1987).

Oswalt, W., *Life cycles and lifeways: An introduction to cultural anthropology.* Palo Alto, CA: Mayfield Publishing (1986).

Overfield, T., *Biologic variations in health and illness.* New York: CRC Press (1995).

Pederson, P., *Counseling across cultures.* Honolulu: University of Hawaii Press (1986).

Rosenthal, M., *Health care in the People's Republic of China.* Boulder, CO: Westview Press (1987).

Spector, R., *Cultural diversity in health and illness* (5th edition). Norwalk, CT: Appleton & Lange (2000).

Spradley, J., *Participant observation.* New York: Holt, Rinehart, & Winston (1980).

Spradley, J., *The ethnographic interview.* New York: Holt, Rinehart, & Winston (1979).

Spradley, J.P., *You owe yourself a drink.* Boston: Little, Brown (1970).

Stewart, E. & Bennett, M., *American cultural patterns* (rev. edition). Yarmouth, ME: Intercultural Press (1991).

Strange, H., Teitelbaum, M., and contributors, *Aging and cultural diversity.* South Hadley, MA: Bergin and Garvey (1987).

Tweddell, C. & Kimball, L.A., *Introduction to the peoples and cultures of Asia.* Englewood Cliffs, NJ: Prentice Hall (1985).

Van Gennep, A., *The rites of passage.* (Translated by M.B. Vizedom & G.L. Caffee). Chicago: University of Chicago Press (1960). Originally published in 1909.

Whiting, B. & Edwards, C., *Children of different worlds: The formation of social behavior.* Cambridge: Harvard University Press (1988).

Whiting, B., *Six cultures.* New York: John Wiley & Sons (1963).

Williams, T., *Cultural anthropology.* Englewood Cliffs, NJ: Prentice Hall (1990).

Wolf, A., *Nurse's work: The sacred and the profane.* Philadelphia: University of Pennsylvania Press (1988).

World Health Organization, *The World Health Report, 1997: Conquering suffering, enriching humanity.* Geneva, Switzerland:WHO (1997).

Worsley, P.W., *The three worlds: Culture and world development.* Chicago: University of Chicago Press (1984).

Young, T., *The health of Native Americans.* New York: Oxford University Press (1994).

Zambrana, R.E., Work, family, and health: Latina women in transition. New York: Fordham University (1982).

Zborowski, M. & Horzog, E., *Life is with people.* New York: International University Press (1952).

CHAPTERS AND ARTICLES

Andrews, M., Transcultural nursing: Transforming the curriculum. *Journal of Transcultural Nursing*, 6(2), 1995, pp. 4–9.

Andrews, M., How to search for information on transcultural nursing and health subjects: Internet and CD-ROM resources. *Journal of Transcultural Nursing*, 10(1), 1999, pp. 69–74.

Baker, S.S. & Burkhalter, N.C., Teaching transcultural nursing in a transcultural setting. *Journal of Transcultural Nursing*, 7(2), 1996, pp. 10–13.

Baldonado, A., Ludwig-Beymer, P., Barnes, K., Stasiak, D., Nemivant, E.B., & Ananas-Ternate, A., Transcultural nursing practice described by registered nurses and baccalaureate nursing students. *Journal of Transcultural Nursing*, 9(2), 1998, pp. 15–25.

Barry, D. & Boyle, J., An ethnohistory of a granny midwife. *Journal of Transcultural Nursing*, 8(1), 1996, pp. 13–18.

Basuray, J., Nurse Miss Sahib: Colonial culture-bound education in India and transcultural nursing. *Journal of Transcultural Nursing*, 9(1), 1997, pp. 14–19.

Bernal, H. & Woman, R., Influences on the cultural self-efficacy of community health nurses. *Journal of Transcultural Nursing*, 4(2), 1993, pp. 24–31.

Berry, A., Mexican-American women's expressions of the meaning of culturally congruent prenatal care. *Journal of Transcultural Nursing*, 10(3), 1999, pp. 203–212.

Bodner, A. and Leininger, M., Transcultural nursing care values, beliefs, and practices of American (USA) gypsies. *Journal of Transcultural Nursing*, 4(1), 1992, 17–28.

Brink, P. & Saunders, J., Cultural shock: Theoretical and applied, in P. Brink (ed.) *Transcultural nursing: A book of readings*. Englewood Cliffs, NJ: Prentice Hall, 1976.

Burkhardt, M.A., Characteristics of spirituality in the lives of women in a rural Appalachian community. *Journal of Transcultural Nursing*, 4(2), 1993, 12–18.

Cabral, H. et al., Foreign born and United States born black women: Differences in health behaviors and birth outcomes. *The American Journal of Public Health*, 80, 1990, pp. 70–72.

Canty-Mitchell, J., The caring needs of African American male juvenile offenders. *Journal of Transcultural Nursing*, 8(1), 1996, pp. 3–12.

Carpio, B. A. & Majumdar, B., Experiential learning: An approach to transcultural education for nursing. *Journal of Transcultural Nursing*, 4(2), 1993, pp. 4–11.

Chmielarczyk, V., Transcultural nursing: Providing culturally congruent care to the Hausa of Northwest Africa. *Journal of Transcultural Nursing*, 3(1), 1991, pp. 15–20.

Chrisman, N., Cultural shock in the operating room: Cultural analysis in transcultural nursing. *Journal of Transcultural Nursing*, 1(2), 1990, pp. 33–39.

Conway, F.J. & Carmona, P.E., Cultural complexity: The hidden stressors. *Journal of Advanced Medical Surgical Nursing*, 1(4), 1989, pp. 65–72.

DeSantia, L. & Thomas, J., The immigrant Haitian mother: Transcultural nursing perspective on preventive health care for children. *Journal of Transcultural Nursing*, 5(2), 1990, pp. 38–41.

Duffy, S., Bonino, K., Gallup, L. & Pontseele, R., The community baby shower as a transcultural nursing intervention. *Journal of Transcultural Nursing*, 5(2), 1994, pp. 38–41.

Eliason, M.J., Cultural diversity in nursing care: The lesbian, gay, or bisexual client. *Journal of Transcultural Nursing*, 5(1), 1993, pp. 14–20.

Field, L., Response to published article: Nursing diagnosis. *Journal of Transcultural Nursing*, 3(1), 1991, pp. 325–330.

Finn, J. & Lee, M., Transcultural nurses reflect on discoveries in China using Leininger's Sunrise Model. *Journal of Transcultural Nursing*, 7(2), 1996, pp. 21–27.

Finn, J., A transcultural nurse's adventures in Costa Rica: Using Leininger's Sunrise Model for transcultural nursing discoveries. *Journal of Transcultural Nursing*, 5(2), 1993, pp. 25–37.

Finn, J., Leininger's model for discoveries at the farm and midwifery services to the Amish. *Journal of Transcultural Nursing*, 7(1), 1995, pp. 28–35.

Foreman, J.T., Susto and the health needs for the Cuban refugee population: Symptoms of depression and withdrawal from moral social activity. *Topics in Clinical Nursing*, 70, 1985, pp. 40–47.

Friede, A., et al., Transmission of hepatitis B virus from adopted Asian children to their American families. *American Journal of Public Health*, 78, 1988, pp. 26–30.

Frye, B.A., The Cambodian refugee patient: Providing culturally sensitive rehabilitation nursing care. *Rehabilitation Nursing*, 15(3), 1990, pp. 156–158.

Gates, M., Transcultural comparison of hospitals as caring environments for dying patients. *Journal of Transcultural Nursing*, 2(2), 1991, pp. 3–15.

George, T., Defining care in the culture of the chronically mentally ill living in the community. *Journal of Transcultural Nursing*, 11(2), 2000, pp. 102–110.

Goforth-Parker, J., The lived experience of Native Americans with diabetes within a transcultural nursing perspective. *Journal of Transcultural Nursing*, 6(1), 1994, pp. 5–11.

Haggstrum, T.M., Norberg, A., & Quang, T., Patients', relatives', nurses' experience of stroke in

Northern Vietnam. *Journal of Transcultural Nursing*, 7(1), 1995, pp. 15–23.

Higgins, B., Puerto Rican cultural beliefs: Influence on infant feeding practices in Western New York. *Journal of Transcultural Nursing*, 11(1), 2000, pp. 19–30.

Hilger, M., Field guide to ethnological study of child life. *Human Relations Area Files: Behavior Science Field Guides*, New Haven, CT, 1960.

Hobus, R., Living in two worlds: A Lakota transcultural nursing experience. *Journal of Transcultural Nursing*, 2(1), 1990, pp. 33–36.

Horn, B., Cultural concepts and postpartal care. *Journal of Transcultural Nursing*, 2(1), 1990, pp. 48–51.

Huttlinger, K. & Wiebe, P., Transcultural nursing care: Achieving understanding in a practice setting. *Journal of Transcultural Nursing*, 1(1), 1989, pp. 17–21.

Huttlinger, K.W. & Tanner, D., The Peyote way: Implications for culture care theory. *Journal of Transcultural Nursing*, 5(2), 1994, pp. 5–11.

Jeffreys, S. & O'Donnell, M., Cultural discovery: An innovative philosophy for creative learning activities. *Journal of Transcultural Nursing*, 8(2), 1997, pp. 17–22.

Kalnins, Z., Nursing in Latvia from the perspective of the oppressed theory. *Journal of Transcultural Nursing*, 4(1), 1992, pp. 11–16.

Kavanaugh, K., Transcultural nursing: Facing the challenges of advocacy and diversity/universality. *Journal of Transcultural Nursing*, 5(1), 1993, pp. 4–13.

Kelley, J. & Frisch, N., Use of selected nursing diagnoses: A transcultural comparison between Mexican and American nurses. *Journal of Transcultural Nursing*, 4(1), 1990, pp. 29–36.

Kendall, K., Maternal and child care in an Iranian village. *Journal of Transcultural Nursing*, 2(1), 1992, pp. 2–15.

Kirkpatrick, S. & Cobb, A., Health beliefs related to diarrhea in Haitian children: Building transcultural nursing knowledge. *Journal of Transcultural Nursing*, 1(2), 1990, pp. 2–12.

Lawson, L.V., Culturally sensitive support for grieving parents. *American Journal of*

Maternal Child Rearing, 15(2), 1990, pp. 76–79.

Leininger, M., Transcultural care principles, human rights, and ethical considerations. *Journal of Transcultural Nursing*, 3(1), 1991, pp. 21–24.

Leininger, M., Current issues, problems, and trends to advance qualitative paradigmatic research methods for the future. *Qualitative Health Research*, 2(4), 1992, pp. 392–414.

Leininger, M., Nursing care of a patient from another culture: A Japanese-American patient. *Nursing Clinics of North America*, 2, 1967, pp. 747–762.

Leininger, M., The culture concept and its relevance to nursing. *The Journal of Nursing Education*, 6(2), 1997, pp. 27–39.

Leininger, M., Cultural differences among staff members and the impact on patient care. *Minnesota League of Nursing Bulletin*, 16(5), 1968, pp. 5–9.

Leininger, M., Ethnoscience: A new and promising research approach for the health sciences. *Image: The Journal of Nursing Scholarship*, 3(1), 1969, pp. 2–8.

Leininger, M., Some cross cultural universal and non-universal functions, beliefs, and practices of food. *Dimensions of Nutrition. Proceedings of the Colorado Dietetic Association Conference.* Fort Collins, CO: Colorado Associated Universities Press, 1970.

Leininger, M., Anthropological approach to adaptation: Case studies from nursing. In *Theoretical Issues in Professional Nursing.* New York: Appleton-Century-Crofts (1971).

Leininger, M., An open health care system model. *Nursing Outlook*, 21(3), 1973, pp. 171–175.

Leininger, M., Anthropological issues related to community mental health programs in the United States. *Community Mental Health Journal*, 7(1), 1973, pp. 50–62.

Leininger, M., Becoming aware of health practitioners and cultural imposition. *American Nurses' Association 48th Annual Convention Proceedings*, 1973, pp. 9–15.

Leininger, M., Nursing in the context of social and cultural systems. In *Concepts Basic to Nursing.* New York: McGraw-Hill (1973), pp. 34–45.

Leininger, M., Witchcraft practices and psychocultural therapy with urban United States families. *Human Organization*, 32(1), 1973, pp. 73–83.

Leininger, M., Humanism, health, and cultural values. In M. Leininger (ed.), *Health Care Issues*. Philadelphia: F.A. Davis, 1974, pp. 37–60.

Leininger, M., Cultural interfaces, communication, and health implications. In *An Adventure in Transcultural Communication and Health (Proceedings of Continuing Education Interdisciplinary Health Professional Workshop, 1974)*. Honolulu: University of Hawaii Press (1976).

Leininger, M., Transcultural nursing: A promising subfield of study for nurse educators and practitioners. In *Current Practice in Family Centered Community Nursing*. St. Louis: Mosby (1976).

Leininger, M., Two strange health tribes: The Gnisrun and Enicidem in the United States. *Human Organization*, 35(3), 1976, pp. 253–261. (See updated chapter in this book.)

Leininger, M., Cultural diversities of health and nursing care. In H. Dietz (ed.) *Nursing Clinics of North America*. Philadelphia: W. B. Saunders, 1977, pp. 5–18.

Leininger, M., Culture and transcultural nursing: Meaning and significance for nurses. In *Cultural Dimensions in Nursing Curriculum (Proceedings of NLN Workshop)*. New York: National League for Nursing Press, 1977.

Leininger, M., Transcultural nursing: Its progress and its future. *Nursing and Health Care*, 2(7), 1981, pp. 365–371.

Leininger, M., Cultural care: An essential goal for nursing and health care. *The American Association of Nephrology Nurses and Technicians (AANNT) Journal*, 10(5), 1983, pp. 11–17.

Leininger, M., Transcultural nursing: An overview. *Nursing Outlook*, 32(2), 1984, pp. 72–73.

Leininger, M., Care facilitation and resistance factors in the culture of nursing. In Z. Wolf (ed.), *Clinical Care in Nursing*. Rockville, MD: Aspen Publications (1986).

Leininger, M., Leininger's theory of nursing: Culture care diversity and universality. *Nursing Science Quarterly*, 2(4), 1988, pp. 152–160.

Leininger, M., Transcultural nurse specialists and generalists: New practitioners in nursing. *Journal of Transcultural Nursing*, 1(1), 1989, pp. 4–16.

Leininger, M., Transcultural nurse specialists: Imperative in today's world. *Nursing and Health Care*, 10(5), 1989, pp. 250–256.

Leininger, M., Transcultural nursing: Quo vadis (Where goeth the field)? *Journal of Transcultural Nursing*, 1(1), 1989, pp. 33–45.

Leininger, M., Ethnomethods: The philosophic and epistemic bases to explicate transcultural nursing knowledge. *Journal of Transcultural Nursing*, 1(2), 1990, pp. 40–51.

Leininger, M., Issues, questions, and concerns related to the nursing diagnosis cultural movement from a transcultural nursing perspective. *Journal of Transcultural Nursing*, 2(1), 1990, pp. 23–32.

Leininger, M., The significance of cultural concepts in nursing. *Journal of Transcultural Nursing*, 2(1), 1990, pp. 52–59.

Leininger, M., Becoming aware of types of health practitioners and cultural imposition. *Journal of Transcultural Nursing*, 2(2), 1991, pp. 32–39.

Leininger, M., Culture care of the Gadsup Akuna of the Eastern Highlands of New Guinea. In M. Leininger (ed.) *Culture care diversity and universality: A theory of nursing*. New York: National League for Nursing Press (1991), pp. 231–280.

Leininger, M., The transcultural nurse specialist: Imperative in today's world. *Perspectives in Family and Community Health*, 17, 1991, pp. 137–144.

Leininger, M., Transcultural nursing. *Pride,* A Kaiser Permanente Publication. Van Nuys, CA: Communication Press (1991).

Leininger, M., Reflection: The need for transcultural nursing. *Second Opinion, April*, 1992, pp. 83–85.

Leininger, M., Quality of life from a transcultural nursing perspective. *Nursing Science Quarterly*, 7(1), 1993, pp. 22–28.

Leininger, M., Evaluation criteria and critique of qualitative research studies. In J. Morse (ed.) *Qualitative nursing research: A contemporary dialogue*. Newbury Park, CA: Sage Publications (1993), pp. 392–414.

Leininger, M., Gadsup of Papua New Guinea revisited: A three decades view. *Journal of Transcultural Nursing*, 5(1), 1993, pp. 21–30.

Leininger, M., Towards conceptualization of transcultural health care systems: Concepts and a model. *Journal of Transcultural Nursing*, 4(2), 1993, pp. 32–40. (Originally published in M. Leininger (ed.), *Health care dimensions.* Philadelphia: F. A. Davis (1976).

Leininger, M., The tribes of nursing in the USA culture of nursing. *Journal of Transcultural Nursing*, 6(1), 1994, pp. 18–23.

Leininger, M., Are nurses prepared to function worldwide? *Journal of Transcultural Nursing,* 5(2), 1994, pp. 2–5.

Leininger, M., Nursing's agenda of health care reform: Regressive or advanced discipline status. *Nursing Science Quarterly*, 7(2), 1994, pp. 93–94.

Leininger, M., Teaching and learning transcultural nursing. In G. Mashaba and H. Brink (eds.), *Nursing education: An international perspective.* Kenwyn, South Africa: Juta & Co. (1994).

Leininger, M., Time to celebrate and reflect on progress with transcultural nursing. *Journal of Transcultural Nursing*, 6(1), 1994, pp. 2–4.

Leininger, M., Transcultural nursing education: A worldwide imperative. *Nursing and Health Care*, 15(5), May 1994, pp. 254–257.

Leininger, M., Reflections: Culturally congruent care: Visible and invisible. *Journal of Transcultural Nursing*, 6(1), 1994, pp. 23–25.

Leininger, M., Editorial: Teaching transcultural nursing to transform nursing in the 21st century. *Journal of Transcultural Nursing*, 6(2), 1995, pp. 2–3.

Leininger, M., Editorial: Time to celebrate and reflect on progress with transcultural nursing. *Journal of Transcultural Nursing*, 6(1), 1995, pp. 2–3.

Leininger, M., Founder's Focus: Nursing theories and cultures: Fit or misfit? *Journal of Transcultural Nursing*, 7(1), 1995, pp. 41–42.

Leininger, M., Teaching transcultural nursing in undergraduate and graduate programs. *Journal of Transcultural Nursing*, 6(2), 1995, pp. 10–21.

Leininger, M., Transcultural nursing: Meaning, relevance, and concerns in a world without boundaries. *Asian Journal of Nursing Science*, 2(4), 1995, pp. 26–34.

Leininger, M. & Cummings, S.H., Nursing's new paradigm is transcultural nursing: An interview with Madeleine Leininger. *Advance Practice Quarterly*, 2(2), 1996, pp. 62–69.

Leininger, M., Quality of life from a transcultural nursing perspective. *Nursing Science Quarterly*, 9(2), 1996, pp. 71–78.

Leininger, M., Founder's Focus: Transcultural nurses and consumers tell their stories. *Journal of Transcultural Nursing*, 7(2), 1996, pp. 32–36.

Leininger, M., Founder's Focus: Transcultural nursing administration: What is it? *Journal of Transcultural Nursing*, 8(1), 1996, pp. 28–33.

Leininger, M., Major directions for transcultural nursing: A journey into the 21st century (keynote address from the 21st Annual Transcultural Nursing Society Conference). *Journal of Transcultural Nursing*, 7(2), 1996, pp. 28–31.

Leininger, M., Founder's Focus: Alternative to what? Generic vs. professional caring, treatments, and healing modes. *Journal of Transcultural Nursing*, 9(1), 1997, pp. 37.

Leininger, M., Founder's Focus: Transcultural nursing: A scientific and humanistic care discipline. *Journal of Transcultural Nursing*, 8(2), 1997, pp. 54–55.

Leininger, M., Overview and reflection of the theory of Culture Care and the ethnonursing research method. *Journal of Transcultural Nursing*, 8(2), 1997, pp. 32–51.

Leininger, M., Understanding cultural pain for improved health care. *Journal of Transcultural Nursing*, 9(1), 1997, pp. 32–35.

Leininger, M., Transcultural spirituality: A comparative care and health focus. In M.S. Roach, *Caring from the heart.* New Jersey: Paulist Press (1997).

Leininger, M., Transcultural nursing research to transform nursing education and practice: 40 years. *Image: Journal of Nursing Scholarship*, 29(4), 1997, pp. 341–347.

Leininger, M., Ethnonursing research method: Essential to discover and advance Asian nursing knowledge. *Japanese Journal of Nursing Research*, 8(2), 1997, pp. 20–32.

Leininger, M., Transcultural nursing as a global care humanizer, diversifier, and unifier. *Hoitotiede*, 9(514), 1997, pp. 219–225.

Leininger, M., Future directions in transcultural nursing in 21st century. *International Nursing Review*, 44(1), 1997, pp. 19–23.

Leininger, M., Special research report: Dominant culture care (emic) meanings and practice findings from Leininger's theory. *Journal of Transcultural Nursing*, 9(2), 1998, pp. 44–47.

Leininger, M. (1999). Response to commentaries on defining transcultural nursing. *Journal of Transcultural Nursing*, 10(3), 1999, pp. 187.

Leininger, M., What is transcultural nursing and culturally competent care? *Journal of Transcultural Nursing*, 10(1), 1999, pp. 9.

Leininger, M., Founder's Focus: Multidiscipline transculturalism and transcultural nursing. *Journal of Transcultural Nursing*, 11(3), 2000, pg. 147.

Leininger, M., Founder's Focus: Transcultural nursing is discovery of self and the world of others. *Journal of Transcultural Nursing*, 11(4), 2000, pp. 312–313.

Leininger, M., Founder's Focus: Theoretical research and clinical critiques to advance transcultural nursing scholarship. *Journal of Transcultural Nursing*, 12(1), 2001, p. 71.

Leininger, M., Transcultural nursing presents an exciting challenge. *The American Nurse*, 5(5), 1974, p. 4.

Leininger, M., Transcultural nursing care in the community. In K. Lundy and S. Janes, *Community health nursing: Caring for the public's health*, Sudbury, Mass: Jones and Bartlett (2001), pp. 218–234.

Ludwig-Beymer, P., From a practice perspective. *Journal of Transcultural Nursing*, 10(3), 1999, pp. 186.

Ludwig-Beymer, P., Transcultural nursing's role in a managed care environment. *Journal of Transcultural Nursing*, 10(4), 1999, pp. 286–287.

Ludwig-Beymer, P., Blankemeier, J., Casas-Byots, C., & Suarez-Balcazar, Y., Community assessment in suburban Hispanic community: A description of method. *Journal of Transcultural Nursing*, 8(1), 1996, pp. 19–27.

Luna, L., Transcultural nursing and Arab Muslims. *Journal of Transcultural Nursing*, 6(1), 1989, pp. 22–23.

Luna, L., Transcultural nursing care of Arab Muslims. *Journal of Transcultural Nursing*, 1(1), 1989, pp. 22–26.

Luna, L., Care and cultural context of Lebanese Muslim immigrants with Leininger's theory. *Journal of Transcultural Nursing*, 5(2), 1994, pp. 12–20.

Luna, L., Culturally competent health care: A challenge for nurses in Saudi Arabia. *Journal of Transcultural Nursing*, 9(2), 1998, pp. 8–14.

MacNeil, J., Use of Culture Care Theory with Baganda women as AIDS caregivers. *Journal of Transcultural Nursing*, 7(2), 1996, pp. 14–20.

Masipa, A., Transcultural nursing in South Africa: Prospects for the 1900s. *Journal of Transcultural Nursing*, 3(1), 1991, p. 34.

McCreary, J.A., The culture of the deaf. *Journal of Transcultural Nursing*, 10(4), 1999, pp. 350–357.

McFarland, M., Editorial: A focus on implementation of transcultural nursing practice. *Journal of Transcultural Nursing*, 7(2), 1996, p. 2.

McFarland, M., Editorial: The concept of culture and the TCN perspective. *Journal of Transcultural Nursing*, 8(1), 1996, p. 2.

McFarland, M., Editorial: Transcultural nursing care of the elderly is a worldwide imperative. *Journal of Transcultural Nursing*, 8(2), 1997, pp. 2–4.

McKenna, M., Twice in need of care: A transcultural nursing analysis of elderly Mexican Americans. *Journal of Transcultural Nursing*, 1(1), 1989, 46–52.

Mead M., Understanding cultural patterns. *Nursing Outlook* 4, 1956, pp. 260–262.

Morgan, M., Pregnancy and childbirth beliefs and practices of American Hare Krishna devotees within transcultural nursing. *Journal of Transcultural Nursing*, 4(1), 1992, pp. 46–52.

Morgan, M., Prenatal care of African American women in selected USA urban and rural cultural contexts. *Journal of Transcultural Nursing*, 7(2), 1996, pp. 3–9.

Muecke, M. & Srisuphan, W., From women in white to scholarship: The new nurse leaders in Thailand. *Journal of Transcultural Nursing*, 1(2), 1990, pp. 21–32.

Nikkonen, M., Changes in psychiatric caring values in Finland. *Journal of Transcultural Nursing*, 6(1), 1994, pp. 12–17.

Omeri, A. & Ahern, M., Utilizing culturally congruent strategies to enhance recruitment and retention of

Australian indigenous nursing students. *Journal of Transcultural Nursing*, 10(2), 1999, pp. 150–155.

Omeri, A., Culture care of Iranian immigrants in New South Wales, Australia: Sharing transcultural nursing knowledge. *Journal of Transcultural Nursing*, 8(2), 1997, pp. 5–16.

Oneha, M.V. & Magyarry, D.L., Transcultural nursing considerations of child abuse/maltreatment in American Samoa and Federated States Micronesia. *Journal of Transcultural Nursing*, 4(2), 1992, pp. 11–17.

Osborne, O.H., Anthropology and nursing: Some common traditions and interests. *Nursing Research*, 18(3), 1969, pp. 251–255.

Pasquale, E.A. The evil eye phenomenon: Its implications for community health nursing. *Home Health Care Nurse*, 2(30), 19–21.

Phillips, S. & Lobar, S., Literature summary of some Navajo child health beliefs and rearing practices within a transcultural nursing framework. *Journal of Transcultural Nursing*, 1(2), 1990, pp. 13–20.

Pickwell, S., The incorporation of family care for Southeast Asian refugees in a community based mental health facility. *Archives of Psychiatric Nursing*, 3(3), 1989, pp. 173–177.

Presswalla, J.L., Insights into Eastern health care: Some transcultural nursing perspectives. *Journal of Transcultural Nursing*, 5(2), 1994, pp. 21–24.

Ray, M., The development of a classification system of institutional caring. In M. Leininger (ed.), *Care: The essence of nursing and health*. Detroit: Wayne State University Press (1988), pp. 93–112.

Ray, M., Political and economic visions. *Journal of Transcultural Nursing*, 1(1), 1989, pp. 17–21.

Reeb, R.M., Granny midwives in Mississippi: A mini ethnonursing study. *Journal of Transcultural Nursing*, 4(2), 1992, pp. 18–27.

Reinert, B.R., The health care beliefs and values of Mexican Americans. *Home Health Care Nurse*, 4(5), 1986, pp. 23, 26–27.

Rosenbaum, J., Cultural care of older Greek Canadian widows within Leininger's theory of Culture Care. *Journal of Transcultural Nursing*, 2(1), 1990, pp. 37–47.

Ross, J.E., Providing health care for Southeast Asian refugees. *Journal of the New York State Nurses' Association*, 20(2), 1989.

Sevcovic, L., Health care for mothers and children in an Indian culture. In *Family Centered Community Nursing*. St. Louis: Mosby (1973).

Smith, D.L., Aspects of the ethnoscience approach to the study of values and needs as perceived by the North American Indian woman in relation to pre-natal care. (Unpublished Master's thesis, University of Washington, Seattle, 1971.)

Smith, S.E., Increasing transcultural awareness: The McMaster-Aga Khan-CIDA Project workshop model. *Journal of Transcultural Nursing*, 8(2), 1997, pp. 23–31.

Sobralske, M.D., Perceptions of health: Navajo Indians. *Topics in Clinical Nursing*, 7(3), 1985, pp. 32–39.

Sohier, R., Gaining awareness of cultural differences: A case example. In M. Leininger (ed.), *Transcultural health care issues and conditions*. Philadelphia: F.A. Davis (1976).

Spangler, Z., Transcultural nursing care values and caregiving practices of Philippine American nurses. *Journal of Transcultural Nursing*, 4(2), 1992, pp. 28–37.

Spector, R., Culture, ethnicity, and nursing. In Potter, P.A. and Perry, A.G. (eds.), *Fundamentals of nursing* (3rd edition). St. Louis: Mosby Yearbook, 1993, pp. 95–116.

Thomas, J.T. & DeSantis, L., Feeding and weaning practices of Cuban and Haitian immigrant mothers. *Journal of Transcultural Nursing*, 6(2), 1995, pp. 34–42.

Tripp-Reimer, T., Cross cultural perspectives on patient teaching. *Nursing Clinics of North America*, 24(3), 1989, pp. 613–619.

Valente, S.M., Overcoming cultural barriers. *California Nurses*, 85(8), 1989, pp. 4–5.

Villarruel, A.M. & Ortis de Montellano, B., Culture and pain: A Meso-American perspective. *Advances in Nursing Science*, 15(1), 1992, pp. 21–32.

Wallace, G., Spiritual care: A reality in nursing education and practice. *The Nurses Lamp*, 21(2), 1979, pp. 1–4.

Wenger, A.F. & Wenger, M., Community and family care patterns of the Old Order Amish. In M. Leininger (ed.), *Care: Discovery and use in clinical community nursing*. Detroit: Wayne State University Press (1988).

Wenger, A.F., Role in context in culture specific care. In L. Chinn (ed.), *Anthology of caring*. New York: National League for Nursing Press (1991), pp. 95–110.

Wenger, A.F., Transcultural Nursing and health care issues in urban and rural contexts. *Journal of Transcultural Nursing*, 4(2), 1992, pp. 4–10.

Wenger, A.F., Cultural context, health, and health care decision making. *Journal of Transcultural Nursing*, 7(1), 1995, pp. 3–14.

Wuest, J., Harmonizing: A North American Indian approach to management for middle ear disease with transcultural nursing implications. *Journal of Transcultural Nursing*, 3(1), 1991, pp. 5–14.

Zborowski, M., Cultural components in response to pain. *Journal of Social Issues*, 8(4), 1952, pp. 16–30.

CLASSIC CULTURE AREA WORKS OF ANTHROPOLOGISTS & SOCIAL SCIENTISTS

Adair, J. & Deuschle, K.W., *The people's health*. New York: Appleton Century Crofts (1970).

Arsensberg, C., *The Irish countrymen*. Garden City, NJ: The Natural History Press (1968).

Benet, S., *Abkhasians: The long living people of the Caucasus*. New York: Holt, Rinehart, and Winston (1974).

Benedict, R., *The chrysanthemum and the sword*. Boston: Boston Press (1956).

Benedict, R., *Patterns of culture*. Boston: Boston Press (1934).

Clark, M., *Health in the Mexican American culture*. Berkeley, CA: University of California Press (1970).

Friedl, E., *Vasilika: A village in modern Greece*. New York: Holt, Rinehart, Winston (1962).

Gans, H.V., *The urban villagers: Group and class in the life of Italian Americans*. New York: The Free Press (1962).

Goodman, M.E., *The culture of childhood*. New York: Teachers College Press (1970).

Gorer, G. & Rickman, J., *The people of Great Russia: A psychological study*. London: Cresset Press (1949).

Hsu, F.L.K., *Americans and Chinese: Two ways of life*. New York: Schuman (1953).

Kiev, A., *Curanderismo: Mexican American folk psychiatry*. New York: The Free Press (1968).

Leacock, E.B., *The culture of poverty: A critique*. New York: Simon & Schuster (1971).

Leininger, M., A Gadsup village experiences its first election. *The Journal of Polynesian Society,* 73(2), 1964, pp. 29–34.

Leininger, M., The Gadsup of New Guinea and early child caring behaviors with nursing care implications. In M. Leininger (ed.), *Transcultural nursing: Concepts, theories and practices*. New York: John Wiley & Sons (1978), pp. 375–398.

Lewis, O., *The children of Sanchez*. New York: Holt, Rinehart, & Winston (1961).

Lewis, O., The culture of poverty. *Scientific American*, 215(4), 1962, pp. 19–25.

Linton, R., *The study of man*. New York: Appleton Century (1936).

Lowie, R.H., *The German people: A social portrait to 1914*. New York: Farrar & Rinehart (1945).

Maclachan, J.M., Cultural factors in health and disease. In E. Gartly Faco (ed.), *Patient, physicians, and illness*. Illinois: Glenco Press (1958).

Mead, M., *Coming of age in Samoa*. New York: New American Library (1929).

Mead, M., *Sex temperament in three primitive societies*. New York: New American Library (1935).

Mead, M., *New lives for old*. New York: Morrow (1956).

Minturn, L. & Lambert, W. W., *Mothers of six cultures*. New York: John Wiley & Sons (1964).

Obeyesekere, G., Pregnancy cravings in relation to social structure and personality in a Sinhalese village. *American Anthropologist*, 65, 1963, pp. 323–341.

Oliver, D., *The Pacific Islands* (3rd edition). Honolulu: University of Hawaii Press (1989).

Paul, B. D., *Health, culture, and community: Case studies of public relations to health programs*. New York: Russell Sage Foundation (1955).

Read, K.E., *The high valley*. New York: Scribners (1965).

Redfield, R., *The little community*. Chicago: University of Chicago Press (1955).

Rebel A.J., Concepts of disease in Mexican American culture. *American Anthropologist*, 62, 1960, pp. 795–814.

Snow, L.F., *Walkin' over medicine*. Boulder, CO: Westview Press (1993).

Spicer, E.H., *Human problems in technological change: A case book*. New York: Russell Sage Foundation (1952).

Spiro, M., *Children of the kibbutz*. New York: Schocken Press (1963).

Stack C., *All our kin: Strategies for survival in a black community*. New York: Harper & Row (1975).

Strutevant, W.C., Studies in ethnoscience. *American Anthropologist*, 66(2), 99–131, 1964.

Thomas, W.L. & Znaniecki, F., *The Polish peasant in Europe and America*. Chicago: University of Chicago Press (1918).

Wallace, A.F., *Culture and personality*. New York: Random House (1970).

Whiting, B., *Six cultures: Studies of child rearing*. New York: John Wiley & Sons (1963).

Whiting, J.W. & Child, I.L., *Child training and personality*. New Haven: Yale University Press (1953).

SELECTED TRANSCULTURAL NURSING AUDIO-VISUALS

Leininger, M., Andrews, M., & McFarland, M., *Transcultural Nursing: Transforming the Profession*. Livonia, MI: Madonna University Audio-Visual Department (34 min. color), 1994.

Leininger, M., Gaut, M., & MacDonald, M. *Human Caring*. Livonia, MI: Madonna University Audio-Visual Department,. (38 min. color), 1994.

Bloch, C. & Bloch, C., *Transcultural Nursing Video*. Produced by Education and Consulting Services, Los Angeles County and University of California Medical Center, 1993.

Leininger, M., *Transcultural Nursing: Discovery and Challenges* (with A. Kulwicki and K. Edmunds), recorded for Madonna Magazine. Livonia, MI: Madonna University, 1992.

Leininger, M., *Leininger's Theory for Cultural Care: Diversity and Universality*. Livonia, MI: Madonna University Audio Visual Department (50 min. color), 1990.

Leininger, M. & Stasiak, D., *Cultural Assessment of American Polish Informant*, Livonia, MI: Madonna University Audio Visual Department (50 min. color), 1990. Available from Insight Media, 2162 Broadway, New York, NY 10024. Phone: 212-721-6313; fax: 917-441-3194.

Leininger, M., *Leininger's Culture Care Theory, Portraits of Excellence of Theorist*. Oakland, CA: ABC Studio, under Dr. David Wallace, (45 min. color), 1989.

Leininger, M., *Care: The Essence of Nursing and Health*. St. Louis, MO: St. Louis University Educational Satellite (40 min. color), 1984.

Leininger, M., *Transcultural Nursing*, St. Louis University, St. Louis, MO: Educational Satellite (30 min. color), 1984.

Leininger, M., *Arab Americans: Cultural Care*. Detroit, MI: Wayne State University (35 min. color), 1983 (available only from the author).

Leininger, M., *Philippine Americans: Culture Care*. Detroit, MI: Wayne State University (40 min. color), 1983 (available only from the author).

Leininger, M., *Polish Americans: Culture Care*. Detroit, MI: Wayne State University (45min. color.), 1983 (available only from the author).

Leininger, M. *Transcultural Nursing: Discovery and Challenges*, 1992.

The Nurse Theorists: Portraits of Excellence—Madeleine Leininger: Transcultural Nursing Care (CD-ROM). FITNE, Inc.,1997.

35

Transcultural Nursing Administration and Consultation

Madeleine Leininger

Knowledgeable and creative ways to provide consultation and administer health care to the culturally different can greatly facilitate human health care services with positive feedback.

As the philosophy, knowledge, and practices of transcultural nursing become an integral part of one's thinking and action modes, transcultural nursing administration and consultation will, of necessity, change to respond appropriately to people and systems of different cultures. To be effective, nurses, physicians, and other health professionals must realize that their administrative and consultation practices need to fit individuals, groups, organizations, and institutions being served. In many respects, while both administration and consultation have different purposes, they are often closely linked together to reinforce similar endeavors. Both administration and consultation can have a profound effect on health care and human services.

In this chapter a brief overview of transcultural nursing administration and consultation will be defined and discussed with a focus on their importance to globalization or particularization of health care. A few transcultural nursing administration and consultation trends, issues, and virtual-reality situations will be identified and briefly discussed. Most importantly, the Theory of Culture Care Diversity and Universality will be used to help the reader realize how valuable and meaningful the theory can be when used for transcultural nursing administration and consultation.

■ Definitions

In general, *transcultural nursing administration refers to the creative and knowledgeable process of assess-ing, planning, and making decisions and policies that will facilitate educational and clinical service goals that take into account cultural caring values, beliefs, symbols, and lifeways of people of diverse and similar cultures for beneficial outcomes.* Effective transcultural nursing administration demonstrates ways of being attentive to different cultural values, beliefs, and lifeways of people while pursuing desired or necessary goals of an institution or service system. A competent transcultural administrator is expected to assess and tailor one's decisions, leadership, policies, and actions so that they reasonably fit the institution and are not offensive and destructive or in great conflict with desired outcomes.[1,2] Transcultural nurse administrators must remain aware that there are diverse cultures when serving people such as the cultures of nursing, hospitals, medicine, and other disciplines, as well as many cultures in the community or region in which one functions. These diverse cultures and subcultures influence administrative, educational, and clinical policies, decisions, and actions. In addition, there are cultural resources to be assessed and considered in arriving at meaningful and appropriate transcultural care administration. Comparative transcultural nursing perspectives in education and clinical services are essential for administrators to use in arriving at sensitive, meaningful, and effective ways to serve or assist human beings.

Considering *transcultural nursing consultation, it refers to the role of an expert well prepared in transcultural nursing and human relationships to assess and offer guidance to individuals, groups, or organizations according to identified desired goals or outcomes.* Transcultural nursing consultation requires a high degree of sensitivity, knowledge, and people competencies. Only recently have nurse administrators and others realized the importance and need for knowledgeable and competent transcultural nursing administrators and consultants to work with diverse cultures over a short or long period.[3] Today and in the future, nurses are challenged to develop and practice transcultural nursing administration and consultation with many diverse cultures in different places in the world and in different work contexts. Transcultural nursing knowledge and skills are essential to communicate, understand, and interact effectively with diverse cultures in clinical, academic, or other settings or institutions. Transcultural nursing administration has become *imperative* to enter and remain in the world of human beings who have different cultural care values, beliefs, and practices that need to be respected and understood for effective outcomes. More and more, a great diversity of human beings are employed or functioning in any typical organization, which challenges administrators to make thoughtful assessments and decisions that are helpful to people and the institution. With the current use of mechanistic and electronic modes of communication and often impersonal tendencies to relate to people, transcultural knowledge, advice, and competencies are extremely important for successful outcomes. In addition, the trend toward global marketing of transcultural services and education makes transcultural knowledge and strategies essential in diverse cultures.

■ Transcultural Knowledge Base

It was in the mid 1950s when I predicted that *all* nurses and health care providers will need to be responsive to people of diverse cultures, but this trend has been slow to take hold until recently.[4] Cultural conflicts, clashes, and tensions among and between staff and especially with nurses and health professionals from diverse world cultures have been evident since World War II, but quite limitedly addressed until recently.[5–8] Nursing administration and education has long needed to become transculturally based with substantive knowledge to respond to growing and conflicting areas related to multicultural practices. Still today, some nurses function in administration and academic institutions without transcultural preparation despite the need to function and understand students, faculty, clients, and staff from diverse cultures in the workplace. Some academic and clinical administrators still rely on a dominant unicultural stance with values, policies, and practices that lead to discrimination, racism, and other problems. There are, however, many rich opportunities for incorporating the talents and values of culturally diverse staff and other people that are often not recognized nor used. Likewise, some nurse consultants remain focused on their dominant unicultural norms and practices to assist people in different countries, despite diverse educational and service institutional needs within a country. Moving nurse administrators and consultants beyond their usual "cultural comfort zone" to accommodate or respond to multicultural needs has been difficult and often met with resistance. Hence, a major and serious deficit exists to make transcultural administration philosophy, practices, and goals an integral part of nursing, administration and consultation.

In the future, academic and clinical nursing service administrators and consultants will be expected to have graduate preparation in transcultural nursing knowledge and competencies to function effectively, successfully, and without racism or discrimination in their work. This will also be necessary to help them grow, expand, and enrich their professional work. Currently, there are less than 1% of doctoral programs and approximately 18% master's degree nursing programs in the United States offering graduate preparation explicitly focused on transcultural nursing administration and consultation, and even less in other countries.[9,10] Currently, many Western nurse administrators and consultants are focused on preparing nurse practitioners, to show cost-benefits and evidence-based outcomes in education and practice. They are also focused on mastering high technologies and electronic communication modes such as the internet for local and distance learning and practices. USA administrators are also focused on managed care in health systems for cost-control practices with nurse practitioners. Nurse administrators and staff prepared in transcultural nursing practices can reduce health costs and expedite consumer recovery and well-being when they provide culturally congruent care. More and more health consumers expect that their health care services and education will become transculturally based to meet their health care expectations and needs in their immediate and growing multicultural world. Also, there are many additional reasons why transcultural nursing needs to be used in nursing administration, some of which have already been discussed in earlier chapters, as well as in other literature sources.

■ Fears and Concerns

Where transcultural nursing administration and consultation have become an integral part of nurses' practices, one will find many benefits and quality-based consumer care in hospitals and community services. Moreover, academic nurse administrators find that they can become confident and able to guide faculty and students with a rapidly growing diverse student population in schools of nursing worldwide. Likewise, nurse consultants who are transculturally grounded discover many new and different ways to help people in education and clinical services. Their services are rewarding to witness with consultees in diverse countries and locally, but there are nurses who fear making changes to accommodate cultural differences or to change attitudes about cultures. These positions are not helpful in nursing education and clinical services and need to be recognized and dealt with to prevent discrimination problems and legal suits. Some administrators fear great chaos will occur with cultural changes and they avoid changes. There is also the unspoken fear that if nurse administrators use transcultural nursing principles, practices, and approaches, they will not be able to control or maintain past policies and practices that they treasure.[11] Some nurse administrators have said that they fear changing to transcultural practices because the medical staff, hospital administrators, and others with whom they work will not accept such changes. They feel it is better to maintain the status quo and please the medical staff and "not rock the boat." These administrators are eager to maintain familiar professional and social ties with colleagues or associates for political reasons.

Amid these attitudes and actions, there are silent ethical and moral voices among academic and service nursing administrators and consultants who recognize the great need for changes to provide cultural diversity education and practices. Some astute nurses have had experiences with cultures in their work or by visiting a country on special assignments, and they clearly see the need for formal preparation in transcultural nursing. It is also interesting that nurse administrators who have degrees in business management, finance, and administration seldom learn about diverse cultures and how to work with diversity factors or how to establish transcultural nursing policies and practices. These nurses often become the leaders and policy-makers in academic and service administration by virtue of being prepared in business and finance. So while some nurse administrators and consultants are realizing the need to shift from unicultural to transcultural nursing, far too few nurse administrators are using transcultural nursing knowledge and skills.

During the past decade there has been an urgent need among academic nurse administrators and some service leaders to establish "international educational exchanges" in a number of foreign countries for students, faculty, and clinicians.[12] Some of these educational and service exchanges have revealed a great need for preparation in transcultural nursing as a result of some unfavorable and negative foreign-exchange outcomes with these students, faculty, and practitioners.[13] Indeed, with many of these exchanges, students, faculty, or clinicians have generally had very limited to no preparation in transcultural nursing or comparative anthropological and social science knowledge to understand cultures and benefit from the so-called exchanges. Many perceptive participants contend they are not truly exchanges but more cultural imposition practices. The current trend is that Western academic nurse administrators and faculty seem driven to get as many international connections, exchanges, and placements for students and faculty as possible, but they fail to prepare students and faculty for meaningful outcomes. However, nursing consultants, faculty, and students who have had preparation in transcultural nursing and mentored transnational experiences abroad are quick to see the importance of prior preparation to make sense out of what they saw or experienced. These nurses use transcultural nursing concepts, practices, and principles to guide their experiences generally and positive outcomes. In general, there is a lack of transcultural nursing knowledge with limitedly prepared nurse faculty, administrators, and consultants in foreign countries. This problem needs to be addressed soon to prevent ongoing and future cultural clashes and "cultural backlash" problems.

 ## Cultural Imperialism

Still another area of concern is about Western nurse consultants, educators, and administrators being especially aware of imposing their "imperialistic," "dominant Western" values, or strong ethnocentric and "unicultural" ideas and practices on non-Western nurses and minority consumers.[14,15] To prevent or lessen such cultural imposition and ethnocentric practices, consultants, as well as faculty and practitioners, need preparation in transcultural nursing *before* going abroad (or even working with diverse cultures within one's homeland). They, too, need mentored field practices with transcultural nurse experts to shape and refine their competencies. Nurse administrators are especially challenged to examine their administrative policies and practices in foreign, local, or other settings to make them positive, safe, and meaningful to clients and to prevent ethical, moral, and legal problems within or between countries.[16] Ethical and moral (especially religious) conflicts, clashes, and negative outcomes can be avoided or lessened when nurses know and are skilled to provide culturally congruent human services. It is an interesting fact that negative and unethical outcomes are seldom expressed by nurses in foreign countries *after* Western consultants, administrators, faculty, or students have returned home. This is especially evident in non-Western cultures as nurses often do not want to offend a "Western expert" and want to be polite to such strangers, which is their cultural value and way of "saving face" as part of their etiquette norms to be upheld. Fear of the unknown about cultures and about encountering very different cultures has handicapped many nurses and has decreased nurses' self-image, confidence, and professional status. Therefore, academicians and nursing service administrators and consultants have a *moral obligation* to be culturally knowledgeable and to have competencies to function effectively with diverse cultures. Andrews has studied and written particularly about international consultation for several decades. She has presented research facts and trends in transcultural and international nurs-

ing for several decades. The reader is encouraged to study her work and viewpoints as a transcultural nurse expert on the subject for several years.[17-19]

Administrative Study Situations

To illustrate the importance of transcultural nursing knowledge for nurse administrators and staff, a few study situations are presented. This first situation illustrates not only the need for transcultural nursing knowledge and competencies, but also the diverse factors to consider to accommodate a large foreign cultural group in a hospital context. Transcultural marketing had already occurred when a Middle Eastern cultural group bought services from a United States health system. This is a reality situation, but has been modified to protect the culture and setting.

Situation One: An honored Arab Muslim from the Middle East was admitted to a large midwestern hospital in the United States for a "diagnostic medical workup." A large Arab group accompanied the client from the Middle East. They sought the services of a renowned physician specialist to assess the client's condition and provide medical services in a well-known hospital. The United States hospital administrators and nursing staff were told of their requests for the Arab Muslim prior to the client's arrival. In a short time the honored Muslim client from Saudi Arabia came to the hospital accompanied with an entourage of about 140 Arab family, friends, and religious support persons. The Arab administrators had made several specific requests in advance, such as the need for a large clinical unit in the hospital to be modified to meet the religious client's and his family's needs. In addition to the clinical unit, the Arab Muslims requested prayer rooms, several hospitality rooms, guest rooms for family staying in the hospital, cooking space, and several other facilities for the 140 family and religious friends. An Arab chef came to the United States to provide their revered client and family with their cultural foods while in the hospital. This was very unusual as the hospital had two excellent hospital chefs. These extensive requests were very unusual and baffling to nursing administrators, staff, and others in the hospital. However, the hospital administrator was supported by the medical administrator to make changes and was reassured of payment for rooms, services, treatment, and care.

Initially, the nursing administrators told me that the multiple and diverse requests stunned the hospital staff and especially a largely Anglo-American administrative and clinical staff. However, the requests were considered, and changes were made in a rather short time span. The nurse administrators had to convert a large acute care unit into an Arab mini-family hospital service with a special room for the client. Rooms were prepared for the client's close kin, friends, and other members of his group. Several nurses, physicians, and other health personnel wondered about the many "strange and unusual requests," and they questioned whether such extensive changes would be given to an American in the Saudi Arabian hospital if needed. Since the hospital changes had to occur very quickly and with limited understanding of "why" and "what for," the nursing staff were busy with the changes, but did not understand cultural reasons for the changes. None of the nursing staff were prepared in transcultural nursing, and so they did not understand this Saudi Arabian culture with its cultural values, religious beliefs, and health care expectations. The nurse administrators, however, were flexible and open to make the necessary changes, but wished they knew more about the culture to facilitate meaningful changes with the staff. Since the nursing staff did not understand the Arab Muslim culture, the nurses said it was very difficult to "make sense out of the changes they were expected to make." Moreover, they did not know about Arab Muslim specific care needs. There were a few staff nurses who resented changing their well-established unit to a completely different one. These nurses believed that the Arabs needed to adjust "to our United States culture and not change our services just for them even though they could pay for the services." Many questions were asked about the culture, and all the people who came with the client. When the Arab client and all his family arrived on the unit and in the large hospital, even more questions arose. "Giving nursing care and performing sound nursing administrative practices was difficult with so many Arabs around." The surrounding hospital community was also shocked to see so many Arabs walking around the area, and some were afraid of them.

I arrived shortly after the Arab Muslim male client and his large accompanying group had entered the hospital. It provided a good opportunity to listen, observe, and talk with the nursing administrators and staff about their concerns and conflict areas. Lectures and discussion group sessions were held with the nurses and many community health nurses. Transcultural nursing research-based knowledge, principles, and care needs were discussed. The nursing and medical staff did their best to meet this major cultural need, but it was a very different experience for them. Most of all, the nurses learned from this experience the critical importance of transcultural nursing to care for the Arab client and his extended family, as well as to prevent cultural clashes and provide culturally congruent care. The Theory of Culture Care was used as a guide to help nurses and administrators care for the Arab Muslims in this situation.

Situation Two: A United States nurse theorist "volunteered" to serve as a theorist and consultant for non-Western nurses "to help the nurses change their traditional practices to modern health care practices and use a nursing theory." The theorist was interested to teach her theory and have the nurses adopt it. She was also interested to visit "a very different non-Western culture from the United States culture." Indeed, this Southeastern Island culture was very different from her culture and was a nontechnological culture. On arrival, the nurse theorist presented her theory, which focused mainly on individualism, on abstract phenomena, and on self-care practices. The local nurses said they listened to this nurse's talk, but did not understand it. These nurses did not ask questions nor raise questions about her ideas. They remained silent. They said they were mainly thinking "where did this nurse come from and what did she want them to do?" The Western nurse consultant left after her two lectures on a 2-day visit. Soon after the local nurses began to ask, "Who was that nurse, and why did she come to talk to us?" Some Island nurses told me, "That visitor's ideas do not fit our people and our nursing care as we do not value individualism and self-care as they are too selfish ideas and so different from our beliefs." Some said individualism would never be possible to use in their home as they must care for the whole extended family and not one individual. Group and family care were important in nursing care plus other values. The Island nurses relied on generic (folk) care and curing practices and seldom used professional services as they were limitedly available in most villages. This situation illustrates that the Western nurse consultant and theorist failed to reach the nurses and their culture, which led to negative and unclear views about her visit. The Island nurses felt they did not want this "foreign nurse" to return again.

From the above two administration and consultant study situations, a few questions need to be considered for critical study and reflections:

1. What happened in Situations One and Two from your viewpoint?
2. What should have been anticipated to help the nurse administrators and nursing staff to prepare for and care for the Arab Muslim client in a strange hospital unit with predominately large Anglo-American female nurses?
3. What factors contributed to the nurse consultant and theorist's unsuccessful visit with the Island nurses? How should the theorist have been prepared before coming as a consultant and theorist to the nurses and the country?
4. If the Culture Care Theory had been used, how might the nurse administrator and the consultant discovered the clients' (nurses') world in both situations?
5. What transcultural nursing research-based knowledge is available that could have helped the nurse administrator and staff and the consultant to be more effective?
6. What did you learn from each situation to help you in your workplace?

The above two study situations show the need for "holding" transcultural nursing knowledge gained through formal study in transcultural nursing to guide nurses toward providing culturally congruent care. Nurse administrators and consultants need transcultural nursing principles, concepts, and research knowledge to guide their decisions and actions in similar ways that they have holding knowledge to care for cardiac clients. In both situations, nurse administrators and consultants need to realize that their effectiveness depends on transcultural nursing knowledge, use, theory, and research to fit the cultures being served. The often-heard philosophy of "just being kind to strangers" has some benefits, but this is not enough for therapeutic and specific outcomes. Culture-specific and holistic care perspectives are essential for quality care practices.

Theory of Culture Care Benefits for Administrators and Consultants

Over the past four decades, the Theory of Culture Care Diversity and Universality has repeatedly been found by nurse users to be "an invaluable guide" to help especially nurse administrators and nurse consultants discover and use *emic* and *etic* research-based findings in their work. (The reader should first review the major tenets and assumptions of the theory with the ethnonursing method in the Sunrise Model in Chapter 3 for the discussion that follows).[20] A few strengths and positive attributes can be highlighted in using the theory for administrators and consultants.

First, the theory can be used in any culture(s), in different organizational health systems, and in educational and service agencies to discover culture care administrative patterns, practices, and needs for decision making or planning. The theory can be used by different health disciplines and by nonhealth agencies to market their services with slight modifications focusing on their specific discipline domains or interests. The theory is comprehensive and holistic to discover worldviews and multiple social structure factors influencing human health services with a caring ethos. Accordingly, the theory has been enormously helpful to nurses in *making comprehensive assessments, in planning for changes, in modifying practices, or in retaining desired practices.* By focusing on the worldview and diverse social structures, features (as well as language expressions, particular environmental and historical factors, and holistic dimensions) can be usually identified. Social structure factors such as political, economic, technology, religion, philosophy, cultural values, beliefs and practices, kinship and social ties, education and legal factors, and other related factors need to become known and used by administrators and consultants. In many Western cultures, political, economic, and technological factors are major interest areas, whereas in non-Western and other cultures, these factors may not be prime factors.[21] More and more social structure factors have become imperative to assess the administrative factors and to grasp an accurate and full picture of the business practices with historical patterns. For without examining social structure factors, administrators and consultants can readily miss critical indicators that influence services and provide only a partial or fragmented view. It is the cultural beliefs, myths, and values that are often critical determinants of whether changes and appropriate decisions can be wisely made within administrative, academic, or clinical organizations. These social structure factors and other dimensions of the theory are depicted in the Sunrise Model, which need to be checked, if one has covered these areas. Neglecting one dimension may lead to false or inaccurate conclusions and poor decisions. More and more legal, political, economic, and technological factors play a major role in administrative decisions and plans in the United States, Canada, and other Westernized health systems. However, one can never assume they have similar relevance in other organizations or cultures. Thus, to change any health or educational system or to be a competent consultant, holistic factors need to be assessed in-depth to discover what factors are relevant. Such facts provide a very sound and reliable basis for administrative or consultation changes or for retaining the best of any services offered.

Second, the Culture Care Theory gives special attention to environmental, linguistic, and ethnohistorical factors related to administration and consultant work. Most assuredly, historical and environmental factors have been increasingly important with administration and in providing quality-based consultation services. Ethnohistorical patterns of how administrative systems have functioned over time and in different environmental contexts are extremely important. The past and current history of any culture, system, or organization should not be slighted. Many indigenous cultures, immigrants, and refugees value their historical roots and want them recognized, as well as their health institutions. Environmental and historical factors are often closely aligned.

It is also important to understand language expressions and to discover the meanings, metaphors, and uses of certain cultural linguistic sayings or terms related to health care and educational systems such as "time is money." What informants say and do may vary, but generally their own words and expressions are important to understand and validate cultural phenomena. In assessing generic (folk) indigenous lifeways or patterns in health care, as well as professional care practices, knowledge of the language is critical to understanding the people. The theorist seeks to discover both differences and similarities to arrive at decisions

or to take action. Discovering caring modalities and any care or cure factors within folk and professional health practices is extremely important to guide decisions and practices.[22] It is also important to emphasize that the concept of care goes beyond the idea of *being per se* to that of understanding *care within a cultural perspective*. Otherwise, care/caring has very little meaning and can lead to questionable conclusions.[23] Nursing administrators and consultants must discover culturally based care patterns and expressions of diverse and similar cultures to make responsible decisions. The diverse and universal care patterns are invaluable in many different contexts as reported in literature sources. Discovering generic care patterns such as *protective care* or *family care* is critical to Mexican and African cultures and other cultures as dominant care constructs. Such dominant culture care themes are important to making sound administrative or consultant decisions or plans. Accordingly, gaps between generic and professional care systems can lead to culture conflicts, racism, cultural biases, and other factors that require attention in administrative services or in consultation. Thus, the Theory of Culture Care gives emphasis to these important dimensions for administrators and consultants, which are often neglected by professional administrators leading to gaps in transcultural care practices.

Third, the Culture Care Theory is especially relevant to discover how academic and clinical administrators, as well as consultants, arrive at their decisions and actions to serve institutions, groups, or individuals. As one focuses on the data being generated from the diverse dimensions depicted in the Sunrise Model, the user will find many explanatory descriptive statements offering sound basis for making decisions and actions related to responsible and congruent care or educational practices. The author has been especially impressed by how valuable the worldview can be for administrators and consultants to arrive at a holistic view and attitudes about changes. Most importantly, the Culture Care Theory has three *built-in theoretical* ways to assess, plan, and develop decisions or actions for culturally congruent, responsible, and beneficial outcomes. While the theory has some abstract features, it also has *very practical ways* to use the data generated from informants to formulate or make concrete decisions or actions. Both *holistic and yet particularistic* features characterize the theory and fit with nursing as both a practical profession and a scientific discipline. Accordingly, the three theoretical modalities of the theory as shown in the Sunrise Model (Chapter 3) become new and invaluable guides for administrative and consultation plans, decisions, actions, or other purposes. The three built-in theoretical modalities are as follows:[24]

1. *Culture care preservation and maintenance* (or what needs to be preserved and maintained within administrative organizations or in consultation work)
2. *Culture care accommodation or negotiation* (or what needs to be accommodated or negotiated in administration or consultation)
3. *Culture care repatterning or restructuring* (or what needs to be reorganized, repatterned, or restructured to make changes)

All modalities are very important for administrative and consultation decisions with groups and individuals. These three modalities can be purposefully considered as one reflects and discusses with key informants their administrative or consultation goals. The three modalities are refreshingly different from the usual or traditional medical treatment or current system *management nursing emphases* with disease entities. These modalities are major breakthroughs in nursing that offer or modify lifeways in education and clinical practices. They are very much needed today to reform or transform health care systems and organizations to become culturally sensitive, appropriate, and meaningful in a rapidly changing multicultural world. Many nurses and other health disciplines such as social workers, dental therapists, and physical therapists are also finding the three modes extremely helpful as they work with consumers and their cultural care needs. Most importantly, the three modes are generally valued by consumers as new ways of helping them preserve their values and lifeways. Several chapters in this book show excellent and specific uses of the three modalities to arrive at culturally congruent, responsible, and meaningful care outcomes in administrative practices.

Hospital Health System Merger Situation

Another example can be highlighted to consider the theory with hospital health system mergers in the United States. With the recent era of reducing or controlling health costs by decentralizing and dismissing nurses and other staff, health care mergers and alliances have occurred in the United States. Some mergers have been done rather suddenly to create one integrated and cost-controlled health care system. In this example, one of the hospitals was a very large health science medical system with a large college of medicine, as well as nursing and other academic health departments. The other hospital was a large private religious hospital that had strong historical roots in the community. The merger was conceived largely by medical and hospital administrators with great promise of benefits to the city and state. The merger included bringing selected physicians, nurses, social workers, and other professionals from the two hospitals into one large academic and service institution for health care in the community. During this time, nearly 138 professional nurses and several nurse administrators were relieved of their positions to "save costs." Seeing this drastic change, many qualified nursing and administrative staff resigned as "they did not find it was possible to practice quality nursing care and to be replaced by less qualified and cheaper staff." A physician leading the merger was the CEO and seemed to deal with many physicians who were vying for key departmental roles to ensure their future security and status within the new organization.

Within one year the merger was declared as "completed," and the CEO resigned. The merger was declared as "successful but troublesome." Many cultural conflicts, clashes, and tensions could be noted and witnessed during the merger process. Limitedly dealt with were client care and nursing issues, as well as confusion about the ultimate goal and perceived benefits. After the CEO had resigned, he commented that the merger was difficult and that he had not realized how different the two institutions were before the merger. It was evident that two very different hospital cultures were suddenly expected to merge and function well together. These two hospitals, one public and one private, were culturally different with different values, norms, and practices. The crux of the problem was that the CEO and other medical staff failed to assess and study the cultural differences *before* the merger was announced and instituted. Had the institutions been assessed with respect to their different philosophies, histories, economics, and cultures with the Culture Care Theory, many differences would have been identified to make meaningful changes and decisions. All dimensions within the Sunrise Model and the theory's tenets would have revealed multiple diverse factors leading to cultural conflicts, clashes, and tensions. The three theoretical modes of the Culture Care Theory would have provided guidelines for a culturally congruent merger of the two hospitals and helped to retain many qualified and valuable nursing care staff. Culture care repatterning and restructuring were clearly needed to identify social structure factors bearing on changes for a congruent merger. Only a few commonalities were evident between the two hospitals to be culturally maintained or preserved. Culture care accommodation and negotiation were also needed to facilitate several unresolved issues among and within health disciplines. None of the merger planners were prepared in transculturalism to assess and understand the different values of the two hospital cultures. The loss of 130 professional nurses and other staff was unfortunate as nurse administrators had spent several years recruiting, preparing, and retaining well-qualified nurses before the merger. Indeed, this is a situation that could have benefitted from a transcultural study before and after and the merger. Transcultural nurses and physician consultants working together and using the Culture Care Theory could have led to beneficial and congruent outcomes. The interface of the Culture Care Theory with health organizations is a new and important advancement in health care research and practice. This situation, with such a costly and large-scale merger, should not have occurred until the cultural care dimensions had been fully studied and analyzed.[25]

Need to Reorganize and Transform Health Care into Transcultural Caring Systems

In many countries and cultures in the world, health care systems often need to be transformed into transculturally caring systems to provide and maintain quality-based health care. The rising costs of health care in most countries, the limited health care access for the poor and minority cultures, and the lack of care to immigrants are indicators to transform health care systems. In the early 1980s I predicted that managed care would not be effective and successful for most health systems in the USA. The major issue was the lack of concern for the underrepresented, the vulnerable, and

those of poor cultures with no insurance or money for health care. Some hospital employers and staff saw managed care to get reimbursements. Generally, however, physicians and nurses have not been too pleased with managed care practices. Granted, managed care offered some needed regulation on health costs, but more study was needed to reach many minorities and other diverse cultures in the United States. Some cultures have rebelled against managed care as they have been denied health care. Other consumers disliked the short hospital stays and the impersonal system operations. Many other problems with insurance companies, HMOs, Medicare and Medicaid, and the paying for certain illnesses and denying payment for others have led to consumer and staff dissatisfaction with managed care practices.

Amid such controversies and cultural disparity issues, national and global health care plans and strategies are being considered by legislators and others. There is also pressure for the globalization and marketing of health care worldwide and for universal health care in the United States. These trends and others will necessitate transcultural health services for very diverse cultures. The culturally congruent care mandate has at last become expressed at the federal, local, and regional levels. I contend that the Theory of Culture Care Diversity and Universality and use of the Sunrise Model and ethnocare research methods can be enormously helpful for transforming and maintaining culturally based caring systems. The theory remains valuable to nurse administrators, nurse consultants, and their leaders in its uses worldwide or for humanistic caring. Already, many nurses who have used the theory have found it most helpful to establish transcultural care practices.[26,27] Transcultural nurse administrators can demonstrate the use of the theory with many beneficial outcomes for transforming nursing and health care services.

Future Expectations

In the future many new and different kinds of health care systems, agencies, centers, institutes, and creative entrepreneur ventures will be developed worldwide. These developments will necessitate that *all* health care practices become transculturally designed and implemented. Transcultural nurse administrators and nurse consultants can play a key leadership role with representatives of other disciplines to transform health care into culturally relevant and effective caring systems. In the future consumers of diverse cultures in democratic countries will become active to plan, control, and establish health care policies, practices, and beneficial outcomes. Health professionals will be expected to serve as *facilitators, active listeners*, and *partners* with consumers and especially in a growing transcultural global world. Many current and dysfunctional health care practices will be replaced by *trusted partnership care agreements, alliances*, and new organizational modes by 2010.[28,29] Nursing's new paradigm in education, research, practice, administration, and consultation will be transcultural nursing.[30] These changes and others will necessitate that nurses become prepared through substantive graduate courses, programs, and multidiscipline research institutes in transcultural nursing. Multidisciplinary transculturalism will dominate many health curricula and clinical services in the next decade. Past unicultural or medically dominated perspectives in nursing and health care will be changed. Fortunately, transcultural nursing leaders anticipating this global trend have been carving new pathways for nearly five decades, and their efforts will be recognized and valued in the near future.

To achieve these desired and futuristic goals, the following summary recommendations merit urgent consideration:

1. Begin immediately to promote, through courses, programs of study, and mentored guidance, preparation of nurses in transcultural nursing, comparative transcultural nursing knowledge and draw on the growing body of transcultural nursing research-based knowledge for practice.
2. Use a theoretical framework such as the Theory of Culture Care Diversity and Universality to discover disparities and use holistic and multiple factors related to transcultural nursing and expressly for transcultural administration and consultation and develop meaningful policies, standards, and practices.
3. Discuss comparative issues, problems, and factors related to transcultural differences and similarities in academic and service organizations and with a global perspective to establish a body of transcultural nursing and health care knowledge.

4. Continue to build and systematically examine the growing body of transcultural nursing (universal and diverse) knowledge to guide future nurses, and especially for those leaders in administration and consultation in different cultures and environmental contexts.
5. Develop innovative models of transcultural nursing administration and consultation that leads to culturally safe, congruent, and meaningful nursing care policies, practices, and educational and research exchange programs.
6. Draw on the expertise, experiences, and research-based knowledge of transcultural nurse experts who have been successful in transcultural nursing practice, administration, and consultation.
7. Identify and publicize through public media the benefits and outcomes of providing culturally congruent caring administration, consultation, and client services in Western and non-Western cultures.
8. Research ethical, moral, and legal issues, problems, and conflicts related to comparative transcultural nursing administration, consultation, and practices in different cultures worldwide for universal patterns.
9. Develop mentorship programs to prepare competent transcultural nursing administrators and consultants as global and local exemplars to promote and support culturally relevant health care reforms, practices, and marketing strategies.
10. Give more attention to comparative culture caring values and practices that are influenced by worldviews, politics, economics, historical issues, technologies, environment, education, gender, and communication modes in different cultures, and especially those bearing on transcultural nursing administration and consultation.
11. Participate with other health and social science disciplines in research practices and in marketing strategies in the ways to reaffirm sound, diverse, and universal transcultural health care knowledge and practices.

In this chapter some important trends, issues, theoretical ideas, and research with futuristic perspectives have been presented related to transcultural nursing administration and consultation as a growing service worldwide.

References

1. Leininger, M., "Transcultural Nursing Administration: An Imperative Worldwide," *Journal of Transcultural Nursing*, July to December 1996a, v. 8, no. 1, pp. 28–33.
2. Leininger, M., *Territoriality, Power and Creative Leadership in Administrative Nursing Contexts. Power: Use It or Lose It*, New York: National League for Nursing Press, 1977, pp. 6–18.
3. Leininger, op. cit., 1996.
4. Leininger, M., *Transcultural Nursing: Concepts, Theories and Practices*, New York: John Wiley & Sons, 1978. (Reprinted Columbus, OH: Greyden Press, 1994.)
5. Leininger, M., *Cultural Differences Among Staff Members and the Impact on Patient Care*, Minnesota League of Nursing Bulletin, 1968, v. 16, no. 5, pp. 5–9.
6. Leininger, M., *Barriers and Facilitators to Quality Health Care*, Philadelphia, PA: F.A. Davis Co., 1975.
7. Leininger, M., "Conflict and Conflict Resolutions in Transcultural Health Care Issues and Conditions," in *Health Care Dimensions*, Philadelphia, PA: F.A. Davis Co., 1976.
8. Leininger, M., "Transcultural Nursing: Administration," in *Transcultural Nursing: Concepts, Theories and Practices*, M. Leininger, ed., Columbus, OH: McGraw-Hill College Custom Series, 1995.
9. Leininger, M., "Future Directions in Transcultural Nursing in the 21st Century," *International Nursing Review*, 1997, v. 44, no. 1, pp. 19–23.
10. Leininger, M., "Survey of Graduate Programs in Transcultural Nursing Offerings," unpublished report, 2000.
11. Leininger, op. cit., 1995.
12. Leininger, M., "Nursing Education Exchanges: Concerns and Realities," *Journal of Transcultural Nursing*, January to June 1998, v. 9, no. 2, pp. 57–63.
13. Ibid.
14. Ibid.
15. Leininger, op. cit., 1995.
16. Leininger, M., *Ethical and Moral Dimensions of Care*, Detroit, MI: Wayne State University Press, 1990.
17. Andrews, M.M., "U.S. Nurse Consultants in the International Marketplace," *Journal of Professional Nursing*, 1985, v. 1, p. 189.
18. Andrews, M.M., "Educational Preparation for International Nursing," *Journal of Professional Nursing*, 1988, v. 1, pp. 430–435.
19. Andrews, M.M., and B.P. Fargotstein, "International Nursing Consultation: A Perspective on Ethical Issues," *Journal of Professional Nursing*, 1986, v. 2, pp. 302–306.
20. Leininger, M., *Cultural Care Diversity and Universality: A Theory of Nursing*, New York: National League for Nursing, 1991.
21. Leininger, op. cit., 1991, pp. 1–74.
22. Leininger, M., *Care: The Essence of Nursing and Health*, Thorofare, NJ: Charles B. Slack, Inc., 1984. (Reprinted in 1990 by Wayne State University Press, Detroit, MI.)
23. Ibid.
24. Leininger, op. cit., 1991, pp. 73–118.
25. Leininger, M., "The Interface of the Culture Care Theory with Health Care Organizations," unpublished paper given at Hennipen Hospital Conference, Minneapolis, MN, September 19, 1999.
26. Uhl, J.E., "Globalization and Nursing Partnership," *Journal of Professional Nursing*, 1991, v. 7, no. 1, pp. 2–3.
27. "Uses of the Culture Care Theory for Nursing Consultation and Administration," personal communications of J. Ehrmin (Ohio Nursing Service), Linda Luna (Saudi Arabia), M. McFarland (Saginaw College), Akram Omeri (Australia), Susan Salmond (Kean University), and J. Uhl, University of Tennessee), and others, 1980–2000.
28. Leininger, op. cit., 1997.
29. Leininger, M., "Major Directions for Transcultural Nursing: A Journey into the 21st Century," *Journal of Transcultural Nursing*, 1996b, v. 7, no. 2, pp. 28–31.
30. Leininger, M., and S.H. Cummings, "Nursing's New Paradigm is Transcultural Nursing: An Interview with Madeleine Leininger," *Advanced Practice Nursing Quarterly*, 1996c, v. 2, no. 2, pp. 62–70.
31. Leininger, M., et al., "Transcultural Nursing Standards, Policies, and Practices." Certification Committee, Transcultural Nursing Society, Livonia, MI, 2001.

SECTION **V**

The Future of
Transcultural Nursing

36

The Future of Transcultural Nursing: A Global Perspective

Madeleine Leininger

The future of nursing is largely contingent on the active advancement and use of transcultural nursing research-based knowledge and practices to serve a rapidly growing multicultural world with cultural care compassion, understanding, and competencies.

Like an eagle spreading its wings and soaring upward and outward to unknown places, transcultural nursing will continue to soar to many places in the world in the 21st century to serve humanity. This century is the Era of Globalization, with nurses realizing that the profession must be viewed with my 1960 motto of "One World with Many Diverse Cultures." Indeed, our world has significantly changed in recent decades to a global perspective in which we live and work with many people from different cultures. Nurses are realizing that what we teach and how we care for people necessitates having transcultural nursing knowledge and skills to be effective and helpful to others. Living in a multicultural world is challenging nurses to understand trends and realities as nurses journey into the 21st century.

Transcultural nurses prepared in transcultural nursing will be expected to give leadership in education, research, and practice to serve people in culturally competent ways. The world will continue to become closely interconnected and intensely multicultural with health professionals scurrying to learn about different cultures and how to function in culturally responsible and effective ways. By the year 2015 the author has predicted that *all health care must be transculturally based to serve people appropriately from many different cultures in the world.*[1] However, this reality will be difficult to fully realize as far too few nurses are prepared to function today as effective practitioners,

researchers, clinicians, and teachers in transcultural nursing. Hence, major crises will prevail as consumers of diverse cultures make demands on health professionals for meaningful and competent care in a changing multicultural world.

With the globalization of transcultural nursing in this century, the nursing profession will gradually be transformed from the past largely unicultural, biomedical, and mind-body emphasis to comparative transcultural caring and healing to prevent illnesses and disabilities and to maintain the health and well-being of people. This transformation will require considerable work with shared research and cooperative interests among health professions. It will require a much broader perspective to understand and use the meanings and values of transculturalism and to make appropriate people-centered decisions. In contrast with other health professions, transcultural nurses will have a head start in transculturalism with several decades of research, teaching, and practice in the past century. By the year 2010, nurses will appreciate and realized the critical importance of transcultural nursing building on existing knowledge and practices. The full transformation process, however, will require many changes in education, teaching, and leadership worldwide to provide culturally competent caring practices. Gradually, nurses will value the author's thesis that "knowing, understanding, and serving people holistically from a transcultural nursing perspective will be the most meaningful professional experience to nurses, and especially to consumers of transcultural nursing practices."

However, to effectively transform nursing and health care systems into transculturally based practice will require many nurses with master's and doctoral preparation in transcultural nursing to function as administrators, educators, researchers and practitioners. To be effective primary, secondary, and tertiary advanced care practitioners and to change health care systems, advanced preparation in transcultural nursing will be essential. Transcultural nurses will be challenged to be mainly *facilitators* of cultural care and to establish different ways to function creatively in schools, hospitals, health agencies, and many new kinds of community settings. By the year 2020 more nurses will be prepared in graduate transcultural nursing programs, which will facilitate meeting consumer expectations and transcultural nursing education and practice goals. Identifying futuristic and specific patterns and lifeways of clients and health centers of diverse cultures will greatly challenge nurses in using not only humanistic and scientific cultural care knowledge, but also appropriate multidisciplinary and interdisciplinary knowledge. Nurses will need to actively learn from other cultures and especially from consumers to generate relevant care decisions and actions. Most importantly, nurses will need to develop creative strategies and different ways to advance and maintain health care to people of diverse and similar cultures. Changing past unicultural policies and administrative practices in education and service to transcultural ones will be a major challenge.

One can also anticipate that, with the increased emphasis on transcultural education and practice, one will find competitive groups and associations developing within and outside of nursing. Already within nursing some nurses have recently established similar global associations such as the "Global Society for Nursing and Health," which has similar goals to the Transcultural Nursing Society established in 1974. From an organizational and public view, establishing similar organizations leads to confusion and the fractionation of nurses' alliances. It limits sharing, advancing, and perfecting knowledge within a major or parent group such as the Transcultural Nursing Society. Multidisciplinary and intradisciplinary groups will increase because of the focus on transculturalism resulting from

consumer needs and expectations. Hopefully, collaboration among such groups will occur to advance transculturalism across disciplines.

Most assuredly, one will find an increased demand for well-prepared transcultural nurses to teach and demonstrate comparative transcultural knowledge and skills. Listening, reflecting, and planning with consumers and other providers and health disciplines will be a dominant emphasis of these experts. Transcultural nurses will need to maintain an open learning attitude and to remain alert to emic and etic cultural data. They will also need to be culturally sensitive to ethical and moral values of consumers in teaching, research, and practice. Transcultural nurses will demonstrate ways to learn from informants by immersion field-study experiences of living in different cultures once they are prepared in advance to study and use transcultural nursing concepts, principles, and general practices. This century will require transcultural nurses to be skilled to work with specific concerns of cultures and to document new ways to facilitate clients' cultural care and health needs in diverse environments. These trends and expectations will greatly contribute to the existing body of transcultural nursing knowledge and competencies with consumer benefits especially for many immigrants.

Future Changes Related to Transcultural Nursing

This new century will be an especially challenging era as nurses learn to function in transcultural organizational structures within different community-based institutions rather than past traditional hospital settings with largely unicultural norms. The new community transcultural nursing paradigm will be essential to teach, practice, and conduct research and for consultation. Promoting wellness by using etic and emic transcultural data in health practices and in community contexts based on comparative knowledge will be essential.[2] This focus can lead to many benefits to consumers and nursing satisfactions. It has been a dream and goal since transcultural nursing was envisioned nearly five decades ago, and it is the new paradigm for this century for a growing and intense multicultural health care world.[3]

In this century there will be major changes in all areas of nursing from hospital to *community-based services*, as well as to establishing new kinds of transcultural and integrative health care centers for diverse populations. Changing nurses, physicians, and other health care providers to a transcultural philosophy and to different practices to accommodate the culturally different in specific ways will be a great challenge. It will mean learning and understanding the cultural care and health patterns, values, and lifeways of people in diverse environmental and community settings. Nurses, as the largest group of health care providers, will be expected to assess and use a broad holistic transcultural caring focus with specific ways to promote the health and well-being of people. Identifying and using culture-specific research-based knowledge that influences the individual and family health and well-being within diverse ecological and community settings will be essential. Those from other cultures will expect nurses and other health professionals to be knowledgeable about their cultures and the environments in which they live, work, function, and have leisure. What leads to illnesses and how to prevent sickness in different cultures and environments will be major areas of study and practice in this century. Ethnocentric and fragmented medical views of clients will be challenged as inadequate for knowing and helping cultures. The totality of living and understanding human beings will be a dominant focus. To grasp a holistic transcultural perspective, nurses and other health professionals will need to become knowledgeable about political, economic, kinship, religious and/or spiritual values, specific cultural beliefs, technologies, and educational factors in their assessments and caring practices. These factors will gradually be seen to influence the health and well-being of clients in different community contexts. Using such knowledge will enable the nurse to make appropriate and meaningful decisions *with* consumers to prevent illnesses, disabilities, and other threats to people's well-being and to assist clients from different cultures in dying.

By the year 2010 *migration* of people from many different cultures and countries will markedly increase in all countries that permit open migration and immigration. It will be difficult to determine who is a cultural minority or majority with such changing populations and frequent resettlement patterns. There are predictions of increased migration waves of people from Latin America, Caribbean, Africa, Southeast Asia, and the Pacific islands to the United States and Canada.[4] Nurses will be expected to understand and work with many of these cultures, as well as cultures from Korea, China, Japan, India, and the Middle East. One can predict, however, that there will be fewer immigrants from Europe to the United States and Canada. Such shifts in the numbers and diversity of people will reaffirm the importance and critical need for transcultural nursing and health care. Nurses and other health care providers will struggle to work with so many different cultures. Language use with cultural understanding will be expected almost overnight in health care. It will be a new major challenge for nurses as they are the ones who usually have the first contact with clients in the community and in other health settings.

Intercultural Internet and person-to-person communication centers will be essential to help immigrants and other newcomers to adjust to different cultural lifeways and changes in home and local community settings. Newcomers will struggle with language as they seek survival and basic needs. New waves of migrants may occur suddenly, giving limited time to prepare for them and their particular needs and expectations. Nurses prepared in transcultural nursing will be able to help these people adjust to cultural changes and to help other nurses and professionals. Transcultural nursing concepts, principles, and theory with research findings of the specific cultures such as Vietnamese, Sudanese, and others will be expected. Nurses with holding culture care knowledge and skills will discover effective ways to care for cultural strangers based on appropriate actions and decisions. Without holding knowledge, nurses will be greatly handicapped and frustrated in providing care to diverse cultures and in preventing culturally offensive actions. Our goal in working with immigrants and newcomers should be to help them become integrated into a community rather than to expect assimilation, alienation, or rejection.[5]

In the future, diverse global and local changes will require nurses to be culturally knowledgeable, sensitive, competent, and responsible nurses. While there will be many modern high-tech electronic devices to use with clients in some places, there may be none to work with the poor, oppressed, homeless, and victimized cultures especially in Third World countries such as Africa. With *high-tech equipment*, clients will expect nurses to show diverse and specific therapeutic caring acts. Building and maintaining trusting relationships with cultures and often without electronic equipment will be essential in homes, nursing centers, hospitals, clinics, disaster areas, and other settings. While many nurses and other health care providers will use high-tech equipment, there will be some cultures that will fear such equipment and may interpret them as harmful spirit intruders or powerful objects to reject or avoid. Nurses must use holding knowledge of a culture to anticipate potential negative or positive consequences to cultures, and especially with x-ray and radar equipment. Nurses need to be aware of such cultural differences with modern technologies and should not assume that all clients know, like, and value technologies. Many fear them.

As nurses travel to many known and unknown places to work and live, their travels will increase in frequency and duration of time. They will see cultures in very extensive poverty and in oppressed situations. There are those that are grossly deprived of health care because of lack of access and money and also because of cultural discrimination practices and policies. Nurses will also see very wealthy people living in secluded and protected environments with lots of material possessions. Seeing and experiencing such contrasts of the cultures of poverty and affluence in the same country will be difficult to understand and accept. Cultural shock, discontent, and deep concern by the nurse will lead to ways to redress such disparities. Knowing ways to help clients in the *culture of poverty* usually requires strategies to repattern past cultural lifeways to promote well-being. Knowledge of economic and political forces along with other social-structure factors will be essential for changes. Also, working directly with the cultures of the poor and wealthy or the "haves and have nots" helps to understand these cultures through their lifeways. Providing care that is focused on what is most important along with areas of potential changes for the poor should be kept in mind. It will be difficult for some Western-oriented nurses who have never experienced the very poor, neglected, and vulnerable. Nurses who value self-care practices rather than group or family care will need to alter such values to work with many non-Western cultures for individualized self-care practices often have less importance for the poor or when other group care is needed.

As nurses become skilled in doing short or extensive kinds of community cultural health care assessments, often different care practices are discovered, especially with rural and urban groups. *Assessing communities for diverse similar patterns of care will require remaining open-minded and drawing on cultural knowledge.* Developing *cooperative trusting partnerships* among cultures will necessitate using political, social, cultural, and other data found with the use of the Culture Care Theory and the Sunrise Model.[6] Discovering unique and common kinds of community nursing care will be a new discovery for many nurses.

Developing interagency and *interdisciplinary* cooperative cultural services with available human and physical resources will characterize future transcultural health care locally, regionally, and worldwide. Nurses well prepared in administrative transcultural health care will be in demand to facilitate transcultural cooperative endeavors.[7] Nurses, physicians, social workers, physical and occupational therapists, pharmacists, dentists, and other health professionals will need to cooperate to provide culturally based transcultural health care. This will not occur until different health disciplines become prepared through substantive transcultural health care education. Interdisciplinary transcultural understandings and practices will be in great demand by 2010. On-line Internet and other transcultural educational programs will be used along with formal courses with faculty mentors. Schools of nursing and other health professions will see the urgent demand for distance transcultural programs, courses, and institutes to hasten interprofessional transcultural education. Field mentorships will be common as more faculty and students become prepared in transcultural nursing and the vital importance of mentoring.

Many ethical and moral problems will arise in this 21st century because of areas of cultural value conflicts and clashes between clients and health care providers. *Transcultural ethical and legal health care* will become a major specialty area for transcultural nurses and others. International and transcultural health laws will become a specialty area to deal with legal and ethical cultural problems. Most lawyers will be generally poorly prepared to deal with the ethical and legal issues of specific cultures. Of course, some lawyers and nurses will proclaim themselves as "transcultural ethicists" but often without preparation about cultures, transcultural nursing, comparative ethics, or theological knowledge, lessening their credibility and effectiveness. Cultural clashes and conflicts with nontherapeutic actions and cultural ignorance will lead to many problems and legal suits, especially with integrative health services. Hence, the demand for in-depth knowledge in transcultural legal, ethical, and moral insights will be important and essential among health care providers, lawyers, and others working with diverse cultures worldwide.

With the rapid increase in demand for culturally competent health services, other academic disciplines such as medical sociologists, medical psychologists, and medical anthropologists will be found in hospitals, clinics, and community agencies. Some of these disciplines will offer their services, but many will be limited in transcultural insights and skills. Anthropologists and sociologists who have worked with transcultural nurses will be more helpful to professional health care providers. Many new disciplines will be conducting research related to different cultures in health care practices, and transcultural education and communication modes will have increased markedly by the year 2010.

With mandatory transcultural care and health competencies and within a community-based perspective, health personnel will scramble to become prepared in comparative health care. Academic and clinical administrators will be seeking transcultural nurse specialists and others to help with transcultural health policies and care practices. Many of these nurse administrators and policy managers will be limitedly prepared in the field, handicapping their efforts to develop and maintain sound health practices.[8] These administrators with their traditional, medical mind-body views will be difficult to change. As a consequence, cultural clashes, racism, and ethnocentrism will lead to legal suits and unethical practices until administrators become prepared in transculturalism and comparative policies. As nursing service administrators gradually become knowledgeable about cultures and differential care practices, they will be able to facilitate quality community care tailored to fit clients' cultural needs within their community and environmental contexts. These administrators who work with transcultural nurse experts and learn how to use ethnonursing, ethnography, narratives, oral and written life histories, and other qualitative research methods will be most effective to repattern traditional nursing and health systems. The use of qualita-

tive methods will be the key to discover rich community culture care data, and these methods will be used more than quantitative reductionistic research methods that limit obtaining emic and etic client and professional data. The ethnonursing, transcultural research method based on the Culture Care Theory will remain in great demand for holistic and in-depth meaningful emic data about cultures and their health needs.

Unfortunately, the 21st century will not see a decrease in *violence, crimes, and overt terrorist acts* largely caused by intercultural misunderstandings, biases, conflicts, racial accusations, and hatred among humans of diverse cultures worldwide. In fact, violence will probably increase in many countries and between countries because of the close linkage of culture to religion, politics, and historical claims to land as seen today in the Middle East. Destructive and impulsive domestic and institutional violence will occur in homes, hospitals, schools, offices, and other places, also caused by ignorance, arrogance, ethnocentrism, and cultural imposition practices. The need for transcultural nursing care concepts, principles, and theories with research-based practices will be greatly needed to alleviate and prevent such domestic, public, and global violence, killings, and intercultural tensions. The current trend of relying largely on dominant Western psychological and physical explanations will be insufficient to understand cultural, political, ethnohistorical, and religious factors related to human violence, terrorists' offenses, and other destructive acts. Understanding the close interrelationship of culture to political, religious, and traditional cultural lifeways of diverse cultural groups will be essential knowledge. Cultural identity, spiritual support, and understanding power struggles must be studied and understood before taking action. In addition, health personnel need to take leadership to shift from the "culture of death and destruction" to the "culture of life" from birth and throughout the life cycle. How people can preserve and maintain healthy lives and live in peace will be the desired goal.

In the future, almost instant electronic communication will be relied on in many places to learn about cultural happenings, health-illness trends, and other new developments. Public educational programs using diverse electronic means will be a major means to learn about diverse cultural information and to deal with cultural conflicts, accidents, and other problems among cultures. Transcultural nurse specialists and general-ists will focus on local, national, and global media to be prepared to deal with daily cultural crises and is-sues. Transcultural nurses, anthropologists, and those of other disciplines with substantive knowledge of cul-tures from historical, geopolitical, and other social structure factors will be much needed. Anthropologists and others can learn much from transcultural nurses with their in-depth direct experiences with clients for beneficial outcomes. The role of cultural caring factors as major influencers of illnesses, violence, health, and death will become publicly recognized as important by the year 2015. Gradually, as intracultural and intercul-tural stresses, conflicts, and lifestyle patterns become known with the transcultural paradigm and explana-tions, there will be new biomedical, DNA, genetics, and cultural knowledge to be integrated into holistic health, illnesses, and acute-chronic conditions. Comparative holistic health and illness with culturally based pat-terned expressions will be the dominant focus to assess and help clients from birth to death. The past and cur-rent roles of transcultural nurses experts working with health providers will greatly increase cultural under-standings and competencies in the public health arenas.

By the year 2010 nurses will be valuing and us-ing culture-specific and some universal transcultural nursing knowledge to guide their teaching, curricula work, and clinical practices. Transcultural nursing care concepts, principles, and research findings from the Culture Care Theory will be especially used.[9] This knowledge along with other research discoveries will greatly strengthen the nurse's ability to provide cultur-ally appropriate, competent, and meaningful care. In the meantime there will be some nurses who will lay claim or try to rename transcultural nursing without ac-knowledging nearly five decades of work by transcul-tural nurse leaders. Interprofessional jealousies, envy, and status recognition along with a lack of professional honesty and integrity can be expected. However, the work of the past and present transcultural nursing lead-ers will ultimately be recognized as an essential and growing global discipline. True scholars and honest users of transcultural nursing knowledge will always value past leaders pioneering contributions in transcul-tural nursing. They will also value classic and substan-tive scholarship of earlier works such as "Quo Vadis" and many transcultural writers for their leadership.[10–12]

The author's Theory of Culture Care Diversity and Universality will be extensively used and a dominant theory worldwide because of its comprehensive, holis-tic, and yet very particularistic ways to help the cultur-ally different or those with similar needs. While the the-ory is not a "Grand" or "Middle-range" theory, nurses will need to abandon such earlier classifications of the-ories. The Culture Care Theory with the use of the Sunrise Model and the ethnonursing method will be-come a major and integral part of most nurses' thinking and action. New and creative ways to discover and use transcultural knowledge worldwide will occur. Other similar models and theories will imitate the Culture Care Theory, but true scholars and users of the origi-nal theory will recognize the source and value its use with the ethnonursing method. More and more "re-search enablers" will be used because they are less of-fensive to cultural informants than traditional research "tools," "instruments," "scales," and other mechanistic intrusive modes of eliciting research data from peo-ple. The idea of discovering universals and diversities about human care in different cultures will markedly grow in use for the body of transcultural nursing science knowledge. It will also be used by other health disci-plines with slight modifications to fit their respective discipline focus and in nonhealth disciplines as educa-tion, politics, religion, and economics. Several nursing theories will become extinct because they will be inad-equate to discover and fully explain complex, holistic, and covert lifeways of cultures. Middle, higher, and lower range theories that fail to recognize cultures and are reductionistic will be limitedly used. Thus by the year 2020, holistic health and comparative human car-ing will prevail to meet many diverse cultural health expectations and benefits. Transcultural nursing will become the dominant focus and arching framework for the past field of nursing. This discipline will be a ma-jor contribution to the world and will provide ongoing, unique or distinct substantive knowledge and practices for the betterment of humanity.

■ Specific Changes for Transcultural Nursing Education and Practice

As transcultural nursing care becomes the central, dominant, and arching framework, major changes in education and practice that are barely known today will slowly occur. Teaching, research, and practice to provide culturally congruent, compassionate, and responsible safe care will, at last, have a high priority in most worldwide nursing education and service settings by the year 2020.[13] Transcultural nursing education will be viewed as *imperative* and require that faculty be well prepared and competent in the discipline. The greatest change will be to help nurses shift from present-day nursing and medical dominant teaching and practice emphasis on diseases, symptom management, and treatment curing modes to holistic and specific cultural healing and caring practices. Helping people to remain well and preventing accidents, illnesses, and chronic diseases will be best understood through a cultural caring lens and will challenge past dominant unicultural knowledge. Undoubtedly, medicine will continue to focus on pathologies, biophysical, and genetic curing modes with clinical experts in these areas and many associates. Nursing and medicine should become *complementary disciplines* rather than *competitive fields* so that human healing and curing can be the goal. Nursing will focus primarily on *caring as healing and well-being*, using broad and specific culture care dimensions as discussed in the Culture Care Theory and depicted in the Sunrise Model.[14] Far more emphasis and credibility will be given to emic-etic caring, cultural values, worldviews, social structure influencers, and other factors influencing health and well-being. Holistic comparative care will provide a distinct and significant contribution to humanity through nurses who are competent.

Comparative Lifeways

With the use of the transcultural nursing paradigm as the major focus, nurses will discover some entirely new ways to become specialists and generalists. They will draw on *selected* biomedical, genetic, environmental, and appropriate nursing knowledge along with other relevant knowledge to provide care. Transcultural nursing will reflect the use of holistic and multidimensional knowledge that is related to theoretical and conceptual perspectives to help individuals, families, and other groups being served. Nurses will function from the client's emic knowledge and life patterns of living but will draw on both broad and specific knowledge from different philosophies, diverse sciences, and

the humanities as the new transcultural nursing and caring science knowledge. Transcultural care knowledge and skills, however, will emphasize patterns and lifestyle ways of living and keeping well within their cultural values' environmental contexts. Culture care and health will be emphasized throughout the entire life span before birth and until elder death. Reinforcing and maintaining patterns of caring to attain and maintain wellness and healing will be stressed. *Comparative life cycle patterns of health care maintenance and prevention of illnesses for infants, children, adolescents, and adults will become the in-depth transcultural areas of study and practice.* Other areas that will be most difficult to master but very importantly will be the spiritual, cultural care values, and historical and environmental factors within diverse community lifeways.

Spiritual Healing

Spiritual healing as caring will be increasingly emphasized in this century amid strong Western secular, materialistic, and technological interests. The *culture of life* and keeping people well through spiritual means will come from cultural clients who want health professionals to recognize and use spirituality as healing. The *culture of death* with abortions, euthanasia, suicides, and homicides will be evident worldwide. The killing of children and the elderly, as well as many deaths caused by war, famine, and destructive acts, will challenge nurses to reverse this trend through a caring ethos. As nurses work with many immigrants, refugees, the poor, oppressed victims of violence, and the homeless in different communities, the search to promote caring as healing will be important using clients' spiritual and religious beliefs. Using caring with AIDS victims and their families, refugees, political victims, the economically deprived, gays, lesbians, and the abused with the three modes of the Culture Care Theory can lead to healthy lifeways. Preventing accidents and acute illnesses and dealing with chronic illnesses in different cultures will necessitate knowing *culture-bound* conditions that do not fit the dominant professional mold of Western illnesses and diseases. Relying on comparative transcultural care knowledge will help nurses worldwide to use approaches different from their past traditional ones with beneficial outcomes. Changing unfavorable human conditions in homes, communities, and work places will be stressed with insights coming from clients' emic perspectives and from social structure and environmental factors. Such new areas and insights that have been limitedly studied in the past in nursing will challenge astute nurses and especially transcultural nurses.

Promoting Well-being

In light of the paradigm shift to transcultural caring to promote and maintain well-being, nurse educators will urgently need to change their teaching content and curricula approaches. Developing truly holistic teaching methods and guiding students into the rich body of comparative culture and care needs will be the future emphasis. Future curricula will need to include far more content on worldview, sociocultural factors, environmental contexts, and historical factors with the already discovered transcultural knowledge. Faculty will need to teach transcultural comparative content such as life-cycle patterns, nutritional needs, and dominant caring and health patterns based on cultural caring and health beliefs and social structure factors. A wealth of new generic (folk) and professional comparative care knowledge within ethnohistorical contexts will characterize the modern nursing curricula by 2015 to provide culturally congruent care outcomes. Some entirely new teaching-learning methods will be encouraged to help students *to discover culture and caring as ways to prevent illnesses, accidents, violence, and death with individuals and groups.* Transcultural nursing instruction will need to be highly innovative with the use of the Internet, films, music, art, and direct-immersion field experiences with families and groups in community and treatment contexts. Faculty will be challenged to know cultures in-depth with comparative research knowledge for students and clients. Feedback experiences should reflect on faculty and theoretical perspectives to facilitate student learning and practices. In fact, faculty who are highly creative, flexible, open-minded, keenly knowledgeable of diverse cultures, and understand their own cultural values and beliefs will be highly sought, retained, and rewarded in schools of nursing. With new transcultural curricula approaches and new ways to teach and mentor students in transcultural nursing, more students will be excited and interested to enter this global and relevant discipline.

They will recognize its importance and necessity to serve many cultures worldwide. It will be a powerful new means to recruit and retain a new generation of nurses for humankind. In fact, it may well turn the critical shortage of nurses into a new professional career, one with global status and respect.

Moral and Legal Decisions

As nurses become more involved in studying transcultural ethical, moral, and legal issues, they will become confident and sensitive to deal with human global conditions. They will also discover ways to integrate religious and ethical values into client care to prevent illness and deal with death and disabilities.[15,16] Nurses will be expected to critically reflect on their own moral and ethical beliefs and values in clinical practices and all human relationships. Discovering ways to help students and clients from diverse cultures to make appropriate ethical and moral decisions will be difficult because of diverse beliefs and values of nurses and clients. To achieve this level of teaching and learning, I contend that nurses will benefit from scholarly self- and other critiques in graduate education. Graduate nursing programs must markedly increase by the year 2010 to provide leadership, scholarship, and competencies in nursing and transcultural nursing. The highly complex nature of this discipline requires depth and breadth of knowledge at the graduate level. Discovering and valuing universal, diverse, and transcendental truths about human beings will require critical study and synthesis of findings with broadly prepared faculty. Secular and materialistic ideas will be challenged in the 21st century by graduate nurses as will the traditional Western and non-Western philosophies of nursing that fail to understand transcultural human conditions, survival, and modes. Graduate students will be interested in theology, law, ethics, and moral issues relating to intense cultural conflicts and global value differences. There will be many lawyers, ethicists, and health theologians in the health field, but few will be prepared in transcultural or international law to arrive at legal and cultural justice or appropriate decisions for clients of diverse cultures.

Holding Knowledge

Most encouraging is that by the year 2020 transcultural nurse experts will have established a substantive body of research-based knowledge that will serve as grounded "holding knowledge" to guide nurses to function in a number of *cultural areas of the world* such as the Middle East, Europe, Australia, Africa, Southeast Asia, South America, the Caribbean, North America, and the Pacific Islands (Oceania). While cultural variability will always exist, common holding knowledge will still help nurses to reflect on, explain, and appropriately respond to people in meaningful ways. Field cultural areas in the world will have been established to work with colleagues and others who value different approaches in teaching, research, and practice. Cultural variations with commonalities among cultures will be recognized and expected by health professions in giving and receiving care. Cultural patterns of changes will occur over time along with stability patterns. Transcultural nurses will be skilled to access and use selected research findings from anthropology, sociology, the arts and humanities, ecology, and computer and space science appropriate to transcultural nursing. In addition, linguistics, communication and historical data will be used as the broad means to grasp the totality of human caring and well-being. Transcultural nurses will also study the impact of acculturation, assimilation, and enculturation processes and phenomena in different care settings with clients. Understanding and working in specific cultural areas such as Africa and Southeast Asia and the sub-Sahara will bring nurses together to share their insights and experiences.

Most of all, nurses will not be expected to *know all cultures* nor to *be skilled in working with every culture*. Instead, nurses will have in-depth knowledge of selected cultures and know how to use general concepts, principles, policies, and research-based knowledge that have *commonalities* across many cultures worldwide and with specific diverse cultures. Both culture-specific and cultural generalities will guide nurses as they serve clients in different environmental and cultural contexts. There will be transcultural nurse experts who will be skilled to know and demonstrate the use of culture-specific care for complex, meaningful, and congruent care. Certified transcultural specialists will be most helpful to other nurses and health care providers. These specialists will be prepared largely in master's, doctoral, and postdoctoral transcultural nursing programs and will serve as role models to others.

Graduate Preparation

As the author has predicted, by the year 2020 most undergraduate nursing programs will have largely disappeared as the profession will realize the need for graduate preparation to become professional, especially in transcultural nursing. Being knowledgeable and competent to work effectively with complex and diverse cultures requires in-depth graduate knowledge in transcultural nursing. As transcultural nursing becomes the dominant focus of nursing, graduate and post-graduate programs will be in great demand by the year 2010. Existing associate and baccalaureate nursing students will be expected to work closely with graduate transcultural nursing experts to ensure cultural competencies and appropriate care decisions. Graduate programs will focus on quality research and relevant theories for therapeutic benefits, outcomes, and rewards in providing culturally competent, safe, and congruent care. The power and effectiveness of human caring within a cultural perspective will become imperative and recognized in time. Postdoctoral programs will increase for nurses seeking advanced global comparative transcultural or international nursing knowledge and practices and for global leadership and consultant roles. Having well-prepared transcultural nurses will be imperative for establishing and maintaining multidisciplinary institutes that will rapidly flourish to meet local, national, and worldwide needs.

Partnership Care

Still another futuristic trend will be what I call *partnership care*. This care practice means nurses and other health care providers will work directly *with clients in open and trusted partnerships* focusing on providing culturally congruent care. Partnership care will be needed among nurses, clients, and others who are working together to discover and maintain wellness for clients that is meaningful and beneficial. To achieve this care, nurses and other health providers need to have *immersion experiences* to discover and understand clients fully to keep them well or to be helpful if dying, disabled, or ill. Transcultural nurses can lead the way to promote true client-nurse partnership care because of their cultural care knowledge and experiences. Understanding different cultures will be essential to care for clients or families over short or long periods even with chronic illnesses and disabilities.[17] The *culture of life* ethos should be promoted from before birth until old age with rewards for wellness in collaborative partnership care practices. With this approach, trust and friendly client-professional relationships will become evident, especially with immigrants. With partnership care, clients, nurses, and other providers will discover together special ways to maintain health and prevent illnesses and accidents and to deal with chronic or acute illnesses, disabilities, and deaths in acceptable cultural ways. A quality of life that is culturally congruent will be valued with partnership care because the efforts are tailored to fit individuals and groups of a culture. Maintaining professional mutual trust, genuine interest, and compassionate care will characterize partnership care that goes beyond a "quick fix," "symptom fix," "mechanistic-object," or "tech" services. Obtaining and blending emic and etic data together in partnership relationships will be a major key to quality and meaningful care to clients and families.

Rural and Urban Differences

In the future far more attention worldwide will be given to differences and similarities between *rural and urban client needs* and human living conditions. In the past, rural communities have often been neglected, taken for granted, or assumed to have the same needs as urban clients. Differences and similarities between rural and urban cultures will help to establish ways to prevent illnesses and to draw on the strengths and assets of people in these rural-urban environmental contexts and different patterns of living. Identifying potential accidents, threats, crime, cultural conflicts, and nonhealthy lifeways in rural contexts will provide different ways to lessen these problems. Immigrants and nonimmigrants living in rural communities often move to large urban areas to seek employment for survival reasons, and for social benefits. Urbanities may move to the rural areas for different reasons. What happens to clients and their health patterns when they move between rural and urban living or the reverse? Where are there examples of healthy rural and urban communities where people live long and stay in good health as a result of their culture care lifeways? What do we know about rural and urban health patterns worldwide? With forced relocation or displacements of people because of wars,

natural disasters, and other reasons, what do we know that favors healthy or unhealthy patterns of living in rural and urban contexts?

Assessing Multicultural Communities

Assessing differences and similarities in lifeways in regions, towns, and countries will be a dominant focus to develop culturally congruent care practices. Discovering how different cultures live and function together will be essential new areas for nurses to discover and plan for care. Conducting culture care assessments for the development of culturally healthy and congruent lifeways will be a strong thrust along with developing guidelines, theories, policies, and practices that fit cultures in diverse community contexts. Most assuredly, the Theory of Culture Care with the Sunrise Model will be a valuable guide to discover community differences and similarities, as well as to assess key factors influencing health or illness lifeways.[18] Community politics and economic struggles along with recognizing and responding to religious, educational, technologic, and cultural factors will be important for quality-based care practices. Acculturation, enculturation, and historical factors must be assessed for accurate data and plans. Prepared transcultural nurses will be essential to assess multicultural communities and to help those not prepared to understand and work effectively with the culturally different. They also can be valuable to transform traditional unicultural communities and accommodate minority and invisible cultures in diverse areas.[19]

Discovering and rethinking about multicultural communities with dominant and minority cultures will be difficult for many nurses unless prepared in transcultural nursing because of subtle and unfamiliar expectations. Identifying major differences and commonalities between Western and non-Western cultures will require "new eyes and ears." For example, Western nurses assessing and working with people in India will find that many people live and function near the Ganges River. The nurses need to realize that the Ganges River is sacred to the people and that it has many uses. The river is used for washing, burying the dead, drinking water, and sacred rituals. Knowledge of the Hindu religion will be essential to understand community culture practices in India and *before* working with the

Hindu people with their unique lifeways about the significance and functions of the Ganges River. Sanitation measures related to improving the people's physical health would today be considered by Western nurses to need drastic repatterning, but understanding the Indian strong religious and cultural values is imperative. Western nurses could experience cultural shock and become impatient to promote sanitation and deal with bathing and other unsanitary uses of the Ganges River. Again, holding knowledge of the Hindu culture is imperative before making any changes. Still another example to challenge nurses to practice *community transcultural nursing* is with the culture of poverty in many non-Western and Western cultures. In many cultures a food supply may be available, but political and tribal groups will not permit the people to have the food. Instead, political groups often sell the food for ammunition and for their own uses. In the meantime, the poor people starve to death. How to help the poor in these cultures requires careful analysis and understanding of historical facts, especially those related to past and present tribal wars, feuds, political interests, economic greed, terrorists' actions, and religious beliefs. In addition, migration patterns and resource persons are essential to know. Knowledge of these cultural and other factors are essential to reach and help the poor, oppressed, and suffering, especially in South Africa and the Caribbean region.

The above future predictions by the author and with some support in the writings by Naisbett,[20] Toffler,[21] and Theobald[22] are important transcultural considerations for nurses. However, as the world conditions change, so will changes occur in administration, research, education, and practice. Drawing on past transcultural nursing knowledge and practices that are meaningful and helpful to cultures is the future trend.

■ Some Current and Predictive Glimpses of Transcultural Nursing Worldwide

In this last section, a few selected glimpses with predictive reflections are in order by the founder of the discipline in moving forward in this new century. Having had the great privilege and opportunity to travel worldwide to study, do research give lectures, teach, and offer consultation over the past 50 years has pro-

vided me with some precious insights over time and in different places.

Now that the discipline of transcultural nursing has been established as a formal area of study and practice, there are still some places where transcultural nursing needs to become fully established and integrated into education, practice, consultation, and research. Today, most perceptive professional nurses view transcultural nursing as imperative and a critical need for nurses to provide culturally congruent and beneficial care to people of diverse cultures. Many wise nurses often say, "There is no way that nurses can practice nursing today without transcultural nursing knowledge and competencies. It is a moral and ethical imperative." One of the greatest challenges, however, is to help nurses gain sufficient in-depth knowledge about cultures and humanistic care to be effective nurses. For without in-depth knowledge and competencies, nurses can be destructive or less beneficial to consumers and in health systems.[23] Hence, a major crisis remains to educate nurses in transcultural nursing so they can be effective and safe with clients. Moreover, such prepared nurses will be able to give care in positive and rewarding ways to those served.

The value and practice of educating nurses before expecting them to care for people has long been a sound philosophy and principle of nursing but also of all respected academic disciplines. Nurses as human beings need to understand phenomena and what one might anticipate to help others and to understand why. To be placed into a client situation without knowledge of the discipline's focus and practices can be destructive with negative consequences. However, one will find some faculty and service personnel casting students and clinical staff into culturally sensitive situations and expecting them to "learn something" without transcultural preparation. Such practices must be eradicated with undergraduate and graduate students and with faculty prepared to teach and help them. Many complaints and unethical practices occur today as students tell about faculty unprepared in transcultural nursing with no courses and no one to mentor them in clinical practices. Faculty preparation is imperative today and the future. For where such courses, programs, and prepared faculty exist, transcultural nursing is a powerful means to help students care for clients and practice transcultural nursing. Although transcultural nursing is complex, it still makes sense and becomes very meaningful to students and clients as beneficiaries of quality transcultural nursing care practices. A firm and imperative commitment is needed worldwide to teach and practice humanistic and scientific transcultural nursing care and to make it a meaningful reality worldwide to those nurses serve.

Establish Graduate Programs

Where established master's, doctoral, and postdoctoral transcultural courses and programs exist, nurses are moving forward with confidence and competencies in their teaching, research, practice, and consultation with many exciting, positive, and significant outcomes.[24] Establishing and maintaining these courses and programs has necessitated considerable leadership efforts and strategic planning. Where sound transcultural educational and certification programs and practices exist worldwide, one can predict less signs of cultural imposition, cultural clashes, and destructive practices with clients, students, faculty, clinical staff, and others.[25] Graduate transcultural education will remain mandatory well into this century for general practices and as a stepping stone to pursue further graduate transcultural studies. Graduate transcultural nursing education will be important to shift nurses and health care systems into the new paradigm focus. Physical and cultural anthropology courses as prerequisites will provide a substantive and broad cultural base for transcultural nursing as discussed in the classic *Nursing and Anthropology* book.[26] Such courses and related ones will help nurses discover the major focus and differences between the disciplines of transcultural nursing and anthropology. While some sociology and psychology courses have been helpful, many have been less helpful to prepare transcultural nurses for global practices because of their Western orientation.

Establish Multidisciplinary Centers

With the critical need for many top scholars in transcultural nursing to meet global needs, *transcultural multidisciplinary health institutes and educational centers* will be needed for transcultural health care. These institutes and/or centers need to be established within institutions of higher education and to offer specific courses and programs for advanced transcultural nurses and with interdisciplinary seminars in teaching, theory, research, and practice. Institute faculty need to be recognized scholars in transculturalism. The purpose, scope, and nature of a true institute must be maintained to achieve its purposes and to focus on in-depth theoretical and research knowledge with renowned multidiscipline scholars in transcultural research and theory. Undergraduate and graduate transcultural offerings should precede the establishment of such institutes because sound preparation is necessary before entering a specific research institute in any discipline. Accordingly, top scholars or faculty experts in transcultural nursing and health care would be reviewed and selectively invited as professors to such multidisciplinary transcultural institutes. Currently, a few institutes in transcultural nursing and multidisciplinary studies are being developed in the United States; however, one can predict that more institutes will be needed to meet global and local needs for competent health care leaders, researchers, and teachers in transcultural health care.

Studying the complex, holistic, and diverse transcultural phenomena necessitates the benefits of intra- and interdisciplinary studies to prepare highly knowledgeable and competent scholars, leaders, teachers, and researchers in a growing and still relatively new discipline for many health care providers. I contend that it is essential for all disciplines (i.e., nursing, medicine, social work, and others) to first be knowledgeable about their *own* discipline focus before participating in multidisciplinary endeavors. Knowing one's own discipline helps when engaging in meaningful dialogue to study and communicate with other disciplines. Being able to debate and share theory and research with another discipline is a growth experience and helps to perfect and refine knowledge with one's own discipline and often in other disciplines. Bringing a discipline perspective "to the table" and not assuming that all disciplines are alike are important in interdisciplinary studies. Of course, some commonalities with the differences will generally occur among disciplines.

Barriers to Progress

Since transcultural nursing has been established as a legitimate and formal academic area of study and practice since the early 1960s and especially in the United States, the new movement is to support transdisciplinary studies to identify commonalities and differences so clients benefit from multidisciplinary knowledge and practices. While this transcultural nursing cultural movement has been slow largely because of cultural biases, ethnocentrism, lack of prepared faculty and practitioners, fears of racism and discrimination, and the lack of visionary leaders, more rapid changes need to occur.[27] Competition and jealousy among nurse leaders since transcultural nursing took hold along with nurse leaders proclaiming that they are the leaders by offering questionable and strange brands of transcultural nursing education needs to be recognized and dealt with for sound progress. Cultural minorities have also asserted their cultural identity and claims as "people of color" to be the experts but without preparation in transcultural nursing. Such interprofessional claims have limited progress and need to be addressed.

The lack of funds, qualified faculty, and academic administrative support have also curtailed transcultural nursing progress in the United States and other places in the world. Interestingly, it has only been since the early 1990s that major nursing organizations in the United States such as the ANA and the American Academy of Nursing have begun to address the need for "culture and care" in nursing education, research, and practice. Several Academy nurse leaders began to identify themselves as authorities in transcultural and international nursing, but again with virtually no formal preparation or substantive knowledge in transcultural nursing and with little interaction with transcultural nurse experts.[28] Such developments have weakened progress, but, despite these hurdles, an active cadre of qualified transcultural nurse leaders and followers through the Transcultural Nursing Society have persistently moved forward in all areas to prepare and promote new leaders and practitioners for tomorrow. During the past four decades, I have educated approximately 30,000 undergraduate and nearly 4000 graduate nursing students and others in the health field professions in specific courses, programs of study, and continuing education modes in transcultural nursing. These nurses and students have been eager and excited to learn transcultural nursing. Through the Transcultural Nursing Society approximately 200 transcultural nurses have been certified and recertified since 1988. Most of these are grad-

uate nurses who have been prepared in the discipline of transcultural nursing and health care and are serving as role models in practice, teaching, research, and consultation. Currently, many undergraduate and graduate students remain extremely interested and committed to learning transcultural nursing. They search daily for courses and mentoring in the United States, Canada, Europe, Philippines, and Southeast Asia. They complain about "an older generation of faculty" who fail to teach, know, or help them learn transcultural nursing. The demand for graduate courses and prepared faculty in the discipline continues to be critical to guide a new generation of nurses for the world. Most students are keenly aware of the many new immigrants, refugees, and others who want help and need nurses who can give culturally competent care.

With nearly one million immigrants and refugees in the United States and in many other countries, nurses and health care providers must respond to these people's needs and lifeways. Countries that support an open transnational migration will continue to get many refugees along with the oppressed, tortured, and poor immigrants. Currently, immigration and migration policies are receiving new attention due to birth decreases in population, especially in Europe, Japan, Canada, and other countries where fertility rates are very low and abortions are high. In fact in some countries as Canada, the abortion rate exceeded live births in 2000.[29] Cultural identity and survival reasons are evident and of deep concern in these countries. Transcultural health care is much needed to meet these shifting immigrations and other factors related to major population changes.

European Trends and Needs

In focusing on Europe with its recent unification of 15 countries, one can anticipate that transcultural nursing and dealing with diversities and commonalities will be very important with limited European resources, money management issues, and other unification concerns. Unfortunately, European countries have been extremely slow to prepare nurses in transcultural nursing. Nurses tend to rely "on their experiences" and past colonialization experiences in many countries. Formal academic preparation and guided field learning in transcultural nursing has been very limited. As a consequence, many European nurses desperately need substantive undergraduate and graduate courses and programs in transcultural nursing to serve people of many different cultures. Immigrants and refugees from Africa, the Middle East, and other countries are generally limitedly understood and cared for in culturally congruent ways. Where many internal cultural clashes, open racism, and violence are reported, as in England and Ireland, there are no graduate transcultural nursing programs offered by nurses prepared in the discipline. Some nurses rely on sociology and anthropology courses but with no conceptualizing or transforming of ideas into transcultural nursing. In the meantime, misconceptions, myths, and misinterpretation of the nature and focus of transcultural nursing and research can be heard among British and Irish nurses. Racism and discrimination practices in the country and in health care are frequently discussed, but are limitedly studied with transcultural nursing theories and practices. Hence, there remains an urgent need for transcultural nursing research and education programs to be established, especially in Britain, Ireland, and other European countries. Wales and Scotland have had conferences on transcultural caring, but they too need graduate courses and faculty in the discipline.

Finland and Sweden   In Finland and Sweden several nurse leaders took active steps in the mid 1980s to teach and practice transcultural nursing in post-RN education. These leaders were quick to recognize the need for formal academic transcultural nursing programs to help with their changing countries. The author and other United States nurses have been active to support these leadership endeavors with major workshops, courses, and conventions over the past two decades. Transcultural nurse leaders such as Dr. Kirsten Gebru, Dr. Pirrko Merilainen, and Anita van Smitten are a few transcultural nursing leaders in these countries who have developed and offered courses in transcultural nursing and conducted research studies with good nursing administrative support. The author has been a consultant and lecturer in the counties since the early 1980s and continues to hear positive outcomes of their nurses' work.

South Africa   In the Republic of South Africa, a few doctorally prepared leaders such as Dr. Hilda Brink,

Dr. Philda Nzimonde, and the late Grace Mashaba have been active supporters of the philosophy and education of the practice of transcultural nursing. However, South African nurses continue to face extremely difficult political, economic, and racial problems in academic and professional settings over the past two decades.[30] While South Africa is trying to move toward promoting democratic cultural and social freedoms, justice, and economic progress, still crime, violence, and a host of other "black-white" issues are evident today, plus the incredible and growing problem of AIDS in the country. Nurses worldwide need to help support African nursing education, leadership, and practices in transcultural nursing for improved health and peaceful intercultural and intertribal relationships across the large continent of Africa, including Samoli, Nigeria, Sudan, Liberia, and other countries.

Australia and New Zealand   In October 2000 the 26th Global Transcultural Nursing Society cosponsored with the Royal College of Nursing, Australia, the annual convention focused on the theme "Transcultural Nurses Lead into the New Millennium." There were important signs that much progress is being made in Australia in transcultural nursing since the author first came into the country in the mid 1980s. With Dr. Akram Omeri's leadership and working with the excellent staff of the Royal College of Nursing Australia, a transcultural chapter has been established encouraging nurses to study and participate in transcultural nursing. Dr. Omeri was the first nurse in Australia with doctoral preparation in transcultural nursing and the first certified transcultural nurse. Still more nurses need similar preparation in the country. Dr. Elizabeth Cameron-Traub is another strong leader to promote the theoretical and practical use of transcultural nursing knowledge using Leininger's Culture Care Theory. Drs. Omeri and Cameron-Traub have now established transcultural nursing courses and research projects in institutions of higher education. Dr. Olga Kanitsaki was an early leader to promote multicultural understanding among nurses in Australia and is now promoting academic study in transcultural nursing in a major institution of higher learning along with a few other nurses. Several transcultural nursing publications and courses are now available in Australia for nurses.[31–33]

Nurses in New Zealand are challenged to work with the Maori and many immigrants. Nurses in Australia are challenged to work with the Australian Aborigines and the Torres Strait Island peoples. In both Australia and New Zealand diligent efforts are being made by nurses to provide congruent, sensitive, and culturally safe care to these indigenous people and their many immigrants. Such reports were presented and discussed at the 2000 Transcultural Nursing Convention in Australia. However, much work lies ahead to provide undergraduate and graduate transcultural nursing courses, to build on existing research knowledge available in transcultural nursing, and to support new studies and courses. Drs. Akram and Cameron-Traub have well demonstrated how effective the Culture Care Theory has been to provide meaningful and appropriate care to non-Aborigines and Aborigines in Australia and immigrants. "Cultural safety," a term coined by Maori nurse leader Ramsden, is a helpful concept valued by some New Zealand nurses, but it is not a theory.[34] Several misconceptions exist about what is transcultural nursing and that safety is an integral part of the Culture Care Theory if accurately taught and understood.[35] Thus, while progress is being made in Australia, far more work is needed to develop undergraduate and graduate programs in transcultural nursing in both New Zealand and Australia.

Southeast Asia Transcultural nursing varies in Southeast Asia, Japan, Korea, China, Taiwan, Borneo, and India. Dr. Basuray has presented the current status of transcultural nursing in India in an earlier chapter. Leininger's visits in many of these countries over the past four decades reveals the continued need for prepared leaders in transcultural nursing and to develop courses for nurses who are so eager to learn about and use transcultural knowledge. Japan was early to value and use transcultural nursing concepts and principles and the Theory of Culture Care largely because of Dr. Fumiaki Inaoka's leadership at the Japanese Red Cross College of Nursing in Tokyo. He and Dr. Sachikl Claus and other nurses have been most helpful to translate the Culture Care Theory and the quantitative method books and other publications into Japanese for nurses' daily use and in research. In addition, these leaders and other nurses in Japan are doing research and teaching transcultural nursing with great enthusiasm and find the Theory of Culture Care and other ideas most meaningful to nurses in their country and with many recent immigrants they care for in Japan.

China In China, Dr. Grayce Roessler, Dr. Joyceen Boyle, and the author began early visits in the 1980s in educating Chinese nurses in transcultural nursing content and practices. While there have been other nurses in these countries, most have not been prepared in transcultural nursing to help Chinese nurses learn transcultural nursing knowledge and competencies. Nevertheless, Chinese nurses have shown a great interest and desire to use transcultural concepts, theories, and practices as they work with many diverse cultures. There are also many outstanding Chinese nurse leaders who are very open to advance transcultural nursing in all Chinese provinces.

Canada and Alaska The current status and future needs in Canada have been presented in an earlier chapter by the author and Dr. Rani Srivastava. The reader is encouraged to read this chapter to get a picture of transcultural nursing in Canada. Alaska has shown interest in transcultural nursing for several decades as the author noted on her visits in the 1970s to Alaska to assess transcultural situations while Dean of Nursing at the University of Washington. Only a few nurses in Alaska have been prepared in the discipline, but cultural anthropologists have been helpful to share their knowledge with nurses and physicians about cultures in Alaska and the Arctic region. Betty Vera is a transcultural nurse who worked with clients and families in the Arctic region for several years. She now is active in promoting transcultural nursing knowledge and practices with mothers and children in England. Dr. Nancy Sanders has recently studied the Inuit in Alaska and developed culture-specific hospital care practices for these people.

Pacific Islands Turning to cultures in the Pacific Islands, the idea of transcultural nursing is limitedly known in Fiji and other small islands in Oceania except for Hawaii. On the big island of Hawaii and on Oahu transcultural nursing has been known since the first transcultural nursing conference was held in 1972 through the University of Hawaii. Loretta Bermosk and myself were facilitators of this successful historical event as the first conference of its kind and before the Transcultural Nursing Society and annual conferences were established. The Hawaii conferences in 1972 and 1995 were overwhelmingly successful largely because Hawaiians historically have been so open to cultural strangers coming and going in their islands. Nurses are also eager to visit this beautiful island, and they often witness first hand that *caring is sharing* as one of the dominant care constructs among Polynesians along with hospitality as caring. During the past two decades, Dr. Genevieve Kinney, the first native Polynesian certified transcultural nurse, has been a most active, enthusiastic, and effective leader to develop a transcultural nursing baccalaureate curriculum. This was one of the first in the country to demonstrate how transcultural nursing is integrated throughout all areas of nursing at the University of Hawaii at Hilo.[36] From the author's perspective, developing transcultural nursing in Hawaii has been "a natural" for teaching and learning research and practice. For the many diverse cultures on the Islands, along with their friendly and caring attitude, transcultural nursing has become meaningful and essential. Dr. Kinney's pioneering work along with her creative strategies have been noteworthy and should continue well into this century.

Papua New Guinea Reflecting on developments in Papua New Guinea, and especially the Gadsup of the Eastern Highlands whom I studied over several decades (see earlier chapter in this book), a few glimpses of interest can be shared. My return visits to the Gadsups have been most valuable to study cultural changes over time and specific transcultural health care practices since my original work in the early 1960s. During my last visit in 1992 to Papua New Guinea, the national nurse organization met with me and held a short conference. These nurse leaders spoke of the importance of all nurses to understand their indigenous people and the newcomers. They wanted foreign nurses to study and live with the people in the village "as Leininger did in the early days." The members of the Papua New Guinea Nurses' Association were keenly aware that I had lived in New Guinea with the people. The President of the Association made this astute comment in 1992 when she introduced me. She said, "*Transcultural nursing actually began in New Guinea when you (Dr. Leininger) first came to this country to study our*

people in the early 1960s. Transcultural nursing will continue to be the focus of our professional care as it is essential to our people and for effective nursing practices."[37]

The Gadsup nurses' interest and commitment to the concept of transcultural nursing was commendable. The nurses hope there will be academic courses at the University of Papua New Guinea in Port Moresby. Since this visit in 1994, I have learned from direct and reliable communication sources that crimes, drug use, theft, AIDS, and distrust of strangers from other countries and from areas within the country are pervasive.[38] The young men called "rascals" are fighting and killing strangers to regain their land and lifeways. Health care services, personnel, and resources have markedly decreased, and care has been very difficult to provide. It has been sad to hear about this development. The reader is encouraged to read the author's early and later work on this first and major longitudinal transcultural nursing study from the 1960s to the present time to see transcultural changes over time.[39,40]

Middle East In the Middle East, Dr. Linda Luna, the first American nurse prepared with a Ph.D. in transcultural nursing, has been conducting research and teaching transcultural nursing at King Faisal General Hospital and Research Center since 1988. She has worked effectively with many expatriated nurses from different Western and non-Western countries in a large hospital context. She has helped these nurses to understand and practice transcultural nursing in Saudi Arabia and wherever cultural differences exist in care. Dr. Barbara Brown, a former American nursing administrator at the Saudi Arabia hospital, was an early advocate and supporter of transcultural nursing. She facilitated understanding and practicing transcultural nursing through conferences and consultation visits. Dr. Luna's recent work in Saudi Arabia is presented in this book, and readers are encouraged to read it. Currently, there are no formal graduate programs in transcultural nursing in the Middle East, but there is some in-service clinical educational mentoring. Dr. Rowaida Al Ma'aitah, a Jordanian nurse leader, has provided several research conferences and international exchange programs in Jordan, but there are no graduate courses *per se* in transcultural nursing in the country. There are also no known courses in transcultural nursing in Iran, Turkey,

Iraq, and Egypt and no prepared transcultural graduate nursing specialists. However, many nurses in these countries are very interested in transcultural nursing and are eager to study this subject matter.

South America and Caribbean In South America and the Caribbean region, the concept of transcultural nursing has been known to nurses since the mid 1980s. Drs. Gloria Wright, Elouise Neves, Dulce Gualda, and Lucie Gonzales were early nurse supporters of transcultural nursing with the Culture Care Theory and qualitative research methods. A few Brazilian nurses have studied transcultural nursing in the United States with the author and are giving leadership in teaching and research in their homeland. Transcultural nursing courses are much needed in these changing and large Latin American countries.

Drs. Jody Glittenberg and Joyceen Boyle were two active transcultural nurse researchers in the Caribbean. They have conducted some sound and outstanding transcultural nursing research studies. Dr. Glittenberg has been active in Caribbean research for several decades, and much of her research publications reflect her keen sensitivity, great insight, and compassion for "her people."[41] In the future, strategies are needed to establish courses and programs of study in transcultural nursing in the Caribbean and other Latin American countries. Guided clinical field practices are important to meet rapidly growing and changing populations in these cultural areas. Nurses working and studying in these cultural areas will undoubtedly need to speak Spanish, Portuguese, and other languages for practice, research, and teaching.

Most assuredly, there are many other places in the world where transcultural nursing leaders and followers are learning about and taking steps to incorporate transcultural nursing into nursing education, practice, and their research. This is a major cultural movement worldwide and an imperative to advance and make transcultural nursing relevant, distinct, and a worldwide contribution.[42] This is a most encouraging movement, but far more transcultural education programs, research, and well-prepared faculty are needed to make transcultural nursing a meaningful global reality. Undoubtedly, students and consumers will continue to remain active to promote and maintain transcultural nursing and health care in this century. These demands will greatly increase and become much more evident in moral and ethical obligations for all health disciplines to provide culturally congruent care in this century. More and more, other health disciplines will see the relevance and importance of transcultural care with respect to life-cycle phenomena, illnesses, accidents, diverse human health states, and death phenomena. Multidisciplinary transcultural education, research, and practices will be a dominant focus in this century with many new discoveries. Transcultural nurses who have already led the way will need to remain active leaders with other disciplines to promote and advance work. Transcultural nurse experts must also be the active leaders worldwide for intra- and for multidisciplinary endeavors and to make transcultural nursing a true global reality.

Most importantly, strategic planning is essential to develop and maintain transcultural nursing worldwide and to work with other disciplines. Transcultural nurse specialists and generalists will need to carry the symbolic "Olympic Torch" to others who need to maintain a big flame for transcultural health care, research, and practices. They will need to promote certification of nurses in transcultural nursing to protect cultures from destructive practices. Moreover, the importance of certification of transcultural nurses will spread to other health disciplines to protect the public and especially for vulnerable cultures and subcultures. Modern electronic communication modes will facilitate learning and obtaining transcultural knowledge for global certification. However, Internet and other electronic information needs to be carefully monitored for accuracy and reliability in professional work to protect clients and nurses. Protecting vulnerable cultures and privacy rights will be of major concern for practicing transcultural nurses and teachers. Getting accurate information from cultures and respecting informant privacy will be a sensitive matter, as well as helping cultures that do not have access to modern technologies, especially poor and oppressed cultures. Ethical and moral problems will prevail and necessitate far more transcultural monitoring to protect clients and health personnel for accurate interpretations of data. Cybernetics and this information age can be a great help in this century for communicating and planning transcultural nursing, but one must remain alert to the nonfavorable aspects by curtailing privacy cultural violations.

Summary: Future Goals

In sum, some important strategic goals and plans for the future in transcultural nursing are the following:

1. Prepare more nurse administrators worldwide in education and service to know, value, and facilitate transcultural nursing
2. Move soon to establish courses, programs, centers, and institutes in transcultural nursing and with multidisciplinary colleagues to meet the critical and growing worldwide needs and demands
3. Actively promote and educate the public through diverse media about the nature, scope, and benefits of transcultural nursing in people care
4. Establish transcultural nursing and health standards and policies for quality congruent and competent nursing and health care services worldwide
5. Obtain funds from various sources to support many more transcultural nursing educational programs and research and more models for transcultural health care
6. Use and build on transcultural nursing knowledge that is already available to nurses in providing culturally competent, safe, and meaningful care for diverse cultures
7. Develop a number of sound transcultural nursing and cooperative research projects worldwide related to advance transcultural nursing globally
8. Develop theoretical models, research strategies, and ways to obtain consumer (emic) and professional (etic) data
9. Identify comparative universals (or commonalities) and the diversities related to cultural congruent care and use this knowledge for a growing body of transcultural nursing and health care discipline practices

In concluding this last book chapter and as the founder and a persistent leader to make transcultural nursing a global human service, it has been most encouraging and rewarding to see transcultural nursing "take roots worldwide" and to see the gradual unfolding of one of the most important disciplines in the health field. One can anticipate that transcultural nursing will be adopted with all health disciplines as an imperative human service. Most of all, transcultural nursing must maintain its comparative focus of human caring as the dominant and central focus of nurses' thinking and actions. When transcultural nursing and other disciplines become fully transculturally focused, then we shall see a new quality of health care services to support the well-being, health, and peaceful relationships among people of diverse and similar cultures worldwide and less violence and destructive human relationships.

References

1. Leininger, M., *Transcultural Nursing: Concepts, Theories, Research and Practice*, Blacklick, Ohio: McGraw-Hill College Custom Series, 1995a.
2. Leininger, M., "Culture Care Theory, Research and Practice," *Nursing Science Quarterly*, 1995b, v. 9, no. 5, pp. 71–78.
3. Leininger, M., *Transcultural Nursing Concepts, Theories and Practices*, New York: John Wiley & Sons, 1978. (Reprint, Columbus, Ohio: Greyden Press, 1994.)
4. Leininger, M., "Major Directions for Transcultural Nursing: A Journey into the 21st Century," *Journal of Transcultural Nursing*, January to June 1996, v. 7, no. 2, pp. 28–31.
5. Leininger, M., *Nursing and Anthropology: Two Worlds to Blend*, New York: John Wiley & Sons, 1970. (Reprint, Columbus, Ohio: Greyden Press, 1994.)
6. Leininger, M., *Culture Care Diversity and Universality: A Theory of Nursing*, New York: National League for Nursing Press, 1991.
7. Leininger, M., "Transcultural Nursing Administration: What Is It?" *Journal of Transcultural Nursing*, 1996, v. 8, no. 1, pp. 28–33.
8. Ibid.
9. Leininger, op. cit., 1991.
10. Leininger, M., "Transcultural Nursing: Quo Vadis (Where Goeth the Field)," in *Transcultural Nursing: Concepts, Theories, Research and Practice*, Blacklick, Ohio: McGraw-Hill, 1995a, Chapter 29, pp. 661–678.
11. Leininger, M., "Transcultural Nursing Research to Transform Nursing Education and Practice: 40 Years," *Image: The Journal of Nursing Scholarship*, 1997, v. 29, no. 4, pp. 341–349.
12. Boyle, J. and M. Andrews, *Transcultural Concepts in Nursing Care*, Philadelphia: Lippincott, 1999.

13. Leininger, M., "Future Directions in Transcultural Nursing in the 21st Century," *International Nursing Review*, Nov–Dec 1996, v. 44, no. 1, pp. 19–23.
14. Leininger, op. cit., 1991.
15. Leininger, M., *Ethical and Moral Dimensions of Care*, Detroit, MI: Wayne State University Press, 1990.
16. Boyle and Andrews, op. cit., 1999.
17. Leininger, op. cit., 1991.
18. Leininger, op. cit., 1996.
19. Leininger, M., "Teaching Transcultural Nursing to Transform Nursing in the 21st Century," *Journal of Transcultural Nursing*, 1995b, v. 6, no. 2, pp. 2–3.
20. Naisbett, J., *Megatrends*, New York: Warner Books, Inc., 1982.
21. Toffler, A., *The Third Wave*, New York: Bantam Books, 1980.
22. Theobald, R., *The Rapids of Change: Social Entrepreneurship in Turbulent Times*, Indianapolis: Knowledge Systems, Inc., 1987.
23. Leininger, op. cit., 1995a.
24. Leininger, op. cit., 1995b.
25. Leininger, op. cit., 1995a.
26. Leininger, op. cit., 1970.
27. Leininger, op. cit., 1995a.
28. Leininger, M., "Rebuttal Excerpts on AAN Culturally Congruent Care Report," *Journal of Transcultural Nursing*, 1993, v. 1, no. 4, pp. 44–48.
29. "European Nations Examine Old Policies on Immigration," *Omaha World Herald Report from United Nations*, published October 19, 2000.
30. Personal communication from Dr. Hilda Brink, 1987 to 2001.
31. Omeri, Akram, *Transcultural Nursing in a Multicultural Australia*, Royal College of Nursing, Australia, 1996.
32. Cameron-Traub, E., "Meeting Health Care Needs in Australia's Diverse Society," in *Contexts of Nursing*, Daly, S., E. Speedy and D. Jackson, eds., Sydney: MacLennan and Petty, 2000.
33. Reid, J., and P. Trompf, *The Health of Aboriginal Australia*, Sydney: Harcourt Brace Jovanovich, 1991.
34. Ramsden, J., "Cultural Safety in Nursing Education in Aotearoa, New Zealand," *Nursing Praxis in New Zealand*, November 1993, v. 1, no. 3, pp. 4–10.
35. Leininger, M., "Leininger's Critique Response to Coup and Ramsden's Article on Cultural Safety and Culturally Congruent Care (Leininger) for Practice," *Nursing Praxis in New Zealand*, 1997, v. 12, no. 1, pp. 17–19.
36. Kinney, G., Personal communication, Hilo, Hawaii, October 1995.
37. Malasa, S., "Introductory Comments to Dr. Leininger for the Papua New Guinea Nurses Association," Personal communication, July 1992, Port Moresby, Papua New Guinea.
38. Orami, John, Letter of personal communication, October 12, 2000.
39. Leininger, M., op. cit., 1978.
40. Leininger, M., "Gadsup of Papua New Guinea Revisited: A Three Decade View," *Journal of Transcultural Nursing*, 1993, v. 5, no. 1, pp. 21–30.
41. Glittenberg, J., *To the Mountain and Back: The Mysteries of Guatemalan Highland Family Life*, Prospect Heights, IL: Waveland Press, Inc., 1994.
42. Leininger, M., "Transcultural Nursing Education: A Worldwide Imperative," *Nursing and Health Care*, May 1994, v. 15, no. 5, pp. 254–257.

■ INDEX ■